Veronica Sheehy
Box 376
Dennisport, Mass
1-394-2568
Box N 68
Westport
636-4890

The Pharmacologic Basis of Patient Care

second edition

Mary K. Asperheim, B.S., M.S., M.D.

House Staff in Pediatrics, Medical University of
South Carolina, Charleston, South Carolina;
Formerly Instructor of Pharmacology, St. Louis University School
of Nursing and Health Services, St. Louis, Missouri

Laurel A. Eisenhauer, R.N., B.S., M.S.N.

Assistant Professor of Medical-Surgical Nursing,
Boston College School of Nursing,
Chestnut Hill, Massachusetts;
Formerly Instructor, Villanova University
College of Nursing,
Villanova, Pennsylvania;
Formerly Instructor,
Boston City Hospital School of Nursing,
Boston, Massachusetts

1973 — W. B. SAUNDERS COMPANY
PHILADELPHIA   LONDON   TORONTO

W. B. Saunders Company: West Washington Square
Philadelphia, Pa. 19105

12 Dyott Street
London, WC1A 1DB

833 Oxford Street
Toronto 18, Ontario

The Pharmacologic Basis of Patient Care

ISBN   7216-1436-1

Print No.:   9   8   7   6   5   4   3   2   1

Preface to the Second Edition

The body of knowledge that is pharmacology is extremely fluid and dynamic, and requires considerable study if one is to remain abreast of current developments. It was with this fact in mind that we have undertaken the second edition of this text, and we have emphasized not only the basic factual knowledge of pharmacology but the nurse's role in drug therapy and her position as a vital member of the health team.

A new chapter entitled "The Role of the Nurse in Drug Therapy" has been added, and the nursing implications have been enlarged throughout the text. In addition, many new drugs representing recent developments in pharmacology have been included, as well as changes in federal drug legislation. Summary charts have been compiled to facilitate the teaching of metabolic and electrolyte imbalance and the dangerous effects of drug interactions. A bibliography has been placed at the end of each chapter, and it includes additional reading references which may be used by the student to enlarge her knowledge of the subject matter.

In response to numerous requests, we have prepared, to accompany this edition, a teachers' manual, which we hope will be of assistance to the teachers of pharmacology at the collegiate nursing level. Included in the manual are various teaching guides, visual aids, currently available films and additional examination questions.

We would like to express our appreciation to Philip Favaro, R.Ph., for his assistance and valuable suggestions in the revision of this text, to Mary Elizabeth Wilcox, R.N., B.S., M.S., Assistant Professor at Northeastern University College of Nursing, for her comments and suggestions for this edition, to Miss Sharon E. Eisenhauer, Mrs. Mary Eisenhauer and Mrs. Sue Pope for their assistance in the preparation of the manuscript and to the faculty and administration of the Boston College School of Nursing who provided support and encouragement during the revision.

MARY KAYE ASPERHEIM FAVARO
LAUREL EISENHAUER

From the Preface to the First Edition

The field of pharmacology has seen a rapid period of growth in the last few decades as a result of extensive research that has provided knowledge of many new drugs and revealed much additional information about older remedies.

In a text intended for nursing students, it would be impractical—if not impossible—to treat each commercial product and combination in detail. The intent of this book has been, therefore, to set forth the mechanisms of action and the symptoms of toxicity that may be expected with each general class of drugs and to discuss in detail only the more commonly used drugs in each class.

With this sort of background, the student can then assimilate information about new products into her general frame of knowledge and more readily understand how each new discovery resembles—or differs from—products already available.

Principles and concepts are emphasized more fully than mere lists of factual information, and a common sense approach to drug usage and administration has been stressed. The nurse should be able to appreciate the correct use of drugs as an invaluable aid in the overall treatment of illness, but at the same time she should retain a healthy regard for the untoward side effects and toxic reactions that are all too frequent with almost every drug in current use.

The chapters of this text are arranged to correspond as much as possible with nursing education in other subject areas. A review of physiology has been included in many chapters when it is necessary to understand the action of drugs.

Each chapter is preceded by a brief outline of the important concepts discussed in that section. The outline is not intended to be all-inclusive, but is merely a guide to the studying of the chapter.

Questions for discussion and review have been included at the end of each chapter. Some questions may be answered only by resorting to outside sources; thus the student is encouraged to enlarge her field of knowledge in pharmacology and related areas.

MARY KAYE ASPERHEIM

Contents

Chapter 1 Introduction to Pharmacology

Important Concepts Discussed

1. *Drugs are derived from animal, vegetable and mineral sources. Until quite recently, most drugs were of vegetable origin.*

2. *Because of unavoidable natural variations in drugs derived from plants, official standards were established to assure uniformity in potency.*

3. *The Federal Food, Drug and Cosmetic Act established restrictions governing the purity, labeling, sale and administration of drugs.*

4. *Federal, state and city laws control all phases of the manufacture, sale and dispensing of narcotics.*

Today's nurse is functioning in an environment that differs in many respects from that of her predecessors. Moreover, the nature of her responsibilities and the way in which she is educated to meet them have changed. New materials, new methods, new attitudes are continuously presenting exciting challenges, and the mere expansion of knowledge in traditional fields makes its own demands on the conscientious student and the competent practitioner.

Examples of these kinds of changes that come readily to mind are the trends toward automation of some hospital functions, and the introduction each year of a staggering number of new drugs or combinations and modifications of older agents. We need to view these innovations in perspective; the dispensing of drugs by a machine in the nursing station certainly eases and modifies some traditional practices of the nurse, but just as certainly it does not reduce her need for thorough understanding of how drugs are prepared and administered. Further, she must still develop the habitual skills of observing patients to assess effectiveness of the medication and to detect untoward effects and begin corrective action. Indeed, the aforementioned rapid increase in the number of drug agents—and especially the increase in the number of agents that are truly potent—makes more necessary than ever the acquisition of real competence in pharmacology.

Pharmacology, the science with which this book is concerned, includes a fascinating range of topics. It is the study of drugs—their sources, chemical and physical properties, physiologic actions, absorption, fate, excretion, and therapeutic uses. Because an overall view of drug therapy as one of the components of total patient care is essential to the nurse, each of the various disciplines involved

1

in pharmacology will be developed in this text to the extent that they contribute to this purpose.

The term pharmacology stems from the Greek words *pharmakon,* meaning drug, and *logos,* meaning a rational discussion. Pharmacology in practice, however, is as old as man. The first primitive man who observed that a leaf he chewed caused diarrhea or somnolence was already concerned with the science of drug therapy. In this simple way, countless drugs have been discovered, only to be forgotten and rediscovered many times. Such agents as opium, belladonna, Rauwolfia, quinine, digitalis and curare were components of ancient remedies long before even the foundations of our modern civilization were laid.

Early Egyptian papyri contained prescriptions including materials still in use today, such as magnesia, lime, soda, iron salts and sulfur. Simple compounds of arsenic and poisons found in plants, for example hemlock and strychnine, were used by the ancient Greeks and Romans. Quinine, an antimalarial drug, was discovered when Peruvian cinchona bark was used to treat the fever and chills of a Spanish officer. The symptoms quickly subsided upon its use, it is said, whereupon it was brought to Europe and used as a drug for fevers of various causes.

Until recent times most of our medicinal agents were portions of plants (roots, bark, leaves and sap), but with the advances in pharmaceutical chemistry, many of the active principles have been isolated and made available in pure form. Furthermore, hundreds of additional drugs are prepared synthetically. The expansion of our knowledge and the increasing complexity of our society have made possible the phenomenal growth of the drug industry. Billions of dollars are spent annually in pharmacologic research.

MODERN ATTITUDES TOWARD USE OF DRUGS

The attitudes toward drug use and the demand for medical personnel are quite different today from those of a few generations past. The average consumer today has read rather extensively of new drugs and scientific advancements in magazines and newspapers, and has heard and seen still more advertisements on the radio and television. As a result he feels qualified to prescribe drugs for himself and to urge physicians to prescribe antibiotics, tranquilizers and other new drugs of which he has read even before their release by the drug companies for general use.

Many qualified persons have become alarmed at this situation and have pointed out the dangers of using drugs promiscuously. Numerous monographs have been written also about the iatrogenic (physician-produced) diseases. Side effects of drugs used to treat illnesses at times can be much more serious than the original conditions. There is no doubt that drug-induced diseases represent one of the most important problems facing medicine today.

A nurse's attitude toward the use of drugs is important; the formation of a correct attitude should be one of the primary aims of any course in pharmacology. *Common sense* is the key word in this connection. The nurse and all others who are concerned with prescribing, administering or dispensing medications must recognize first and foremost that the normal body functions optimally when it is supplied with a balanced diet and an adequate amount of rest and recreation. Under circumstances of abnormal emotional stress or physical or functional abnormalities, however, supportive therapy must be given temporarily to restore, at least in part, normal body processes. The "miracle drugs," although often life-saving, may well be a two-edged sword, because they can produce serious and even permanent damage if used unwisely.

Even in her personal life the nurse must be convinced of the extreme importance of taking drugs only when absolutely necessary. Since she has constant access to potent, habit-forming and dangerous drugs, the temptation may well arise to use them indiscriminately herself. Dexamyl Spansules are *not* necessary every time she wants to lose five pounds; Darvon capsules are *not* necessary for a simple headache; sleeping capsules are *not* necessary for daytime sleeping after a night shift. The fact that nurses rate high among drug addicts in the medical field is unfortunate, for in most instances the serious consequences could easily have been avoided by the maintenance of a proper respect for drugs. An intelligent appreciation of the life-saving properties of drugs is necessary; so also is a healthy awareness of the serious side effects that may be produced if drugs are misused.

TERMS USED IN PHARMACOLOGY

Drug. The term "drug" has been defined by the Federal Food, Drug and Cosmetic Act as applying to: (1) articles recognized in the official pharmaceutical standards such as *The United States Pharmacopeia,* the *National Formulary,* the *British Pharmacopoeia,* the *Pharmacopoeia Internationalis;* or other such official volumes; (2) articles intended for use in the diagnosis, cure, mitigation, treatment or prevention of disease in man or animals; (3) articles other than food which are intended to affect the structure or any function of the body of man or animals; and (4) articles intended for use as a component of any article specified in clauses (1), (2) or (3).

Pharmacodynamic agent. A drug classified as a pharmacodynamic agent can stimulate or depress either biochemical or physiologic functions and thus either relieve the symptoms or alter the course of the disease.

Chemotherapeutic agent. Chemotherapeutic agents are intended primarily to inhibit or destroy aberrant cells, such as cancer cells, or microbial parasites that cause disease; while at the same time having minimal effect on healthy living tissue.

Pharmacology. Pharmacology is the study of the responses of living organisms to chemical stimuli. This is a broad definition and includes virtually all the biologic disciplines; pharmacology comprises chiefly the sciences of pharmacodynamics, pharmacotherapeutics, pharmacognosy, pharmacy and toxicology. The science of pharmacology involves specific knowledge of the sources of drugs, their physical and chemical properties, their physiologic actions in the body and their metabolic fate and therapeutic uses.

Pharmacodynamics. The study of the biochemical and physiologic effects of drugs and their mechanisms of action is given the name pharmacodynamics. Much of the subject matter of this science involves biochemistry, microbiology, physiology and pathology. The study is unique in that its focal point is the action of drugs—their absorption, distribution, biotransformation and excretion. Structure-activity relationships, or the prediction of drug action on the basis of chemical structure, have recently become an important phase of pharmacodynamics. The synthesis of many new drugs has resulted from research performed in this area.

Pharmacotherapeutics. Pharmacotherapeutics is the branch of pharmacology concerned only with the use of drugs in the treatment of disease. In this study the therapeutic effects of one agent are compared with those of another on the basis of ability to halt a disease or disease process.

Pharmacognosy. Pharmacognosy, a term derived from the Greek words *pharmakon,* meaning drug, and *gnosis,* meaning knowledge, is concerned with the history, production, commerce, selection, identification, preservation and use of drugs of plant and animal origin.

Pharmacy. Pharmacy involves knowledge of the physical and chemical properties of drugs and available dosage forms. The pharmacist is concerned primarily with preparing, compounding and dispensing medicines upon the written order of a licensed practitioner.

Toxicology. The science of toxicology deals with the noxious effects of drugs. This study involves not only the natural and synthetic compounds used in therapy, but also the numerous other substances that may be responsible for toxic reactions.

Naming drugs

Chemical name—The chemical name describes the drug's structural formula.

Official name—The U.S.P. and/or N.F. designate an official name for the drug. The official name is often identical with the generic name.

Generic name—The laboratory or company that first develops the drug usually assigns a generic name, which is often an abbreviation of the chemical name.

Trade name—each manufacturer may assign a trade or brand name to the drug.

SOURCES OF DRUGS

Drugs are obtained from the animal, vegetable and mineral kingdoms. They may be used in the crude or raw form, or as dried or fresh organs or organisms and their natural exudations; or the active ingredients, such as the various alkaloids, glycosides, alcohols, esters or aldehydes, may be isolated from these crude substances and employed for various therapeutic purposes.

Many drugs that were formerly obtained only from natural sources are now prepared synthetically; this method is generally more satisfactory when it can be used. Synthetic procedures have contributed greatly to the advancement of pharmacology, and are responsible for the great majority of the new "miracle drugs" in present use. Very often only a slight alteration in chemical structure can greatly change the action of a drug in the body. Drugs can be given a more selective action and the number of undesirable side effects can be greatly reduced by such slight changes.

Following are a few examples of drugs obtained from the various sources:

Animal kingdom. Drugs obtained from the animal kingdom vary greatly in their pharmaceutical applications. Many drugs are prepared from the glands of animals (e.g., thyroid hormone, insulin, and sex hormones); other drugs may be prepared from shells and exoskeletons (e.g., prepared chalk), or from substances such as beeswax and cobra venom, which are extruded from animals.

Vegetable kingdom. Until relatively re-

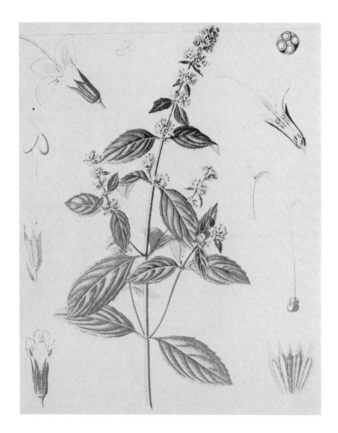

FIGURE 1. *Mentha piperita*, the source of peppermint oil. (From Claus: Pharmacognosy, 4th Ed. Lea and Febiger, 1961.)

cent times, most of the substances used as drugs were of vegetable origin. Almost every part of the plant has been used for pharmaceutical or healing purposes: roots (digitalis, glycyrrhiza or licorice, sarsaparilla); rhizomes (aspidium, iris); barks (cinchona, sassafras, wild cherry); leaves (hyoscyamus, belladonna, digitalis, peppermint, senna); fruits (*Rhamnus cathartica,* colocynth, caraway, juniper berries); flowers (clove, corn silk); and seeds (flaxseed, black mustard, castor oil).

Mineral kingdom. Only a few minerals in their pure forms are used in current therapy. These would include copper sulfate, magnesium sulfate, and aluminum.

Synthetic drugs. In addition to active ingredients of plant and animal drugs that are now prepared synthetically, hundreds of drugs that are classified as corticosteroids, tranquilizers, psychic energizers, chemotherapeutic agents and germicides are prepared by synthetic chemical procedures.

DEVELOPMENT AND EVALUATION OF NEW DRUGS

PROCEDURE

In the United States the development and use of new drugs for interstate commerce is controlled by regulations administered by the Food and Drug Administration (F.D.A.). Clinical data that have been developed during the investigation of the drug must be submitted.

The investigational phase is controlled by F.D.A. regulations and involves the thorough investigation and study of the pharmacologic effects of the drug in animals in order to find evidence that the drug has some effectiveness and is sufficiently safe to warrant further testing in studies on man. Early studies are done on all actions and effects of the drug, dosage, chemical properties, metabolism, side effects and acute and chronic toxicity. From this data, the drug's safety margin is estimated, i.e., the ratio between the dose causing the desirable effect and the dose causing toxic effects. The drug's therapeutic index — its relative safety

in comparison to standard drugs — is also determined and is considered in the decision to conduct further studies. Further studies are conducted on animals in order to determine chronic toxic effects on organs and tissues, especially the kidney, liver, bone marrow, blood and fetus of pregnant female animals.

Initially in human studies, the new drug is administered carefully to normal, healthy volunteers and to patients. Except under unusual circumstances, all persons involved give their consent to participate in the experiment. Ethical and moral aspects of such human investigations have been specified by F.D.A. guidelines.

If the experiments with patients give indications that the drug may have some effectiveness, further pharmacologic studies and controlled clinical studies are done to determine the new drug's efficacy and safety.

In clinical studies it may be necessary for the nature of the medication to be concealed from the patient (single-blind experiment) or from both the patient and all persons involved in the conduct and administration of the study (double-blind experiment). The "blind" experiments are necessary particularly when the subjective aspects of the drug's effect, such as relief from pain or anxiety, are being evaluated. These studies attempt to reduce the possibility that the patient's response may be from conscious or unconscious suggestions made by the staff or from the psychologic effect on the patient of receiving "a medication" rather than from the specific action of the drug.

In some studies a placebo, or another drug used for comparison, may be given to certain patients in the study rather than the experimental drug. Usually the agent administered to an individual patient is identified only by a code number so that those involved in the study do not know which agent is the actual drug being tested until data have been collected and analyzed. This is intended to give greater objectivity to the study and is also helpful in distinguishing drug effect from possible spontaneous remission of a disease.

The evaluation of a drug's effectiveness and safety continues even after it is in general clinical use. Reports of adverse effects and other clinical experience and data must be submitted by the manufacturer to the Food and Drug Administration. The F.D.A. has responsibility for the continuous evaluation of the toxicity and effectiveness of drugs in general use, and can remove from the market any drug found to be too dangerous in comparison to its therapeutic usefulness. The F.D.A. may also require changes in the labeling of certain drugs or the deletion of claims made by the drug's manufacturer.

NURSE'S ROLE

If the nurse finds herself participating in a clinical study of an investigational drug or caring for the patient involved, she may need to adapt her nursing care to some degree. The nurse must become acquainted with the research methodology in order to give good nursing care to the patient, while working within the framework and specifications of the research.

Depending on the research design and her degree of participation, the nurse should determine from the physician or investigator the nature of the drug, its actions, effects and uses, dosage forms and strengths available and the observations she should make in relation to effect and toxicity. She should also determine what action she should take if toxicity should develop.

The nurse should determine from the investigator the patient's degree of knowledge about the drug and its effect, and whether his informed consent has been obtained. In caring for a patient receiving an experimental drug, the nurse should avoid influencing, either postively or negatively, the patient's attitude toward the drug or the study. She should refer the patient's or family's questions to the physician or investigator, so that the greatest amount of objectivity is maintained while the patient's needs are met and rights are respected.

DOSAGE FORMS

Drugs may be administered in many ways. Very often the dosage form and the mode of administration determine to a great extent the therapeutic efficacy of the drug. After a compound is isolated and its pharmacologic properties are evaluated, much additional time and research are devoted to the preparation of palatable and effective dosage forms.

Listed here are the more common pharmaceutical preparations.

Solutions: liquid preparations containing one or more substances completely dissolved. Every solution has two parts—the solute (dissolved substance) and the solvent (the liquid in which it is dissolved).

Waters: saturated solutions of volatile oils (e.g., peppermint water, camphor water).

Syrups: aqueous solutions of a sugar. These may or may not have medicinal substances added (e.g., ipecac syrup, simple syrup).

Spirits: alcoholic solutions of volatile substances, also known as essences (e.g., essence of peppermint, camphor spirit).

Mucilages: aqueous preparations containing viscous substances such as gums and starches. These are used mostly as suspending agents (e.g., tragacanth mucilage).

Elixirs: solutions containing alcohol, sugar and water (e.g., terpin hydrate elixir, phenobarbital elixir). They may or may not be aromatic and may or may not have active medicinals. Most frequently they are used as flavoring agents or solvents.

Tinctures: alcoholic or hydroalcoholic solutions prepared from drugs (e.g., iodine tincture, digitalis tincture).

Fluidextracts: alcoholic liquid extracts, of drugs made by percolation so that 1 cc. of the fluidextract contains 1 Gm. of the drug (e.g., glycyrrhiza fluidextract). Only vegetable drugs are used.

Emulsions: dispersions of fat globules in water (or water globules in fat) prepared with the aid of an emulsifying agent (e.g., Haley's M-O, Petrogalar).

Liniments: mixtures of drugs with oil, soap, water or alcohol and intended for external application with rubbing (e.g., camphor liniment, chloroform liniment).

Lotions: aqueous preparations containing suspended materials and intended for soothing local application. Most are patted on rather than rubbed (e.g., calamine lotion, Caladryl lotion).

FIGURE 2. Actual sizes of empty gelatin capsules. (Lyman: *American Pharmacy.* 5th Ed., J. B. Lippincott Co., 1960.)

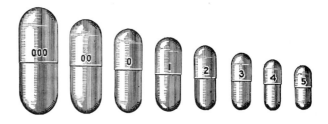

Powders: single dose quantities of a drug or mixture of drugs in powdered form; wrapped separately in powder papers (e.g., Seidlitz powder).

Tablets: single dose units made by compressing powdered drugs into a suitable mold (e.g., aspirin tablets).

Pills: single dose units made by mixing the powdered drug with a liquid such as syrup, and rolling the mixture into a round or oval shape (e.g., Hinkle's pills). These are largely replaced by other dosage forms today.

Capsules: powdered drugs within a gelatin container (e.g., Benadryl capsules). Liquids may be placed in soft gelatin capsules (e.g., cod liver oil capsules).

Suppositories: mixtures of drugs with some firm base such as cocoa butter, to be molded into shape for insertion into a body orifice. Rectal, vaginal and urethral suppositories are the most common types (e.g., Dulcolax suppositories, Furacin vaginal suppositories), but nasal or otic suppositories can be made.

Ointments: mixtures of drugs with a fatty base for external application, usually with rubbing (e.g., zinc oxide ointment, bengué ointment).

DRUG STANDARDS

Before the standardization of drugs became requisite, variations in potency led to many unnecessary ill effects. Differences in the strain of plant used, growing conditions and various other environmental circumstances can drastically alter the amount of active ingredient contained in a plant drug. One gram of the crude drug from one source may have little or no effect, whereas the same amount from another source could contain a near lethal dose. Official drug standards have now been established to limit the variability of active ingredients in subsequent doses of drugs.

American Drug Standards

In the United States the two official volumes of drug standards are *The United States Pharmacopeia* and the *National Formulary;* all drugs recognized as official in this country

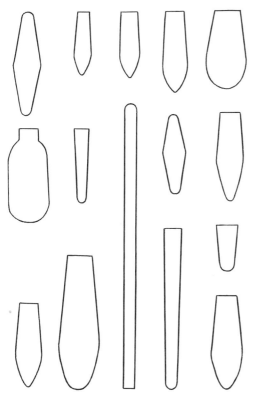

FIGURE 3. Variety of sizes and shapes of suppositories.

are described in these books. A third book, the *Homeopathic Pharmacopoeia*, though still official, is seldom used today. Many other reliable and excellent reference books are also available if more detailed pharmacologic information is desired.

The United States Pharmacopeia (U.S.P.). The object of the U.S.P. is to provide standards for drugs and medicines of therapeutic usefulness or pharmaceutical necessity. The approved therapeutic agents used in medical practice are described and defined in this publication with respect to source, chemistry, physical properties, tests for identity, tests for purity, assay, method of storage and average therapeutic dose. Most of the preparations detailed in the U.S.P. are single drugs rather than compound mixtures. Directions are given, however, for the preparation of those drugs that must be compounded.

When seen after a drug name, U.S.P. designates a drug whose strength and quality are up to official standards.

The first pharmacopeia in the United States was published in 1820, and since that time numerous revisions have appeared. It is now the practice to revise the *Pharmacopeia* at five-year intervals, to publish a bound supplement midway between revisions, and to issue interim revision announcements or sheet supplements whenever required. In this manner the *Pharmacopeia* is kept abreast of rapid advances in pharmacotherapeutics.

National Formulary (N.F.). The *National Formulary* was first published in 1888 as the *National Formulary of Unofficial Preparations.* At that time it contained only formulas for preparations of drug mixtures. Standards for those drugs not listed in the U.S.P. were included in the N.F.

The publication became an official drug standard when so designated by the Pure Food and Drugs Act of 1906, after which its title was shortened to the present form.

The N.F. lists drugs on the basis of demand as well as therapeutic value. Many drugs which have been deleted from the U.S.P. appear in the N.F. The *National Formulary* differs also from the *Pharmacopeia* in that it contains many more formulas for drug mixtures than does the U.S.P.

New Drugs. In 1965 the American Medical Association began publication of *New Drugs,* a replacement for the former *New and Nonofficial Drugs* (N.N.D.). Whereas listing in N.N.D. implied approval by the Council on Drugs of the A.M.A, the new publication lists drugs whether or not they have been approved by the Council. The inclusion of any particular drug does not imply endorsement or acceptance by the A.M.A. *New Drugs* is an annual publication containing information on drugs introduced during the past ten years. It is organized according to therapeutic indications, and the information provided is based on evaluations of new drugs by the Council on Drugs and its consultants.

British and Canadian Drug Standards

British Pharmacopoeia (B.P.). Like *The United States Pharmacopeia,* this book contains official standards for drugs that are official in the United Kingdom, the British dominions and the Crown colonies.

The B.P. is published by the British Pharmacopoeia Commission under the direction of the General Medical Council. Doses of the drugs included are expressed chiefly in the metric system, although the imperial system is used in some instances.

British Pharmaceutical Codex (B.P.C.). The Pharmaceutical Society of Great Britain publishes this text, which is similar in scope and content to the *National Formulary.*

Canadian Formulary (C.F.). The *Canadian Formulary* is published by the Canadian Pharmaceutical Association and was given official status by the Canadian Food and Drug Act. It contains formulas for many pharmaceutical preparations that are used frequently in Canada and in addition has standards for new Canadian drugs that are not included in the *British Pharmacopoeia.*

Physician's Formulary. Published by the Canadian Medical Association, the *Physician's Formulary* contains formulas for many pharmaceutical preparations used frequently in Canadian medical practice. It is similar to *New Drugs* published by the A.M.A. in the United States.

International Standards

Many nations of the world publish their own compendia of drug standards—e.g., Germany, France, Czechoslovakia, Turkey and Poland. In South America, however, a Spanish translation of *The United States Pharmacopeia* is used as the official standard. The *Pharmacopoeia Internationalis* is recognized as official in many countries.

Pharmacopoeia Internationalis (I.P.). Because of the many and varied standards and systems of nomenclature used by the different national pharmacopeias, a desire for greater uniformity of terms, strengths and composition of drugs led to the publication of the *International Pharmacopoeia* by the World Health Organization in 1951. The nomenclature of the *Pharmacopoeia* is in Latin; the doses are in the metric system.

Although published in English, French and Spanish, the *Pharmacopoeia* is not designed to have official status in any country unless it is specifically adopted by the national pharmacopeial authorities. Many drugs official in other national pharmacopeias are included, as well as long-established drugs and newer agents that have not been accepted as yet by the various national pharmacopeias. An unusual feature of the I.P. is the inclusion of tables of doses for children up to five years of age.

Additional Reference Sources

The following books do not have official status; however, they are useful adjuncts to the official volumes when more specific information is desired.

United States Dispensatory. The *Dispensatory* is a general reference text that contains information of a botanical, chemical and pharmaceutical nature as well as the general therapeutic indications for drugs.

In addition to information on drugs included in the U.S.P. and N.F., the *Dispensatory* also lists drugs included in the *British Pharmacopoeia* and the *Pharmacopoeia Internationalis* as well as many nonofficial drugs in use at the present time.

Physicians' Desk Reference (PDR). Physicians' Desk Reference is published annually by Medical Economics, Inc., with the cooperation of most of the pharmaceutical manufacturers in the United States. Each product description is prepared by the manufacturer and edited by his medical department before it is included in PDR.

Even though the amount of information contained in PDR falls far short of that which would be desirable for a thorough acquaintance with the various medicinal agents it describes, this book has proved to be one of the most widely used reference sources available today. This is probably because of its convenient arrangement. It is divided into six sections, each printed on paper of a different color. In the various sections the drugs are listed alphabetically by brand name, then by groups of drugs with similar content, then by therapeutic indication. The main body of the book contains summaries of the composition, action and uses, mode of administration, dosage, side effects and contraindications of commercial pharmaceutical products.

Hospital Formulary. The *Hospital Formulary,* published by the American Society of Hospital Pharmacists, contains a collection of drug monographs and additional information on the various classes of drugs, such as antibiotics, tranquilizers and corticosteroids. The *Formulary* is intended for use by physicians, nurses and allied medical personnel and is an excellent reference source. It supplies much more information on medicinal agents than can be found in the PDR. Because of its loose-leaf arrangement, supplements can be added every few months to keep the *Formulary* as up-to-date as possible for a reference text. The *Hospital Formulary* is somewhat formidable in appearance, which is probably the reason it is not utilized to a greater extent.

The *Formulary* is divided into sections based upon drug action—e.g., central nervous system drugs, expectorants and cough preparations, etc. The sections are then subdivided; the section on central nervous system drugs, for instance, is divided into the subsections general anesthetics, respiratory and cerebral stimulants and so forth. Within each subsection the drugs are listed alphabetically by generic name. Drugs may be found in the index under either trade name or generic name.

The small amount of time it takes to become familiar with the *Hospital Formulary* is well worth the effort when concise and comprehensive information on therapeutic agents is desired.

Remington's Pharmaceutical Sciences. Although *Remington's Pharmaceutical Sciences* is a text primarily for pharmacists, it provides sufficient information on both official and nonofficial old and new drugs to be a useful reference for any of the allied medical professions.

Drugs are listed in the index by their trade, generic and common names. Information is included on the physical and chemical properties of drugs, their solubility, general uses, incompatibilities, doses and mode of administration.

American Drug Index. The *American Drug Index* includes in outline form the ingredients of various trademarked drugs, as well as the names of their manufacturers, general uses and doses. It is a useful reference for the ingredients of commercial preparations, but it is not intended to convey pharmacologic or toxicologic information.

In addition, many hospitals have their own formularies, which in some cases are valuable sources of drug information.

DRUG LEGISLATION IN THE UNITED STATES

The principal laws that affect medications in the United States are the Federal Food, Drug, and Cosmetic Act of 1938 and the narcotic laws.

FEDERAL FOOD, DRUG, AND COSMETIC ACT. The current Federal Food, Drug, and Cosmetic Act became law in 1938. The act is designed for the protection of public health, but it also serves to protect the physician from unethical practices of irresponsible drug manufacturers. Enforcement of the law is entrusted to the Food and Drug Administration of the Department of Health, Education, and Welfare. Features of the act that are of particular interest to the medical professions and that apply to drugs are as follows:

1. Drugs used in the diagnosis of disease and drugs intended to affect the structure or any function of the body are under governmental control.

2. The law prohibits traffic in drugs and devices that are dangerous to health under conditions of use prescribed on the label.

3. Traffic in new drugs is prohibited unless such drugs have been adequately tested to show that they are safe for use under the conditions of use prescribed in their labeling. Exemption from this requirement is granted solely to drugs intended for investigational use by qualified scientific experts.

4. Drugs intended for human use must bear labels warning against habit formation if they contain any of the listed narcotic or hypnotic habit-forming substances or any derivative of such substances that possess the same properties.

5. The labels of nonofficial drugs must list the active ingredients and indicate the quantity of certain specified ingredients.

6. The labels of drugs and devices must bear warnings against use in pathologic conditions or by children when such use may be dangerous to health.

7. The labels of official drugs must indicate any differences from the official standards of strength, quality or purity.

8. Official drugs must be packaged and labeled as prescribed by the U.S.P. and N.F.

9. The act declares nonofficial drugs illegal if the standard of purity or quality falls below the standard claimed.

10. The act requires that drugs listed as antiseptics possess germicidal power.

The food and drug laws assist the physician in that they rigidly control the standards, purity and composition of drugs and drug mixtures. In the last analysis, the law is designed to protect the layman who insists on indulging in self-medication, but its effects cannot compare with the protection afforded by proper medical care on the part of a physician.

NARCOTIC AND DANGEROUS DRUG LAWS.
On May 1, 1971 the Controlled Substances Act become effective, listing new requirements for the control of the manufacture, sale and dispensing of narcotics and dangerous drugs. New additions and/or reclassifications of drugs may be made as often as every six months thereafter.

There are established five schedules of controlled substances, to be known as schedules I, II, III, IV and V, defined as follows:

Schedule I
  A. The drug has a high potential for abuse.
  B. There is no currently accepted medical use for the drug or other substance in the United States.
  C. There is a lack of accepted safety for use of the drug or other substance under medical supervision.

Some examples of drugs in this schedule are heroin, marihuana, LSD, peyote and mescaline.

Schedule II
  A. The drug has a high potential for abuse.
  B. There is a currently accepted medical use in treatment in the United States, or a currently accepted medical use with severe restrictions.
  C. Abuse of the drug or other substance may lead to severe psychologic or physical dependence.

Some examples are opium, morphine, codeine, dihydromorphinone (Dilaudid), methadone (Dolophine), Pantopon, meperidine (Demerol), cocaine, oxycodone (Percodan), anileridine (Leritine), oxymorphone (Numorphan) and oral and injectable amphetamines.

Schedule III
  A. The drug has a potential for abuse less than the drugs in Schedules I and II.
  B. There is a currently accepted medical use in the United States.
  C. Abuse of the drug may lead to moderate or low physical dependence or high psychologic dependence.

Examples are glutethimide (Doriden), phenmetrazine (Preludin), Paregoric, methyprylon (Noludar), methylphenidate (Ritalin), and barbiturates *except* phenobarbital, methylphenobarbital and barbital.

Schedule IV
  A. The drug or other substance has a low potential for abuse relative to the above classes.
  B. There is a currently accepted medical use in the United States.
  C. Abuse may lead to limited physical dependence or psychologic dependence relative to drugs in Schedule III.

Examples are phenobarbital, methylphenobarbital, barbital, chloral betaine (Beta Chlor), Chloral hydrate, ethchlorvynol (Placidyl), ethinamate (Valmid), meprobamate (Equinil, Miltown) and paraldehyde.

Schedule V
  A. The drug has a low potential for abuse relative to substances in Schedule IV.
  B. The drug has a currently accepted medical use in treatment in the United States.
  C. Abuse may lead to limited physical dependence or psychological dependence relative to the drugs in Schedule IV.

The drugs in this class are the drugs formerly treated as exempt narcotics. They generally are narcotic substances containing one or more nonnarcotics in mixture form. Many cough preparations are in this schedule as is Lomotil.

It must be remembered that these federal regulations may be made more stringent by individual state narcotic and dangerous drug laws. In any case, the stricter of the two laws must be obeyed. Some states may require that drugs listed on the lower federal schedules be treated as schedule II or III drugs, for instance, and there may be some intrastate variation governing the amount of narcotic drug permitted for a compound to be listed as a Schedule V, or nonprescription drug.

CANADIAN DRUG LEGISLATION

Food and drug control in Canada has been operative on a national basis since 1874 when the Parliament of Canada passed a law preventing the sale of adulterated foods and drugs.

At the present time the Food and Drug

Directorate of the Department of National Health and Welfare enforces the Food and Drugs Act, the Patent Medicine Act and the Narcotic Control Act, although the last is enforced largely by the Royal Canadian Mounted Police.

CANADIAN FOOD AND DRUGS ACT. The Canadian Food and Drugs Act exerts a considerable influence upon the lives and habits of the Canadian people as well as upon the agricultural and industrial interests of Canada. Although many of the statutes deal with general problems such as the production, manufacture and distribution of a food or drug, others deal exclusively with one food (e.g., the Maple Products Industry Act). Restrictions are at both federal and provincial levels. There is considerable duplication of legislation at these two governmental levels; however, the statutes are presented from different points of view and each has a particular purpose. The Food and Drugs Act empowers the Governor in Council to prescribe the standards of quality and to fix the limits of variation in any food or drug that is not described in the law.

According to the law, a food or drug must be correctly labeled and unadulterated according to standards set in the statutes. There must be no deceptive marks or designs on the package regarding the ingredients therein. Section 7 of the Act creates a form of statutory misbranding if an article is advertised as a treatment for certain specific diseases listed in schedule A. The list of 36 diseases includes such ailments as gangrene, appendicitis, influenza, sexual impotence and alcoholism. The law states also that unless a drug is clearly labeled to be otherwise, it must comply with the standards of the recognized pharmacopeias and formularies listed in schedule B.

Schedule F of the Food and Drugs Act lists drugs that must be sold only on prescription. A prescription for any of these drugs must not be refilled unless the practitioner so directs and specifies the number of times that it may be refilled. Indictment proceedings are instituted in serious violations of this statute. New drugs are added to schedule F as they are marketed.

Schedule G lists the controlled drugs, amphetamines, barbiturates, benzphetamine, methamphetamine and their salts and derivatives, which must be obtained only through firms licensed to deal in controlled drugs. A signed requisition is required before the medicine may be released, and records of all transactions must be maintained.

Schedule H was added to an amendment to the Act in 1962, and prohibits the sale of thalidomide and lysergic acid diethylamide. Amendments to the Act enable the Council to withdraw from the market any drug that is considered to be too toxic for general use.

CANADIAN NARCOTIC CONTROL ACT. The Narcotic Control Act states, "Except as authorized by this Act or the regulations, no person shall have a narcotic in his possession. No person shall traffic in a narcotic, or export or import into Canada any narcotic except under the provisions of the Act. In addition, no person shall cultivate opium poppy or marihuana except under the authority of and in accordance with a license issued to him by the Minister of National Health and Welfare."

A person who has obtained a narcotic pursuant to the regulations of the Narcotic Control Act is authorized to be in possession of that narcotic if he is a licensed dealer, a practitioner, a pharmacist or a hospital administrator, if he has obtained a narcotic prescription or if he is authorized by the Minister to be in possession of narcotics.

A 1966 amendment states that any individual for whom a narcotic prescription has been issued shall not seek or receive another prescription for a narcotic from a different practitioner without disclosing to that practitioner the particulars of every prescription or narcotic that he has obtained within the previous 30 days.

Everyone authorized to possess narcotics must keep an official record of all narcotics received, the name and address of the supplier, and the date received; he must keep also a similar record concerning all persons for whom the narcotic was supplied. All records must be retained for at least two years.

A signed and dated prescription by a qualified practitioner must be received by the pharmacist before he may legally dispense a drug governed by the Narcotic Control Act. Drugs included are opium, coca (cocaine), *Cannabis sativa* (marihuana), and all synthetic addicting drugs.

Exempt narcotics. A pharmacist may, without a prescription, sell a preparation containing $\frac{1}{8}$ grain or less codeine per tablet or other solid form, or $\frac{1}{3}$ grain or less per fluid ounce in liquid preparations if the narcotic is combined with one or more non-narcotic medicinal ingredients. Such medications must have affixed to the container a caution label stating that the preparation contains codeine and should not be administered to children except on the advice of a physician.

Hospital regulations. Specific narcotic regulations that apply to hospitals are as follows. A person in charge of a hospital shall enter in a book, register or other record maintained for such purposes the following information:

1. the name and quantity of any narcotic received;

2. the name and address of the person from whom the narcotic is received and the date it is received;

3. the name and quantity of any narcotic used in the manufacture of drugs received;

4. the name of any narcotic manufacturer whose drugs are used and the date of manufacture of these drugs;

5. the name of patients for whom a narcotic other than an oral prescription narcotic is dispensed;

6. the name of the practitioner ordering or prescribing a narcotic other than an oral prescription narcotic;

7. the date a narcotic other than an oral prescription narcotic is ordered or prescribed and the form and quantity thereof.

The above records shall be retained for a period of not less than two years. The hospital administrator shall take all necessary steps to protect narcotics in the hospital against loss or theft, and report to the Minister any loss or theft of narcotics within ten days of his discovery thereof.

A person in charge of a hospital shall furthermore furnish any information, in such form and at such times as the Minister may require, respecting the use of narcotics in that hospital. He shall produce to an inspector any books, records or documents required by these regulations, and permit an inspector to make copies thereof or take extracts from them. He shall also permit an inspector to check all stock of narcotics in the hospital.

Finally, a person in charge of any narcotic in a hospital shall dispense this narcotic only to a person or animal under treatment as an inpatient or outpatient, and only upon the written order or prescription of a medical practitioner.

NURSING IMPLICATIONS

Regulations related to narcotics and other dangerous drugs are carried out within the hospital or health care agency by the institution's policies. Many of these policies and procedures affect the nurse. Although these policies and procedures may vary from institution to institution, there are many common features.

Narcotics and controlled drugs are kept under double lock, i.e., these drugs are kept within a locked closet within the locked medicine closet or room. The medication keys must be on the nurse's person at all times.

Special forms and records are usually required. They ordinarily involve recording data, in a special book or record, about each narcotic dose used. Orders for narcotic and other controlled drugs are valid for a certain number of hours as determined by the hospital's policy. The nurse must therefore check the physician's order carefully to be sure it has not expired before she administers the drug.

Narcotics and other controlled drugs must be accounted for at all times. These drugs must be counted and checked by the nursing staff at each change of shift. Any discrepancies must be reported to the pharmacist and/or the nursing supervisor.

Hospital policies may also include procedures to be followed for the disposal of a drug that is not administered or is accidentally contaminated. Some hospitals may also have special policies concerning the administration of narcotics by nursing students.

The nurse should be thoroughly familiar with the policies and regulations in effect at the hospital or health care facility in which she is administering medications.

QUESTIONS FOR DISCUSSION AND REVIEW

1. What is the difference between a capsule, a tablet and a pill?
2. What makes a drug "official"? Why is it important that a drug correspond to official standards?
3. Look up the official standards for:

    a. phenobarbital   c. tetracycline
    b. digitalis   d. acetylsalicylic acid

4. How does the N.N.D. differ from the U.S.P.?
5. Do you believe that federal drug control will always be necessary? Why or why not?
6. May every physician prescribe narcotics? Why do you think restrictions of this sort are necessary?
7. Do you think self-medication in general is a good idea? What basic principles could you outline as a "rule of thumb" to determine when self-medication is advisable and when it is not?
8. What does U.S.P. on a drug label signify?
9. What sources of drug information are available in your clinical setting? Does the hospital have its own formulary?
10. What are the nurse's responsibilities in relation to narcotics and other controlled drugs in your hospital? What are the hospital's policies and regulations? What special policies, if any, apply to nursing students?

BIBLIOGRAPHY

American Medical Association: *New and Non-Official Drugs.* Philadelphia, J. B. Lippincott Co., 1965.
American Medical Association Council on Drugs: *AMA Drug Evaluations.* Chicago, American Medical Association, 1971.
American Pharmaceutical Association: *National Formulary.* 12th Ed. Washington, D.C., 1965.
Cutting, W. C.: *Handbook of Pharmacology.* 4th Ed. New York, Appleton-Century-Crofts, 1969.
Faddis, M. O.: Drugs, drugs, and more drugs. *Amer. J. Nurs., 62*:64, (July) 1962.
Goodman, L. S., and Gilman, A.: *Pharmacologic Basis of Therapeutics.* 4th Ed. New York, Macmillan Co., 1970.

Hospital Formulary. Washington, D.C., American Hospital Formulary Service, 1964.

Lewis, J. R.: Drug evaluation by Council on Drugs. *J.A.M.A., 185*:256, 1963.

Lorber, G.: Sources of drug information. *Amer. J. Nurs., 63*:101–103, (December) 1963.

Martin, E. W. (ed.): *Husa's Pharmaceutical Dispensing.* 5th Ed. St. Louis, C. V. Mosby Co., 1959.

Modell, W.: Safety in new drugs. *J.A.M.A., 190*:141, 1964.

Osol, A., Farrar, G. E. and Pratt, R.: *The Dispensatory of the United States of America.* Philadelphia, J. B. Lippincott Co., 1960.

Remington's Practice of Pharmacy. 12th Ed. Easton, Pa., Mack Publishing Co., 1961.

Smith, R. G.: The development and control of new drugs. *Amer. J. Nurs., 62*:56–58, (July) 1962.

The Merck Manual of Diagnosis and Therapy. 11th Ed. Rahway, N. J., Merck, Sharpe and Dohme Research Laboratories, 1966.

Chapter 2 The Role of the Nurse in Drug Therapy

Important Concepts Discussed

1. *Drug therapy is an important and integral part of the patient's medical and nursing care plan.*
2. *Nursing observations during patient assessment should be directed toward indications of drug effectiveness as well as side effects.*
3. *Nursing measures should be designed to promote drug effect and to reduce side effects of drug therapy.*
4. *Teaching the patient, family and general public about drug use and the dangers of self-medication is an important nursing role.*

THE ROLE OF THE NURSE

The nurse's role and responsibilities in drug therapy are changing as nursing and the health care system changes and adapts in response to the health needs of society and technologic advances. The health team membership is growing and becoming more complex. New members with new or specialized functions are joining the health team. The roles of many members are expanding and overlapping.

Traditionally the registered nurse has been the one who administers most medications to the patient after the physician has prescribed the drug and the pharmacist has dispensed it. Changes are occurring in which this breakdown of functions is no longer as clearly delineated. Licensed practical nurses are widely used in the administration of medications. In certain settings the pharmacist has become more involved in the clinical aspects of drug therapy and in the actual administration of drugs to the patient. In some hospitals drugs may be prepared and administered from a centralized drug room rather than by the nursing staff on the patient care unit.

Computerization has been developed for many aspects of this intricate process, from the prescribing of a drug by the physician to the administration, recording and billing of the drug. Other approaches and systems of drug distribution have been developed to improve the safety and efficiency of the process and to reduce the financial costs involved. Some of these trends are discussed further in Chapter 3.

Whether or not the nurse herself actually administers a particular drug, she must have a knowledge and understanding of pharmacology in order to provide intelligent and competent nursing care. A drug is given to a person and that person remains the center and focus of nursing. Drug therapy cannot be viewed in isolation from the patient, his illness or other aspects of his care. Drug therapy is an important and often vital part of the patient's care, but in order for the drug therapy to be effective and safe, it should be integrated with all other aspects of the patient's medical and nursing care plan.

Since an important role of the nurse is her continual assessment of the patient, the nurse should have a sufficient knowledge of the pharmacology of the drugs the patient is receiving in order to observe for indications of drug effectiveness as well as signs of toxicity. An understanding of the pathophysiology of the patient's illness and the relationship of drug action and effect to the illness is also essential for the nurse. Nursing interventions to promote and evaluate drug effectiveness should be designed and implemented as part of the nursing care plan for the patient.

KNOWLEDGE AND UNDERSTANDING NEEDED BY THE NURSE

The types of knowledge that the nurse needs about the pharmacology of a drug are numerous. The nurse must understand where and how a drug acts and the ways in which bodily mechanisms are altered. This understanding will enable her to give intelligent nursing care and also facilitate her understanding of the drug effect in relation to the patient's pathophysiologic state. Conversely, the nurse needs an understanding of the pathophysiology of the patient's disease in order to understand drug action and effects. These understandings will also enable the nurse to recognize conditions or situations in which a drug is contraindicated.

The nurse needs to know the effects produced by the drug, both the desired or intended effect and the side effects. Since a particular drug may be used in a variety of conditions for different reasons and different effects, the nurse should be aware of the effect desired by the physician for a particular patient.

Knowledge of the usual range of dosage and the factors which affect drug dosage are needed by the nurse in order for her to detect erroneous dosage orders. In some instances, the effect of the drug depends on the dosage in which it is given. For example, milk of magnesia is used as an antacid in a dosage of 4 ml., but it is used as a laxative in a dosage of 30 ml.

Knowledge of the route by which a drug should be administered is important in order to prevent harm to the patient by the use of an incorrect route. Some drugs can be given only by a certain route and are ineffective or dangerous if given by another route. The nurse must also know how to give drugs correctly by each route of administration in order to insure optimal drug absorption and effect. Incorrect technique may be harmful and even fatal. As will be discussed in Chapter 3, intramuscular injection technique must be done correctly in order to prevent the drug from being injected into a blood vessel, nerves or subcutaneous tissue.

The nurse should also be familiar with the possible interactions that a drug may have with food or other drugs the patient is receiving. The nurse is often in a position to detect the possibility of such interactions occurring. If a new drug is ordered for a patient, the nurse's knowledge of other drugs the patient is receiving should enable her to predict or detect interactions which should be brought to the physician's attention.

An understanding of the patient as an individual is essential to the total plan of care. Just as the physiologic aspects of the patient's condition must be understood in relation to drug action, the psychologic and emotional aspects of drug therapy must also be considered.

Although a particular drug is known to produce certain effects, the effects of that drug in an individual patient are not always predictable. Physiologic reasons may be a factor, but the psychologic aspects of the drug therapy should not be underestimated. As was discussed earlier in Chapter 1, the power of suggestion is of sufficient significance in drug response that clinical studies of drugs often must be conducted under special circumstances in order to reduce the influence of suggestion on the patients.

The nurse should consider the meaning of the drug therapy to the patient. Drug therapy may assume great importance to the patient in that the giving of the drug may represent a positive concrete action taken by the health team for him. Perhaps too often the patient sees the nurse only at the times that his medications are administered. The scheduling of medications often provides the patient with his sense of time and the framework for daily activities. Such a patient may become rather distressed by a delayed or omitted dose.

The administration of a drug may be seen by the patient as a cure for his symptoms and problems, or it may be viewed as an indication that he is severely ill. The type of attitude, of course, depends a great deal on the patient, his actual illness and his perception of it, the particular drug and the patient's previous knowledge or experience with the drug. The influence of the patient's attitude toward drug therapy will be discussed further in relation to meeting the learning needs of the patient.

THE NURSE AND DRUG EFFECT

With her knowledge of a drug's action and intended effect, the nurse should make observations to evaluate drug effect, and should initiate nursing measures to promote the effect intended. Nursing interventions should be used to prevent or reduce a patient's need for certain types of drugs. Because of the usual close relationship of the drug action to the patient's underlying disease or condition, the nursing care should be designed to meet the total needs of the patient and to support the effectiveness of all therapeutic measures prescribed.

The administration of a drug should not be viewed as a substitute for the nursing care of the patient. The needs of a patient should not be considered met by drug therapy alone. The drug therapy should be integrated with nursing interventions that are based on the nurse's knowledge of her patient and the reason why the drug was prescribed. For example, a sedative or tranquilizer should not be used in place of efforts to determine the source of a patient's anxiety or the basis for his behavior. When these drugs are used, the nurse should also strive to increase the therapeutic use of the nurse-patient relationship in order to determine and meet the patient's needs. Good nursing care often can alleviate or greatly reduce a patient's need for certain types of drugs.

There are several approaches available to the nurse in collecting data used in the evaluation of drug effectiveness. The patient's subjective response is an important criterion in most instances. It is important, therefore, that the patient be asked directly or indirectly for his evaluation of the drug's effectiveness.

The nurse's observations are essential in the evaluation of drug effectiveness. Systematic and directed observations based on a knowledge of the drug's pharmacology and the individual patient are necessary. Methods of collecting data for evaluating drug effect should be incorporated into the plan of care. The monitoring of vital signs, intake and output records and the patient's weight are examples of methods used to measure drug effect and the patient's overall response to the medical and nursing plan of care.

Table 1 gives examples of nursing measures that promote drug effect or reduce a person's need for a drug and some of the methods by which the effectiveness of the drug therapy and nursing interventions can be evaluated.

The results of the patient's laboratory tests may support or give direction to the nurse's observations of both drug effect and the development of side effects. Certain laboratory tests are specific in evaluating drug response, while others are more general indices of changes in the patient's physical condition. An example of a laboratory test for evaluating drug effect is the prothrombin time. The

TABLE 1 Examples of Nursing Interventions to Promote and Evaluate Drug Effect

INTENDED EFFECT	MEASURES TO PROMOTE EFFECT AND/OR REDUCE THE NEED FOR THE DRUG	EVALUATION OF THE EFFECTIVENESS OF DRUG ACTION AND NURSING MEASURES
Analgesia	Assess through observation and interview: the nature of the pain, the meaning of the pain, and the patient's reaction. Change of position to relieve pressure, lessen edema. Tell patient of the analgesic drug effect. Diversion and other measures, to produce general relaxation.	Subjective patient response. Decreased muscular tension and general relaxation. Increased mobility of affected part.
Antacid	Administer antacid promptly at frequency ordered. Instruct patient to avoid obviously irritating foods; bland diet if ordered; small frequent feedings. Reduce anxiety and emotional stress as much as possible. Provide quiet restful environment.	Decrease in nausea Decreased pain and "heartburn." Decreased or absence of melena if previously present.
Antihistamine	Prevent occurrence of allergic response by careful checking for drug or food allergies; education of patient about his allergy and sources of allergens. Avoid vasodilation from external heat or physical activity if urticaria is present. Supportive measures depending on the type and severity of allergic response.	Decrease or absence of signs and symptoms of allergic response, e.g., hayfever, coryza, urticaria and other skin eruptions, pruritus, asthma, wheezing.
Antihypertensive	Reduce factors promoting hypertension. Quiet restful environment. Avoid use of stimulants, e.g., caffeine, nicotine. Determine source of anxiety and stress.	Decrease in blood pressure. Decrease in headache, dizziness and other symptoms related to hypertension.
Anti-infective	Good nutritional intake. Sufficient rest. Adequate fluid intake. Appropriate use of techniques and principles of medical and surgical asepsis. General cleanliness and hygiene.	Decrease in fever, malaise, white blood cell count, culture results, signs and symptoms of infection.
Antitussive and Expectorant	Frequent change of position. Promote adequate hydration. Promote deep breathing and coughing. Elevate head of bed if possible. Hard candy to soothe pharynx.	Decrease in occurrence of cough. Productive cough. More restful sleep. Decrease in rales.
Cathartic and Laxative	Determine patient's usual pattern of elimination: frequency, usual time of day, previous use of cathartics. Adequate fluid intake and bulk in diet. Sufficient exercise. Offer bedpan frequently, especially after meals. Insure privacy during elimination.	Regular elimination of soft formed stool. Daily or routine check on bowel elimination. Absence of abdominal distention, fecal impaction.
Hypnotic	Determine patient's usual bedtime ritual and sleeping pattern. Provide usual ritual as much as possible. Provide quiet comfortable environment. Promote physical comfort: back and skin care, positioning, clean smooth bed. Determine any basis for difficulty in sleeping. Promote physical activity and wakefulness during the day.	Subjective patient response. Observe patient frequently to determine length and depth of sleep, restlessness.

results of this blood test reflect the degree of blood coagulability and are a vital tool in measuring the effect of certain anticoagulants as well as in indicating the development of overdosage.

The beneficial or detrimental effects of a drug on bone marrow and the hematopoietic system are reflected in the results of such blood tests as white cell counts and platelet counts. The nurse therefore should be familiar with the results and meaning of various laboratory tests in relation to the drug therapy and the patient's general condition.

The nurse also should be aware of the drugs which can affect the results of certain laboratory tests. Some drugs may cause false or misleading results. For example, certain drugs can affect the results of urine testing for glycosuria. A false positive result could be dangerous if insulin dosage is prescribed on the basis of this result. It usually is necessary to use a different type of testing agent, depending on the particular drug the patient is receiving.

THE NURSE AND DRUG SIDE EFFECTS

Since the nurse has an important role in observing the patient for drug side effects, she needs to know what side effects are commonly caused by a particular drug. Some side effects, those which indicate toxicity to the patient, require immediate nursing intervention such as using emergency drugs or discontinuing the drug and notifying the physician. Other side effects develop more slowly and require close observation by the nurse.

In later chapters of this book the therapeutic actions, toxic effects and less severe side effects of groups of drugs and of individual drugs are presented. Because many drugs have similar side effects, for which the medical and nursing responses are similar, it may be valuable to include here a chart summarizing the major side effects commonly produced by drugs in general. It is intended to guide the nurse as to what ob-

servations she should make when she knows that a drug is likely to produce a certain side effect. The column headed "Nursing Implications" gives nursing actions that will help prevent the side effects whenever possible, as well as suggestions for dealing with the effects once they occur.

Some of the effects listed are simple side effects, that is, effects other than the principal action desired. These usually cannot be avoided, and nursing action is directed at alleviating the symptoms. Other effects are considered actually toxic, and symptoms must be reported immediately.

It is hoped that the chart can be used as a reference for observations and nursing action with future drugs as well as drugs now in use.

THE NURSE AND ALLERGIC REACTIONS

Allergic reactions to a drug are an ever-present possibility, even though certain drugs are more likely to produce an allergic response and certain patients are more prone to develop an allergic reaction. The nurse has an important role in helping to prevent the occurrence of allergic reactions. During the admission interview or the nursing history, the nurse should question the patient about allergies to foods, drugs and other substances. The nurse should use other approaches in addition to a direct question about allergies. Some patients may not be familiar with the term or meaning of "allergy" and may respond more accurately to questions about drugs or foods they "can't take" or which "bother" them, past episodes of rashes or hives, hayfever or wheezing.

Once it is determined that a patient has or is suspected of having an allergy, the nurse should report this to the physician and also make appropriate notation of the allergy on the nursing Kardex and care plan, the front of the patient's chart, the physician's order sheet and other places as indicated by hospital policy.

The patient who is unconscious or unable to communicate should be checked carefully for the presence of a Medic Alert or similar tag on his person and for an identification card in his belongings. These may indicate the presence of an allergy or other important medical condition. All nursing and health personnel should be familiar with the universal medical identification symbol which was designed and promoted by the American Medical Association and endorsed by the World Medical Association as a standard universal symbol.

The Medic Alert Foundation International is a nonprofit, charitable organization which makes available a special identification tag to be worn by persons with a medical condition that should be known in an emergency. The Medic Alert symbol appears on one side and the other side has a brief statement of the person's problem and a telephone number which can be called for further information about the person's condition and treatment. The names and location of the person's nearest relatives and personal physician can also be obtained from this source. This information is available 24 hours a day

NURSING RESPONSIBILITIES IN DRUG SIDE EFFECTS

SIDE EFFECT	OBSERVE FOR:	NURSING IMPLICATIONS
Allergic reactions:		
a. anaphylaxis	a. decreased blood pressure, local edema, prickling feeling in throat, edema of face and hands, cyanosis, choking cough and violent asthma, weak pulse.	a. *This is an emergency*: emergency drugs and equipment should be readily available. Sera should be given only by a physician and only after a sensitivity test has been done. Nurse can help prevent occurrence by asking patient carefully about allergies, checking carefully for Medic Alert tags. Apply tourniquet if drug injected in a limb.
b. urticaria	b. edematous pinkish elevations that itch and smart; may occur on any part of body.	b. Laryngeal edema and obstruction of trachea are possible. If allergy suspected, withhold medication until physician can be consulted. After appearance of urticaria, avoid vasodilation for patient's comfort: tepid or cool bath, cool environment, light bedclothes. Lotions and other measures may be indicated to reduce itching.
Atropine-like side effects	Dryness of mouth and nose, flushing and dryness of skin, tachycardia, urinary retention, blurring of vision.	Patient may need to be reassured that effects will disappear when drug is withdrawn. Chewing gum or hard candy may alleviate dryness of mouth. Check should be made on patient's voiding. Patient should not operate dangerous machinery. Supervision of ambulation may be indicated. Drugs producing these side effects would be contraindicated for patient with glaucoma.

Table continued on following page.

NURSING RESPONSIBILITIES IN DRUG SIDE EFFECTS (Continued)

Liver damage

Jaundice, especially in sclerae of eyes: hemorrhages under skin; dark urine that forms when container is shaken.

Liver function studies may be indicated.
Pruritus from jaundice may be alleviated by good skin care, complete removal of soap. Fingernails may have to be cut to prevent scratches and infection.
Many drugs are detoxified by the liver and may become harmful if liver damage is present for any reason.

Renal or kidney damage

Anuria, oliguria, hematuria, crystalluria, albuminuria; indications of fluid and electrolyte imbalance.

Accurate recording and intelligent evaluation of intake and output.
Urine that is smoky in appearance may indicate hematuria.
Frequent urinalyses, blood chemistry studies, and tests of renal function may be indicated.
If kidney function is decreased for any reason, excretion of drugs is impaired, and toxic and cumulative effects of any drug the patient is receiving is possible.

Cardiovascular effects:

a. Arrhythmias

a. Any change in rate, rhythm, volume, or character of pulse, EKG changes.

a. Frequent vital signs. Count pulse for one full minute to detect irregularities.
Apical pulse and apical radial pulse may be more accurate.
General observation of cardiac status indicated.

b. Hypotension

b. Decrease in blood pressure, dizziness, syncope, shock.

b. Check blood pressure before and after administration of drug with this potential effect.
Orthostatic or postural hypotension: patient should be recumbent for 20–30 minutes after drug given, and should regain upright position gradually.
Bedside rails and supervision and/or restriction of ambulation may be needed. If hypotension is severe, vasopressor drugs and other emergency drugs and equipment may be needed.

c. Hypertension

c. Elevated blood pressure, epistaxis, emotional irritability, headache, visual disturbances, dizziness.

c. Frequent vital signs. Reduce emotional and environmental tensions as much as possible. Promote rest.
Hypotensive drugs may be needed.

Blood dyscrasias:

Frequent blood studies indicated for early detection of blood dyscrasias. Education of public essential: to refrain from taking drugs without physician's supervision, discard old prescriptions.
Nurse can help prevent prolonged and unnecessary use of drugs by consulting with physician about a patient's continued need for a particular drug.

a. Aplastic anemia

a. Pallor, weakness, dyspnea, anorexia, fever, headache, bleeding from mucous membranes.

a. *All* of bone marrow function may be affected in aplastic anemia.
Frequent vital signs. Conserve strength as much as possible. Encourage adequate nutrition.

NURSING RESPONSIBILITIES IN DRUG SIDE EFFECTS

Blood dyscrasias (continued):

b. Thrombo-
cytopenia

b. Purpura, petechiae, melena, epistaxis, hematuria, symptoms of internal bleeding.

b. Frequent vital signs. Avoid pressure and irritation of skin. Use soft toothbrush. Use small gauge needle if parenteral injection necessary. Careful, gentle handling.

c. Agranulocytosis, leukopenia

c. Chills, fever, sore throat, cough, malaise, lesions of mouth.

c. Patients receiving drugs likely to cause this effect should be instructed to report any symptoms immediately.
Mouth should be checked periodically for lesions. Frequent vital signs.
When leukopenia occurs, patient must be protected from infection. Contact with visitors and personnel should be restricted; isolation techniques may be needed.
Prophylactic antibiotics may be indicated.

Central nervous system effects:

a. Extrapyramidal effects

a. Abnormal involuntary movements: tremor, athetosis, chorea, dystonia. Alterations in muscle tone. Difficulty in preserving equilibrium in erect and sitting position.

a. Depending on particular drug, effects generally disappear upon withdrawal of drug. Consult with physician; patient may need reassurance. Bedside rails, and supervision and/or restriction of ambulation may be indicated. Anti-Parkinsonian drugs may be prescribed.

b. Stimulation of C.N.S.

b. Anxiety, nervousness, insomnia.

b. Avoid giving last daily dose of drug too close to bedtime to reduce possibility of insomnia. Reduce environmental stimulation as much as possible.
Stimulation of C.N.S. may precipitate convulsions, especially if patient has history of epilepsy.

c. Depression of C.N.S.

c. Dizziness, vertigo, drowsiness, decrease in pulse or respiration, decreasing level of consciousness.

c. Person should not operate car or dangerous machinery. Bedside rails, and supervision and/or restriction of ambulation may be needed. .
Check vital signs, especially before giving additional doses of drugs producing this effect. Caution patient about use of other drugs which may produce further C.N.S. depression.

Gastrointestinal effects:

a. Irritation of gastric mucosa

a. Nausea, vomiting, anorexia.

a. Give drug with or after meals, or with milk or antacid if ordered unless absorption of the drug would be impaired. Drug may be contraindicated if patient has history of peptic ulcer.
Investigate possibility of using enteric-coated preparation.
Small, frequent and attractive meals may help in dealing with anorexia.

b. Small bowel ulceration

b. Abdominal pain, melena, distention, diarrhea.

b. Frequent vital signs. Observe stools and test for occult blood.
Consult with physician for medication to control diarrhea.

c. Constipation

c. Decrease in frequency of stools, hardness of stools.

c. Careful, systematic check on patient's bowel movements. Insure adequate bulk and fluid in diet. Encourage exercise if possible. Laxatives and enemas as ordered by physician.

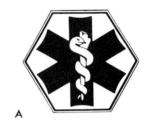

A

BRACELETS:

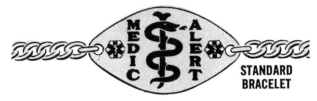

STANDARD
BRACELET

SMALL BRACELET
(Children's and Ladies')

DISCS:

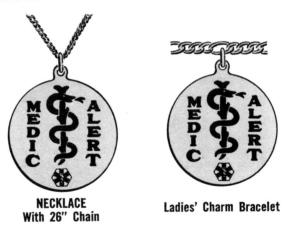

NECKLACE
With 26" Chain

Ladies' Charm Bracelet

B

FIGURE 4. *A,* Devised by the AMA as the universal emergency medical identification symbol, this 6-pointed figure means: "Look for medical information that can protect life." The person displaying this symbol carries upon his person information which should be known to anyone helping him during an accident or sudden illness. (From the American Medical Association, Department of Health Education, Communications Division, Chicago, Illinois 60610.) *B,* Medic alert emblems shown actual size. (From Medic Alert Foundation International, Turlock, California 95380.)

by collect telephone call to the California headquarters. The person also carries an identification card which lists his major medical problems and the persons to be contacted in an emergency.

The nurse often is in a position to inform patients of their need for some type of medical identification and of the availability of the services of Medic Alert. Patients who could benefit from having their medical problem known in an emergency include: those persons who have known allergies or other undesirable reactions to substances used in first aid, such as penicillin, antitoxins and opium derivatives; persons whose medical conditions may create an emergency, such as in hemophilia, the use of contact lenses, tracheostomy, diabetes or epilepsy; those who need a particular medication routinely, such as anticoagulant, glucocorticosteroids, insulin; and persons who have some problem in communicating, such as those who are deaf, aphasic, mute or who speak only a foreign language.

THE TEACHING ROLE OF THE NURSE

Teaching patients, their families, and the general public is an increasing responsibility of the nurse. This includes teaching related to drugs and drug therapy as well as teaching about the person's disease and other aspects of his care. By her teaching effectiveness in health promotion, the nurse may have an important role in the prevention of illness and the reduction of the need for certain types of drugs.

Usually, the patient should be told at least the general purpose of the drugs he is receiving. The increasing knowledge of the general public about diseases and drugs necessitates a fuller and more detailed explanation to most patients.

Although teaching patients about drug therapy is advocated by the American Medical Association, there are situations in which the initiation of a detailed explanation to the patient is not considered the role of the nurse.

An example is when the drug therapy cannot be explained to a patient without a discussion of a diagnosis which is not known or has not been divulged to him. Some physicians, fortunately only a few, are opposed to teaching by the nurse and consider teaching about drug therapy to be the role of the physician only. Such a situation, however, does not relieve the nurse of any responsibility since she should establish communication with the physician about the patient's specific questions or concerns in order to plan with the physician how best to meet the patient's learning needs.

Teaching opportunities are numerous within the hospital setting, in the home and in the community. In her development and implementation of a teaching plan for individuals or groups, the nurse must utilize her knowledge of the principles of learning and teaching.

Instructing the patient and his family about drug therapy is of particular importance when a patient is taking a drug at home or over an extended period of time.

Factors affecting teaching

Before initiating any teaching, the nurse should determine the patient's understanding and attitude toward his condition, his drug therapy and other aspects of his care. This is essential to promoting his optimal participation in his plan of care. A patient who doubts or does not understand his need for a drug is not as likely to take his medication correctly as a patient who understands the reasons why a drug is needed and what it is expected to do for him. Patients with an inadequate understanding of their conditions or the drug therapy may be inclined to stop taking a drug when their symptoms recede and they feel better.

A patient's attitude toward his condition and his degree of acceptance of his illness and resulting limitations are primary considerations. His receptivity to learning and his readiness for learning will be affected by these factors. A patient's omission of drug doses may be a way of denying to himself and others that he is ill.

Other factors which will affect the teaching approach and process are the person's intellectual ability, degree of literacy, level of language ability and vocabulary, his previous knowledge and experience with the drug or other drugs, his level of motivation and physical factors such as impaired vision.

The success of the teaching plan in insuring that the patient take drugs safely and as prescribed may be affected by additional factors. Forgetfulness is often a problem, especially with the elderly. Measures which may help are the association of the pill-taking with daily events, such as immediately after breakfast, or devising a charting method for the patient to record each dose. Some patients reduce or omit drug doses in an attempt to be thrifty. Investigation into the socioeconomic needs of the patient may be indicated.

With some medical conditions, the patient adjusts his drug dosage by himself, under certain circumstances as indicated by his physician. This type of patient should be thoroughly familiar with the signs, symptoms and circumstances under which he should do this. For example, a person who has diabetes mellitus may be instructed to take a specified dose of insulin when his urine testing for glycosuria is positive.

It should be insured that the patient take the correct drug in the prescribed manner. A patient may become confused about the identity of a particular drug, especially if he is taking several medications. Fortunately, more and more physicians are directing the pharmacist to put the name of the drug on the prescription label

The physician's instructions on the prescription label should be clarified and reviewed with the patient. The patient should be told how a drug is to be taken, such as with a full glass of water or before meals.

Additional instruction will be needed if the drug is to be administered by a route with which the patient is not familiar, e.g., sublingually or as a rectal suppository.

If injection technique must be taught, the teaching plan must include the principles of asepsis involved, the care and handling of the equipment used, the rotation of injection sites and the other aspects and precautions involved in injection technique. The psychologic stress of self-injection is a primary consideration throughout the process of instruction. Often a family member or neighbor is included in this instruction in order to be prepared in the event that the patient should become unable to administer the drug himself.

DRUG SIDE EFFECTS. Although it is probably unwise to detail all the possible side effects of a drug, the patient should be told the signs and symptoms that should be reported to his physician. This includes symptoms of the side effects more commonly caused by a particular drug as well as indications that the drug is not producing the desired effects. For example, a person who is taking an antibiotic at home should be told to notify his physician if he develops a sore throat, sores in his mouth, a tendency to bruise easily or other indications of a blood dyscrasia. He should also be instructed to notify his physician if he continues to have a fever or other symptoms indicating that the antibiotic is not effective against the infecting organism.

Side effects which are expected but which may be alarming to a patient usually should be explained before they occur. Side effects, such as the blackening of stools from iron preparations and the discolorations of urine by various drugs, may be quite alarming to an uninformed patient. Patients who are receiving drugs which may produce drowsiness should be advised against driving, using dangerous machinery or engaging in other activities which may require alertness and quick response.

If a drug the patient is receiving is likely to interact with other drugs or foods that he may ingest, he should be made aware of these interactions. Patients may inadvertently purchase nonprescription medicines that contain drugs which interact with the prescribed drug. The ingestion of alcohol when a person is receiving certain drugs causes an exaggeration of central nervous system depression which can result in death.

An example of this type of interaction occurs when a person combines barbiturates with alcohol.

STORING DRUGS. Instructing the patient and his family in the proper storage of drugs is necessary in order to insure that the patient does not take drugs which have deteriorated. Some drugs become physiologically harmful because of chemical changes which occur as they deteriorate. The loss of a drug's effectiveness through its deterioration may be quite dangerous in many situations. The patient and the physician may have difficulty in determining the basis or reason for the return of the patient's symptoms. Patients should be instructed not to use any drug which has changed in color or appearance.

If a drug is to be refrigerated, the nurse should be sure that the patient understands that the drug is to be kept in the refrigeration area, not frozen in the freezer compartment. If a drug is sensitive to air or moisture, it should be kept in a tightly sealed container and should not be kept in the humid atmosphere of the bathroom. Such medication should not be carried or stored for extended periods of time in pillboxes or other containers that are not airtight. Patients should be instructed to avoid leaving medicines on windowsills or other areas where they may decompose on exposure to light. Usually, drugs which are particularly sensitive to light are dispensed in dark brown containers to decrease the penetration of light; these drugs should not be transferred to other containers.

Patients, as well as the general public, should be told to discard all medicines after they are no longer needed. This is important in order to prevent the ingestion of outdated drugs, and also serves to emphasize the dangers of self-medication or offering medications to another person. Drugs should be discarded into the sewer system whenever possible, rather than into the trash or garbage where they may be found by curious children or hungry pets.

If children are present in the home or are likely to be visitors, drugs should be stored in an area that is inaccessible to them. Finding such a place often is much easier said than done. Various commercial medicine cabinets and containers have been developed in an attempt to deal with the problem of keeping drugs away from curious children.

PROPER USE OF DRUGS. The nurse should provide anticipatory guidance to parents concerning their approaches to their children about drug use. Parents should help their children to understand that medications should be taken when they are sick and only when a doctor tells them to do so. Children should not be told that medicine is candy since they then may consider all medicines as candy to be eaten freely. Disguising medications in foods in order to persuade or trick a child into taking a drug should be avoided. In addition to the possibility of the child's developing an aversion to the particular food used, the child invariably is quite aware that the drug is in the food and that deception is being practiced.

Education of the public about the proper use of drugs is a vital role of the nurse in this era when drugs are so widely used for legitimate and illegitimate reasons. The widespread advertising found everyday on television, radio, in magazines and newspapers advocates the use of various nonprescription drugs for all kinds of pains and stresses of daily living. Many people have come to feel that some type of medication is an essential part of their lives. Although some drugs are necessary to some persons, other people may need to learn alternative ways of reducing or coping with the stresses of their lives.

Consumer education is also needed in order that people may properly assess the various claims of the different drug preparations that are available without prescription. The nurse is often in a position to provide this type of information along with other aspects of health promotion. She may also be able to provide guidance in helping the patient in the purchase of a nonprescription drug brand that is less expensive yet just as effective as a higher priced brand.

The dangers of self-medication should be

taught to all patients and the general public whenever the opportunity arises. Treating oneself with drugs raises the possibility of inducing a toxic or other dangerous drug response. More importantly, self-medication and treatment delays a person's being diagnosed and appropriately treated in the early stages of a disease when a cure is more likely and treatment is more effective. For example, a person who decides to take vitamin pills because he feels tired may not be diagnosed as having cancer until such a late stage that the chances of a cure are greatly reduced.

Through health counseling, the nurse can play a most vital role in promoting the optimal health of patients, families and the general public. She should encourage and explain the necessity of prompt and adequate medical supervision. Within this framework, the development of a healthy and sensible respect for the use of drugs should be encouraged by the nurse.

QUESTIONS FOR DISCUSSION AND REVIEW

1. Analyze commercials and advertisements for their potential impact on the general public?

2. Why is it important for the nurse to understand: drug action? effect? dosage? route? side effects? contraindications? the individual patient?

3. Identify nursing measures you could use to promote the following types of drug effect: analgesia? hypnosis? antihistamine? How would you know if your nursing measures were effective?

4. What are the nursing implications if a drug is likely to cause the following side effects: atropine-like effects? blood dyscrasias? extrapyramidal effects? C.N.S. depression?

5. Review the principles of learning and identify how they may be applied to teaching a patient about his drug therapy.

6. Outline a teaching plan concerning the dangers of self-medication for a patient for whom you have cared.

BIBLIOGRAPHY

Berblinger, K. W.: The influence of personalities on drug therapy. *Amer. J. Nurs., 59:*1130, 1959.

Billars, K. S.: You have pain? I think this will help. *Amer. J. Nurs., 70:* 2143, (October) 1970.

Chambers, W. G. and Price, G. G.: Influence of the nurse upon effects of analgesics administered. *Nurs. Res., 16:*228 (Summer) 1967.

Conway, B., et al.: The seventh right. *Amer. J. Nurs., 70:*1040, (May) 1970.

Dlouhy, A., et al.: What patients want to know about their diagnostic tests. *Nurs. Outlook, 11:*265, 1963.

Finn, A.: Patients should know procedures to be followed when taking medications. *Mod. Nurs. Home, 23:*57, (November-December) 1969.

Gurski, B. M.: Rationale of nursing care for patients with blood dyscrasias. *Nurs. Clin. N. Amer., 1*:23, (March) 1966.

Hecht, A. B.: Self-medication, inaccuracy and what can be done. *Nurs.
Outlook, 18*:30, (April) 1970.

Hopkins, S. J.: The storage of drugs. *Nurs. Times, 65*:459, (April 10)
1969.

Kron, T.: Stepping beyond the five rights in administering drugs. *Amer.
J. Nurs., 62*:62, (July) 1962.

Leary, J. A., Vessela, D. M. and Yeaw, E. M.: Self-administered medications. *Amer. J. Nurs., 71*:1193 (June) 1971.

Levine, M. E.: Breaking through the medications mystique. *Amer. J.
Nurs., 70*:799, (April) 1970.

Libow, L. S., et al.: Self-administration of medications by patients in
hospital or extended care facilities. *J. Amer. Geriat. Soc., 18*:81,
(January) 1970.

Lineham, D. T.: What does the patient want to know? *Amer. J. Nurs.,
66*:1066, (May) 1966.

Mills, D. H.: Soliciting drug information from newly admitted patients.
Hospitals, 39:75, (March) 1965.

Neely, E., et al.: Problems of aged persons taking medications at home.
Nurs. Res., 17:52, (January-February) 1968.

Parker, P. F.: Drugs and people. *Amer. J. Hosp. Pharm., 24*:351, 1967.

Schwartz, D.: Medication errors made by aged patients. *Amer. J. Nurs.,
62*:51, (August) 1962.

Shawn, Sister Mary: Teaching a patient. *Amer. J. Nurs., 64*:126, (April)
1964.

Streeter, V.: The nurse's responsibility for teaching patients. *Amer. J.
Nurs., 53*:818, (July) 1953.

Webb, C.: Tactics to reduce a child's fear of pain. *Amer. J. Nurs., 66*:2698,
(December) 1966.

Wu, R.: Explaining treatments to young children. *Amer. J. Nurs., 65*:71,
(July) 1965.

Chapter 3 The Administration of Medications

Important Concepts Discussed

1. *Depending upon their mode of administra-tration, drugs may exert a local or systemic effect.*
2. *The mode of administration affects the rate of onset of action as well as the thera-peutic efficacy of a drug.*
3. *The nurse should be alert for untoward effects of drugs. Warning symptoms should be carefully noted and reported to the physician.*
4. *A standard procedure for administering drugs and intelligent concentration by the nurse can be safe-guards against the occurrence of medication errors.*

The administration of medications has become one of the most important responsibilities of the professional nurse, and as such should be performed with the utmost care and precision at all times.

A nurse should never administer a drug until she has first become thoroughly familiar with it as regards its therapeutic intent, dosage, mode of administration and potential side effects. The rapid introduction of many new therapeutic agents makes this learning experience time-consuming and difficult, but it is nevertheless of the utmost importance if the nurse is to fulfill her professional and legal responsibilities and maintain the trust placed in her by both the patients in her care and the prescribing physician.

Since information on new drugs is rarely found in the standard reference texts, even as a student the nurse should become acquainted with the drug information files in the hospital pharmacy or enlist the help of the hospital pharmacist in the location of new drug literature.

Medications understandably are extremely important from the patient's point of view. To him they often represent the only positive steps that he takes toward recovery during his hospital day. Accordingly, since he has little opportunity for distraction by other pressing problems, he can become seriously disturbed by delays in receiving his regular medications—or by a wait of six to eight hours for the first dose of a new drug that his physician had prescribed on early morning rounds. Although it is probably inevitable that unforeseen interruptions in the nurse's schedule may occasionally cause delay in the giving of medication, every effort should be made to eliminate these occurrences, and there can be no excuse for the "forgetting" or total omission of a medication dose.

A patient's remark about his "new" medication or a pill that "looks different this time" should always be taken as a warning of a possible medication error. Needless to say, the dose in question should be withheld until the order can be verified.

A slightly different approach should be taken when administering injectable rather than oral medications. It is no secret that even the strongest and most self-sufficient man can become a terrified youngster when approached with a syringe and needle. As a first—and very important—point, injections should never be referred to as "shots," as this term may conjure up a host of unpleasant specters in the mind of the patient. Instead, the injection should always be introduced as the "medicine your doctor ordered for you." A few minutes used to explain the procedure briefly are always well worth while and greatly simplify the procedure by promoting relaxation and cooperation on the part of most patients.

MEDICATION ORDERS

LEGAL ASPECTS

The nurse administers medications upon the order of a licensed physician. She does not carry out the order automatically, but is legally and morally responsible for the patient's safety. The physician should be questioned about an order if any portion of it is unclear, if the drug ordered would seem to be harmful to the patient, if the dosage is outside of the usual range or if the route of administration ordered is not correct. After the physician has been questioned, and if there is still a doubt in the nurse's mind about administering the drug as prescribed, the nurse should contact her nursing supervisor. The nurse may and should refuse to administer the drug as prescribed if she believes that it will result in harm to the patient.

A fairly common misconception is that the physician alone, rather than the nurse, is legally responsible for the results of an erroneous order. The physician is responsible, but the nurse is also legally responsible for her own acts. The nurse who administers a drug upon an erroneous order can be held legally responsible for any harm resulting to the patient. It is evident, therefore, that the nurse must have a thorough knowledge of the pharmacologic aspects of the drug ordered. She must be accurate in interpreting physician's orders and in using techniques in administering medications.

Medication orders by law must be written and signed by a physician. Only in an emergency may a nurse act on an oral order for a medication, and under these circumstances a written order signed by the physician must follow within 24 hours. The validity of telephone orders is determined by hospital policy.

Each medication order must include the name of the drug, the dose of the drug, the route of administration and the dosage schedule to be followed. The nurse must know the correct interpretations of abbreviations commonly used in writing prescriptions, and the hospital's time schedule for drug administration. Any question concerning these directions must be clarified with the physician before the drug is administered. Countless serious medication errors could have been avoided easily if a nurse had taken the few minutes required to question the spelling of a drug name or the dose of a medication.

Most hospitals have in effect a system of automatic "stop orders" for all medications. The standard time that medications may be administered without being reordered by the physician varies greatly among different institutions, but in most instances it is from three to seven days. In some hospitals only certain types of drugs, such as antibiotics have automatic stop dates. Preoperative orders are considered automatically cancelled after the patient has had surgery.

Routine or p.r.n. orders may in certain cases be written in advance by physicians for medications always prescribed for patients with a particular diagnosis. E.g., the laxatives, antiseptics and ointments used for hemorrhoidectomies are often classed as routine orders by proctologists. Orders for these may be entered on the medication chart by the nurse and later signed by the physician. In this type of situation, the nurse has a great responsibility in assessing the patient's condition and his need for a "routine" drug. She may need to consult the physician, rather than carry out the order as prescribed.

Routine orders may never be given for narcotics, however. Narcotics must always be ordered for each individual patient by the physician in charge. Ordinarily, there is a 72-hour automatic stop order for narcotics in a hospital. At the end of this time a completely new order must be written and signed by the physician before additional narcotics may be administered.

The policies of the hospital may specify drugs which may not be administered by the nurse. The nurse should be thoroughly familiar with those policies concerning the administration of medications.

PREVENTING MEDICATION ERRORS

In spite of the detailed procedures and regulations regarding the administration of medications which will be described below, medication errors occur with disconcerting frequency. A drug that is given in the wrong dose, or at the wrong time, or is not given at all can produce sequelae that are just as serious as those created by giving the wrong drug altogether.

Many errors occur because the nurse has not followed the prescribed procedure for drug administration, or has taken short-cuts to save a few steps or a precious moment of time. Lack of concentration, likewise, is a too-frequent source of error. The administration of medications is one responsibility that must never become a routine. To be sure, with time a nurse may become highly skilled and efficient in this task, but when she becomes skilled to the point of being unthinking and mechanical, she can unwittingly make serious and even lethal errors.

Inadequate communication between the physician and the nurse is a great offender. The small inconvenience of calling back even the most irascible physician is incomparably slight when compared to the safety of the patients in the nurse's care. Instances of nurses filling out a drug order for "Metergan Cystic" following an oral order for "Mepergan–60," or of improperly transcribing a hastily written order for "Theragran" as "Thorazine" are a matter of record. Inade-

quate knowledge of medications is a constant source of danger when taking oral medication orders. Most physicians would be only too happy to spell the name of an unfamiliar drug, and they should always be asked to do so whenever the slightest doubt exists.

Because many drugs have similar names and often do not differ greatly in appearance, the name of the drug should be verified with the medicine card three times during the preparation of any dose. It should be checked before the bottle is taken from the shelf, when pouring the medication, and before replacing the bottle.

Correctly identifying the patient for whom the medication is prepared is also extremely important. Before administering the medication the nurse should always check his hospital identification band, or ask him to give his name. Since many patients will respond to an incorrect name, it is unwise to rely only on the patient's response when his name is called. The hospital wrist band or other identification aid should always be checked if the patient is incoherent or comatose.

ROUTES OF ADMINISTRATION OF DRUGS

The route of administration is highly important in determining the action of drugs. In certain cases the effect of the drug is entirely different from that intended if it is administered by the incorrect route. Cocaine, for example, is quite effective as a local anesthetic when applied topically. However, if it is given orally or injected, its predominant effect is central nervous system stimulation and euphoria.

Other drugs may be actually harmful if given by the incorrect route. Aminophylline, corticosteroids, hormone preparations and many other agents are prepared in two or more parenteral forms—one for intravenous use and one or more for intramuscular administration. Intramuscular preparations generally are more concentrated or more insoluble than the corresponding intravenous medication, and serious harm can come to the patient if they are given intravenously.

Consequently, the correct route is almost as important as the correct drug if optimal therapeutic effects are to be achieved. The proper route will be insured if the correct technique for administering a drug by the route specified is used.

ADMINISTRATION FOR LOCAL EFFECTS

Drugs may exert local effects if applied topically to the skin or mucous membranes, or in some instances if they are injected into the subcutaneous tissues or the lower spinal cord.

APPLICATION TO THE SKIN

The skin as a general rule absorbs drugs only slightly; thus for the most part agents applied to intact skin exert only a local effect. An important exception to this rule of non-absorption is observed if the skin is broken or denuded over a relatively large area. Many otherwise innocuous substances then are able to enter the body fluids and are absorbed systemically, sometimes with serious results. Examples of these potentially toxic substances are methyl salicylate and boric acid; these agents should never be applied to large areas of denuded skin or applied repeatedly for prolonged periods of time.

The drugs and types of pharmaceutical preparations designed for topical application are discussed in Chapters 8 and 18. The nursing implications involved in applying drugs to the skin also are discussed in Chapter 18.

APPLICATION TO THE MUCOUS MEMBRANES

Drugs may be applied to almost all the various mucous membranes of the body, including those of the eye, nose, throat, mouth, rectum and respiratory and genitourinary tracts. Drugs for application to these sensitive tissues assume many forms—from topical preparations resembling those for application to the skin, to suppositories, powders for insufflation and solutions for irrigation or instillation.

Because of the aqueous nature of the mucous membrane secretions, and the moist surfaces of the membranes which are constantly bathed in body fluids, most medications are more readily absorbed through the mucous membranes than through intact skin. The range of drugs that may be safely applied to these tissues is thus limited to those nontoxic when absorbed. The absorptive properties of the mucous membranes are at the same time beneficial, however, since they provide a means by which drugs may be applied topically for systemic use.

SUPPOSITORIES

Drugs in the form of suppositories may be inserted into any of the body orifices, for example, the rectum, urethra, vagina, or more rarely into the nose or ear. Depending upon the nature of the drug and the suppository base employed, these agents may exert a local or systemic effect.

ENEMAS

Enemas likewise may be administered for a local or systemic effect. When the latter effect is desired, retention enemas are employed and the drug stays in contact with the rectal mucous membranes until absorbed.

NASAL ADMINISTRATION

Drugs applied to the nasal mucous membranes may be in oily or aqueous solutions, or powdered medications may be blown upon the surfaces by means of a nasal insufflator. The use of oily substances, such as mineral oil, in the nose has declined greatly in recent years since the possibility has become appreciated that small droplets of the oil will be aspirated into the lungs, producing a lipid pneumonia. Mineral oil is extremely inert in the body and will not be absorbed from the lung tissues even after many years of contact at the site, thus a constant source of irritation is present. The danger of lipid pneumonia is especially great when mineral oil nose drops are administered to small children since they aspirate the liquid more readily than adults.

In administering nose drops to a patient, the nurse should be sure that the patient's nasal passages are clear, so that the drug to be instilled will come in contact with the mucous membranes of the nose. The patient should be positioned with his head tilted backwards. The solution is drawn into the dropper. Care should be taken that the solution is not allowed to run into the bulb of the dropper since this could result in the contamination of the solution with particles of rubber. The dropper is placed just within the nares and the prescribed number of drops is inserted. Contact of the dropper with the mucous membrane itself should be avoided since this may stimulate sneezing and also contaminate the dropper. Contamination of the dropper is avoided because of the possibility of introducing bacteria into the medication container, which may provide an excellent environment for bacterial growth. Any solution remaining in the dropper should be discarded and should not be returned to the container.

Medications may also be delivered to the mucous membranes of the nose by the use of atomizers or nasal sprays. Essentially the same principles apply as in the administration of nose drops. Special care should be taken to avoid exerting too great a force on the spray since this may result in the drug's entering the sinuses or eustachian tubes. Nasal spray nozzles should be cleansed thoroughly after each use in order to prevent bacterial growth on the nozzle or within the container. Because of the likelihood of bacterial contamination, nasal sprays should never be used by more than one person. Patients should be cautioned against excessive use of these sprays since systemic absorption can occur, especially if excess amounts are swallowed into the stomach.

LOZENGES OR TROCHES

Lozenges or troches are used for their local effect on the mouth and throat. For optimal effectiveness, they should be allowed to dissolve gradually in the mouth and should not be chewed or swallowed whole. Systemic effects may occur from the portion that is swallowed.

INHALATION

Certain drugs may be inhaled into the respiratory tract for their local effect on the bronchial tree or on the secretions within the lung. Drugs must be in vapor form in order to be inhaled. This is accomplished by the use of a nebulizer or steam which carries the drug into the lung. A further discussion of this route of administration and the nursing implications involved can be found in Chapter 16.

EAR DROPS

Drugs may be instilled into the auditory canal for local effects such as local anesthesia or a local antiseptic action. Sterile technique is not essential provided that the tympanic membrane is intact. The patient is positioned so that the affected ear is uppermost. After the auditory canal has been straightened, the prescribed solution is dropped onto the side of the canal. The solution should be at or near body temperature. The patient should remain in the same position for a sufficient length of time to insure that the drug will not escape from the auditory canal when the head is held upright.

OPHTHALMIC PREPARATIONS

Drugs may be administered in the eye for their local effect on the conjunctiva of the eye or for their effect within the anterior eye chamber. Because of the sensitivity of the eye and the dangers of infection, drugs or solutions applied to the eye should be sterile. The principles of aseptic technique should be utilized during their administration. The label of the eye preparation should be carefully checked in order to be sure of the correct drug and strength, and to be sure that the preparation is intended for ophthalmic use. Solutions should be carefully checked for any indications of deterioration.

When eye drops are to be instilled into the eye, they are placed into the conjunctival sac, and should never be placed directly on the cornea. The patient should be positioned with his head back and tilted toward the same side as the eye in which the drug is to be placed. This is done to prevent the drug from flowing by gravity into the tear duct near the inner canthus of the eye or out of the affected eye into the unaffected eye. In addition to the decrease of effect in the eye, a medication which enters the tear duct may reach the nasal cavity and pharynx and may then produce systemic effects which could prove dangerous. Applying pressure over the inner canthus immediately after the instillation of the drug is another method of decreasing the loss of medication through the tear duct.

The eyelids and lashes should be cleansed prior to the instillation of the eye drops; be careful to wipe from the inner canthus outward to the outer canthus. The lower lid is pulled down with the finger of one hand and the patient is instructed to look up. The drug is then dropped into the exposed lower lid. Precautions should be taken to prevent the tip of the dropper from touching or injuring the eye. Patients are particularly apt to blink or move suddenly when a drop makes contact with the conjunctiva. During the instillation, the nurse should rest the side of her hand that is holding the dropper on the patient's forehead so that her hand and the dropper will be more likely to move with the patient if he should suddenly move his head or body.

After the drops have been instilled, the lower lid should be released and gentle pressure should be placed on the inner canthus. The patient should be instructed to close his eyes gently and to rotate his eyeballs in order to distribute the drug over the surface of the eye. Excess medication left in the dropper should be discarded and not returned to the bottle. If the dropper has not been contaminated, it may be returned to the bottle. Droppers should be used for one type of drug only; each patient should have his own supply of medication and droppers.

Ophthalmic ointments are applied to the eye in a similar manner. The label on the ointment should indicate that it is for ophthalmic use. The eyelids are cleansed as in the instillation of eye drops. The ointment is squeezed from the tip of the tube onto the inverted lower eyelid; take care that the tip does not come in contact with the eye. The patient gently closes his eyelid. The ointment dissolves from the heat of the body and is distributed over the eye surface by the patient's eyeball movements.

ADMINISTRATION FOR SYSTEMIC EFFECTS

Drugs may be administered by all known routes for systemic effects. Although all drugs are not absorbed equally well using all routes of administration, oral, sublingual, parenteral, rectal and topical application to the skin and mucous membranes may be employed for general or systemic absorption of a drug.

ORAL ADMINISTRATION

Administration of a drug by the oral route is by far the most convenient and most acceptable method of systemic administration. It has the disadvantage of being relatively slow in onset of action, however, so that in most cases it may not be used in emergency situations when immediate action of the drug is mandatory. Since drugs must be in solution form before they can be absorbed, the administration of oral medications with at least a half-glass of water or other liquid will help to increase the rate of absorption. Even with recent advances in methods of preparing oral medications, 30 to 45 minutes is usually required before the drug is absorbed in sufficient amounts to have any therapeutic effect. Often 1 to 1½ hours is required for peak effects. This time span is of little consequence in most medications, but is of concern if a patient is in acute pain, cardiac arrest, status asthmaticus or similar emergency circumstances.

Oral administration may not be used when the patient is nauseated, vomiting, having gastric suction, semiconscious or has any condition in which the gag and swallowing reflexes are diminished or absent.

Drugs that are irritating to the mucous membranes of the stomach and thus may cause vomiting or discomfort (e.g., iron salts or salicylates) may be administered in the form of enteric-coated tablets, which are prepared to remain intact while in the acid medium of the stomach but disintegrate in the neutral or alkaline juices of the intestine. Preparations of this type should not be crushed before administering and the patient should be instructed not to chew the tablets before swallowing them.

Liquid medications usually have accelerated action and are more predictable in their absorption than are the solid or tablet forms. Many drugs cannot be prepared in liquid form, however, because of their instability in solution, or because of their bitter or unpleasant taste. When a disagreeable liquid must be administered to a patient, every effort must be made to make the preparation more palatable. Ice may be given to numb the taste buds prior to taking the medication, and the dose may be followed by a drink of water, or the use of a mouthwash or hard candy. Fruit juices or other beverages may be used as vehicles for the administration of some medications, while others, such as castor oil, are more acceptable if simply chilled in the refrigerator before they are given.

Some liquids, such as hydrochloric acid and liquid iron preparations, are harmful to the tooth enamel, and should always be given, diluted, through a glass drinking straw placed in back of the teeth.

Liquid cough syrups should not be diluted or followed by water since part of their effect is related to a local action on the pharyngeal mucous membranes.

SUBLINGUAL ADMINISTRATION

Only a few drugs can be absorbed from the sublingual mucous membranes in amounts sufficient to render this an acceptable mode of administration. When administered in this way, the tablet is retained under the tongue until it is completely dissolved and the drug absorbed by the capillaries present in the mucous membranes. The patient should be carefully instructed in this route of administration in order to prevent his swallowing the drug.

Nitroglycerine, proteolytic enzymes and certain male hormones are among the few drugs that are effective when given sublingually.

BUCCAL ADMINISTRATION

In buccal administration, as in sublingual administration, the patient holds the tablet in contact with the mucous membranes until it is dissolved. In this case, however, the tablet is placed between the teeth and the mucous membranes of the cheek rather than under the tongue. The full cooperation of the patient must be assured for the effective use of this mode of administration, since patients are likely to swallow tablets held in this position.

Only a few hormonal and enzyme preparations are administered buccally at the present time.

RECTAL ADMINISTRATION

As previously noted, drugs may be administered rectally for local or systemic effect. The rectal route is often chosen for systemic effects if the patient is nauseated, comatose or uncooperative, or if the medication has a taste and/or odor that would be objectionable if given orally.

Generally, absorption from the rectal site is slower and less predictable than when medications are taken orally. For this reason larger doses are used when the drug is administered rectally. Drugs are administered rectally as suppositories or as retention enemas.

The rectal route is often preferred when administering medications to infants or very young children.

Suppositories, which usually contain glycerine, lanolin or other substances which melt at body temperature, should be stored under refrigeration. The patient is placed on his side and is well draped. The buttocks are separated to expose the anus. The suppository should be lubricated and inserted into the anus and beyond the anal sphincters by the forefinger. A rubber or plastic glove or finger cot should be used to protect the finger. Immediately after insertion the buttocks should be held together firmly, in case peristalsis has been stimulated by the insertion of the suppository. Depending on the circumstances, patients may be taught to insert suppositories themselves; however, it should be determined whether the patient is able to insert the suppository beyond the anal sphincters. The drug must reach the rectum in order to be absorbed and produce its effects.

When medications are given rectally in the form of retention enemas, certain adaptations in the technique of administering an enema are needed in order to decrease the likelihood of stimulating peristaltic activity which would expel the drug. The volume of the solution in which the drug is dissolved should be small, usually no more than 150 cc. A rectal tube or catheter with a small diameter should be used to decrease stimulation of the anal sphincters. The solution should be close to body temperature and should be allowed to flow in slowly. Since peristalsis in the colon is stimulated reflexively by the presence of food in the stomach, the scheduling of rectal administration of drugs should be planned before meals whenever this is possible.

INHALATION

General anesthetic gases are the chief category of drugs that may be administered effectively for systemic effect via the respiratory tract. Few liquid or solid medications are solubilized or absorbed sufficiently well to permit their administration by this route. Exceptions are amyl nitrite, some asthma preparations and a few hormones, e.g., posterior pituitary extract, all of which may be absorbed in sufficient quantities to render them effective following inhalation.

PARENTERAL ADMINISTRATION

Parenteral medications are those given with a hypodermic needle. These preparations may be injected intradermally, subcutaneously, intramuscularly or intravenously.

Although the parenteral administration of drugs is, with few exceptions, the most effective and most rapid form of systemic therapy, it is at the same time the most dangerous. Since the onset of action is rapid, untoward effects may be precipitated, sometimes almost irreversibly. This is especially true when drugs are injected intravenously, and it is for this reason that in many hospitals only physicians are permitted to administer intravenous medications. In many cases this regulation is not interpreted to apply to drugs that are contained in large amounts of solution for intravenous infusion, for in this case the drug is quite diluted, and a closer control can be kept on the effects of the drug since the rate of infusion can readily be decreased or halted should untoward symptoms develop.

Aseptic technique is an absolute necessity whenever the skin is broken in the administration of medications since local abscesses or even generalized infections may result from contamination. Hypodermic tablets must never be poured into the hands prior to dissolving them in a syringe, and great care must be taken to avoid contamination of syringes and needles. The needle, the inside of the syringe barrel and the outside of the plunger which comes in contact with the inside of the syringe must be kept sterile. Cleansing of the skin at the site of injection is advocated, using an anti-infective to cleanse in a circular motion outward from the injection site.

Medications for injection are prepared in the form of single dose and multiple dose vials. The single dose containers are always employed for intravenous medications since the risk of contamination upon reentry into the vial is too great to be permitted in intravenous therapy. The multiple dose containers

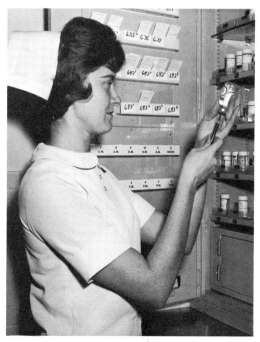

FIGURE 5. Aseptic technique must be maintained when medications for injection are prepared.

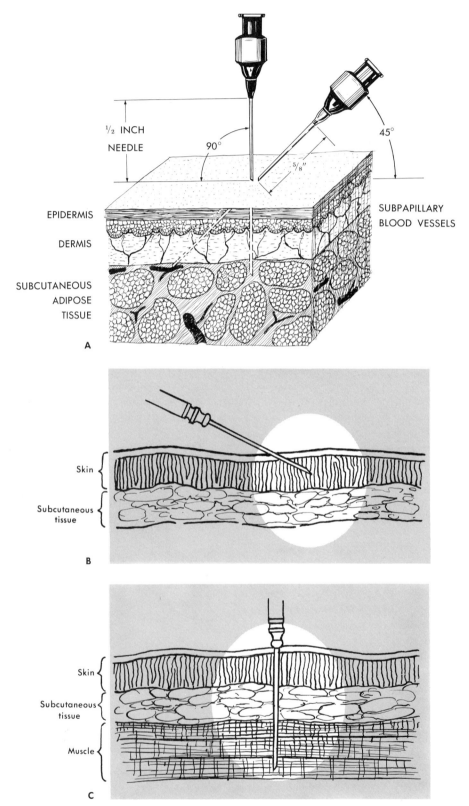

1/2 INCH
NEEDLE

90°

45°

5/8"

EPIDERMIS

DERMIS

SUBCUTANEOUS
ADIPOSE
TISSUE

SUBPAPILLARY
BLOOD VESSELS

A

Skin

Subcutaneous
tissue

B

Skin

Subcutaneous
tissue

Muscle

C

FIGURE 6.   Three types of injections—A, B, C. (From DuGas: *Kozier-DuGas' Introduction to Patient Care.*
Ed. 2. W. B. Saunders Co., Philadelphia, 1972.)

may be used for subcutaneous or intramuscular administration, however, if aseptic technique is employed. If any sign of precipitation, cloudiness or color change occurs in the multiple dose vial it should be discarded immediately. Expiration dates should be checked carefully, and the manufacturer's directions for reconstitution and storage of parenteral drugs should be followed closely.

Many parenteral preparations now are supplied in the form of disposable syringes which certainly are more convenient and greatly reduce the risk of contamination.

INTRADERMAL INJECTION. Intradermal or intracutaneous injections are those made into the layers of the skin itself (Fig. 6, A). The needle is inserted into the skin at an angle almost parallel to the skin surface.

Intradermal administration of drugs has quite a limited use since the route may be employed only for very small amounts of medication which will not be irritating to the tissues. Systemic absorption is relatively slow. Intradermal administration is used primarily for diagnostic skin tests. Areas of the body where the skin is thin, such as the inner surface of the forearm and the middle back, are usually chosen for intradermal injection.

SUBCUTANEOUS INJECTION. The subcutaneous or hypodermic injection is given beneath the skin into the fat or connective tissue immediately underlying the dermis.

Although any subcutaneous tissue may be used, the common sites for injection are the upper lateral portion of the arms, the anterior thigh, and the abdomen. The subcutaneous tissue in the buttocks may also be used. Sites which are tender, red, edematous, or pruritic should not be used. If the patient is receiving repeated injections, a plan for rotating the sites of injection should be made in writing and consulted before each injection.

A 25-gauge needle is usually used, with the length varying from $3/8$ to $5/8$ inch. The choice of needle length will depend on the depth of the patient's subcutaneous tissue and the angle to be used during the injection (Fig. 6, B). A 45 degree angle of the needle to the skin is usually used for subcutaneous injection. With a shorter needle, a 90 degree angle may be used and is advocated in some

situations, as when administering insulin or heparin subcutaneously.

The skin over the injection site is cleansed with an anti-infective, and the subcutaneous tissue is gently grasped and lifted from the muscle. After the needle has been inserted, the grasp is released before the drug is injected. In an obese person it may be necessary to spread the skin taut between two fingers before injection. Some authorities, however, advocate leaving the skin in its natural state rather than grasping or stretching the skin.

After the needle has been placed in the subcutaneous tissue, aspiration should be done to insure that the needle is not within a blood vessel. The plunger of the syringe should be withdrawn slightly and the lower portion of the syringe checked for the presence of blood. If no blood is present, the medication should be injected at a slow steady rate. The needle should be withdrawn at the same angle at which it was inserted in order to prevent further tissue damage. Firm pressure with an alcohol sponge should be applied at the point of injection and the area should usually be massaged to stimulate the circulation to the area and thus promote absorption of the drug.

The volume of medication that may be given by subcutaneous injection is limited to 2 cc. in most circumstances; however, larger volumes may be administered if the enzyme hyaluronidase is first infiltrated into the injection site. Hyaluronidase solubilizes or liquefies hyaluronic acid, the chief component of the interstitial cellular "cement," and thus greatly facilitates absorption of even large volumes of fluid. Hypodermoclysis, the infiltration of large volumes subcutaneously, is often employed to administer fluids to infants or to adults when it is impossible to administer intravenous fluids for one reason or another. Only very soluble and nonirritating drugs may be administered in this way.

INTRAMUSCULAR INJECTION. Injection of medications may be made directly into the muscular elements of the body (Fig. 6, C). In this type of injection a 1 to 3 inch needle is inserted directly at a 90 degree angle.

The volume of fluid that may be given in-

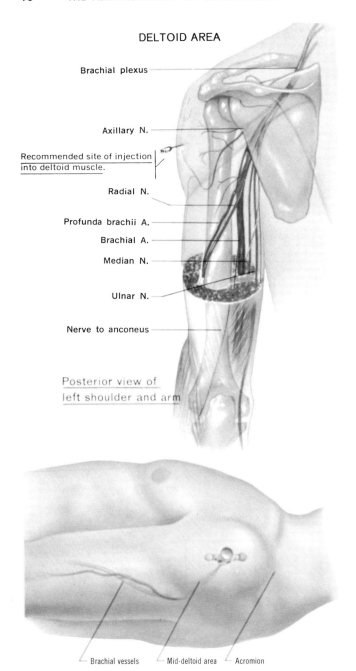

DELTOID AREA

Brachial plexus

Axillary N.

Recommended site of injection
into deltoid muscle.

Radial N.

Profunda brachii A.

Brachial A.

Median N.

Ulnar N.

Nerve to anconeus

Posterior view of
left shoulder and arm

Brachial vessels   Mid-deltoid area   Acromion

FIGURE 7. *A*, The deltoid site for intramuscular injection. (From *How to Give an Intramuscular Injection.* Pfizer Laboratories, Professional Service Department. New York, N.Y.) *B*, The deltoid site for intramuscular injection. (Courtesy of Wyeth Laboratories, Philadelphia, Pennsylvania.)

tramuscularly into one muscle is theoretically 1 to 5 cc. If more than 5 cc. is to be injected, less pain and tissue trauma are produced if two injection sites are used. Again, care should be taken not to insert the medication into a blood vessel. Intramuscular injection presents the added danger of injury to nerves and bones. These dangers can be reduced by the correct selection of the site of intramuscular injection.

Preferable sites for intramuscular injection include the deltoid muscle in the upper arm, the vastus lateralis muscle in the anterolateral portion of the thigh, and the gluteal muscles.

Deltoid. The site for injection into the

deltoid muscle should be chosen carefully because of the dangers of injection into blood vessels and injury to bone and nerves. The injection site should be within a rectangular area bounded on the top by the lower edge of the acromium and on the bottom by the point on the lateral aspect of the arm that is opposite the axilla. The width of the rectangle should be the middle third of the lateral aspect of the upper arm. (See Figure 7.) For accurate site selection, it is important that the entire upper arm be exposed. Patients should remove their clothing rather than just rolling up their sleeves.

Dorsogluteal site. When the gluteal muscles are used for intramuscular injection, great care must be taken that the site is chosen correctly because of the danger of injury to the sciatic nerve and to blood vessels in the area. The upper outer portions of the gluteus maximus or gluteus medius are used. The selection of the site may be accomplished by different methods.

One method of determining the site is to divide the gluteal area into quadrants. The gluteal area *is not limited to the buttock or "cheek";* the gluteal area extends upward to the iliac crest. The quadrants should be determined by using the iliac crest, not the portion of the "cheek," as a boundary. After the quadrants are determined, the site of injection is selected in the upper, outer quadrant. (See Figure 8.)

An alternative method of determining this site is to drawn an imaginary line from the posterior superior iliac spine to the greater trochanter. The injection should be made in the area that is lateral and superior to the line.

As can be seen, the patient's buttock and gluteal area should be fully exposed in order to locate the anatomical landmarks needed to insure the selection of the correct site. The patient should be lying down, since the gluteal muscles are contracted when a person is standing. Besides being painful, an injection into a contracted muscle may result in the leakage of the drug into the subcutaneous tissue. The best position for injection into this site is having the patient prone with his arms over the side of the bed and his toes inverted inward. The position promotes maximal relaxation of the gluteal muscles as well as relaxation of the patient generally. If the patient is lying on his side, dorsiflexion of the feet will help to promote relaxation of the gluteal muscles.

Ventrogluteal site. The ventrogluteal site, also known as von Hochstetter's site, has increased in popularity. It is advocated because of its distance from major nerves or vessels; the density of the gluteus medius and minimus is usually adequate in this area, even in emaciated patients. Another advantage is that the injection may be given while the patient is lying on his back, al-

FIGURE 8. Intramuscular injection in the gluteal area. (Courtesy of Wyeth Laboratories, Philadelphia, Pennsylvania.)

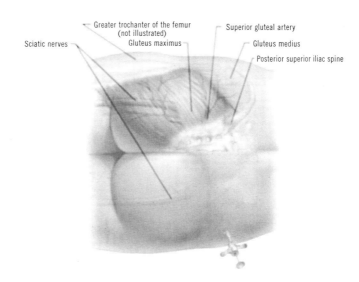

Sciatic nerves

Greater trochanter of the femur (not illustrated)

Gluteus maximus

Superior gluteal artery

Gluteus medius

Posterior superior iliac spine

VENTROGLUTEAL SITE

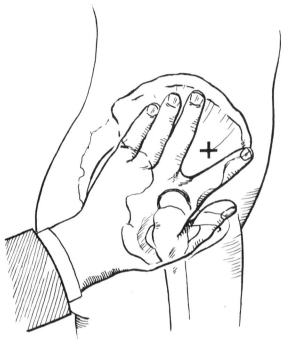

FIGURE 9. The injection is made between the index and middle fingers, spread as far as possible, forming a V. (Courtesy of Abbott Laboratories.)

though this site also can be used when a patient is sitting, lying prone, or on his side. A disadvantage to the use of this site may be that the patient can observe the injection being given.

The greater trochanter, the anterior superior iliac spine and the iliac crest are located by palpation. When injecting into the patient's right side, place the palm of the left hand over the greater trochanter with the fingers pointing to the patient's head. (Care should be taken that the greater trochanter is not mistakenly identified as the anterior superior iliac crest since the site thus resulting may involve the sciatic nerve.) The index finger is placed on the anterior superior iliac spine. The middle finger should be spread posteriorly as far as possible to form a V-shaped area. The site of injection should be in the center of the triangle, and the needle should be directed slightly upward toward the area immediately below the iliac crest. (See Figure 9.)

Vastus lateralis. The site for injection into the vastus lateralis is within the area between the midanterior aspect of the thigh and the midlateral aspect of the thigh. The length of the area extends from a hand's width below the greater trochanter to the same distance above the knee. (See Figure 10.)

Intramuscular injections in children. Administering injections to children requires special adaptation in techniques and approaches. Needle lengths are usually shorter than those used in adults. Children and infants will need to be restrained to some degree because of the dangers of movement during the injection.

The dorsogluteal area may be used, but is not advocated by many authorities because the gluteal muscles are not fully developed until the child has begun to walk and has assumed an upright posture. The vastus lateralis is a common site for intramuscular injection in infants. With the infant on his back, the anterolateral aspect of the thigh is grasped and the muscle tissue compressed in one hand. This helps to prevent leg movement by the infant and also localizes the muscle tissue. The needle is injected to a depth of no more than one inch in an antero-

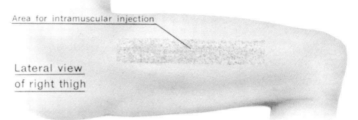

VASTUS LATERALIS

FIGURE 10. Vastus lateralis. (From *How to Give an Intramuscular Injection.* Pfizer Laboratories, Professional Service Department, New York, N.Y.)

posterior direction. The anterolateral portion of the upper thigh may be used if the needle is inserted at a 45 degree angle, with the needle pointing toward the infant's toes. (See Figure 11.) The ventrogluteal site may also be used.

Technique of intramuscular injection. After the drug has been prepared and measured, and before it is injected, about 0.2 cc. of air should be pulled into the syringe. When the syringe is inverted for injection, the air rises to the top near the plunger and serves to push all of the medication out of the syringe and needle. In addition to insuring that the patient receives all of the medication, this also helps to prevent the medication entering the subcutaneous tissue as the needle is being withdrawn. This is of particular importance when a drug is known to be irritating or damaging to subcutaneous tissues.

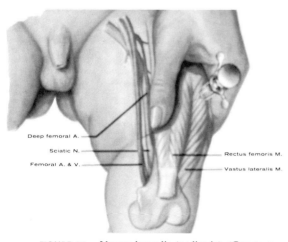

FIGURE 11. Vastus lateralis (pediatric). (Courtesy of Wyeth Laboratories, Philadelphia, Pennsylvania.)

The site chosen for the injection should be palpated in order to detect areas of induration or trigger zones, which will result in pain if the injection is made in this area. Before inserting the needle, it is wise to check to be sure that the lumen of the needle has not become occluded by the medication, since some drugs tend to solidify on contact with air.

The skin at the site of injection is cleansed with alcohol or other anti-infective. The cleansing should be done in a circular manner from the site of injection outward. When injecting a medication into a relatively thin person or a child, the skin and muscle should be pinched before the needle is inserted. In an obese person, or when injecting into the dorsogluteal area, it is often better to stretch the skin between two fingers prior to injection. Individual adaptations in techniques and needle length and angle must be made in order to insure that the drug is injected into the center of the muscle.

The needle is usually injected at a 90 degree angle. Generally, it should not be inserted to its full length; allow a portion of the needle to remain outside the skin in the event that the needle should break off from the hub. The chance of this occurring is greatly reduced with the use of disposable needles. Needles that are resterilized and used repeatedly may become weakened and are more likely to break. Any type of needle that has been inadvertently bent during the preparation of the drug should not be used for the actual injection. If the needle should break while it is in the patient and it cannot be readily removed by pulling on the exposed portion of the needle, the site of insertion should be circled immediately with a pen mark and the physician notified.

After the skin has been cleansed and the needle has been inserted to the appropriate depth, aspiration must be done to insure that the needle is not within a blood vessel. The plunger of the syringe should be withdrawn slightly to create suction and the lower end of the syringe should be checked carefully for the presence of blood. It is recommended that the needle be withdrawn slightly during aspiration in order to insure that the needle bevel is not against the wall of a blood vessel, in which case the blood would not enter the syringe even though the needle was in the blood vessel. Greater suction should be exerted if the drug is thick or oily in nature or if a small gauge needle is used. Very careful observation is needed when the medication is dark or red in color since the blood entering the syringe will be more difficult to detect.

If the needle is determined to be in a blood vessel, the best course of action would be to prepare a new dose of the drug using a new needle and syringe. If this is impractical for a serious reason, another needle should be used and the injection given in another site. Careful observation is essential when aspirating at the second site since blood is already present in the syringe from the first injection attempt.

The drug should be injected always into the muscle to allow for the dispersion of the drug into the muscle tissues. Care should be taken that the needle is withdrawn at the same angle as it was inserted in order to prevent further tissue damage. Pressure should be applied to the injection site and the area massaged in order to promote the distribution and absorption of the drug. The site used for the injection should be recorded, particularly if the patient is receiving repeated injections.

A relatively new technique, the "Z" technique, is used with medications such as iron preparations which tend to discolor the skin or irritate subcutaneous tissue if there is any leakage from the muscle injection site. In this technique the upper outer quadrant of the buttock is used. A separate needle is used to withdraw the medication from the vial along with 0.5 cc. of air. This needle is then replaced with a longer intramuscular needle. The skin is pulled to one side over the intended injection site and the injection of the medicine is made, followed by the 0.5 cc. of air then 10 seconds is allowed for the dispersal of the medication before the needle is removed. As the stretched skin returns to its original position, the path of the needle to the injection site is sealed with subcutaneous connective tissue.

INTRAVENOUS INJECTION. Intravenous injection is employed to administer medications, especially in emergency situations, when a rapid onset of action is desired. In this procedure medications are injected directly into the blood stream through a vein, thus avoiding the loss of time involved in absorption of the drug from other parenteral sites. The median basilic or median cephalic vein at the bend of the elbow is most often used. The subclavian vein is now used for the infusion of intravenous fluids. The patient should be observed closely during insertion of the intravenous catheter and during the therapy since pneumothorax and hydrothorax have been known to occur. Both therapeutic and untoward effects occur with extreme rapidity, however, and caution must be employed when administering drugs intravenously.

In addition to the obvious advantage of rapid action, intravenous therapy is also extremely useful for the administration of irritating drugs which could not be administered by any other parenteral route because of the tissue damage they would produce. The intima or endothelial lining of the blood vessels is quite resistant to the corrosive action of these drugs. Many of the new antineoplastic drugs can only be administered intravenously because of their necrotizing effects on other tissues.

As mentioned previously, the administration of medications intravenously usually is considered a function of the physician rather than of the nurse. Depending on the provisions of state laws and hospital policy, the registered nurse with specialized preparation may be allowed to give certain specified drugs intravenously. These nurses usually carry out this function within specialized patient care units in which the policies and procedures concerning this method of drug administration by the nurse are clearly defined.

In some situations, again depending on hospital policy and legal restrictions, nurses may administer certain types of drugs, such as antibiotics, intravenously by inserting the drug into a certain amount of intravenous infusion solution, which then flows by intravenous drip into the patient's venous system. The volume of the intravenous solution into which the drug is added may vary. An intravenous solution into which a drug has been added must be clearly labeled with the name of the drug added, the dosage, time the drug was added and the name of the person who added the drug.

Incompatibility of a drug with the intravenous solution or other drugs is a major problem in giving drugs intravenously. Although certain drugs are known to be incompatible with certain types of solutions, incompatibilities are often unpredictable. This is because incompatibilities may be related to such variables as the pH of the solution, the temperature of the solution at the time the drug is added and the sequence in which drugs are added to the solution. Any solution in which a precipitate forms should not be used; the flow should be halted immediately if this occurs during the infusion.

The intravenous route is also used for the administration of large volumes of fluids by infusion (venoclysis). Such fluids may contain electrolytes, dextrose or other sugars, proteins, vitamins, or occasionally specific drugs, and are given to combat dehydration, to increase blood volume, to treat electrolyte deficiencies and to supply nourishment when the oral route cannot be used. The fluids should be isotonic with normal body fluids, or nearly so, to avoid damage to blood cells.

In intravenous infusion the solution flows into the vein by gravity from a large glass flask through tubing, with a clamp on the tubing to control the flow. An adapter tip connects the tubing to a standard needle which is taped to the site. Occasionally an intravenous catheter (Intracath) may be employed to facilitate continuous fluid administration. The Intracath consists of a slender needle within a flexible plastic cylinder about the width of a small vein. After the needle is inserted into the vein it may be withdrawn through the center of the plastic tubing leaving only the flexible tubing within the vein. This method greatly increases the comfort of the patient since he may move around quite freely during the administration of fluids. In addition, the Intracath considerably reduces the incidence of extravasation of fluids during administration.

Other similar types of intravenous catheters have been developed; they usually vary in the length of tubing which remains within the patient's vein. When an intravenous catheter is removed, it should be inspected carefully to be sure that it is still intact and that a portion of it has not been left within the vein.

When a patient is receiving intravenous infusion therapy, the nurse has several areas of responsibility. If a drug has been added to the infusion, the patient must be observed carefully because of the rapidity with which effect and toxic effects can occur. The rate of flow of the infusion should be maintained at the rate indicated by the physician. Chapter 4 discusses methods of calculating infusion rates. In addition to mechanical regulation, the rate of flow of the infusion may be affected by other factors. The position of the needle within the vein may affect flow rate; the rate may be slowed or stopped by the bevel of the needle being against the lining of the vein. This often results from a change in the patient's position, especially if the needle is near a moving joint.

The response of the patient to the intravenous infusion should be carefully observed and noted. An increase in the pulse rate may indicate too rapid infusion. This may result in congestive heart failure, particularly in children and the elderly, or others who have a poor cardiac reserve.

The area around the site of the intravenous injection should be observed for redness and swelling or other signs of inflammation which might indicate the development of phlebitis.

Insuring that the needle remains within the

vein is another nursing responsibility. The area should be protected from pressure and from movement if the site is at or near a movable joint.

The area around the intravenous site should be observed for indications of infiltration, i.e., the fluid is flowing into the subcutaneous tissue rather than into the vein. Swelling, pain and coldness of the swollen area in comparison to the surrounding tissues are indications that the fluid has infiltrated. The rate of flow of the infusion may have slowed or stopped completely. Lowering the bottle of intravenous fluid below the level of the vein produces a siphoning action. If blood flows into the tubing, the needle is patent and is within the vein. The absence of blood in the tubing during siphoning usually, but not always, indicates that the needle is not within the vein. It also may indicate that there is a clot within the needle.

When the infusion is to be discontinued, the dressing around the intravenous site should be carefully removed until the needle or intravenous catheter is viewed. The needle or catheter is then removed and firm pressure with an alcohol sponge is exerted over the site for at least a minute in order to prevent extravasation of blood from the vein into the surrounding tissues.

An accurate system of recording intravenous infusion therapy should be used in order to prevent errors and to provide an accurate assessment of the patient's fluid and electrolyte status. Observations of the patient's reactions to the intravenous therapy and drug therapy, if any, should be included in the nursing assessment of the patient and should be recorded in the nurses' notes.

INTRA-ARTERIAL INJECTION. A recently introduced method of drug administration is that of intra-arterial administration. Certain antineoplastic drugs are presently administered intra-arterially through a specially adapted administration set. When the drug is inserted directly into the artery leading to the cancerous tissue or organ, it can exert a maximal effect on the diseased part, and at the same time produce fewer toxic systemic side reactions because of the lower dosage that can be employed.

Continuous low dose therapy may be continued on an outpatient basis using the intra-arterial route. Patients may be discharged with arterial catheters in place and with a month's supply of the antineoplastic drug in small plastic containers prepared for self-administration by the patient. In this procedure a pressure apparatus similar to a blood pressure cuff is attached to the arm of the patient, and is placed around the plastic container of medicine which the patient has attached to the free end of the arterial catheter. The apparatus is calibrated to deliver small doses of the drug continually over 24 hours. Each morning the patient merely replaces the empty plastic bag with a full one. It is the current belief of some practitioners that continuous low dose cancer therapy is more efficacious and produces fewer side effects than intermittent high dose treatment.

PROCEDURES FOR THE ADMINISTRATION OF MEDICATIONS

Every hospital has a standard procedure for the administration of medications. These procedures may vary greatly from institution to institution, and regulations may be changed or added to continually as a result of particular experiences within the institution. Consequently, although certain general guidelines and policies are likely to be followed by many institutions, there is no one standard procedure for drug administration. It is, therefore, of the utmost importance to learn and to follow the regulations of the individual hospital carefully and exactly.

Bearing in mind these individual differences, it is possible to outline here some typical procedures and general considerations that are relatively uniform in most institutions. Most of the following are based on legal implications and are intended to promote the safety of the patient.

1. A nurse should administer only medications that she herself has prepared.

2. Conversations or other distractions should be avoided while preparing medications.

3. The medicine cabinet should be in a

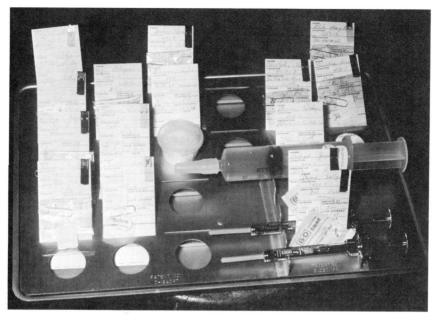

FIGURE 12.   Medicine tray prepared for the administration of various forms of medication.

room not accessible to the public and should be kept locked at all times except when medications are being prepared.

4. In hospitals in which a medication nurse gives all the medications, she is responsible for the keys to the medicine cabinet at all times. In certain hospitals, in accordance with the concept of total patient care, each staff nurse administers medications to the patients for whom she is responsible. In any event, a system of restricted access to medications must be developed.

5. Medicines for individual patients should be kept separated in a special section of the cupboard.

6. All stock supplies should be stored in an orderly manner, with separate storage areas for medications intended for internal and external use.

7. Refrigeration should be available for medications which are perishable at room temperature.

8. The labels of all medicine bottles should be neat and legible. The nurse may never relabel a medication bottle. It must be sent to the pharmacy if relabeling is necessary.

9. Errors of omission, dosage or type of medication must be reported at once to the head nurse and an incident report filled out.

10. The medicine must be charted as soon as it is given. This responsibility cannot be delegated to anyone else by the nurse who gives the medication.

PROCEDURE FOR THE ADMINISTRATION OF ORAL MEDICATIONS.   Keeping in mind that many of these principles apply to the administration of medications by other routes as well, a sample procedure for the administration of oral medications will be outlined in full.

1. Before a medication is administered, the nurse must have a written order by the physician clearly stating the medication, dosage, route and frequency of administration. If a verbal order is taken by the nurse, the physician must authenticate the order by his signature within 24 hours. The nurse should check to be sure that the medication has not been given and that the order is still valid. She should also check to be sure the patient is not N.P.O. for surgery, tests or some other reason.

2. A separate medication card should be filled out for every medication and should contain the name of the patient, the room number, and the name, dosage, frequency

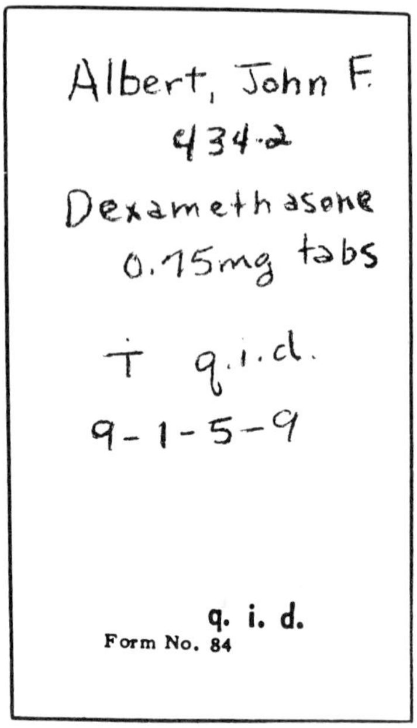

Albert, John F.
434·2
Dexamethasone
0.75mg tabs

T̄ q.i.d.
9-1-5-9

q. i. d.
Form No. 84

FIGURE 13. A sample medicine card bearing information necessary for the administration of the medication.

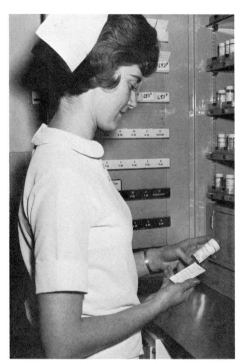

FIGURE 14. The label of the medication bottle should be checked carefully with the medication card.

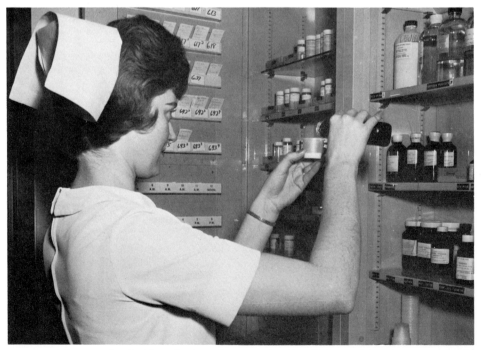

FIGURE 15. When pouring liquid medications the nurse should hold the medicine glass at eye level and her thumb should mark the volume to be measured.

and route of administration of the medication (Fig. 13). In addition the duration of the order, the current date and the initials of the nurse who transcribed the order should be added.

3. The identity of the medication should be verified three times with the medication card: when taking the container from the shelf, before pouring it, and before putting it back on the shelf (Fig. 14).

4. Shake the bottle well if the medication is a liquid. When pouring liquids avoid soiling the label by holding the bottle with the label in the palm of the hand. The bottle should be wiped clean with a damp cloth or towel following each use. The rim of the bottle should be wiped before and after the medication is poured. This prevents the drug from becoming concentrated and falling into the solution or into the container, thereby increasing the strength of the medication. Fluid medications should be measured by reading the fluid level at the bottom of the meniscus when the medicine glass or graduate is held at eye level (Fig. 15).

5. Tablets and capsules should be handled in such a way that the fingers do not come in contact with them. The cap of the medication bottle, or a separate medication cup, may be used to drop the tablet or capsule into the medicine cup (Fig. 16).

6. Place the medicine with the identifying card in the medicine tray. The medicine tray or cart should never be left unattended when it is outside of the medicine closet.

7. Identify the patient by checking his wristband.

8. Take any special nursing action indicated, such as checking the patient's pulse, before administering the drug.

9. Remain with the patient until the medicine is swallowed.

10. Chart the medication immediately. Narcotic medications also must be recorded on the appropriate Harrison Act narcotic sheets. Certain drugs, such as insulin, cardiac drugs and anticoagulants, may be recorded on additional records.

11. Record in the nurses' notes observations related to drug effect and side effects.

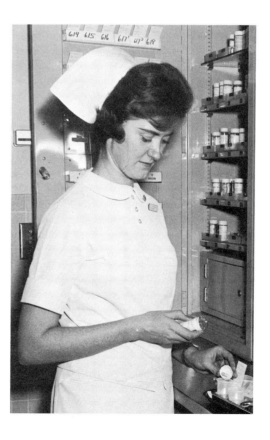

FIGURE 16. Oral medications should be prepared in such a way that they are not touched by the fingers.

MODERN TRENDS IN DRUG ADMINISTRATION

UNIT DOSE DISPENSING. Many experts in the field of drug administration are of the opinion that much valuable nursing time could be conserved if medications were dispensed using a decentralized hospital pharmacy and the unit dose system. Accordingly, several of the larger hospitals throughout the country are presently working with various forms of this plan.

In this system, small pharmacy sub-stations are installed on the nursing units and a pharmacist is on the floor at all times to transcribe medication orders directly from the patient charts, to add medications to intravenous solutions, to dilute and draw up any injectable medications and to prepare each dose of medication as it is ordered. The medicine trays for regularly scheduled doses of drugs are prepared throughout the day by the pharmacist for administration by a nurse (Figs. 17, 18).

Although in general the system is quite successful and has been readily accepted by physicians, nurses and pharmacists, a few practical problems can be foreseen. Since one pharmacist may be responsible for two or three nursing units, he may not always be immediately available for p.r.n. medications. This difficulty may be overcome by preparing the p.r.n. medications in advance and leaving them in a cupboard designated for this purpose. Medication cards are filled out with the patient's name and the name and dosage of the drug, and one dose of the drug is then attached to the card. The dose may be administered by the nurse as needed and the card placed in a refill box for replacement by the pharmacist.

The advantages of the unit dose system are obvious and manifold. Since all written records of drugs, including the Harrison narcotic sheets and the patient charges, are kept by the pharmacist, the nurse is consequently able to devote much valuable time to other aspects of patient care.

In addition, the presence of a pharmacist on the nursing unit makes him more readily available to physicians, nurses, students and

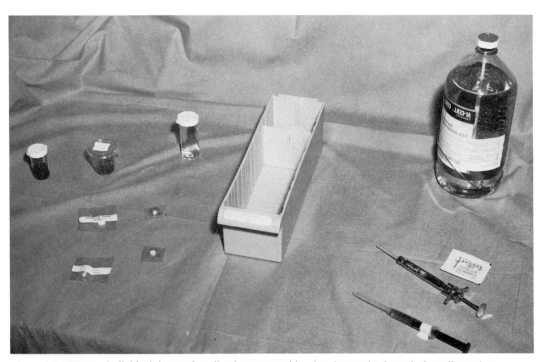

FIGURE 17.   Individual doses of medication prepared by the pharmacist for unit dose dispensing.

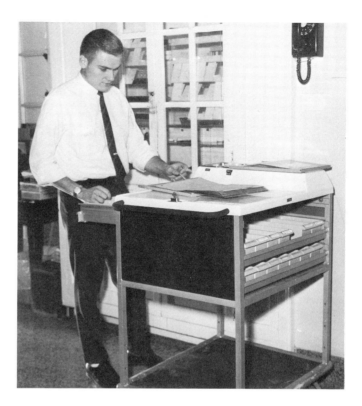

FIGURE 18. In unit, dose dispensing the pharmacist prepares and labels each dose of medicine and places it in the patient's drawer in the medicine cart.

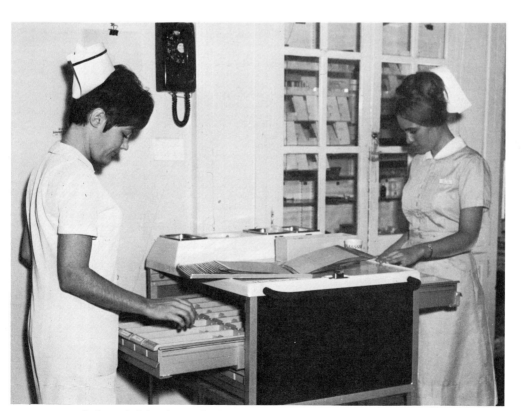

FIGURE 19. Before administering medication the nurse checks each dose with her medication orders.

allied medical personnel for consultation on the various aspects of drug therapy and enables a closer check on the total drug therapy being given to each patient. Therapeutic incompatibilities, possible adverse drug reactions from combination therapy and incorrect doses can more readily be foreseen and prevented under these circumstances than would be possible if all patient orders were filled in a central pharmacy by a large staff of pharmacists.

It seems highly probable that the unit dose system of drug administration will gain rapid acceptance among hospital and medical personnel and will probably be incorporated into many hospitals in the near future.

AUTOMATED SYSTEMS OF DRUG DISPENSING. In a few hospitals drugs are now dispensed by an automatic system employing electronic tape to record all drug transactions. Dispensing machines are located in the nursing units, and an accompanying drug cart is used for actual administration of medications. The pharmacy staff is responsible for keeping the dispensing machines stocked, and the nurse simply withdraws from the machine the specific medication required for each patient. This system is felt by participating hospitals

to be efficient and record-keeping is simplified. This system has the disadvantage of being somewhat prone to error, however, and no double check is provided for unsafe doses of the medications or for dangerous combinations of drugs, which may not be recognized by the nurse.

THE PRESCRIPTION

The prescription has an obscure origin in the beginnings of civilized man. Many Egyptian records have been preserved which contain a variety of medical formulas cut on stone or written on papyrus. The Ebers Papyrus, which was written about the sixteenth century B.C., is considered to be an unofficial formulary or private recipe book. It contains, in addition to specific recipes for medications, many invocations for driving away the evil spirits of disease from the body.

The modern prescription is an order for medication written by a physician, dentist, veterinarian or some other licensed medical practitioner. While osteopaths may legally write prescriptions, chiropractors and opticians may not.

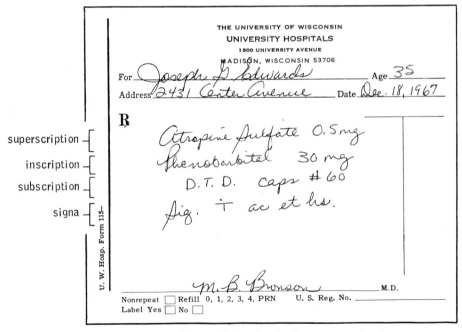

FIGURE 20. A sample prescription showing the component parts.

There are six components in a prescription:

1. The current date and the patient's name and address.
2. The superscription, which consists of the symbol "℞," meaning "Take thou."
3. The inscription, which states the names and quantities of ingredients.
4. The subscription, which gives directions to the pharmacist.
5. The signature, designated (Sig.), which gives the directions to the patient and is embodied in the directions on the label of the filled prescription.
6. The signature of the physician, his address and registry number.

The prescription is usually written in English, although a combination of Latin and English may still be used by some physicians, even in the same prescription. Quantities may be expressed in either the apothecaries' or metric system. Figure 20 shows an example of a prescription with numbers to indicate the various parts.

In the hospital, medicine orders written by nurses often replace the prescription. The nurse copies the physician's order on the medicine order and sends it to the pharmacist. This procedure is a poor one at best, despite its common acceptance. Many errors are made daily from misspelled, misread and hasty transcription of drug orders. Unfortunately, it would be practically impossible for the physician to write each medication order and refill request for his patients. This area is one in which the nurse must exercise the greatest care, and she must be extremely accurate in transcribing the physician's order to the medication blank.

ABBREVIATIONS USED IN PRESCRIPTIONS

Abbreviation	Meaning	Abbreviation	Meaning
aa.	of each	o.u.	both eyes
a.c.	before meals	part. aeq.	equal parts
ad	to, up to	p.c.	after meals
ad lib.	as much as desired	pil.	pill
alt. hor.	every other hour	p.o.	by mouth
aq. dest.	distilled water	p.r.n.	as needed
b.i.d.	twice daily	pulv.	powder
$\bar{c}$.	with	$\bar{q}$.	every
caps.	capsule	$\bar{q}$. h.	every hour
cc.	cubic centimeter	q.i.d.	four times daily
d.t.d.	give such doses	q.s.	as much as required
elix.	elixir	qt.	quart
et	and	℞	take
ext.	extract	$\bar{s}$	without
fl. or fld.	fluid	sol.	solution
ft.	make	s.o.s.	if needed (for one time)
Gm.	gram	sp. or spir.	spirit
gr.	grain	sp. frumenti	whiskey
gtt.	a drop	$\overline{ss}$	half
h.s.	at bedtime	stat.	immediately
H.T.	hypodermic tablet	syr.	syrup
L.	liter	tab.	tablet or tablets
liq.	liquid, solution	t.i.d	three times daily
M.	mix.	tr.	tincture
mist.	mixture	ung.	ointment
ml.	milliliter	ut dict.	as directed
non rep.	not to be repeated	vin.	wine
O.	pint	ℨ	dram
o.d.	right eye	♏	minim
ol.	oil	℥	ounce
o.s.	left eye	℈	scruple

QUESTIONS FOR DISCUSSION AND REVIEW

1. How can errors in drug administration be minimized?

2. Which mode of administration would be used to obtain the most rapid effect? Which mode would probably give the slowest? Why?

3. What precautions must be taken when administering intramuscular injections in the dorsogluteal area? Why?

4. Must a prescription always be written on a physician's special prescription pad? Is a prescription legal no matter what it is written on? What would constitute legality in a prescription?

5. What routine is used for administering medications in your hospital? What are the hospital's policies concerning:
   a. verbal orders
   b. telephone orders
   c. automatic stop dates
   d. drugs which may not be administered by the nurse
   e. intravenous administration of drugs by nurses?

6. How could you help to minimize the discomfort from a drug which is disagreeable in taste?

7. What are the advantages of the ventrogluteal site for intramuscular injection?

8. Outline a teaching plan for a patient who must administer a drug to himself subcutaneously.

9. Why should precautions be taken to prevent eye drops from reaching the tear duct immediately after instillation?

10. What are the nurse's legal responsibilities in the administration of medications?

BIBLIOGRAPHY

Abbott Laboratories. *Parenteral Administration* (booklet). North Chicago, 1970.

Adriani, J.: Venipuncture. *Amer. J. Nurs., 62*:66, (March) 1962.

Baker, K. N. and McConnell, W. E.: How to detect medication errors. *Mod. Hosp., 99*:95 passim, (July) 1962.

Block, B.: Site of injection of penicillin. *J.A.M.A., 188*:95, 1964.

Bowles, G. C., Jr.: The pharmacist could help the nurse more if the law let him. *Mod. Hosp., 113*:136 (December) 1969.

Brunner, L. S., et al.: *Textbook of Medical-Surgical Nursing.* 2nd Ed. Philadelphia, J. B. Lippincott Co., 1970.

Coates, F. C. and Fabrykant, M.: Insulin injection technique for preventing skin reactions. *Amer. J. Nurs., 65*:127, (February) 1965.

Dann, T. C.: Routine skin preparation before injection—is it necessary? *Nurs. Times, 62*:1121, (August 26) 1966.

Drew, J. A. and Blumberg, M. S.: What happens to medication orders? *Amer. J. Nurs., 62*:59, (July) 1962.

Du Gas, B. W.: Kozier-Du Gas' *Introduction to Patient Care.* 2nd Ed. Philadelphia, W. B. Saunders Co., 1972.

Fogg, J.: Patients, drugs, and nurses. *Nurs. Times,* (April 8, 1966), p. 473.

Fuerst, E. V. and Wolff, L.: *Fundamentals of Nursing.* 4th Ed. Philadelphia, J. B. Lippincott Co., 1969.

Gragg, S. H. and Rees, O. M.: *Scientific Principles in Nursing.* 6th Ed. St. Louis, C. V. Mosby Co., 1970.

Hanson, D.: Intramuscular injections. Injuries and complications. *Amer. J. Nurs., 63*:99, (April) 1963.

Haward, L. R.: Some psychological aspects of intramuscular injection. *J. Ment. Sci., 108*:843, 1962.

Hershey, N.: The apparently erroneous order. *Amer. J. Nurs., 64*:111, (January) 1964.

Hershey, N.: He can't take the responsibility. *Amer. J. Nurs., 66*:1053, (May) 1966.

Hershey, N.: Question that drug order. *Amer. J. Nurs., 63*:96, (January) 1963.

Hopkins, S. J.: The storage of drugs. *Nurs. Times, 65*:459, (April 10) 1969.

Hosford, R. F.: Automatic drug dispensing. *Hospitals, 37*:96, (January 16) 1963.

Hospital medication errors. *J.A.M.A., 195*:31, 1966.

How to give an intramuscular injection (pamphlet). New York, Pfizer Laboratories, 1971.

Hoynak, R. M.: Promoting medication safety. *Nurs. Outlook, 11*:497, (July) 1963.

Intramuscular Injections (booklet). 3rd rev. ed. New York, Wyeth Laboratories, 1970.

Kern, M. S.: New ideas about drug systems. *Amer. J. Nurs., 68*:1251, (June) 1968.

Kernicki, J.: Needle puncture; health asset or menace. *Nurs. Clin. N. Amer., 1*:269, (June) 1966.

Kron, T.: Stepping beyond the five rights in administering drugs. *Amer. J. Nurs., 62*:62, (July) 1962.

Levine, M. E.: Breaking through the medications mystique. *Amer. J. Nurs., 70*:799, (April) 1970.

Lorber, G.: Sources of drug information. *Amer. J. Nurs., 63*:101, 1963.

Martin, E. W. (ed.): *Husa's Pharmaceutical Dispensing.* 5th Ed. Easton, Pa., Mack Publishing Co., 1959.

Pitel, M.: The subcutaneous injection. *Amer. J. Nurs., 71*:76, (January) 1971.

Pitel, M. and Wemett, M.: The intramuscular injection. *Amer. J. Nurs., 64*:104, (April) 1964.

Regan, W. A.: The new standing orders and their legal pitfalls. *R.N., 31*:38, (April) 1968.

Regan, W. A.: You, doctors and hospital: equals before the law. *R.N., 28*:86, (October) 1965.

Slonacker, M. R.: Administering drugs from a central drug room. *Amer. H. Nurs., 62*:108, (December) 1962.

Thomas, S.: Medication errors can be prevented. *Canad. Nurse, 65*:50, (May) 1969.

Travell, J.: Factors affecting pain of injection. *J.A.M.A., 158*:368, (June 4) 1955.

Webb, C.: Tactics to reduce a child's fear of pain. *Amer. J. Nurs., 66*:2698, (December) 1966.

Wempe, B. M.: The new and old intramuscular injection sites. *Amer. J. Nurs., 61*:56, (September) 1961.

Willig, S.: Drug-dispensing/administering. *Amer. J. Nurs., 64*:126 (June) 1964.

Chapter 4 Mathematical Principles of Drug Therapy

Important Concepts Discussed

1. *Two systems of weight and measurement are used in pharmacy: the apothecaries' system and the metric system.*

2. *The inverted stock rule is used to calculate parenteral doses from hypodermic tablets.*

3. *Children's doses are reduced from adult doses according to rules based on age or weight.*

4. *Solutions may be prepared from pure drugs or from dispensing tablets. The metric system is ordinarily used in determining ratio and percentage strengths of solutions.*

5. *The alligation method is employed for dilutions of strong solutions.*

It is essential that the nurse have a working knowledge of the fundamental principles of arithmetic in order to make the accurate calculations necessary for the administration of medications. The mechanics involved are no more complicated than addition, subtraction, multiplication and division, but it is necessary to become familiar with the systems of weight and measure used in medicine.

ARITHMETIC REVIEW

ROMAN NUMERALS

The system of Roman numerals uses letters to designate numbers. Roman numerals are retained in the apothecaries' system of measures and they are often used in writing prescriptions and stating doses of drugs.

Basic Roman numerals are expressed as follows:

Roman numeral	Arabic numeral
I	1
V	5
X	10
L	50
C	100
D	500
M	1000

A few basic rules are used in combining the numerals:

1. When a Roman numeral precedes one of larger value, its value is subtracted from the larger. When a numeral follows one of larger value, its value is added to the larger.

EXAMPLES:
(a) IX = (10 − 1) = 9
(b) XI = (10 + 1) = 11

2. When two numerals of identical value are repeated in sequence, their values are added. (Numerals may never be repeated more than three times in sequence.)

EXAMPLES:
(a) III = 3
(b) MMMCCIII = 3203

3. When a numeral is placed between two numerals of a greater value, the lesser is subtracted from the numeral following it.

EXAMPLES:
(a) MCM = 1900
(b) CXLIX = 149

EXERCISES

A. Express the following in Roman numerals:
1. 54 _____
2. 1649 _____
3. 47 _____
4. 94 _____
5. 301 _____
6. 1950 _____
7. Your age _____
8. The current year _____

B. Express the following in Arabic numbers:
1. MCMXLIX _____
2. XLVIII _____
3. CIII _____
4. XIX _____
5. LVIII _____
6. CCLVIII _____
7. IX _____
8. XC _____

FRACTIONS

A fraction is a portion of a whole. When expressed numerically it indicates the number of equal parts into which the whole has been divided, and how many of these equal parts are being considered.

For example, the fraction $\frac{2}{3}$ means 2 of 3 equal parts. It could also be written $2 \div 3$ since it indicates division into 3 equal parts. The numbers 2 and 3 are called the "terms of the fraction." The lower number is the denominator, or the divisor, and tells into how many parts the unit is divided. The upper number of the fraction, or the numerator, is also the dividend and tells how many parts of the unit are taken.

Proper fraction. A proper fraction is one having a numerator less than the denominator, such as $\frac{1}{4}$, $\frac{3}{8}$.

Improper fraction. An improper fraction is one having a numerator greater than the denominator, such as $\frac{7}{5}$, $\frac{5}{3}$.

An improper fraction designates a quantity greater than one unit.

Complex fraction. A complex fraction is one whose numerator or denominator, or both, are fractions, such as $\frac{\frac{1}{2}}{3}$, $\frac{\frac{3}{4}}{\frac{2}{3}}$.

Mixed number. A mixed number consists of a whole number and a fraction, such as $3\frac{2}{7}$.

CHANGING AN IMPROPER FRACTION TO A MIXED NUMBER

1. Divide the numerator by the denominator.
2. Write the remainder, if any, as a fraction reduced to the lowest terms.

EXAMPLES:
(a) $\frac{11}{7} = 1\frac{4}{7}$
(b) $\frac{24}{5} = 4\frac{4}{5}$

CHANGING MIXED NUMBERS TO IMPROPER FRACTIONS

1. Multiply the whole number by the denominator of the fraction.
2. Add this product to the numerator of the fraction.
3. Write the sum as the numerator of the improper fraction; the denominator remains the same.

EXAMPLES: (a) $3\frac{2}{5} = \frac{15+2}{5} = \frac{17}{5}$
(b) $4\frac{2}{3} = \frac{12+2}{3} = \frac{14}{3}$

EXERCISES

A. Change the following to whole or mixed numbers:

$\frac{12}{4}$ _____

$\frac{9}{4}$ _____

$\frac{27}{13}$ _____

$\frac{127}{12}$ _____

$\frac{42}{6}$ _____

B. Change the following to improper fractions:

2 _____

$3\frac{1}{2}$ _____

$4\frac{1}{8}$ _____

$1\frac{1}{10}$ _____

5 _____

REDUCING FRACTIONS. Fractions are reduced to their lowest or simplest terms by dividing both the numerator and the denominator by the greatest number that is contained in them evenly (greatest common divisor). When both the numerator and denominator are divided by the same number, the value of the fraction does not change. Fractions are usually written in their lowest terms.

EXERCISES

A. Reduce the following fractions to their lowest terms:

$\frac{6}{24}$ _____

$\frac{9}{27}$ _____

$\frac{1}{3}$ _____

$\frac{2}{8}$ _____

$\frac{2}{4}$ _____

B. Change the following fractions to higher terms:

$\frac{1}{2}$ _____

$\frac{3}{4}$ _____

$\frac{1}{8}$ _____

$\frac{2}{7}$ _____

$\frac{4}{16}$ _____

ADDITION OF FRACTIONS

1. If the fractions have the same denominator, add the numerators, write the sum over the common denominator and reduce the fraction to lowest terms.
2. If the fractions have unlike denominators, first find their lowest common denominator; add the numerators as described.
3. To add mixed numbers, first add the fractions, then add the sum of the whole numbers.

EXAMPLES:

(a) $\frac{2}{3}$
$+ \frac{1}{3}$
$\frac{3}{3} = 1$

(b) $\frac{3}{4} = \frac{3}{4}$
$+ \frac{1}{2} = \frac{2}{4}$
$\frac{5}{4} = 1\frac{1}{4}$

(c) $1\frac{1}{2} = 1\frac{2}{4}$
$+ 2\frac{3}{4} = 2\frac{3}{4}$
$3 + \frac{5}{4} = 4\frac{1}{4}$

EXERCISES

Add the following numbers:

$1\frac{1}{2} + \frac{2}{3} =$ _____

$\frac{3}{4} + \frac{2}{8} =$ _____

$1\frac{2}{3} + 2\frac{1}{7} =$ _____

$2\frac{1}{8} + 1\frac{2}{7} =$ _____

$\frac{3}{7} + \frac{1}{8} =$ _____

SUBTRACTION OF FRACTIONS

1. If the fractions have the same denominator, find the difference between the numerators and write it over the common denominator. Reduce to lowest terms.
2. If the fractions have unlike denominators, first find the lowest common denominator, then proceed as described.
3. To subtract mixed numbers, first subtract the fractions as described; then find the difference between the whole numbers. If the fraction in the subtrahend (lower number) is larger than the fraction in the minuend (top number), it is necesary to borrow from the whole number before subtracting the fractions.

EXAMPLES:

(a) $\frac{4}{3}$
$- \frac{2}{3}$
$\frac{2}{3}$

(b) $\frac{7}{8} = \frac{7}{8}$
$- \frac{1}{4} = \frac{2}{8}$
$\frac{5}{8}$

(c) $4\frac{1}{2} = 4\frac{3}{6} = 3\frac{6+3}{6}$
$- 1\frac{2}{3} = 1\frac{4}{6} = 1\frac{4}{6}$
$2\frac{5}{6}$

EXERCISES

Subtract the following:

$\frac{4}{7} - \frac{1}{3} =$ _____

$4\frac{2}{3} - 1\frac{3}{4} =$ _____

$1\frac{2}{7} - \frac{1}{7} =$ _____

$13\frac{1}{2} - 7\frac{7}{8} =$ _____

$1\frac{2}{3} - \frac{4}{3} =$ _____

MULTIPLICATION OF FRACTIONS AND MIXED NUMBERS

1. Change mixed numbers to improper fractions.
2. Cancel if possible by dividing any numerator and denominator by the largest number contained in each.

3. Multiply remaining numerators to find the numerator of the answer.
4. Multiply the remaining denominator to find the denominator of the answer.

EXAMPLES:

(a) $1\frac{1}{2} \times \frac{2}{3} = \frac{3}{2} \times \frac{2}{3} = 1$

(b) $\frac{1}{2} \times \frac{5}{16} \times \frac{1}{4} \times \frac{8}{5} = \frac{1}{64}$

(c) $2\frac{1}{8} \times \frac{3}{4} = \frac{17}{8} \times \frac{3}{4} = \frac{51}{32} = 1\frac{19}{32}$

EXERCISES

Multiply the following:

$\frac{1}{2} \times \frac{3}{4} =$ _____

$2\frac{1}{7} \times \frac{3}{21} =$ _____

$\frac{6}{18} \times 1\frac{3}{6} \times \frac{1}{2} =$ _____

$\frac{3}{8} \times 4\frac{1}{2} =$ _____

$\frac{4}{12} \times \frac{1}{3} \times \frac{3}{16} \times \frac{12}{24} =$ _____

DIVISION OF FRACTIONS AND MIXED NUMBERS

1. Change mixed numbers to improper fractions.
2. Invert the divisor (the number after the division sign).
3. Follow steps for multiplication of fractions.

EXAMPLES:

(a) $\frac{1}{2} \div 1\frac{1}{6} = \frac{1}{2} \div \frac{7}{6}; \frac{1}{2} \times \frac{6}{7} = \frac{3}{7}$

(b) $3\frac{1}{2} \div \frac{1}{2} = \frac{7}{2} \div \frac{1}{2}; \frac{7}{2} \times \frac{2}{1} = 7$

EXERCISES

Divide the following:

$\frac{1}{2} \div 3 =$ _____

$\frac{2}{3} \div \frac{1}{3} =$ _____

$4\frac{1}{2} \div \frac{1}{2} =$ _____

$6 \div \frac{3}{2} =$ _____

$2\frac{1}{4} \div \frac{1}{8} =$ _____

RATIO. A ratio indicates the relationship of one quantity to another. It indicates division and may be correctly expressed in fraction form. For example, the ratio 1:2 may be written as $\frac{1}{2}$.

PROPORTION. A proportion shows the relationship between two equal ratios. A proportion may be expressed as:

$1 : 2 : : 2 : 4$ or

$1 : 2 = 2 : 4$ or

$\frac{1}{2} = \frac{2}{4}$

In a proportion the first and fourth terms are called the extremes, the second and third terms are the means. In a proportion, the product of the means equals the product of the extremes. Since this is always true, if one of the terms in the proportion is unknown, it can be determined by substituting x for the unknown term and solving the proportion, using the following steps:

1. Multiply the means and the extremes, letting x signify the unknown term.
2. Divide the known product by the coefficient of x to solve for the unknown term.

EXAMPLES:

(a) $2 : 4 : : x : 8$

$4x = 16$

$x = \frac{16}{4} = 4$

(b) $\frac{3}{8} = \frac{x}{16}$ $8x = 48$ $x = 6$

EXERCISES

$\frac{2}{3} = \frac{x}{9}$ _____

$\frac{3}{9} = \frac{4}{x}$ _____

$x : 24 : : 1 : 6$ _____

$\frac{3}{x} = \frac{100}{1000}$ _____

$3 : 9 : : 27 : x$ _____

DECIMAL FRACTIONS

A decimal fraction is a fraction whose denominator is 10 or any multiple of 10, as 100, 1000, and so forth. It differs from a common fraction in that the denominator is not written, but is expressed by the proper placement of the decimal point. Usually decimal fractions and mixed decimals are called simply "decimals."

READING AND WRITING DECIMALS

1. Observe the scale below. All whole numbers are to the left of the decimal point, all fractions are to the right.

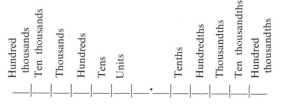

2. In reading a decimal fraction, read the number to the right of the decimal point, and use the name that applies to the "place value" of the last figure.

Example: 0.393 = three hundred ninety-three thousandths.

3. In reading a mixed decimal, first read the whole number, then the decimal fraction. The word "and" shows the place of the decimal point.

Example: 57.057 = fifty-seven and fifty-seven thousandths.

EXERCISES

A. Read the following:
   1. 1.007
   2. 39.1
   3. 375.0027
   4. 125.21
   5. 10,001.0001

B. Express the following as decimal fractions:
   1. Thirty-three and seven thousandths.
   2. Fifty thousand and one tenth.
   3. Four and one hundredth.
   4. Six hundred and one ten-thousandth.
   5. Five and twenty-seven hundred-thousandths.

ADDITION AND SUBTRACTION OF DECIMALS

1. Write the decimals in a column placing the decimal points directly under each other.
2. Add or subtract as indicated.
3. Place the decimal point in the answer directly under the decimal point in the original numbers.

EXERCISES

A. Add the following:

   27.1 + 3.007 =   _____

   127 + 0.1 =   _____

   3.4 + 1 =   _____

   6.9 + 1.745 =   _____

   10.9 + 0.0075 =   _____

B. Subtract the following:

   27.9 − 0.3 =   _____

   375.4 − 1.7542 =   _____

   10 − 0.001 =   _____

   9.5 − 0.3 =   _____

   675.2 − 3 =   _____

MULTIPLICATION OF DECIMALS

1. Multiply as in the multiplication of whole numbers.

2. Find the total number of decimal places in the multiplier and multiplicand.
3. Point off in the product, starting from the right, this total number of decimal places.
4. If the product contains fewer figures than the required decimal places, prefix as many zeros as are necessary.

EXAMPLES:

$$
\begin{array}{r}
\text{(a)}\quad 21.3 \\
\times\ 0.04 \\
\hline
.852
\end{array}
\qquad
\begin{array}{r}
\text{(b)}\quad 10 \\
\times\ .00027 \\
\hline
70 \\
20 \\
\hline
.00270
\end{array}
$$

EXERCISES

Multiply the following:

   3.1 × 1.75 =   _____

   10 × 0.1 =   _____

   6.97 × 1.34 =   _____

   6 × 0.003 =   _____

   125 × 1.0 =   _____

DIVISION OF DECIMALS

1. If the divisor is a whole number, divide as in the division of whole numbers and place the decimal point in the quotient directly above the decimal point in the dividend.
2. If the divisor is a decimal, make it a whole number by moving the decimal point to the right of the last number in the divisor. Move the decimal point in the dividend the same number of places and proceed with division as in step 1. (If the dividend contains fewer places than required, zeros may be added.)

EXAMPLES:

(a) 3.10 ÷ 2

$$
\begin{array}{r}
1.55 \\
2\overline{)3.10}
\end{array} = 1.55
$$

(b) 6.875 ÷ 0.32

$$
\begin{array}{r}
21.48 \\
0.32\overline{)6.87\ 50} = 21.48 \\
\underline{64\ \ \ } \\
47 \\
\underline{32} \\
155 \\
\underline{128} \\
270
\end{array}
$$

EXERCISES

Divide the following and carry the answer to the third decimal place:

34.2 ÷ 0.18 _____

36 ÷ 0.0075 _____

100 ÷ 1.75 _____

42.75 ÷ 1.2 _____

0.0075 ÷ 5 _____

CHANGING DECIMALS TO FRACTIONS

1. Express the decimal as it is written in fraction form.
2. Reduce to lowest terms.

EXAMPLES:

(a) $0.1 = \frac{1}{10}$

(b) $0.75 = \frac{75}{100} = \frac{3}{4}$

CHANGING COMMON FRACTIONS TO DECIMALS

1. Divide the numerator by the denominator.
2. Place decimal point in the proper position.

EXAMPLES:

(a) $\frac{1}{2} = 2)\overline{1.00}^{.50} = 0.5$

(b) $\frac{7}{8} = 8)\overline{7.000}^{.875} = 0.875$

EXERCISES

A. Change the following to decimals:

$\frac{18}{20}$ _____

$\frac{2}{3}$ _____

$\frac{9}{10}$ _____

$\frac{3}{4}$ _____

$1\frac{2}{6}$ _____

B. Change the following to fractions:

0.5 _____

0.125 _____

0.56 _____

0.3 _____

0.95 _____

PERCENTAGE

The term per cent and its symbol % mean parts per hundred. A per cent number is a fraction whose numerator is expressed and whose denominator is understood to be 100. It can be changed to a decimal by moving the decimal point two places to the left to signify hundredths, or to a fraction by expressing the denominator as 100.

EXAMPLES:

(a) 95% = 95. = 0.95

(b) 37% = 37. = 0.37

(c) 210% = 210. = 2.10

EXERCISES

Complete the following:

Fraction	Decimal	Per cent
$\frac{2}{3}$	_____	_____
_____	0.67	_____
$\frac{9}{10}$	_____	_____
_____	1.45	_____
_____	_____	45%
$\frac{1}{3}$	_____	_____
_____		50%
$\frac{3}{3}$	_____	_____
_____	0.75	_____
_____	_____	14%

FINDING PER CENT OF A NUMBER

1. Change the per cent to a decimal or common fraction.
2. Multiply the number by this decimal.

EXAMPLES:

(a) What is 10% of 50?

50 × 0.10 = 5.0

(b) What is 25% of 250?

250 × 0.25 = 62.5

EXERCISES

1. How many apples would constitute 25% of a dozen?
2. $33\frac{1}{3}$% of a gross income of $9000 would be what amount?
3. A manufacturer foresees a loss of 10% of his product in packaging. If the original weight were 4500 lb., what would be the net weight he will market?

4. If taxes on a net income of $10,000 were calculated at 25% on the first $8000 of income and 40% of income over $8000, what would be the annual tax paid?
5. An alloy is 25% silver. How much silver would be contained in 4 tons of the alloy?

FINDING WHAT PER CENT ONE NUMBER IS OF ANOTHER

1. Make a fraction of the two numbers, using the number after the word "of" as a denominator.
2. Reduce fraction to lowest terms.
3. Change the reduced fraction to a per cent.

EXAMPLES:
(a) 25 is what per cent of 100?
$$\frac{25}{100} = \frac{1}{4} = 25\%$$

(b) 3 is what per cent of 9?
$$\frac{3}{9} = \frac{1}{3} = 33\frac{1}{3}\%$$

EXERCISES

1. 16 is what per cent of 24?
2. What per cent of water (H_2O) is oxygen? (m.wt. hydrogen = 1; m.wt. oxygen = 16)
3. What per cent of salt is contained in a mixture if 1 pound salt is mixed with 5 pounds sugar?
4. What per cent of a candy mixture is gum drops if 3 pounds gum drops are mixed with 6 pounds other candy?
5. What per cent of a cake is chocolate if 1 ounce chocolate is contained in pound of batter?

WEIGHTS AND MEASURES

The systems of weights and measures commonly used in medicine are the metric and apothecaries' systems. Because both systems may be used in reference to a single drug or prescription, it is essential to become familiar with them and to be able to convert rapidly from one to the other whenever necessary.

THE METRIC SYSTEM. The metric system is now being used exclusively in the *United States Pharmacopeia.* Undoubtedly it will completely replace the apothecaries' system in the foreseeable future. Arabic numbers and decimals are used with the metric system.

The units used are:
Liter for volume (fluids)
Gram for weight (solids)
Meter for linear measure (length)

The basic units are multiplied and divided by a multiple of ten to form the entire system. Only a few equivalents are used in medicine, however. These are:

Volume
1000 milliliter (ml.) = 1 liter (L.)

Weight
1000 micrograms (mcg.) = 1 milligram (mg.)
1000 milligrams (mg.) = 1 gram (Gm.)
1000 grams (Gm.) = 1 kilogram (kg.)

The milliliter (ml.) is essentially equivalent to a cubic centimeter (cc.), and for all practical purposes these units may be used interchangeably. Hence even though we are not adhering strictly to the metric system, it is correct to say:

1000 cc. = 1 liter

THE APOTHECARIES' SYSTEM. The apothecaries' system is much older than the metric system and is based on the weights of materials familiar to relatively primitive cultures. Hence a "grain" in the apothecary system originally meant the weight of a grain of wheat.

The apothecaries' system today is employed chiefly with older drugs. When the apothecaries' system symbols or abbreviations (e.g., ℥, gr.) are used, especially in prescription writing, some physicians and pharmacists still employ the conventional form in which small Roman numerals are used and the unit is written ahead of the quantity. That is, 20 grains would be written: gr. xx. Sometimes a line is drawn over the numerals—as, gr. x̄x̄—and often the numeral i is dotted to distinguish it from the Roman numeral l, for 50. Thus 13 grains would be written: gr. xı̇̄ı̇̄ı̇̄.

The apothecaries' measurements most

commonly used in medicine are the following:

Volume

60 minims (♍)	=	1 fluid dram (ʒ)
8 fl. drams	=	1 fluid ounce (ʒ)
16 fl. ounces	=	1 pint (0.1 or pt.)

Weight

20 grains (gr.)	=	1 scruple (Э)
3 scruples	=	1 dram (ʒ)
8 drams	=	1 ounce (ʒ)
12 ounces	=	1 pound (lb.)

(Note: In the avoirdupois system of weights and measures commonly used in the U.S.A. there are 16 ounces in 1 pound; hence an apothecaries' pound is not equivalent to an avoirdupois pound)

An apothecaries' minim is roughly equivalent to one drop. This equivalence is sufficiently accurate to regulate intravenous feedings and the like, but for precise procedures or the measurement of a dose in drops, a calibrated dropper must be used, for there is a great variety in the size of drops, depending on the diameter of the dropper, the viscosity of the liquid, and so forth.

CONVERSION BETWEEN THE METRIC AND APOTHECARIES' SYSTEMS. In order to convert from one system to another, some essential equivalents must be learned. A tabulation of the most commonly used equivalents follows.

Weight	Volume
60 mg. = 1 grain	1 cc. = 16 minims
1 Gm. = 15 grains	30 cc. = 1 ounce
30 Gm. = 1 ounce	500 cc. = 1 pint
2.2 lb. = 1 kg.	1000 cc. = 1 quart

Volume

1 teaspoonful	= 1 dram	= 4 or 5 ml.
1 tablespoonful	= ½ ounce = 4 drams	= 15 ml.
1 teacupful	= 6 ounces	= 180 ml.
1 glassful	= 8 ounces	= 240 ml.

The proportion method is the simplest way to carry out conversions.

EXAMPLE:

Convert 100 mg. to grains

100 mg. = 0.100 gram; 1 gram = 15 grains

$$\frac{1 \text{ gram}}{0.100 \text{ gram}} = \frac{15 \text{ grains}}{x}$$

$$1x = 1.5$$

$$x = 1.5 \text{ grains}$$

EXERCISES

1. Convert 1 L. to quarts.
2. Convert 1 grain to milligrams.
3. Convert 1 ʒ to Grams.
4. How many drams in 1 Gram?
5. Convert 1 ʒ to grains.
6. How many milliliters in 1 fl. ʒ?
7. Convert 1 lb. to kilograms.
8. Convert 1½ pints to milliliters.

SOLUTIONS

Solutions are used constantly in nursing. They are used as disinfectants and antiseptics, and are administered parenterally in large amounts, usually by the intravenous route. Smaller doses of solid or liquid drugs also may be administered parenterally in solution form.

Although the task of preparing solutions does not ordinarily fall to the nurse in modern hospitals, she should nevertheless understand the basic principles of their preparation and be able to prepare them should the occasion arise.

A solution is a clear, homogeneous liquid with no tendency to settle out upon standing. It results from dissolving one or more substances in a liquid, usually water. The parts of a solution are the *solvent* (the liquid in which the solute is dissolved) and the *solute* (the substance dissolved).

TYPES OF SOLUTIONS. The strength of a solution may be expressed as a percentage. Depending on the way the solution is prepared, the percentage strength may represent (1) weight in weight (W/W), that is, the weight of the solute compared to that of the total solution. Or (2), the percentage may be that of weight in volume (W/V), that is, the weight of the solute compared to the volume of total solution. (3) In volume in volume solution (V/V) the volume of solute is compared to the volume of total solution.

The strength of a solution also is frequently expressed as a ratio. A 1:250 solution contains one part of solute to 250 parts of total solution.

PREPARING SOLUTIONS

Solutions can be made from pure drugs, tablets or stock solutions. *Pure drugs* are solid or liquid substances in unadulterated form. Sodium chloride, sodium bicarbonate and boric acid are among such substances often used in making solutions. Alcohol is a liquid substance also classed as a pure drug, and synthetic and natural antibiotics such as penicillin, which are marketed in vials for injection purposes, also fall into this category. *Tablets* are preparations of pure drugs containing a specific quantity of drug per tablet. *Stock solutions* are relatively strong solutions containing a specified amount of drugs in solution, and are usually diluted as needed in particular instances.

SOLUTIONS EXPRESSED IN PERCENTAGE STRENGTH. Solutions expressed in percentage strength may be most easily compounded using metric units. Because 1 cc. of water (the most commonly used solvent) weighs 1 Gm., for all practical purposes Gm. and cc. may be used interchangeably when calculating solution strengths. Therefore a percentage (weight-volume) solution may be prepared by dissolving the required number of grams of drug in enough water to make 100 cc. of solution. Thus a 10% solution would contain 10 Gm. of drug (solute) in 100 cc. (ml.) of solution.

EXAMPLES:

(a) Prepare 250 cc. of a 4% solution of boric acid.

(A 4% solution is equivalent to 4 Gm. boric acid in 100 cc. water.) Therefore, in terms of proportion:

4 Gm. : x :: 100 cc. : 250 cc.

$$\frac{4 \text{ Gm.}}{\text{x Gm.}} = \frac{100 \text{ cc.}}{250 \text{ cc.}}$$

$$100 \text{ x} = 1000$$

$$\text{x} = \frac{1000}{100} \text{ or } 10 \text{ Gm.}$$

The solution needed will contain 10 Gm. boric acid in 250 cc. water.

(b) If 153 Gm. of sucrose is dissolved in enough water to make an 85% solution, how many cc. of syrup is made?

$$\frac{85 \text{ Gm.}}{153 \text{ Gm.}} = \frac{100 \text{ cc.}}{\text{x}}$$

$$85 \text{ x} = 15300$$

$$\text{x} = \frac{15300}{85} = 180 \text{ cc.}$$

EXERCISES

1. How many grams of Neo-Silvol is required to make 50 ml. of a 5% solution?
2. How many ounces of a chemical are required to prepare 8.5 liters of a 10% solution?
3. How much salt must be added to one liter of solution to make normal saline solution? (Normal saline solution is 0.9% sodium chloride solution.)
4. How many grains of mercuric chloride are needed to prepare 1 quart of a 0.25% solution?
5. How many ml. of 4% boric acid solution can be prepared from 1 ounce of boric acid?
6. What is the per cent of active ingredient in a solution that contains 25 ml. of drug in 200 ml. of solution?
7. What per cent solution would be prepared if 4 drams of drug are added to 100 cc. solution?
8. How many fluid drams of Lysol are contained in 1000 cc. of a 9% solution?
9. How much drug is needed to make 3 gallons of 5% solution?
10. How much sodium chloride is needed to prepare 150 ml. of a 16% solution?

RATIO SOLUTIONS. When the strength of a solution is expressed in terms of a ratio, again the terms may be expressed in grams and cubic centimeters. That is, a 1:500 solution may be thought of as containing 1 Gm. of drug in 500 cc. of water.

EXAMPLE:

How much mercuric chloride is required to prepare 1 liter of a 1:2000 solution?

1 Gm. : x : : 2000 cc. : 1000 cc.

$$\frac{1 \text{ Gm.}}{x} = \frac{2000 \text{ cc.}}{1000 \text{ cc.}}$$

$$2000\,x = 1000$$
$$x = \frac{1000}{2000} \text{ or } 0.5 \text{ Gm.}$$

EXERCISES

1. How much drug is contained in 100 cc. of a 1:1000 solution?
2. What weight (in grains) is needed to prepare 500 cc. of a 1:250 solution?
3. How many grams of drug would be needed for problem No. 2?
4. Express the following in terms of percentage solutions:
   (a) 3:1000   (b) 6:100   (c) 2:350
5. How much sodium chloride is needed to make 1 liter of a 9:1000 solution?
6. How much acetone is needed to make a gallon of a 1:150 solution?
7. How much 1:1000 solution could be made from 55 Gm. of drug?
8. How much drug would be contained in a quart of 1:1000 solution?
9. How many grams of a 1:100 mixture of sugar in sand can be made from 1 ounce of sugar?

10. Express a 7.5% solution in terms of a ratio.

DILUTIONS FROM STRONG SOLUTIONS. To prepare a dilute solution from a strong stock solution, a simple and rapid method for determining the aliquot parts is the alligation method.

Procedure

1. Express solution strengths in percentages.
2. In the left column place the per cent strength of the strong stock solution at the top; at the bottom place the per cent strength of the diluent (e.g., water = 0%).
3. In the center column place the per cent strength of the desired solution.
4. Diagonally subtract the smaller from the larger number in *each case* and place the difference at the end of the diagonal line.
5. The differences now indicate the number of parts of each strength of solution that must be used to prepare the desired quantity in the desired strength.
6. Directly convert the parts to ounces, cc., quarts, gallons and so forth, to obtain the desired amount of solution.

EXAMPLES:

(a) Prepare 500 cc. of a 2% solution from a 10% solution.

```
10%        2    2 parts (cc.) of 10% (× 50) = 100 cc. of 10% solution
      2%
0%         8    8 parts (cc.) of water   (× 50) = 400 cc. water
               ─────────────────        ──────────────────────────
               10 parts (cc.) total      (× 50) = 500 cc. desired total
```

The basic "formula" for the solution is 2 parts of the 10% solution to 8 parts of water, giving 10 parts of total solution. Since 500 cc. of solution is needed, the parts may be considered as cc. and the formula enlarged 50 times to give 500 cc. of solution.

(b) How much 1:20 solution is needed to prepare 1 liter of a 2% solution?

Change 1:20 to per cent $\frac{1}{20} = 0.05 = 5\%$ solution.

```
5%         2    2 parts (cc.) of 5%    (× 200) = 400 cc. of 5% solution
      2%
0%         3    3 parts (cc.) of water (× 200) = 600 cc. of water
               ───────────────────     ──────────────────────────────
               5 parts (cc.) total      (× 200) = 1000 cc. of desired total
```

(c) How much 1:5000 solution may be made from 1 ounce of 1:100 solution?

Change to per cents 1:5000 = 0.02%

1:100 = 1%

| 1% | | 0.02 | 0.02 part (equiv. to) 2 parts | (× 15) = | 30 cc. of 1% solution |

0.02%

0%   0.98   0.98 part (equiv. to)   98 parts   (× 15) = 1470 cc. water

1.00 part (equiv. to) 100 parts   (× 15) = 1500 cc. desired total

This problem differs from the others in that the volume of the strong stock solution is the known quantity instead of the desired total volume. Since 1 ounce = 30 cc., this volume is placed in the formula and the number of times the other quantities must be enlarged is determined.

EXERCISES

1. How much 1:50 solution can be made from 200 cc. of a 25% solution?
2. How much water must be added to 150 ml. of a 1:20 solution to make a 1% solution?
3. How much 1:200 solution is needed to make 1 pint of a 1:500 solution?
4. How much 7% iodine solution is needed to make 1 quart of a 2% solution?
5. How much 10% mercurochrome solution is required to make 4 ounces of a 2% solution?
6. How much 10% silver nitrate solution is needed to prepare one gallon of a 1:1000 solution?
7. How much 50% magnesium sulfate solution must be used to make 8 ounces of a 10% solution?
8. How much 1:10 Lysol solution must be used to make 1 quart of a 1:1000 solution?
9. How much 12.5% Zephiran solution is needed to make 1 gallon of 1:1000 solution?
10. How much 95% alcohol solution is needed to make 1 quart of 70% solution?

DOSAGES

ORAL DOSAGE FROM STOCK SOLUTIONS.   Stock solutions of drugs either are prepared commercially or may be compounded in the pharmacy. In either case they contain a specified amount of drug as stated on the label. The proportion method is used to calculate the amount of the stock solution that is required to give the desired dose.

EXAMPLE:

(a) How much of a sodium bromide solution labeled 0.5 gram/5 cc. is required to administer 15 grains of the drug?

$$15 \text{ grains} = 1 \text{ gram}$$

$$\frac{0.5 \text{ Gm.}}{1 \text{ Gm.}} = \frac{5 \text{ cc.}}{x}$$

$$0.5 \, x = 5$$

$$x = \frac{5}{0.5} \text{ or } 10 \text{ cc.}$$

(b) How much of a 15% solution is required to give 100 mg. of drug?

1000 mg. = 1 Gm., thus 100 mg. = 0.1 Gm.

$$\frac{15 \text{ Gm.}}{0.1 \text{ Gm.}} = \frac{100 \text{ cc.}}{x}$$

$$15 \, x = 10$$

$$x = \frac{10}{15} \text{ or } 0.67 \text{ cc.}$$

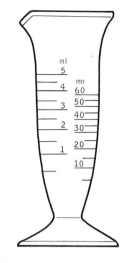

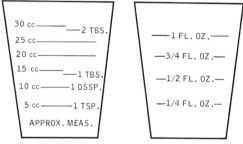

FIGURE 21. Conical graduate and medicine glass.

Since 0.67 cc. is too small a volume to measure accurately for oral administration, a small amount of the stock solution may be first diluted to 1/10 its strength (i.e. by adding 9 cc. of water to 1 cc. of stock solution) and 6.7 cc. (0.67 × 10) administered orally as the dose.

PARENTERAL DOSAGE FROM AMPULES OR VIALS. Drugs intended for parenteral use often are commercially prepared in the form of ampules or vials, and may be in liquid or powder form. It is often necessary to give doses smaller than the total dose contained in the ampule or vial, particularly in the case of antibiotics such as penicillin. The proportion method again is used to perform these calculations.

EXAMPLES:

(a) How many cc. should be withdrawn to obtain 250,000 units of penicillin from a vial labeled 600,000 units/cc.?

$$\frac{600,000 \text{ units}}{250,000 \text{ units}} = \frac{1 \text{ cc.}}{x}$$

$$600,000 \ x = 250,000$$

$$x = \frac{250,000}{600,000} \text{ or } 0.42 \text{ cc.}$$

As above, since 0.42 cc. is too small an amount to be measured accurately, dilution may be performed in the syringe using a small quantity of the original solution in order to obtain a slightly larger dose for administration. E.g., 1 cc. of the original solution may be mixed with 3 cc. of water, yielding 4 times the original volume. The amount given to the patient then would be 1.68 (0.42 × 4) cc.

(b) From a dry powder form of penicillin, which is supplied in vials containing 5 million units each, prepare a solution containing 500,000 units/cc.

$$\frac{500,000 \text{ units}}{5,000,000 \text{ units}} = \frac{1 \text{ cc.}}{x \text{ cc.}}$$

$$500,000 \ x = 5,000,000$$

$$x = \frac{5,000,000}{500,000} \text{ or } 10 \text{ cc.}$$

Thus, considering the powder volume, enough water must be added to the vial to produce a total volume of 10 cc.

EXERCISES

1. How much of a 200 gr./fluid dram stock solution is required to give a 300 gr. dose?

2. From a solution of penicillin containing 300,00 units/cc. how much is required to give a 150,000 unit dose?

3. From a streptomycin solution containing 1 gram/2.5 cc. prepare a 0.25 Gm. dose.

4. What volume of solution must be prepared in a vial containing 1 Gm. of drug in order to have a concentration 0.2 gram/cc.?

5. How much phenobarbital solution labeled 10 gr./dram is needed to give 0.5 Gm. of drug?

6. How much of a 10% solution is needed to give 1 gram of drug?

7. How much of a 20% solution is needed to give 15 grains of drug?
8. What per cent solution is prepared if 5 cc. of water is added to 200 mg. of a powdered drug? (Assume the drug does not add volume to the solution.)
9. What is the per cent strength of a solution labeled 1 mg./cc.?
10. How much solution is needed to give 10 Gm. of a drug from a solution labeled 12.5 Gm./50 cc.?

PARENTERAL DOSAGE FROM HYPODERMIC TABLETS. Drugs to be used parenterally may be prepared in the form of sterile hypodermic tablets (H.T.), which are dissolved and administered by injection. A volume of between 8 and 16 minims (0.5–1 cc.) is generally chosen as the amount of diluent for a hypodermic tablet, since the desired volume to be injected is usually within this range.

When it is necessary to give doses larger or smaller than the size of hypodermic tablets in stock, a convenient rule to follow is the Inverted Stock Rule:

$$\frac{\text{dose ordered}}{1} \times \frac{1}{\text{dose on hand (tablet size)}} \times$$

diluent per tablet = volume for patient.

EXAMPLES:

(a) Prepare a 20 mg. dose of a drug from 15 mg. H.T.
$$\frac{20}{1} \times \frac{1}{15} \times 15 \text{ minims} = 20 \text{ minims}$$

(b) Prepare a $\frac{1}{60}$ gr. dose from a $\frac{1}{40}$ gr. H.T.
$$\frac{\frac{1}{60}}{1} \times \frac{1}{\frac{1}{40}} \times 15 \text{ minims} =$$
$$\frac{1}{60} \times \frac{40}{1} \times 15 \text{ minims} = 10 \text{ minims}$$

NOTE: In example (a) the final volume is obviously larger than the amount needed to dissolve each tablet. Hence, *more than one* tablet is needed to administer the ordered dose. When more than one tablet is required, the amount of diluent chosen (15 minims) is used *for each tablet.* The dose is administered by dissolving 2 tablets in 30 minims of water for injection and administering 20 minims to the patient. The additional volume (10

minims) needed to dissolve the tablets is discarded before the drug is given to the patient.

If unusually large or small doses are ordered the amount of diluent must be adjusted accordingly to keep the administered volume within normal limits: e.g., if 5 hypodermic tablets are required for a given dose, 5 minims of diluent for each tablet may be chosen instead of the more usual 15 minims.

EXERCISES:

1. Prepare an injection of 10 mg. morphine from 15 mg. hypodermic tablets.
2. A dose of 0.5 mg. atropine is ordered. The tablets in stock contain $\frac{1}{60}$ grain.
3. Prepare $\frac{1}{300}$ gr. atropine from $\frac{1}{200}$ gr. hypodermic tablets.
4. Prepare 30 mg. phenobarbital from 1 gr. tablets.
5. Prepare $\frac{1}{6}$ gr. codeine from $\frac{1}{2}$ gr. tablets.
6. Prepare $\frac{2}{3}$ gr. Pantopon from $\frac{1}{3}$ gr. tablets.
7. Prepare $\frac{1}{120}$ gr. atropine from 1 mg. tablets.
8. The physician orders $\frac{3}{4}$ gr. codeine. On hand are $\frac{1}{2}$ gr. tablets.
9. The ordered dose of dihydromorphonone is $\frac{1}{30}$ gr.; on hand are 2 mg. tablets.
10. Prepare $\frac{1}{6}$ gr. Luminal from 1 gr. tablets.

INSULIN DOSAGE

Insulin, like many other drugs obtained from certain animal and plant sources, is standardized in units based on its potency, rather than on weight measures such as milligrams or grams. Insulin is supplied in 10 cc. vials labeled according to the number of units per cc. Thus U-40 insulin designates a strength of 40 units/cc.

The simplest and most accurate way to measure insulin is with an insulin syringe (Fig. 22). The most common type is calibrated on one side for U-40 insulin and on the other side for U-80 insulin. The prescribed number of units is merely drawn up into the syringe.

If an insulin syringe is not available, a tuberculin syringe may be used and the unit dosage may be converted to the equivalent number of minims or cc. using the proportion method.

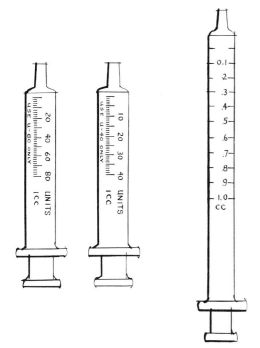

both types. What would be the dose of each in minims?

5. What would be the dose of each type of insulin in the above problem if U-80 insulin were used?

CHILDREN'S DOSAGE

Children as a general rule are not able to tolerate adult doses of drugs. There are several formulas for graduating dosage for children according to their age or weight. Two useful formulas are:

Young's Rule:

$$\frac{\text{age of child}}{\text{age of child} + 12} \times \text{average adult dose}$$
$$= \text{child's dose}$$

Clark's Rule:

$$\frac{\text{weight of child}}{150 \text{ lb.}} \times \text{average adult dose}$$
$$= \text{child's dose}$$

Fried's Rule:

$$\frac{\text{age in months}}{150 \text{ months}} \times \text{average adult dose}$$
$$= \text{child's dose}$$

EXAMPLE:

(a) Calculate the dose of phenobarbital (adult dose = 30 mg.) for a 30 lb. infant.

$$\frac{30 \text{ lb.}}{150 \text{ lb.}} \times 30 \text{ mg.} = 6 \text{ mg.}$$

(b) Calculate the dose of tetracycline (adult dose = 250 mg.) for a 2 year old child.

$$\frac{2}{2 + 12} \times 250 \text{ mg.} = 35.9 \text{ or } 36 \text{ mg.}$$

(c) Calculate the dose of morphine for a 10 month old child (adult dose = 15 mg.).

$$\frac{10}{150} \times 15 = 1 \text{ mg.}$$

EXERCISES

1. Cheracol contains $\frac{1}{6}$ gr. of codeine in each teaspoonful (5 ml.). If the usual adult dose of codeine is $\frac{1}{4}$ gr., what volume of Cheracol should be given to a 4 year old child?

2. The average adult dose of paregoric is 80 minims. What is the dose for a 30 pound child?

FIGURE 22. Insulin syringes. (Sutton, A. L.: *Bedside Nursing Techniques in Medicine and Surgery.* Ed. 2. W. B. Saunders Co., Philadelphia, 1969.)

EXAMPLE:

What would be the dose in minims for an order of 30 units of insulin using U-40 regular insulin?

$$16 \text{ minims} = 1 \text{ cc.}$$
$$\frac{40 \text{ units}}{30 \text{ units}} = \frac{16 \text{ minims}}{x}$$
$$40 x = 480$$
$$x = \frac{480}{40} \text{ or } 12 \text{ minims}$$

EXERCISES

1. What would be the dose in cc. if 35 units of insulin is given using (a) U-40 insulin; (b) U-80 insulin?

2. How many minims would be required in each case for the above doses?

3. What would be the dose in minims if 60 units of insulin is prescribed using U-80 insulin? What is the dose in cc.?

4. The physician orders 10 units regular insulin to be mixed with 30 units NPH insulin. On hand are U-40 strengths of

	Adult Dose	Age or Weight of Child	Child's Dose
Ipecac syrup	2 tbsp.	10 months	
Penicillin	600,000 units	60 lb.	
Aspirin	650 mg.	2 years	
Menadione	1 mg.	8 years	

3. The average adult dose of dihydromorphinone is 2 mg. What would be the dose for a 6 year old child?
4. The average adult dose of a drug is 15 mg. Calculate the dose in grains for an 8 year old child.
5. The adult dose of TAO is 250 mg. four times daily. What would be the daily dose for a 60 lb. child?
6. Antepar syrup contains 100 mg./ml. of piperazine citrate. What volume of syrup should be given to a 6 year old child if the adult dose is 1.5 grams?
7. Calculate children's doses for the above table.

THE RATE OF INTRAVENOUS INFUSIONS

The nurse may be required to use mathematical calculations in certain situations involving the flow rate of intravenous infusions. Optimally, the rate of flow in drops per minute should be specified by the physician; however, the rate often is indicated as the volume to be absorbed in a certain number of hours or minutes.

The equipment used for intravenous infusions is available with various bores which provide drops of a certain size. Therefore, the usual apothecary to metric system conversion equivalent of 15 minims = 1 cc. should *not* be used unless the equipment being used is calibrated in this equivalent. Certain types of intravenous equipment deliver drops of such a size that 10 drops = 1 cc. Other equipment or attachments to the intravenous infusion sets provide much smaller drops, so that one cubic centimeter may contain 60 or 100 drops. It is essential that the nurse know the calibration of the intravenous equipment being used on a particular patient.

One type of calculation involves determining the rate of flow in drops per minute according to the number of cc.'s the patient is to receive in a certain amount of time.

EXAMPLE:

(a) If 1200 cc.'s of intravenous fluid is ordered to be absorbed in 10 hours, and the equipment is calibrated so that 15 drops = 1 cc., what should be the rate of flow in drops per minute?
1. Determine the number of cc.'s per hour:
   1200 cc. : 10 hrs. : : x cc. : 1 hr.
   $$10 x = 1200$$
   $$x = 120 \text{ cc./hr.}$$
2. Convert the cc./hr. to cc./minute:
   120 cc. : 60 minutes : : x cc. : 1 minute
   $$60 x = 120$$
   $$x = 2 \text{ cc./minute}$$
3. Convert cc.'s to drops:
   1 cc. : 15 drops : : 2 cc. : x drops
   $$x = 30 \text{ drops}$$
4. Answer: 30 drops per minute
Alternate Method of Calculation:
(See below)

$$\frac{\text{total cc.'s}}{\text{time in minutes}} = \text{cc./minute} \times \text{set calibration} = \text{drops/minute}$$

$$\frac{1200 \text{ cc.}}{600 \text{ minutes}} = 2 \text{ cc./minute} \times 15 = 30 \text{ drops per minute}$$

Another application of these calculations involves determining the estimated length of time it will take for an infusion to be absorbed if it is flowing at a predetermined rate. This involves calculations in the reverse order from that used in the previous types of problems.

EXAMPLE:

(b) How long will it take for 1000 cc.'s of I.V. fluid to be absorbed if it is flowing at 30 drops per minute, and the set is calibrated so that 15 drops = 1 cc.?

1. Convert drops to cc.'s to determine the number of cc.'s/minute:
   15 drops : 1 cc. : : 30 drops : x cc.
   $$15\,x = 30$$
   $$x = 2 \text{ drops per minute}$$

2. Determine how many minutes it will take for 1000 cc. to be absorbed:
   1000 cc. : $\times$ minutes : : 2 cc. : 1 minute
   $$2\,x = 1000$$
   $$x = 500 \text{ minutes}$$

3. Convert minutes to hours (if necessary):
   60 minutes : 1 hour : : 500 minutes: $\times$ hours
   $$60\,x = 500$$
   $$x = 8.33 \text{ hours or 8 hours and 20 minutes}$$

(Note that 8.33 hours is 8⅓ hours, not 8 hours and 33 minutes)

EXERCISES

1. What should the rate be in drops per minute if 500 cc. of fluid is to be absorbed in 4 hours, and the set is calibrated for 10 drops = 1 cc.?

2. If an I.V. set is calibrated for 100 drops = 1 cc. and 1000 cc. of fluid is to be absorbed in 20 hours, what should be the rate of flow in drops per minute?

3. If an I.V. infusion of 1500 cc. is to be ababsorbed in 15 hours, what should the rate of flow be if the I.V. set is calibrated so that:
   a.) 1 cc. = 15 drops
   b.) 1 cc. = 10 drops
   c.) 1 cc. = 60 drops

4. If an I.V. infusion is running at 40 drops per minute and the set is calibrated so that 10 drops = 1 cc., how long should it take for 2000 cc. to be absorbed?

5. How long will it take 1200 cc. of fluid to be absorbed if the I.V. infusion is running at 40 drops per minute and the set delivers 60 drops per ml.?

6. If an I.V. set is calibrated for 100 drops = 1 cc., how long will it take an infusion of 1000 cc. flowing at 30 drops per minute to be absorbed?

EQUIVALENT WEIGHTS AND NORMAL SOLUTIONS

To understand equivalent weights or more often millequivalents (mEq.) as they are used in medicine, it is necessary to have a fundamental knowledge of a few basic chemical definitions.

Atomic weight—The number that represents the weight of an atom of an element as compared to 16, which is arbitrarily selected to represent the weight of an atom of oxygen.

Molecular weight—The molecular weight of a compound is the sum of the weights of the atoms of which it is composed.

Equivalent weight—That weight which is equivalent in reacting power to 1 Gm. of hydrogen or 8 Gm. (one-half atom) of oxygen.

Thus the equivalent weight of HCl would equal its molecular weight since it contains one hydrogen atom. The equivalent weight of sulfuric acid or H_2SO_4 would be ½ the molecular weight since there are two hydrogen atoms.

Computing the equivalent weights of salts follows the same principle. The equivalent weight of NaCl or KCl would be equal to the molecular weight since the single sodium or potassium ion could be replaced by only one hydrogen. The equivalent weight of sodium carbonate or Na_2CO_3 would be ½ the molecular weight since the two sodium ions could be replaced by two hydrogen ions.

Millequivalent—One-thousandth of an equivalent weight, similar to the relationship between milligrams and Grams. Millequivalents are sometimes conveniently used to designate dosage in medicine.

Normal solution—A normal solution is one containing one equivalent weight of a compound per 1000 cc. solution. A 1 normal solution of sodium chloride, then, would have one molecular weight (58.5 Gm.) per 1000 cc. solution.

N.B. This must not be confused with the common application of the term "normal saline" which is commonly used in medicine to designate a solution which is isotonic with human body fluids. Normal saline contains 0.9% sodium chloride, or 9 Grams per 1000 cc.

Molar solution—A 1 molar solution is one which has one molecular weight of a compound per 1000 cc. (regardless of equivalent weights or other factors).

BIBLIOGRAPHY

Anderson, E. M.: *Workbook of Solutions and Dosage of Drugs, Including Arithmetic.* 8th Ed. St. Louis, C. V. Mosby Company, 1968.

Blume, D. E.: *Dosage and Solutions.* Philadelphia, F. A. Davis Company, 1969.

Cook, A. C. and Macaw, K. D.: *A Mathematical Guide to Dosage and Solutions.* Philadelphia, W. B. Saunders Company, 1962.

Hart, L. K.: *The Arithmetic of Dosages and Solutions: A Programmed Presentation.* 2nd Ed. St. Louis, C. V. Mosby Company, 1969.

Jessee, R. W.: *Self-teaching Tests in Arithmetic for Nurses.* 8th Ed. St. Louis, C. V. Mosby Company, 1971.

Keane, C. B., and Fletcher, S. M.: *Drugs and Solutions.* 2nd Ed. Philadelphia, W. B. Saunders Company, 1970.

Plein, J. B. and Plein, E. M.: *Fundamentals of Medications: A Test-Workbook of Dosage, Solutions, Mathematics and Introductory Pharmacology.* Philadelphia, J. B. Lippincott Company, 1967.

Sackheim, G. I. and Robins, L.: *Programmed Mathematics for Nurses.* 2nd Ed. New York, The MacMillan Co., 1969.

Saxton, D. F. and Walters, J. F.: *Programmed Instruction in Arithmetic, Dosages, and Solutions.* 2nd Ed. St. Louis, C. V. Mosby Company, 1970.

Thingstad, J. E.: *Mathematics for Pharmacy Students.* New York, John Wiley and Sons, Inc., 1964.

Chapter 5 The Action of Drugs in the Body

Important Concepts Discussed

1. *The physiologic effect of a drug is closely related to its chemical structure. Even slight chemical alterations can greatly change the therapeutic efficiency of a drug.*

2. *A drug produces a pharmacological effect when the concentration at the site of activity attains a critical level.*

3. *Drug action depends upon individual rates of absorption, distribution, detoxification and elimination. These factors may vary greatly even among "normal" adults, but the variance may be critical in the child and in the elderly individual.*

4. *Absorption of drugs from a parenteral site is a combination of diffusion and filtration.*

5. *Many drugs undergo a chemical transformation within the body before they are converted to active compounds.*

6. *The detoxification mechanism of the body in many cases involves the chemical transformation of a drug before it is eliminated. These transformation reactions may be divided into oxidations, reductions, hydrolyses and syntheses.*

7. *Many drugs used concurrently or in too rapid sequence have untoward or fatal effects.*

THE NATURE OF DRUG ACTION

The mechanism by which a given drug produces a desired pharmacologic effect, that is, its action, is basically a matter of cellular physiochemistry. The action of all drugs is at the cellular level, where the drug either acts on the cell surface, reacts within the cell membrane or combines chemically with the internal components of the cell. Although the details of drug action are not yet completely understood, it is believed that in most cases the mechanism is one of chemical combination with enzymes or other essential cellular components.

The cell component on which a drug exerts

its action is often called its *receptor,* and the locus of action is known as the *receptor site.* Receptors are believed to be specific chemical groupings such as carboxyl, amino, sulfhydryl and phosphate groups which are responsible for the activity of enzymes and also take part in cellular oxidation processes and other aspects of cellular metabolism. By chemical combination with these groupings a drug may act on the cell by interfering with its utilization of essential substances—a process known as *competitive inhibition.* The anticancer drugs referred to as antimetabolites, for example amethopterin and mercaptopurine, act by preventing the synthesis of DNA, the basic building block material of the cell.

Other drugs exert an effect on the permeability of the cell membrane, thereby altering the nature of the cellular components that pass through the membrane. And still others act on the transport systems that carry material from the cell surface to the nucleus. There is an ever-widening spectrum of ways in which individual drugs are known to act on the cell and its function, sometimes by purely physical means involving such effects as osmosis, but more often by chemical combination.

CHEMICAL STRUCTURE AND DRUG ACTIVITY

As may be inferred from the foregoing discussion, the characteristic action of a drug is intimately related to its chemical structure. The study of the relationship between chemical structure and pharmacologic action (structure-activity relationship) has led to the synthesis of many valuable agents.

Sometimes this relationship is a very broad one. For example, it has been shown in study of the local anesthetics that although certain basic structural features seemingly are associated with anesthetic activity, many variations of this basic structure can be introduced without a loss of characteristic pharmacologic properties.

On the other hand, some drugs lose their

activity completely if the slightest change is made in the configuration of the molecule. In some instances specificity of structure is of such fundamental importance that optical isomers differs in their pharmacologic action.

Although it is tempting to attribute the action of a drug to its specific chemical configuration, there are many instances of drugs of totally different chemical structures that possess similar actions.

The discovery that some drugs can affect body cells or microorganisms because they are chemically similar to cellular constituents has helped somewhat to clarify the problem of structure-activity relationship. For example, compounds possessing structural similarity to the vitamins can produce symptoms of avitaminosis by competitive inhibition. These compounds are sufficiently similar to the vitamins to replace them as components of enzymes, the only difference being that the enzyme is unable to function with this "pseudovitamin." Antivitamins of this type, e.g., the folic acid inhibitors, are currently being used as cancer drugs since tissue growth is greatly impeded by their presence.

It is not necessary for the nurse to be able to identify the specific structural groups associated with pharmacological activity; it is sufficient to know that such relationships exist and, in general, that changes in pharmacologic activity may be wrought by even slight changes in the structure.

DRUG PATHWAYS IN THE BODY

After administration, a drug is distributed by the body fluids and ultimately arrives at the site of action. There are a number of barriers that the drug must surmount before it can achieve an effective concentration at the site of activity. These are chiefly a succession of membranes such as the skin, the lining of the gastrointestinal tract, the lining of the respiratory tract, the membranes enclosing the blood and other body fluids, the membranes surrounding individual cells, and also those about the various intracellular structures.

Body membranes are of three types: (1) those, like the skin, composed of several layers of cells, (2) those composed of a single layer of cells, and (3) those of less than one cell in thickness, such as the membrane of a single cell. The mechanisms by which substances may move across a membrane fall into three general types: simple diffusion, pinocytosis (or phagocytosis) and carrier-mediated transport.

Since body membranes are composed of a combination of lipids and proteins, fat-soluble substances are able to *diffuse* across them quite readily in most instances. The driving force in this case is merely the diffusion gradient—that is, the higher concentration of the substance on one side of the membrane. Water-soluble substances are not able to diffuse as readily, but they are able to move through the pores in the membrane.

Pinocytosis and phagocytosis are processes whereby particulate material such as dye particles, zymogen granules and perhaps proteins cross the cell membranes. In *phagocytosis* the cell membrane merely closes around the particle in ameboid fashion. *Pinocytosis* is slightly different, however. When the cell is carrying on pinocytotic activity the membrane appears to have a series of spherical indentations or "bubbles." When these indentations reach a certain size the outer cell membrane merely fuses around them and the small sphere containing the ingested substance is within the cell. Reverse pinocytosis can occur also, and small spheres or "bubbles" of material can be pinched off the cell membranes.

Carrier-mediated transport is the most widely accepted mechanism for the transport of substances such as sodium, potassium, sugars and amino acids across cell membranes. This theory postulates the presence of a carrier within the membrane itself which combines with the substance to be transported, moves across the membrane, and releases the transported material on the other side of the membrane. This process involves more energy than either of the other two, and this energy is obtained from the adenosine triphosphate (ATP) stored in the cell.

ABSORPTION OF DRUGS

ABSORPTION FROM THE GASTROINTESTINAL TRACT. The absorption of drugs and other foreign substances across the lining of the gastrointestinal tract is largely explained on the basis of simple diffusion. It appears that the lipid solubility of non-ionized forms of drugs is the most important factor determining the passage of most drugs across the membrane. Other factors of importance include the surface area, the rate of passage through the intestine and the amount of blood flow through the portion of the intestine concerned.

In most instances the stomach is considered to be of limited importance in the absorption of drugs. The stomach has been found to be permeable to fat-soluble, non-ionized forms of drugs and to be relatively impermeable to the ionized forms. Weak acids such as the salicylates and barbiturates which are largely un-ionized in the acid medium of the stomach are readily absorbed. There is no appreciable absorption here of highly ionized drugs such as potassium chloride or sodium iodide, however.

Available evidence indicates that absorption from the intestine is largely like that from the stomach, with ready absorption of lipid-soluble non-ionized substances and hindered absorption of highly ionized substances.

Although it is true that most drugs and foreign organic compounds appear to cross the intestinal membranes by a process of simple diffusion, there is evidence that a drug can be absorbed by one of the specialized transport systems. These are exceptions to the rule, however, and are not of great pharmacological importance.

ABSORPTION FROM PARENTERAL SITES. The absorption of drugs from subcutaneous sites is a combination of diffusion and filtration. The capillary wall is a membrane which behaves like the cell membranes previously described. Lipid-soluble substances penetrate the membrane at rates which vary according to their solubility and seem to penetrate along the entire surface of the membrane. Water-soluble materials penetrate the membrane at rates that are inversely related to their molecular size, since they must pass through the small pores in the surface. All substances are capable of crossing the capillary membranes, however.

Some drugs are capable of modifying the rate of absorption from subcutaneous sites. For instance, epinephrine will delay absorption by causing constriction of the blood vessels in the zone of absorption, with the net result being a depression of blood flow through the area and reduced absorption.

As mentioned in the previous chapter, when large volumes of fluid are administered subcutaneously, the enzyme hyaluronidase is often given concurrently. Since the principle component of the intercellular "cement" is hyaluronic acid, this enzyme facilitates diffusion by breaking up the large hyaluronic acid molecules and thus reducing the viscosity of the intercellular fluid.

ABSORPTION THROUGH THE SKIN. Penetration of drugs through the skin may be via the epidermis, the sweat glands, the sebaceous glands or the hair follicles. The drugs seem to pass through a lipid-like barrier in all these structures.

DISTRIBUTION OF DRUGS

After absorption into the blood stream, drugs are distributed throughout the body and penetrate into various tissues. Once in the blood stream, the rate of penetration of drugs into most tissues is not a major factor limiting drug activity since an equilibrium takes place rather rapidly in most organs. Exceptions to this rule are bone and adipose tissue, which are relatively poorly supplied with blood vessels; therefore, a longer period of time is required to achieve equilibrium in these areas. The blood-brain barrier poses a further problem in drug absorption and many agents are unable to gain access to the brain even after entering the blood stream.

A drug produces a pharmacologic effect when the concentration of the agent at the tissue site attains some critical minimum level. The magnitude of the effect is determined by four factors:

1. The affinity between the drug and tissue receptors.
2. The intrinsic potential of the drug to cause an effect.
3. The state of responsiveness of the target tissue to the changes.
4. The effectiveness of cellular and systemic reflexes in resisting or modifying the changes induced by the drug.

DELAY IN ONSET OF ACTION

There are a number of possible explanations for delay in onset of action after the administration of what has been considered to be an effective dose of a drug.

One explanation may be that the drug has to undergo metabolic transformation, being converted from an inactive form to an active one. A second possibility is that the drug has been administered in a form in which it is not absorbed, or has been given by an unsuitable route.

Drugs may also be given in a form in which they will be stored in the body in various sites or bound to proteins, thus intentionally providing a slow release of the active ingredient and prolonging the therapeutic effect. To achieve this, drugs may be implanted under the skin as pellets or injected in the form of compounds with low solubility. The obvious benefit of this prolonged action is the reduction in the number of injections necessary to maintain an effective blood level of the drug. In addition, a more constant blood level of the drug is attained in this manner, which is advantageous in many types of therapy.

FACTORS MODIFYING DRUG ACTION

Many factors modify the actions of drugs and must be taken into account in the therapeutic use of medicinal agents.

1. *Dose.* Obviously the dose of a drug greatly influences its actions. The amount of a drug that causes untoward reactions in the average individual is known as the "toxic dose"; the amount that kills, the "fatal dose." The "lethal dose," as ascertained experimentally under controlled conditions, repre-

sents the amount of a drug that is fatal in a certain percentage of animals. It is usually expressed in terms of the percentage of animals killed—designated by the suffix after the abbreviation LD (lethal dose). The LD_{50}, then, would represent the lethal dose for 50% of the test animals. The figure can be applied to humans on a proportional basis based on body weight.

The LD_{50} divided by the effective therapeutic dose for 50% of the subjects (ED_{50}) gives the therapeutic index (TI).

$$TI = \frac{LD_{50}}{ED_{50}}$$

For example, if the lethal dose was 9 grams and the effective dose 1 gram, the therapeutic index would be $\frac{9}{1}$ or 9. For a drug for which the lethal dose was 6 grams but the effective dose 4 grams, the therapeutic index would be considerably lower—1.5. The higher the therapeutic index, the safer the drug.

2. *Age.* As a rule, children are more sensitive to drugs than are adults, and there are certain agents, such as central depressants, to which very young children are abnormally sensitive. Formulas for calculating the doses for children have been discussed in Chapter 4. The aged also are apparently more susceptible to certain drugs, for example endocrine compounds, opiates and general anesthetics. It is frequently desirable to modify drug dosage in older patients.

3. *Body weight.* The ratio between body weight and the amount of drug given determines the concentration that can be attained in the body. For this reason the average dose of a drug should be altered if prescribing for an abnormally light or heavy individual.

4. *Sex.* Women are more susceptible to the action of certain compounds than are men, and in some instances this increase in responsiveness is sufficient to demand reduction in dosage.

5. *Time of administration.* The time at which a drug is administered sometimes influences dosage. This is especially true for oral therapy in relation to meals. Absorption proceeds more rapidly if the stomach and upper portion of the intestinal tract are free of food, and a dose of drug which is adequate before a meal may be ineffective if given after a meal. In the case of irritating drugs, however, much larger amounts can be tolerated if food is present in the stomach.

6. *Route of administration.* Inasmuch as rate and extent of absorption differ with the route of administration, dosage must be adjusted to take this factor into account. The intravenous dose of a drug is often smaller than the subcutaneous, and this in turn is smaller than the oral dose.

7. *Rate of excretion.* Particularly when long-term medication is necessary, the rate of excretion or destruction of a drug must be taken into account when the dosage is determined. If a drug is repeatedly given and absorbed at a more rapid rate than it can be destroyed or excreted, the concentration in the body will rise and toxic symptoms may appear. This is known as *cumulative action.* Often it is desirable to maintain an even concentration of a drug in the body in order to obtain a constant level of therapeutic effect. Once this level is attained, the so-called "maintenance dose" can be determined.

8. *Drug combinations.* When drugs having the same type of action are given in combination, the average dose of each should be reduced. When the combined effect of two drugs administered at the same time is equal to the sum of their individual effects, the response is known as *summation.* If the combined action of the two is greater than that which can be anticipated from the sum of their individual actions, the result is referred to as *potentiation* or a *synergistic effect.*

9. *Tolerance.* When a drug is taken repeatedly over a long period, tolerance to its action may develop. That is, it may be necessary to increase the dose in order to obtain the desired therapeutic response. This phenomenon is particularly likely to occur with addictive drugs such as narcotics.

10. *Idiosyncrasy and hypersensitivity.* An idiosyncrasy is an abnormal or unusual response to a drug, while hypersensitivity refers to an allergic reaction to a drug. These reactions may take many different forms which range from mild skin reactions to severe

disorders which may even be fatal. For the most part these reactions cannot be predicted, so that they must be dealt with as they arise. Very often the dose of a drug must be decreased, or it must be discontinued altogether if the reactions are severe.

FATE OF DRUGS IN THE BODY

Once a drug is absorbed, the manner in which it is altered within a living organism is of great importance in determining whether the compound will exert the desired effect and have the desired duration of action, or whether it will have toxic or other undesirable effects on the body. In the past, the metabolic changes of foreign compounds in the body have been referred to as "detoxification mechanisms," but since there are many instances in which a foreign compound is converted to a more toxic substance, this term cannot be used in the strict sense to cover all the reactions of such compounds.

Some compounds are not metabolized in the body and are excreted unchanged. We may refer to these as being biochemically inert, although they are pharmacologically active.

The majority of foreign organic compounds undergo chemical changes in the body, however, resulting in the excretion, usually by the kidney, of specific metabolites. Excretion by other channels such as the expired air, and the bile, feces, saliva and skin may also occur.

The type of change that occurs in the body depends primarily upon the structure of the compound, but the other factors such as the route of administration, diet and individual idiosyncrasies also may be involved. These changes, which are sometimes referred to as "bio-transformations," can be divided into four types: oxidations, reductions, hydrolyses and syntheses. The oxidations, reductions and hydrolyses are many and varied, but in general, compounds of similiar structure are oxidized, reduced or hydrolyzed in quantitatively similar manner. The syntheses, or conjugation processes as they are often called, involve chiefly carbohydrates, amino acids, sulfur and various other substances that are modified in the body by

alkylation and acylation reactions—that is, the body manufactures a chemical side-group which is attached to the original drug molecule and which greatly affects its pharmacological action.

The detailed study of the biotransformations of the various types of drugs does not lie within the scope of this text. Suffice it to say that these reactions by and large occur through drug-metabolizing enzymes, the activity of which has been shown to be either depressed or stimulated by many circumstances.

In summary, then, it is possible to see that a number of factors are involved in the pharmacologic action of a drug. As the study of the metabolic pathways continues and our knowledge of metabolism increases, it conceivably will some day be possible to "direct" the action of a drug to an intended site by chemical alterations and to foresee and eliminate factors that interfere with optimal drug activity.

DRUG INTERACTIONS

As more and more potent drugs appear on the market, it has become increasingly evident that severe and even fatal consequences may occur as a result of drug interactions. Dangerous interactions may happen when two or more agents are used simultaneously, when insufficient time has elapsed between discontinuing one drug and instituting therapy with another or when drugs are combined with certain foods and alcohol.

Drug interactions generally fall into the following categories:

1. Additive or synergistic effects when two drugs with the same pharmacologic action are taken.

2. Inhibition of both drugs when agents with antagonistic effects are taken.

3. Interference in the absorption, distribution or excretion of one compound by another.

4. Alteration of metabolism of a drug by stimulation or depression of the microsomal enzyme system of the liver.

The following table of drug interactions is by no means complete, but it presents many of the more well known interactions.

TABLE 2 Drug Interactions

CLASSIFICATION	DRUG	COMBINED WITH	CONSEQUENCE

	Ethyl alcohol	Amitryptyline (Elavil)
		Antihistamines
		Barbiturates
		Chloral hydrate
		Chlordiazepoxide (Librium)
		Codeine
		Desipramine (Norpramin)
		Diazepam (Valium)
		Hydroxyzine (Atarax, Vistaril)
		Imipramine (Tofranil)
		MAO inhibitors
		   Phenelzine (Nardil)
		   Tranylcypromine (Parnate)
		Meprobamate (Equanil, Miltown)
		Morphine
		Nortriptyline (Aventyl)
		Phenothiazine tranquilizers
		   Chlorpromazine (Thorazine)
		   Prochlorperazine (Compazine)
		   Thioridazine (Mellaril)
			Increased central nervous system depression

		Disulfiram (Antabuse)
		Metronidazole (Flagyl)
		Nitrofurans
		   Furazolidone (Furoxone)
		   Nitrofurantoin (Furadantin)
		Quinacine (Atabrine)
		Sulfonylureas
		   Chlorpropamide (Diabinese)
		   Acetohexamide (Dymelor)
		   Tolbutamide (Orinase)
			Abdominal cramps, flushing, vomiting, malaise due to interference in detoxication of alcohol

		Insulin	Higher doses required
		Mecamylamine (Inversine) Methyldopa (Aldomet) Nitrates, nitrites Nitroglycerin	Increased hypotensive effect

Amphetamines
 	
Appetite suppresants
		Antidepressants, tricyclic
		   Amitriptyline (Elavil)
		   Desipramine (Norpramin)
		   Imipramine (Tofranil)
		   Nortriptyline (Aventyl)
		   Protriptyline (Vivactyl)
		MAO inhibitors
		   Phenelzine (Nardril)
		   Tranylcypromine (Parnate)
			Hypertensive crisis

		Methyldopa (Aldomet) Reserpine Inversine	Inhibit antihypertensive effects

Anesthetics	In general	Hypotensive agents
		   Reserpine
		   Inversine
		   Phenothiazine tranquilizers
			Potentiate hypotensive effect

		Antibiotics
		   Kanamycin
		   Neomycin
		   Streptomycin
			Respiratory depression, Neuromuscular paralysis

	Chloroform	Epinephrine Norepinephrine	Ventricular tachycardia or fibrillation
	Cyclopropane Halothane	Epinephrine Norepinephrine	Ventricular tachycardia or fibrillation

Table continued on following page.

TABLE 2 Drug Interactions—*Continued*

CLASSIFICATION	DRUG	COMBINED WITH	CONSEQUENCE
Anesthetics (*Continued*)	Ether	Tubocurarine Propanolol Tubocurarine	Potentiation of tubocurarine Myocardial depression Potentiation of tubocurarine
Antibiotics	Neomycin	Tubocurarine General anesthetics	Enhanced muscular relaxation and respiratory paralysis
	Streptomycin	Tubocurarine General anesthetics	Enhanced muscular relaxation and respiratory paralysis
	Kanamycin	Tubocurarine General anesthetics	Enhanced muscular relaxation and respiratory paralysis
	Penicillin	Antacids	Inhibits penicillin
		Chloramphenicol (Chloromycetin) Tetracycline (Achromycin)	Inhibits antibiotic activity of both
		P-aminobenzoic acid (Pabalate) Salicylates	Potentiates penicillin due to interference with excretion
	Tetracyclines	Penicillin Anticoagulants Iron compounds Milk, antacids	Inhibit activity Potentiate anticoagulation Block absorption
	Chloramphenicol	Anticoagulants	Potentiates anticoagulant

Anticholinergics	In general	Analgesics
		Narcotics
		Antihistamines
		Nitrites, nitrates
		Phenothiazine tranquilizers
		Methylphenidate (Ritalin)
		Procainamide (Pronestyl)
		Quinidine
		MAO inhibitors
		    Phenelzine (Nardil)
		    Tranylcypromine (Parnate)
		Antidepressants, tricyclic
		    Amitriptyline (Elavil)
		    Desipramine (Norpramin)
		    Imipramine (Tofranil)
		    Nortriptyline (Aventyl)
		    Protriptyline (Vivactyl)
			Potentiate anticholinergic effects

Anticoagulants	Bishydroxycoumarin
	    (Dicumarol)
	Warfarin (Coumadin)
	Phenindione
	    (Danilone)
		Anesthetics
		Antibiotics
		  tetracycline
		  chloramphenicol
		  neomycin
		Chlorpromazine (Thorazine)
		Diazepam (Valium)
		Hydroxyzine (Vistaril)
		Indomethacin (Indocine)
		Isoniazid (INH)
		Methyldopa (Aldomet)
		Phenylbutazine (Butazolidin)
		Quinine
		Quinacrine (Atabrine)
		Salicylates
		Sulfonylureas
		    Chlorpropamide (Diabinese)
		    Acetohexamide (Dymelor)
		    Tolbutamide (Orinase)
			Increased anticoagulant activity

Table continued on opposite page.

TABLE 2 Drug Interactions—*Continued*

CLASSIFICATION	DRUG	COMBINED WITH	CONSEQUENCE
Anticoagulants (*Continued*)		Antihistamines Aminocaproic acid (Amicar) Barbiturates Chloral hydrate Contraceptives, oral Ethchlorvynol (Placidyl) Glutethimide (Doriden) Griseofulvin (Grisactin)	Decreased anticoagulant activity
Anticonvulsants	In general	Phenothiazines Reserpine	Inhibit anticonvulsants
	Diphenylhydantoin (Dilantin)	Aminosalicylic acid (PAS) Chloramphenicol (Chloromycetin) Disulfiram Isoniazid Phenylbutazine (Butazolidine) Salicylates	Potentiates diphenylhydantoin
	Ethotoin (Peganone)	Phenacemide (Phenurone)	Symptoms of paranoia
Antidepressants, tricyclic	Amitriptyline (Elavil) Despramine (Norpramin) Imipramine (Tofranil) Nortriptyline (Aventyl) Protriptyline (Vivactyl)	Guanethidine (Ismelin) MAO inhibitors Amphetamines Epinephrine	Decrease antihypertensive effect Hyperpyrexia, convulsions N.B. A lapse of 14 to 21 days should occur between administration of these two classes of drugs. Hypertensive crisis Hypertensive crisis
Antidepressants, MAO inhibitors	Phenelzine (Nardil) Tranylcypromine (Parnate)	Alcohol Barbiturates Narcotics Amphetamines Levodopa Ephedrine Doxepine (Sinequan) Neosynephrine Tyramine-containing foods–i.e. cheese, wine, beer, sherry, yogurt, chicken liver, pickled herring, yeast extract, chocolate	Increased central nervous system depression Hypertensive crisis
Antihistamines	In general	Anticoagulants Alcohol Anticholinergics Hypnotics Reserpine Narcotics Tranquilizers Barbiturates	Inhibit anticoagulants Increased central nervous system depression Inhibit each other

Table continued on following page.

TABLE 2   Drug Interactions (*Continued*)

CLASSIFICATION	DRUG	COMBINED WITH	CONSEQUENCE
Antihypertensives	Guanethidine (Ismelin)	Tricyclic antidepressants Amphetamines Ephedrine	Inhibits antihypertensive effect
		Alcohol Anesthetics Reserpine Thiazide diuretics	Enhances antihypertensive effect
	Hydralazine (Apresoline)	Thiazide diuretics Epinephrine	Enhances antihypertensive effect Inhibits pressor effect of epinephrine
	Methyldopa (Aldomet)	Amphetamines Tricyclic antidepressants	Inhibits antihypertensive effect
		Triazide diuretics Alcohol	Enhances antihypertensive effect
		MAO inhibitors	Headache, hypertension
	Reserpine (Serpasil)	Anesthetics	Enhances antihypertensive effect
		Digitalis Quinidine	Cardiac arrthymias Cardiac arrest
	Inversine	Amphetamines Thiazide diuretics	Inhibits antihypertensive effect Enhances antihypertensive effect
Antineoplastics	In general	Other antineoplastics Irradiation	Mutual potentiation and increased toxicity
	Azathioprine	Allopurinol (Zyloprim)	Potentiation
	Cyclophosphamide (Cytoxan)	Corticosteroids Chloramphenicol	Mutual inhibition Increased bone marrow depression
	Mercaptopurine (Purinethol)	Allopurinol (Zyloprim)	Potentiation
	Amethopterin	P-aminobenzoic acid Salicylates Sulfonamides Barbiturates Tranquilizers Diphenylhydantoin (Dilantin)	Increased toxicity and bone marrow depression
	Thio-tepa	Chloramphenicol Sulfonamides	Increased bone marrow depression
Barbiturates	In general	Alcohol MAO inhibitors Narcotics Hypnotics Phenothiazine tranquilizers Salicylates Reserpine	Increased central nervous system depression
		Anticoagulants, oral	Diminished anticoagulant effect
		Hydrocortisone	Lessens effect of hydrocortisone
		Antihistamines	Mutual inhibition

Table continued on opposite page.

TABLE 2   Drug Interactions—*Continued*

CLASSIFICATION	DRUG	COMBINED WITH	CONSEQUENCE
Cardiac drugs	Propanolol (Inderal)	Chloroform Ether	Myocardial depression
		Digitalis	Bradycardia
		Quinidine	Potentiates cardiac depression
		Diphenylhydantoin (Dilantin)	Potentiates propanolol
		Reserpine	Increased sympathetic nervous system depression
		Insulin Oral hypoglycemics }	Increased hypoglycemia, early signs of hypoglycemia may be masked
	Quinidine	Anticoagulants	Potentiates anticoagulant
		Muscle relaxants	Potentiates muscle relaxation
		Reserpine	Cardiac arrhythmia
		Propanolol	Potentiates cardiac depression
		Diphenylhydantoin (Dilantin)	Potentiates quinidine
	Procainamide (Pronestyl)	Muscle relaxants } Magnesium	Increased neuromuscular blockade
		Anticholinergics	Increased anticholinergic effect
		Thiazide diuretics	Potentiates hypotensive effect
	Digitalis	Diuretics	Hypokalemia and resultant increased digitalis effect and toxicity
		Calcium salts	Increased digitalis effect. Heart may arrest in systole
		Reserpine Guanethidine (Ismelin) } Isoproterenol	Arrhythmia, bradycardia
		Diphenylhydantoin (Dilantin) } Quinidine Procaine	Digitalis potentiation and bradycardia

Diuretics	Ethacrynic acid (Edecrine)
	Furosemide (Lasix)
		Antihypertensive agents
		Digitalis
		Uricosuric agents
		  Allopurinol (Zyloprim)
		  Probenecid (Benemid)
			Increased hypotension
			Increased digitalis effects
			Inhibit uricosuric effect

	Mercurials	Urine acidifiers
		  (Ammonium chloride)
		Chloride salts
		Urine alkalinizing agents
		  (Sod. bicarbonate)
			Enhance diuresis
			Enhance diuresis
			Inhibit diuresis

	Spironolactone (Aldactone)	Antihypertensives	Enhances antihypertensive effect
	Thiazide diuretics	Antihypertensives Digitalis Norepinephrine Phenothiazines Uricosuric agents	Enhance antihypertensive effect Enhance digitalis effect Inhibit antihypertensive effect Increase antihypertensive effect Inhibit uricosurics

Hypoglycemics	Sulfonylureas
	  Tolbutamide
	   (Orinase)
	  Acetohexamide
	   (Dymelor)
	  Chlorpropamide
	   (Diabinese)
		Alcohol
		Anticoagulants
		MAO inhibitors
		Sulfonamides }
			Increase hypoglycemic effect

Table continued on following page.

TABLE 2   Drug Interactions—*Continued*

CLASSIFICATION	DRUG	COMBINED WITH	CONSEQUENCE
		Corticosteroids Diuretics Isoniazid Nicotinic acid Oral contraceptives	Inhibit hypoglycemic effect
		Barbiturates Sedatives Hypnotics	Increased central nervous system depression
	Insulin	Alcohol	
		Bishydroxycoumarin Chloramphenicol Guanethidine Oxyphenbutazone Probenecid Pyrazinamide Salicylates Sulfonamides Propanolol	Increased hypoglycemic effect
		Corticosteroids Diuretics Isoniazid Nicotinic acid Oral contraceptives	Inhibited hypoglycemic effect

Tranquilizers	In general	Central depressants
		  alcohol
		  barbiturates
		  narcotics
		  sedatives
		  hyponotics
		  antihistamines
		  anesthetics
			Potentiate sedation

	Phenothiazines	Anticholinergics	Potentiate anticholinergic
		Epinephrine	Often severe hypotensive effect
		Hypotensive agents	Potentiate hypotensive effect
		Thiazide diuretics	Hypotensive effect increase
Uricosurics	Allopurinol (Zyloprim)	Acetohexamide (Dymelor) Probenecid (Benemid)	Enhances uricosuric effect
		Ethacrynic acid Furosemide Thiazide diuretics Xanthine diuretics	Inhibits uricosuric effect
		Azathioprine (Imuran)	Increased antimetabolite effect
	Probenecid (Benemid)	Indomethacine (Indocin)	Enhances uricosuria
		Penicillin Erythromycin	Higher antibiotic levels in blood
		Salicylates Xanthine diuretics	Prevents uricosuria

QUESTIONS FOR DISCUSSION AND REVIEW

1. What factors determine the fate of a drug in the body?

2. Is it ever desirable to have a delay in onset of action of a drug? Can you think of an example?

3. Why would lipid solubility be a factor in permitting drugs to cross cell membranes?

4. Why would prolonged action be advantageous in drug therapy?

5. When is prolonged action of a drug a disadvantage?

6. Explain the difference between pinocytosis and carrier-mediated transport.

7. What is the significance of a low therapeutic index, e.g., a TI of 3?

8. Give a theory that would explain variation in action of a drug on different parts of the body even though the dose that is administered is carried equally to all organs and tissues of the body.

BIBLIOGRAPHY

Aaron, H.: Drugs, some adverse interactions. *Amer. J. Nurs., 66*:1545, 1966.

Baer, R. L. and Harber, L. C.: Photosensitivity induced by drugs. *J.A.M.A., 192*:989, 1965.

Beecher, H. K.: The powerful placebo. *J.A.M.A., 159*:1602, 1955.

Berblinger, K. W.: The influence of personalities on drug therapy. *Amer. J. Nurs., 59*:1130, 1959.

Beutler, E.: Drug-induced blood dyscrasias. III. Hemolytic anemia. *J.A.M.A., 189*:143, 1964.

Bush, M. T. and Sanders, E.: Metabolic fate of drugs: barbiturates and closely related drugs. *Ann. Rev. Pharmacol., 7*:57, 1967

Campbell, J. A. and Morrison, A. B.: Oral prolonged medication. *J.A.M.A., 181*:102, 1962.

Carlin, H. S. and Perkins, A. J.: Predicting pharmaceutical incompatibilities of parenteral medications. *Amer. J. Hosp. Pharm., 25*:270, 1968.

Crosby, W. H. and Kaufman, R. M.: Drug-induced blood dyscrasias. IV. Thrombocytopenia. *J.A.M.A., 189*:417, 1964.

DiPalma, J. R.: What to do about adverse drug reactions. *R.N., 28*:57, (October) 1965.

DiPalma, J. R.: The why and how of drug interactions. *R.N., 33*:63, (March) 1970.

Doll, R.: Recognition of unwanted drug effects. *Nurs. Times, 65*:1328, (October 16) 1969.

Donn, R.: Intravenous solution manual and incompatibility file. Its use in a community hospital. *Amer. J. Hosp. Pharm., 24*:459, 1967.

Drug Interactions, (booklet). Oradell, New Jersey, R.N. Magazine, Medical Economics, Inc., 1970.

Edward, M., Sr.: pH—an important factor in the incompatibility of additives in intravenous therapy. *Amer. J. Hosp. Pharm., 24*:440, 1967.

Erslev, A. J.: Drug-induced blood dyscrasia—Aplastic anemia. *J.A.M.A., 188*:531, 1964.

Fischer, H. K. and Olin, B.: The dynamics of placebo therapy. *Amer. J. Med. Sci., 232*:504, 1956.

Fouts, J. R.: Drug interactions: effects of drugs and chemicals on drug metabolism. *Gastroent., 46*:486, 1964.

Fowler, T. J.: Some incompatibilities of intravenous admixtures. *Amer. J. Hosp. Pharm., 24*:450–457, (August) 1967.

Gaddum, J. H., et al.: Symposium on drug antagonism. *Pharmacol. Rev., 9*:211, 1957.

Gallelli, J. F.: Stability studies of drugs used in intravenous solutions Part I. *Amer. J. Hosp. Pharm., 24*:1, 1967.

Goodman, L. S. and Gilman, A.: *Pharmacological Basis of Therapeutics.* 4th Ed. New York, Macmillan Co., 1970.

Holzel, A.: Drug toxicity in children. *The Practitioner, 194*:98, 1965.

Huguley, C. M.: Drug-induced blood dyscrasia. II. Agranulocytosis. *J.A.M.A., 188*:817, 1964.

Interactions of Drugs. *The Medical Letter, 12*:23 (Issue 309), (November 13) 1970.

Kern, R. A.: Anaphylactic drug reactions. *J.A.M.A., 179*:20, 1962.

King, T. M. and Burgard, J. K.: Drug interactions. *Amer. J. Obstet. and Gynec., 98*:128, 1967.

Lasagna, L.: Placebos. *Sci. Amer., 193*:68, 1955.

Little, W. A.: Drugs in pregnancy. *Amer. J. Nurs., 66*:1303, 1966.

Meyers, E. L.: Extemporaneous mixing of parenteral medications. *Hosp. Formulary Mgmt., 2*:32, 1967.

Parker, E. A.: Solution additive chemical incompatibility. *Amer. J. Hosp. Pharm., 24*:434, 1967.

Salicylates and increased Pro Time. *J.A.M.A., 214*:11, (December) 1970.

Shirkey, H. C.: Drug dosage for infants and children. *J.A.M.A., 193*:443, 1965.

Weiner, I. M.: Mechanisms of drug absorption and excretion. *Ann. Rev. Pharmacol., 7*:39, 1967.

Williams, T. R.: *Detoxification Mechanisms.* 2nd Ed. New York, John Wiley and Sons, Inc., 1959.

Chapter 6 Vitamins and Minerals

Important Concepts Discussed

1. *Vitamins are organic compounds that are not synthesized by the body and must be supplied in the diet.*

2. *The fallacies associated with vitamin therapy often are the result of misleading advertising which has little or no foundation in scientific fact.*

3. *Minerals, although often required only in minute amounts, play an important part in body metabolism.*

4. *The education of the patient and family concerning principles of good nutrition is an important part of the nursing role.*

VITAMINS

Diseases of the human organism caused by a deficiency of vitamins probably are as old as the human race. Among the uncovered skeletons of prehistoric man are some that show definite signs of rickets (vitamin D deficiency) and of scurvy (vitamin C deficiency). The symptoms of these diseases, of beriberi (Vitamin B_1 deficiency) and of night blindness (vitamin A deficiency) were known to early physicians and are described in various manuscripts dating from the first thousand years A. D.

The early Greek, Roman and Arabic physicians recommended internal and external therapy with the livers of goats to overcome night blindness. In the middle of the sixteenth century, citrus fruits were recommended as a cure for scurvy, a disease which had long plagued sailors on voyages without a supply of fresh fruits and vegetables.

It was not until the early part of the twentieth century, however, that animal experiments demonstrated the requirements for certain preformed organic materials in the diet. These compounds were at first believed to be amines, hence the name "vital amines," which was later shortened to "vitamins."

Vitamins are organic compounds, present in minute amounts in natural foods. They are not synthesized by the human body, but must be supplied preformed in the diet to promote normal growth, development, nutrition and maintenance of life.

As a group, vitamins are extremely unstable to heat, light, oxygen and changes in acidity. Extreme conditions in cooking and storage of foods may very well destroy the greater part of the vitamin content. Overcooking vegetables, allowing cut citrus fruits to be exposed to air for a period of time or soaking peeled vegetables may render the food almost useless as a source of vitamins.

FALLACIES CONNECTED WITH VITAMIN THERAPY

Although false advertising is becoming more and more rigidly controlled by government agencies, many implied misconceptions are still commonly found in vitamin advertisements—and consequently in the public attitude.

Contrary to popular belief, vitamins do *not* prevent colds, they do *not* arrest that tired rundown-feeling, they contribute nothing toward the cure of that enigmatic and highly questionable syndrome of "tired blood," and they are of no use whatsoever in increasing resistance to disease in well-nourished individuals.

Admittedly, a person in poor health is more susceptible to various ills than a normal, healthy person, but especially in a society such as ours, where the average person is almost always adequately nourished —if not overnourished—supplemental vitamins are a waste of time and money.

There are, of course, exceptions to this statement: conditions such as pregnancy, childhood or old age may require an additional dietary supplement if eating habits are not adequate to meet daily nutritional needs. Fad diets often may lead to serious nutritional deficiencies. Drug addicts and alcoholics often develop deficiencies since appetite may be depressed by the drugs. There may be other factors involved also. Who will deny psychotherapeutic effect on an aged or even not-so-aged patient who finds in his teaspoonful of liquid or bright red capsule the added lift to begin another day? The psychologic effect of medication is not to be taken lightly, and vitamins, because they are nontoxic with a few exceptions, are frequent ingredients of placebo medications of this sort.

There is, however, a pharmacological basis for vitamin therapy under certain circumstances, and our study will consider the vitamins from that standpoint.

THE STANDARDIZATION OF VITAMIN POTENCY

As mentioned, early studies of vitamins utilized experimental animals, and the measurement of their activity was based on their ability to prevent or cure specific diseases in such animals. This *bioassay* method resulted in the measurements of

vitamin activity being expressed in terms of units. Standard units of all vitamins were determined under the auspices of the *U.S. Pharmacopeia* and the World Health Organization. More recently, however, it has been felt that the expression of vitamin potency in terms of milligrams is more accurate than the use of units, and at present the potencies of all vitamins except A and D are expressed in milligrams.

DAILY REQUIREMENTS OF VITAMINS

The minimum daily requirements (MDR) of normal persons for each vitamin now are generally agreed upon by most nutritional experts, except in the case of a few vitamins to be noted later. The Food and Nutrition Board of the National Research Council has established a set of Recommended Daily Dietary Allowances giving standards for the daily intake of vitamins and other essential dietary components. The minimum daily requirements cited throughout this chapter are in agreement with these standards.

NURSING IMPLICATIONS

Once it has been determined that a vitamin deficiency is present, steps should be taken to determine its cause. Although the deficiency may be from an underlying pathology, it often is based on insufficient amounts of the vitamin being ingested by the patient. This will involve assessment of the patient's eating and nutritional patterns in order to determine the reason for the dietary insufficiency. Factors, such as poor condition of the teeth or gums, absence of teeth, faulty dentures and socioeconomic problems, may be involved. It may be necessary to teach the patient the basic principles of good nutrition and the preparation of foods to insure the retention of vitamins and other nutrients. Patients may also need to be taught economical methods of purchasing and preparing food, and the importance of reading and assessing food labels for nutritional value.

In some instances, much of this assessment and teaching may be done by the nutritionist or dietician; however, the nurse must be knowledgeable in these areas in order to reinforce and assess the effects of the teaching.

If a patient is placed on vitamin drug therapy, the patient and the nurse should not overlook the necessity of insuring an adequate dietary intake, unless the patient's condition makes this impossible, as when the patient is being maintained by intravenous infusions. Nursing observations should be directed toward the effectiveness of the vitamin drug therapy in preventing vitamin deficiency, as well as any signs of toxicity that may occur.

The nurse should utilize opportunities for teaching the principles of good nutrition in order to prevent the occurrence of a vitamin deficiency. Opportunities often arise in the hospital setting when the nurse observes or assists the patient in menu selection. Other opportunities arise when providing anticipatory guidance to parents, when dealing with children's food fads.

The general public should be aware of the dangers of the overuse of vitamins, and the necessity of seeking medical help rather than self-medication with vitamins and other drugs which might delay diagnosis and early treatment of serious diseases.

Fat-Soluble Vitamins

Vitamin A, U.S.P.

Vitamin A is a fat-soluble, unsaturated alcohol which is unstable and readily destroyed by oxidation when heated in the presence of air. It occurs in esterified form in blood and in storage depots in the body, especially the liver, and is quite resistant to destruction under these conditions.

Several highly colored substances, called carotenes, which occur in nature, are precursors of vitamin A. The chemical structures of about thirty of these carotenes are known; however only four have vitamin A activity: alpha, beta and gamma carotenes and cryptoxanthin. Familiar carotenoid pigments are the red coloring matter of tomatoes, the red pigment of lobsters, the yellow of buttercups and dandelions, the red of paprika and pimiento and the yellow of the corpus luteum.

The biologic function of vitamin A is apparently very complex and it seems to be a factor necessary for the physiologic integrity of many organs. In general, however, it may be considered chiefly as a regulator of the growth and activity of epithelial tissues. Since the liver can store enough vitamin A to meet bodily requirements for as long as a year, the rate of development of deficiency symptoms is slow.

Vitamin A deficiency. Skin changes are induced in the deficiency state. Keratinization occurs along with dryness and roughness followed by hyperkeratosis of the hair follicles. There is often a generalized increase in skin pigmentation. These changes are usually seen first on the lateral aspects of the thighs, followed by eruptions on virtually all of the body surface.

In the eye various changes occur. Vitamin A is known to be necessary for formation of one of the major retinal pigments, and one of the earliest symptoms of vitamin A deficiency is night blindness, or a diminished efficiency in adapting to a changed intensity of light. Later stages of deficiency are accompanied by a severe eye disease known as xerophthalmia in which the eyeball dries and atrophies. If the condition progresses it leads to permanent blindness.

Toxicity. In recent years attention has been drawn to the fact that a surplus of vitamin A can cause definite toxic symptoms. Since it is stored in the liver, continued doses above the daily requirement can after a period of time mount to toxic proportions. Overdosage with vitamin A has been reported to produce a hemorrhagic state suggestive of scurvy, skin changes that resemble those of vitamin A deficiency, and suppression of the menses, along with rarefaction of the bones and cranial hyperostosis (hypertrophy of the bone) in infants.

If given with or after meals, the occurrence of flatulence or eructation may be reduced.

sources. Fish liver oils, milk, eggs, butter, leafy green and yellow vegetables, liver.

MINIMUM DAILY REQUIREMENT (MDR.) 5000 units.

COMMERCIAL PREPARATIONS. Aquasol A, Stabil-A (see also under vitamin D).

AVERAGE THERAPEUTIC DOSE. 15,000 to 25,000 units orally daily.

VITAMIN D

At present there are about ten distinct chemical compounds that are known to possess vitamin D activity. The greater number of these are of theoretical interest only, but a few are of practical importance because of their application to the relief of vitamin D deficiency in man.

Each of these compounds has a corresponding inactive precursor on which potency is conferred by chemical or physical means. Thus, ergosterol, when activated by ultraviolet light, either in the animal body or outside, is converted into calciferol (also known as viosterol or vitamin D_2). In a similar manner 7-dehydrocholesterol, a normal constituent of the natural oils of the skin, is activated by exposure to ultraviolet radiation with the production of a substance of antirachitic potency called vitamin D_3.

EFFECTS, DEFICIENCY STATES AND THERAPEUTIC USES. Vitamin D regulates the metabolism of calcium and phosphorus in the body, maintaining concentrations of these elements in the blood that will permit deposition of calcium salts, and thus it affects the proper formation of bones and teeth. Because of this relationship, it would be natural to expect that the need for this vitamin is

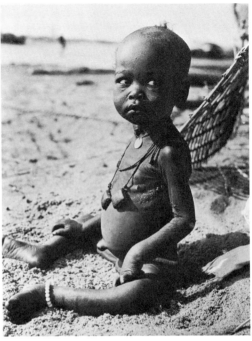

FIGURE 23.   Rickets in a child in French Sudan. (Courtesy World Health Organization; photo by Dr. Holstein.)

highest at that period of life when the formation of bone from the calcium and phosphorus of food is in its most active stage. This period naturally occurs during infancy and early childhood, and it is at this time that the characteristic vitamin D deficiency condition, *rickets,* develops. The disease may occur at any time in the growing period, but most cases develop before two years of age.

Although far less common than the infantile form, an adult deficiency state does exist. Known as *osteomalacia,* it is

carotene   vitamin A

marked by an increasing softening of the bones so that they become flexible and twisted leading to deformities. If treated in the early stages, it is readily amenable to vitamin therapy.

Because of the capacity of humans to provide their own antirachitic factor through ultraviolet irradiation, a serious grade of vitamin D deficiency usually develops only in individuals who not only need moderately large amounts of the vitamin, but in addition have practically no exposure to daylight except that filtered through window glass. Pregnancy will often bring on a vitamin D deficiency if supplemental vitamins are not administered.

The capacity of vitamin D to raise the blood calcium level has caused its preparations to come into wide use in the treatment of hypoparathyroidism, a condition in which the blood calcium is low. However, a closely related sterol, dihydrotachysterol or A.T.10, which has a marked blood calcium–raising action with little or no antirachitic activity, has come to be a drug of choice for this condition.

TOXICITY. In toxic amounts vitamin D frees calcium and phosphorus from the bones and redeposits it in soft tissues, principally in the walls of the blood vessels, but also in the kidney tubules, bronchi and heart. Vitamin D toxicity has even been fatal on occasion. Preliminary symptoms of toxicity include anorexia, thirst, urinary urgency, vomiting and diarrhea. Serum calcium levels should be measured in order to determine dosage levels.

Preparations should be stored in a cool place and protected from light.

SOURCES.   Ultraviolet irradiation, fish liver oils, milk and milk products, eggs, liver.

MDR.   400 units.

COMMERCIAL PREPARATIONS:

Ergocalciferol, U.S.P. (Calciferol, B.P., Drisdol, Vitamin D_3) Synthetic Oleovitamin D (Viosterol in Oil) Dihydrotachysterol, U.S.P. (Hytak-

erol, A.T.10)—Dose: 0.125–1 mg. daily

Combination products:

Oleum Percomorpheum—This concentrate of percomorph and other fish oils provides 6250 units of vitamin A and 900 units of vitamin D per 5-drop dose.

Dical-D—Each tablet contains 500 mg. of dicalcium phosphate and 333 units of vitamin D.

Os-Cal—In addition to several other vitamins and minerals each tablet contains 1668 units of vitamin A and 167 units of vitamin D.

AVERAGE THERAPEUTIC DOSE.   600 to 900 units orally daily.

VITAMIN E

Although it is known as the "fertility vitamin," the exact importance of vitamin E to humans has not as yet been proved. Animal experimentation in rats has shown that, when fed a diet free of vitamin E, rats are able to initiate pregnancy in a normal fashion, but early in gestation the fetuses die and are resorbed. In the male rat, deficiency leads to an irreversible degeneration of the seminal epithelium of the testes, resulting in permanent sterility. Studies on guinea pigs and certain other animals have shown degenerative changes in the nervous system and skeletal musculature resulting in muscular dystrophy.

Our knowledge of vitamin E is very incomplete at the present time. One theory has proposed that many of the effects of the vitamin may be due at least in part to its ability to act as an antioxidant.

Although it is fat-soluble, vitamin E is poorly stored in the body and toxic symptoms have not been reported. There is some evidence that very large doses may mobilize phosphorus and produce decalcification of the bony structures of the body.

SOURCES.   Green leafy vegetables, vegetable oils, wheat germ oil.

MDR.   Unknown.

COMMERCIAL PREPARATIONS.   Tocopherex, Epsilan-M, Eprolin.

VITAMIN K

The existence of only two naturally occurring vitamins K of high activity, vitamin K_1 and K_2, has been proved with certainty. It has been shown, however, that certain synthetic chemical compounds having similar but less complex structures also show vitamin K activity and have the added advantage of water solubility.

menadione sodium bisulfite

Menadione sodium bisulfite and menadiol sodium diphosphate are the chief synthetic analogues of vitamin K that are used commercially. The natural vitamin K is fat-soluble, and the presence of bile salts in the intestinal fluid is needed to emulsify and thus reduce the size of fat particles prior to absorption. In the event of an obstruction of the bile duct, then, the natural vitamin K would not be of benefit if administered orally. The water-soluble synthetic analogues are generally the preferred form for oral administration in any case.

vitamin K_1

DEFICIENCY STATES.   Vitamin K, which is known as the antihemorrhagic vitamin, is necessary for the maintenance of normal blood coagulation by aiding in the formation of prothrombin by the liver. Deficiency states are characterized by hypoprothrombinemia, prolonged blood clotting time and hemorrhagic tendencies.

Since this vitamin is synthesized by microorganisms that are normally present in the intestinal tract of humans, a true deficiency state in an adult is quite rare. After prolonged oral therapy with broad-spectrum antibiotics the gastrointestinal flora is reduced in number and modified to the extent that a deficiency of this vitamin may possibly develop. Prolonged diarrhea, sprue, celiac disease and ulcerative colitis may also interfere with absorption of vitamin K. In these conditions parenteral administration is usually of more benefit than any type of oral vitamin K therapy.

A deficiency state does occur with relative frequency in the newborn since very young infants do not as yet have the intestinal flora to manufacture the vitamin. Vitamin K_1 oxide is the preferred treatment for prophylaxis of hemorrhagic disease of the newborn. At the time of delivery it is often injected directly into the umbilical vein (usual dose is 5 mg.). If the mother has been receiving anticoagulant therapy, larger doses may be necessary. The synthetic analogs of vitamin K were used quite extensively at one time for prophylaxis in the newborn, but the incidence of kernicterus (severe jaundice in which there are degenerative changes in certain brain centers) has been found to be higher when the water-soluble derivatives are used than when the natural vitamin K is administered.

Prothrombin deficiencies, including those produced by anticoagulant therapy, respond favorably to either synthetic or natural vitamin K therapy. Parenteral forms of vitamin K should be available as an emergency drug in the event of anticoagulant overdose. A higher dose of anticoagulant may be needed when therapy is resumed after the administration of vitamin K.

Patients with severe liver damage respond poorly to any type of vitamin K therapy because the liver is unable to synthesize prothrombin from the vitamin even when it is available in sufficient quantities.

SOURCES.   Microorganisms in the intestinal tract, green leafy vegetables, tomatoes, liver, milk, eggs, wheat bran and others.

MDR.   1 mg.

Phytonadione, U.S.P. (Phytomenadione, B.P., Vitamin K_1, Mephyton, Konakion). This form may be given orally or intravenously. Dose: 10 mg. I.V.; 5 mg. three times daily orally.

Phytonadione Colloidal Solution (Aqua-Mephyton)—Because of the smaller particle size of this injectable preparation, it may be administered subcutaneously, intramuscularly or intravenously. Dose: 1–5 mg.

Water-soluble preparations:
Menadione Sodium Bisulfite, N.F. (Menaphthone Sodium Bisulphite, B.P., Hykinone). Dose: 1–5 mg. subcutaneously, intramuscularly or intravenously.

Menadiol Sodium Diphosphate, U.S.P. (Synkayvite). Dose: 5 mg. 1–3 times daily orally, subcutaneously, intramuscularly or intravenously.

Water-Soluble Vitamins

Unlike the fat-soluble vitamins, the water-soluble vitamins are not stored in the body. Thus, what is not used is excreted daily. Toxic levels cannot be accumulated, but neither is the body able to hold a supply in reserve for future use.

Many of the water-soluble vitamins are members of the group known as the *vitamin B complex*. Originally it was thought that these were a single vitamin—vitamin B—but research has gradually shown that there are several separate factors often found together in food but having different functions.

THIAMINE HYDROCHLORIDE, U.S.P. (ANEURINE HYDROCHLORIDE, B.P., VITAMIN B_1)

Thiamine, known as the antiberiberi or antineuritic vitamin, apparently acts as a coenzyme in the intermediate steps of carbohydrate metabolism. Failure of this essential action is believed to be associated with the clinical symptoms of the deficiency states.

THIAMINE DEFICIENCY. The deficiency state as it occurs in man is called *beriberi* and is characterized by accumulation of pyruvic acid and lactic acid particularly in the blood and brain, and by impairment of the cardiovascular, nervous and gastrointestinal systems. Severe neurologic lesions can result from a thiamine deficiency.

Classic beriberi is endemic in areas where the prevalent diet consists of decorticated rice, that is, chiefly in Asia, and has been known there since earliest recorded times. The disease occurs in two forms: wet beriberi, characterized by edema and cardiovascular symptoms, and dry beriberi, characterized by peripheral neuritis, paralysis and atrophy of the muscles. Mixed cases are common.

The edema of wet beriberi begins in the legs and in severe cases may become generalized with ascites, hydrothorax and hydropericardium. The primary feature is congestive heart failure which does not respond to usual digitalis therapy.

Dry beriberi is characterized by ascending, bilateral and symmetrical polyneuritis. There is a tenderness of the muscles followed by loss of vibratory sense and anesthesia. Toe and foot drop may occur and the calf muscles may atrophy. Disturbances of the higher nervous centers, nystagmus and ophthalmoplegia are frequent. In advanced stages there is general muscular atrophy, ataxia and mental confusion.

Beriberi is uncommon in the United States, especially since the practice of enriching white flour with thiamine has come into use, but borderline cases of mild deficiency are often seen. Chronic thiamine deficiency, or subclinical beriberi, is difficult to diagnose because its symptoms are primarily subjective: fatigue, dizziness, headache, insomnia, irritability, poor memory, personality changes. There may also be slight indigestion, palpitation, shortness of breath, swelling of the ankles, sensory disturbances and neuritic pains of various sorts.

SOURCES. Yeast, germ layers and outer portions of cereal grains, beef, liver, pork, legumes, nuts, eggs.

MDR. 0.5 mg.

COMMERCIAL PREPARATIONS. Betalin S. Bewon Elixir.

AVERAGE THERAPEUTIC DOSE. 25 to 100 mg. orally three times daily.

RIBOFLAVIN, U.S.P., B.P. (VITAMIN B₂)

The exact mechanism of action of riboflavin is unknown, but it is known to be a constituent of the enzymes responsible for cellular respiration, and plays a role in both carbohydrate and protein metabolism.

RIBOFLAVIN DEFICIENCY. The most frequently reported manifestation is vascularization of the cornea. In advanced cases capillaries may invade the entire cornea and there may be ulceration and secondary infection. There are often lip lesions and cracking at the corners of the mouth. The tongue may be painful and may develop a characteristic magenta color along with a pebbly appearance. Dermatoses are frequent, beginning with seborrheic lesions about the nose, on the cheeks and chin and sometimes on the ears, hands and scrotum.

Riboflavin deficiency rarely is seen as an individual entity. The usual picture is a combination of thiamine and riboflavin deficiencies, and often deficiency of other nutritional factors as well.

SOURCES. Eggs, enriched bread and cereals, leafy green vegetables, lean meats, dried yeast and milk.

MDR. 1.5–2.5 mg.

COMMERCIAL PREPARATIONS. Riboflavin or lactoflavin tablets.

AVERAGE THERAPEUTIC DOSE. 10–15 mg. orally daily.

PYRIDOXINE HYDROCHLORIDE, U.S.P., B.P. (VITAMIN B₆)

Vitamin B₆ is a complex of three closely related chemical compounds—pyridoxine, pyridoxamine and pyridoxal. Pyridoxine hydrochloride is the form used therapeutically.

Pyridoxine functions in converting tryptophan to nicotinic acid derivatives and is important as a coenzyme in the metabolism of amino acids, and also in the utilization of essential fatty acids.

Deficiencies of this vitamin in humans have been chiefly seen in infants fed an unsupplemented liquid formula in which the pyridoxine has been destroyed by heating. Convulsions are the principal symptoms noted. Deficiencies have also been noted in patients receiving the antitubercular drug, isoniazid, since this agent interferes with the action of vitamin B₆. Supplemented doses are usually given to patients receiving isoniazid over a long period of time.

Adults fed a pyridoxine-deficient diet develop seborrheic dermatitis along with clinical signs similar to those of other vitamin B deficiencies, such as glossitis, cheilosis and polyneuritis, all of which are reversible by pyridoxine administration.

SOURCES. Wheat germ, vegetables, dried yeast, meat, whole grain cereals.

MDR. 1–2 mg. (not definitely determined yet).

COMMERCIAL PREPARATIONS. Sold as pyridoxine.

AVERAGE THERAPEUTIC DOSE. 10–25 mg. orally three times daily.

NIACIN, N.F. (NICOTINIC ACID, B.P.)

Niacin is part of the coenzyme system that is concerned with oxidation within the living cell. These coenzymes act as hydrogen transporters and are active in the metabolism of carbohydrates. The amide of niacin (niacinamide or nicotinamide) is actually the active form of the vitamin within the body and is often the form prescribed therapeutically. Niacin has been used orally as a vasodilator for many peripheral vascular diseases, although it is not used extensively for this purpose presently. However, it must be remembered that the vascular effects of flushing and pruritus accompany administration of niacin.

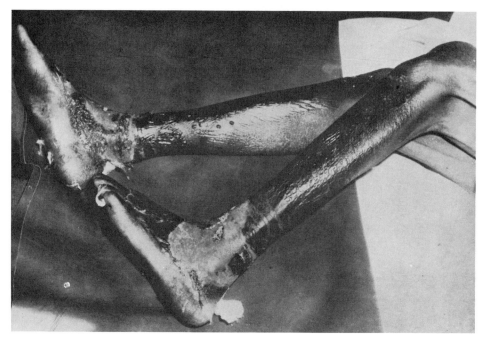

FIGURE 24. Severe case of acute pellagra. (Courtesy World Health Organization.)

NIACIN DEFICIENCY. *Pellagra* in man is primarily a nicotinamide deficiency, although a deficiency of the amino acid tryptophan, a precursor of niacin in the body, also may be involved. Early symptoms include glossitis, stomatitis, insomnia, anorexia, abdominal pain, diarrhea, forgetfulness, morbid fears and vertigo. The dermatitis that accompanies the condition is especially prominent on the exposed areas of the body—the face, neck, hands, forearms, feet, elbows, etc. The precipitating factors are sunlight, heat and friction.

> **SOURCE.** Lean meats, liver, dried yeast, enriched bread and cereals, eggs.
> **MDR.** 10–18 mg.
> **COMMERCIAL PREPARATIONS.** As niacin or nicotinamide. Combinations containing niacin are: Berocca-C, Mytinic Liquid.
>
> **AVERAGE THERAPEUTIC DOSE.** 50 mg. orally three times daily.

CYANOCOBALAMIN, U.S.P., B.P. (VITAMIN B₁₂)

Vitamin B_{12} is a very important antianemic vitamin. A deficiency in the body produces the formerly incurable blood dis-

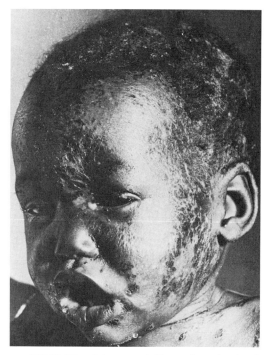

FIGURE 25. A boy, aged 13 months, who developed kwashiorkor as a result of a tea and sugar diet. (Courtesy World Health Organization; photo by Dr. R. F. A. Dean.)

order, pernicious anemia. In this condition there are drastically reduced numbers of blood cells in the peripheral blood, and progressive neurologic symptoms. If untreated, the condition is fatal. It is important for the patient to understand that continued treatment for the rest of his life will be needed if irreversible neurological damage is to be prevented.

The basic functions of vitamin B_{12} are still not clear. It is known to play a role in the synthesis of nucleic acids and thereby in red blood cell formation. It also has a part in the metabolism of nerve tissue, and in iron metabolism. Adequate amounts of vitamin B_{12} are usually present in a normal diet since it is so widely distributed in nature, and if it is lacking in the diet, there is sufficient formation of the vitamin by the normal bacterial flora of the intestinal tract to supply the normal person with this vitamin. A clinical vitamin B_{12} deficiency is seldom if ever due to a lack of the vitamin; rather it is due to an inability on the part of the individual to absorb it. Certain cells of the stomach normally produce what is known as the "intrinsic factor," which appears to be necessary for vitamin B_{12} absorption. If this intrinsic factor is missing, no amount of the vitamin taken orally will correct the deficiency state. For this reason therapeutic doses of vitamin B_{12} are almost always administered parenterally. Since preparations are red in color, careful observation is needed during injection when checking to be sure the needle is not in a blood vessel.

Certain preparations intended for oral use attempt to supply the intrinsic factor as well as the "extrinsic factor"—vitamin B_{12}. The intrinsic factor is ordinarily supplied in the form of pulverized hogs' stomachs. It is of limited value only.

SOURCE. Intestinal microorganisms, liver, kidney, milk, salt water fish, oysters, lean meat, food of animal origin in general.

MDR. Not known, because of microorganism synthesis.

COMMERCIAL PREPARATIONS. Rubramin, Redisol.

AVERAGE THERAPEUTIC DOSE. 500–1000 mcg. I.M. once daily. Patients are often maintained on a weekly dose of 1000 mcg.

FOLIC ACID, U.S.P., B.P.

Folic acid, also known as folacin and pteroylglutamic acid, is an essential factor in blood cell formation in humans, and its action is related to that of vitamin B_{12}, though the relationships are not yet clear. Folic acid functions as a coenzyme, and is concerned in the formation of nucleoproteins.

Folic acid produces a response in blood which is similar to that of vitamin B_{12}. The concentrations of hemoglobin and red cells increase to normal and the bone marrow gradually returns to its normal state. However, folic acid alone does not maintain normal blood values indefinitely and furthermore it does not arrest or reverse the neurologic manifestations of pernicious anemia, even though it corrects the blood disorder. The masking of the blood symptoms by folic acid treatment may delay the diagnosis of pernicious anemia until more extensive neurologic damage has been done. For this reason the inclusion of folic acid in the numerous proprietary vitamin preparations has been forbidden by law.

Certain other macrocytic anemias respond to folic acid when purified liver extracts and vitamin B_{12} are ineffective. Neurologic involvement rarely, if ever, occurs with these anemias. There is generally free hydrochloric acid in the gastric juice (in contrast to pernicious anemia), and gastric secretion need not be signficantly disturbed. Diarrhea, steatorrhea and impaired absorption are common, however. Glossitis is also a frequent symptom of folic acid deficiency.

The biologically active form of folic acid is actually folinic acid, also known as the citrovorum factor, which is found in crude liver extract. Folinic acid, as calcium leucovorin, U.S.P. (3 to 6 mg. a day), may be used in the treatment of megoblastic anemias and as an antidote for the toxicity of folic acid antagonists used in cancer chemotherapy. Ascorbic acid (see below) is involved with the synthesis of folinic acid, and a deficiency of ascorbic acid is thought to be responsible for some cases of megaloblastic anemia in infancy and pregnancy. In the presence of adequate ascorbic acid, folic acid and folinic acid are about equal therapeutically.

SOURCE. Leafy green vegetables, yeast, meats.

MDR. 0.2–0.4 mg.

COMMERCIAL PREPARATIONS. Folvite.

AVERAGE THERAPEUTIC DOSE. 5 mg. orally three times daily.

PANTOTHENIC ACID (CALCIUM PANTOTHENATE, U.S.P.)

Pantothenic acid, so named (from the Greek *pantos* meaning "all") because of its universal distribution in living tissues, apparently plays an important role in metabolism, but no human deficiency syndrome has been recognized and its therapeutic use is not clear. Pantothenic acid is a component of coenzyme A, which is concerned with many acetylation reactions in tissues.

Symptoms of deficiency in the chick include keratitis, dermatitis, fatty liver, lesions of the spinal cord and involution of the thymus.

SOURCE. Liver and muscle tissues, cereal, milk, eggs.

MDR. Not determined.

COMMERCIAL PREPARATIONS. Calcium pantothenate.

USUAL THERAPEUTIC DOSE. 10 mg. orally daily.

BIOTIN

Biotin, a substance essential to all cellular life, probably acts as a coenzyme in metabolic reactions. It is readily manufactured by intestinal microorganisms. Biotin deficiency may be induced only by inhibiting the growth of all intestinal bacteria or by feeding diets containing excessive amounts of raw egg white. The protein avidin, present in egg white, forms a stable compound with the biotin and prevents its absorption.

In the rat, deficiency symptoms include loss in weight, a generalized dermatitis, and progressive spastic paralysis.

SOURCE. Egg yolk and liver, many other foods.

MDR. 150–300 mcg.

COMMERCIAL PREPARATIONS. In combinations such as Berocca-C, and Super Plenamins.

USUAL THERAPEUTIC DOSE. 0.2 mg. orally daily (rarely used therapeutically).

ASCORBIC ACID, U.S.P., B.P. (CEVITAMINIC ACID, VITAMIN C)

The exact mechanism of action of ascorbic acid (vitamin C) is not clearly understood. It is thought to function as an enzyme or coenzyme in oxidation-reduction reactions in the cell. It is known to be essential for growth, and in particular for the production and maintenance of the collagen in all fibrous tissue. It is thus needed for the formation of teeth and bone. It also maintains the intercellular cement substance, thereby preserving capillary integrity, and it promotes the repair of damaged tissue and the healing of wounds.

ascorbic acid

Ascorbic acid is easily destroyed by heat, oxidation and alkalis and much of it is lost from food in cooking. Mothers should be taught not to heat orange juice, or add vitamins before heating formulas. It is stored in the body to some extent, but excess amounts ingested are excreted in the urine. It should be incorporated into the diet daily.

ASCORBIC ACID DEFICIENCY. Capillary fragility, as might be expected, is one of the principal effects of vitamin C deficiency, and the symptoms of severe deficiency are chiefly related to this effect. These include bleeding of the gums and hemorrhagic lesions about the joints or other areas subject to stress. The teeth may be loose, and there may be fatigue and pallor, resulting from anemia.

Scurvy, the clinical disease caused by severe vitamin C deficiency, is rarely seen today in its classic form. The disease is easily diagnosed, the first indications often being pain and tenderness of the extremities. The next most frequent symptom is enlargement of the costochondral junction.

Milder types of vitamin C deficiency are fairly common in those with an inadequate diet. In addition to the symptoms already mentioned, dental caries, pyorrhea and infections of the mouth are thought to be related to a deficiency of this vitamin.

SOURCES. Citrus fruits, tomatoes, cabbage, green vegetables, peppers, raw potatoes.

MDR. 70–75 mg.

COMMERCIAL PREPARATIONS. Ce-vi-sol, ascorbic acid, U.S.P.

USUAL THERAPEUTIC DOSE. 100–500 mg. orally daily.

MINERALS

CALCIUM AND PHOSPHORUS

Primary calcium and phosphorus deficiencies from inadequate intake are rare. The organism needs only to replace the small amounts of these minerals lost from the skeleton as a result of daily wear and tear. This amounts to a few hundred milligrams per day, and there is scarcely a diet that does not contain this quantity of calcium and phosphorus. However, when the calcium-phosphorus balance is upset, the normal calcification of the skeleton is disturbed. Such conditioned calcium and phosphorus deficiency can give rise to the following clinical syndromes:

1. *Rickets* and *osteomalacia* due to a vitamin D deficiency in which insufficient calcium is absorbed from the intestine.

2. *Osteoporosis,* in which calcium and phosphorus are absorbed but fail to be deposited in the skeleton. This condition is a result of decreased formation of bone matrix and is caused by any circumstances whereby the synthesis of protein is impaired, e.g., senility, semi-starvation, etc.

3. *Hyperparathyroidism,* in which calcium and phosphorus are too rapidly removed from the skeleton.

4. *Renal osteopathy,* in which acidosis causes excessive calcium and phosphorus absorption from the bones and subsequent loss in the urine.

5. *Tetany,* which may be precipitated by hypocalcemia or alkalosis or both. It is seen postoperatively when there has been excessive damage or removal of the parathyroid glands during thyroid surgery. The lowered serum calcium results in increased excitability of peripheral nerves and ganglia leading to cramps of individual muscles followed by tonic contractions of muscle groups. Gastric pain, nausea, vomiting, generalized convulsions and slowing of the heart may occur. On electrocardiogram there is a typical prolonged Q-T interval.

CALCIUM LACTATE, N.F., B.P. Calcium lactate is an excellent oral source of calcium ion for the treatment of calcium deficiency. It is seldom used intravenously. The lactate salt is less likely to irritate the gastric mucosa than calcium chloride when given orally.

DOSE. 5 Gm. orally three times daily.

CALCIUM GLUCONATE, U.S.P., B.P. Calcium gluconate is especially useful as a parenteral source of calcium in the treatment of tetany. It is less irritating than calcium chloride and may be given orally, intramuscularly or intravenously.

DOSE. Oral—4–15 Gm. daily.

I.V.—10 cc. of 10% solution.

CALCIUM CHLORIDE, U.S.P., B.P. In addition to providing an immediate source of calcium ions for treatment of tetany, calcium chloride also acts as an antispasmodic for smooth muscle and is of special value in the treatment of colic arising from lead poisoning. Calcium chloride is the specific antidote for the treatment of magnesium poisoning.

Because the calcium ion is excreted by the bowel or deposited in bone leaving the chloride ion free to combine with fixed base in the body, this salt acts as an acid-forming diuretic, although it has largely been replaced clinically by newer synthetic drugs. As a diuretic it is used for the same purposes and in the same dosage as ammonium chloride. It is irritating to the tissues, however, and its parenteral use is restricted chiefly to intravenous administration.

Intravenous administration of calcium must be given slowly to prevent too great a calcium concentration which could induce prolonged muscle contraction, with a particularly serious effect on heart muscle. Because of its irritating effects on tissues, care must be taken to avoid extravasation which could cause sloughing of subcutaneous tissue.

DOSE. Intravenous—5 to 20 ml. of a 5% solution.

CALCIUM GALACTOGLUCONATE (NEOCALGLUCON). Calcium galactogluconate is the most soluble of the nonirritating calcium salts. Since absorption of a calcium salt is in direct proportion to its solubility, this preparation is often the one of choice for oral administration. It is often given during pregnancy, lactation, and periods of growth, for the treatment of leg cramps and any other condition in which calcium supplements are indicated.

Each 5 cc. of this compound in syrup form contains the calcium equivalent of 20 grains of calcium gluconate.

DOSE. 15 cc. orally two or three times daily.

IRON

The importance of iron as a component of blood hemoglobin is generally appreciated. That it is an essential constituent of all other cells is less commonly realized, however.

The amount of iron required by the cells of the body in general is relatively small, amounting probably to not more than 0.3 Gm. in a 70 kg. adult. This iron is essential, however, for metabolism of the cell and is unavailable for blood formation; it is con-

served by the body and, like the iron of muscle hemoglobin, is probably not decreased even in states of severe iron deficiency. It is the iron contained in blood hemoglobin and in the stores of the spleen, liver and bone marrow—which may amount to 4 Gm. or more in adults—that is depleted in patients with an iron deficiency.

The development of hypochromic anemia is the most prominent and often the only distinctive manifestation of an iron deficiency. The condition is readily reversible when adequate amounts of available iron are added to the diet.

The actual needs for iron could be easily met if all of the iron in food could be absorbed. Only a portion of that ingested is utilized, however, the greater part being excreted largely unchanged in the stool. For this reason the daily iron intake must greatly exceed the actual daily requirement of the body.

The presence of iron in the stools causes them to have a tarry appearance which the patient may mistake for evidence of intestinal bleeding if he is not warned of this in advance.

Oral iron preparations are absorbed more completely if given between meals or on an empty stomach; however, gastric irritation and discomfort may necessitate administering the drug with or after meals. Many drugs are poorly absorbed if the patient is taking iron salts concurrently (see table of drug interactions in Chapter 5).

Liquid iron preparations should be well-diluted and given with a straw placed in back of the teeth in order to prevent damage to tooth enamel. Iron preparations should not be given with milk or antacids.

The importance of foods high in iron in the diet, as well as principles of good nutrition should be included when teaching the patient. He should be instructed to report the occurrence of diarrhea or constipation. Parents should understand the danger of overdosage to children if iron preparations are accidentally ingested.

SOURCES: Meat, eggs, green vegetables, legumes, fruits, cereals.

FERROUS SULFATE, U.S.P., B.P. (FEOSOL).
Ferrous sulfate is the most commonly employed hematinic preparation and is used to treat iron deficiency anemias. The drug is most commonly dispensed in tablet form, although liquid forms are available.

DOSE. 325 mg. orally three times daily.

FERROUS GLUCONATE, N.F., B.P. (FERGON).
When used orally as a hematinic agent, ferrous gluconate causes fewer side effects—especially gastric distress—than does ferrous sulfate.

DOSE. 300 mg. orally three times daily.

FERROUS FUMARATE, U.S.P. (IRCON). Although the efficacy of ferrous fumarate is comparable to that of ferrous sulfate when used to treat iron deficiency anemias the untoward gastric effects are somewhat less severe. This drug may often be employed without difficulty in patients who cannot tolerate other preparations of iron. When side effects occur, they include anorexia, nausea, vomiting, cramping and constipation or diarrhea. The effects generally subside as therapy is continued.

DOSE. 200 mg. orally three times daily.

DEXTRIFERRON, N.D. (ASTRAFER). Dextriferron is a water-soluble iron preparation in which iron is fixed to a carbohydrate compound. It differs from other parenteral iron preparations in that it is not irritating to the intima of blood vessels, and is designed for intravenous administration.

This preparation should not be used when administration of iron by the oral route is possible, and is ordinarily restricted to use in patients who are intolerant or resistant to oral iron therapy. It is occasionally used in late pregnancy when there is severe iron deficiency anemia and insufficient time to obtain an adequate response from administration of oral iron preparations.

Dextriferron should be administered intravenously by the physician, and the I.V. infusion rate should not exceed 5 cc. per two minutes.

TOXICITY. Systemic side effects such as fainting, transient elevation of temperature, nausea, vomiting, abdominal pain and diarrhea have been reported. Extreme precautions should be taken to prevent overdosage of iron by this route. Therapy should be discontinued if the expected results are not obtained following administration of the calculated dose of dextriferron. A second course of therapy is not indicated except in the case of proven massive intercurrent hemorrhage. It is contraindicated in pernicious anemias and anemia associated with chronic leukemia or bone marrow depression due to any cause. It is contraindicated in hemolytic anemias such as thalassemia, sickle-cell anemia, the anemia of pyridoxine deficiency and hemochromatosis. It should not be given when there is evidence of liver damage, and has been shown to be ineffective in the anemias of chronic infection or inflammatory conditions.

DOSE. The dose is calculated according to the severity of the anemia. Approximately 150 mg. of iron in women or 200 mg. in men are required to raise the hemoglobin level by 1 Gram per 100 cc. blood. In addition to this, approximately 1000 mg. of iron is needed for storage depots. A trial dose of 1.5 cc. (30 mg. iron) should be given before administration of the therapeutic dose to preclude untoward effects.

IRON SORBITEX, N.D. (JECTOFER). Iron sorbitex is a complex composed of iron and a sorbitol-citric acid complex. It should only be administered intramuscularly, never intravenously, and is given only in cases where oral iron preparations are not tolerated. It may be given late in pregnancy in cases of severe iron deficiency anemia and in some patients who cannot be relied upon to take oral iron preparations such as geriatric, psychiatric and occasionally obstetric patients. It is not recommended for use in pediatric patients.

It should be given deep I.M. into the upper outer quadrant of the buttock using the

Z-tract technique to help prevent irritation and brown discoloration of the skin. Temporary local discomfort may be experienced following the intramuscular injection. It is important to withdraw the plunger of the syringe slightly prior to injection to prevent the injection of the iron compound into a blood vessel.

TOXICITY. A transient alteration in taste perception has been noted in some patients which lasts 10 to 12 hours after the injection. Systemic reactions may occur, such as headache, dizziness, flushing, nausea and vomiting as well as precordial pressure sensations, generalized pain and hypotension. Hypotensive effects have also been noted when the parenteral preparation is administered concurrently with an oral iron preparation. When systemic effects occur, they generally appear within 30 to 120 minutes after the injection and subside within a few hours. Chronic administration of the preparation may produce frequency of micturition, hematuria and albuminuria, all of which subside within two to four days following cessation of therapy. It is used only in simple iron deficiency anemia and is contraindicated in all other anemias, such as thalassemia, sickle-cell anemia, pernicious anemia, bone marrow depression and the anemia of infection or chronic inflammation. It is also contraindicated in patients with a history of renal failure, a history of prior to present genitourinary infections, liver damage or hemochromatosis.

DOSE. The dose is calculated on the basis of the patient's anemia. Ordinarily 225 mg. of the preparation is required to raise the hemoglobin concentration by 1 Gram per 100 cc. blood. Precautions should be taken to avoid overdosage of iron.

IRON DEXTRAN INJECTION (IMFERON). This solution binds iron in an organic complex which provides an equivalent of 50 mg. of elemental iron per cc. solution. It is administered intramuscularly in the treatment of severe iron deficiency anemia, but only when the oral administration of iron is impossible or impractical. Patients in this category may include women in the last trimester of pregnancy, patients with gastrointestinal disease, or recovering from gastrointestinal surgery and in certain selected additional cases.

Imferon should be given deep I.M. into the upper outer quadrant of the buttock, using the Z-tract technique to help prevent irritation and brown discoloration of the skin. Pain may be experienced at the site of injection. Because of the dark color of the preparation, careful observation is needed during aspiration to be sure the needle is not in a blood vessel.

TOXICITY. A few deaths have resulted from anaphylactic reactions incurred as a result of the use of parenteral iron, thus it should be administered with caution. Without the protective natural barrier of the stomach, overdosage of iron is easy to obtain. Excessive amounts of iron may cause hemosiderosis. Fever, urticaria and headache may occur, as may staining of the skin at the injection site.

Initial test doses of 0.5 cc. are advisable prior to beginning therapy.

DOSE. 2 to 5 cc. I.M. every other day. Doses are individually calculated according to weight. Administration should be by the Z technique to minimize staining of the skin.

IRON CHOLINE CITRATE (FERROLIP, CHEL-IRON, KELEX). Because the iron is held in complex with organic compounds, the ferrous ion of these compounds is released at a slower rate and the gastric symptoms are often less severe than with ferrous sulfate.

DOSE. 330 mg. orally three times daily.

SODIUM, POTASSIUM AND CHLORIDE

All living things contain large amounts of water and varying amounts of inorganic materials including the chlorides and other salts of sodium and potassium. Although these substances are essential constituents of all tissues, water and salts are not ordinarily thought of as foodstuffs in the strict sense of the term. They undergo no essential change in the body and are excreted in the same form as that in which they are ingested.

All the complicated biochemical and biophysical reactions constantly going on in an individual, and which in essence constitute life, proceed normally only when the temperature, water and electrolyte concentrations, osmotic pressure, hydrogen ion concentration and other properties of the interstitial fluids that bathe every living cell are kept within very narrow limits. The main functions of *sodium* and *chloride* in the body are related to the regulation of body water and the control of plasma volume, the regulation of osmotic pressures of the extracellular fluids and the mechanisms associated with the buffer reactions of the body. A further discussion of fluid and electrolyte balance can be found in Chapter 19.

Potassium is the principal cation within the tissue cells and probably plays a part similar to that of sodium in the extracellular fluid. It has other functions, however, which are related to neuromuscular transmission of nerve impulses, to muscular contraction, to the processes of phosphorylation and the deposition of glycogen as well as additional functions that are not fully understood at the present time.

Potassium salts are indicated in the treatment of diabetic acidosis, potassium loss due to diarrhea or vomiting, and surgical conditions accompanied by nitrogen loss, and in increased urinary excretion of potassium such as occurs during diuretic administration.

The symptoms of hypokalemia include anorexia, malaise, decreased tone of the gastrointestinal tract resulting in gaseous distention, vomiting and silent intestinal ileus, generalized weakness and muscle tremors. Severe hypokalemia can result in paresthesias and flaccid paralysis of the extremities. The effect on cardiac function may be indicated by a weak pulse and changes in the electrocardiogram and can result in heart block or cardiac arrest. It is important, therefore, that this deficiency be detected by careful observation and periodic determination of serum potassium levels.

In addition to their use as replacement solutions, potassium salts possess weak diuretic properties, but are not routinely employed for this purpose. They should be administered only when the renal function is normal. Orally administered preparations should be given with at least one-half glass of water in order to prevent a saline cathartic effect which could cause further potassium loss.

Fresh oranges and bananas are excellent sources of potassium, and supplemental orange juice in the diet of persons on prolonged diuretic therapy is beneficial in many instances in preventing the development of hypokalemia.

Toxicity. Potassium salts should be given with caution to avoid potassium toxicity, especial care being employed if they are given intravenously. They should not be given if there is evidence of renal disease, in Addison's disease, or on the first postoperative day unless serum potassium is low.

Careful observation for hyperkalemia should be made whenever potassium is administered. If given intravenously, the rate of the infusion must be carefully monitored so that the patient receives no more than 20 mEq. per hour.

Symptoms of hyperkalemia include irritability, intestinal colic and diarrhea, oliguria progressing to anuria, lowered blood pressure, electrocardiographic changes and cardiac arrhythmias which can lead to cardiac arrest.

POTASSIUM CITRATE, N.F., B.P. Potassium citrate is used as an expectorant and as a systemic alkalizer. It also has diuretic properties but is seldom employed for this purpose.

> **DOSE.** 1–2 Gm. orally every few hours diluted with ½ glassful water.

POTASSIUM CHLORIDE, U.S.P., B.P. This is the salt most frequently employed when a potassium supplement is desired. In addition to its diuretic properties, it is also of benefit in the relief of familial periodic paralysis, a rare disease characterized by recurrent attacks of muscular weakness. On occasion it has been found useful in the relief of Meniere's disease.

The use of enteric-coated tablets reduces the gastric irritation produced when potassium chloride is administered orally. Small bowel perforations have been reported following oral potassium chloride administration.

When given intravenously, potassium chloride should be administered in isotonic balanced electrolyte injection or isotonic sodium chloride injection. It should not be given alone or in a solution containing dextrose. The rate of flow of the solution should be carefully checked so that no more than 20 mEq. per hour is absorbed.

It should be kept in mind that potassium chloride is an ingredient of certain commercial intravenous solutions such as Ringer's solution, Darrow's solution and Hartmann's solution.

> **DOSE.** 6–10 Gm. orally daily in divided doses. 1–3 Gm. I.V.

KAON ELIXIR. This palatable oral preparation of potassium gluconate is often employed for oral potassium therapy. It is especially useful when administered along with diuretics to replace potassium losses. It may be used with digitalis to reduce cardiac toxicity, and as a treatment for primary digitalis intoxication.

With this preparation, incidences of bowel ulceration have not occurred as they have with the enteric-coated potassium chloride tablets.

Kaon elixir is contraindicated—as are all potassium salts—in inadequate urinary output, in untreated Addison's disease and in hyperadrenalism due to the adrenogenital syndrome.

> **DOSE.** 15 cc. (40 mEq. potassium) orally three times daily after meals.

POTASSIUM TRIPLEX. Each 5 cc. of this preparation supplies 15 mEq. potassium in the form of 0.5 Gm. each of potassium acetate, potassium bicarbonate and potassium citrate. It is used to treat potassium deficiencies especially from long-term diuretic therapy, digitalis intoxication, low dietary intake of potassium, potassium loss due to vomiting and diarrhea, diabetic acidosis, metabolic alkalosis, corticosteroid therapy and familial periodic paralysis.

> **DOSE.** 5 cc. (15 mEq. potassium) orally three times daily.

IODINE

Iodine is an essential component of the thyroid hormone (see also Chapter 15). A deficiency of this mineral leads to an inability of the body to manufacture the hormone and to consequent hypothyroidism. Conversely, a relatively high dose of iodine will inhibit the thyroid gland. It is sometimes administered for this purpose prior to surgery in hyperthyroid individuals to make them better surgical risks.

The use of iodine as a topical anti-infective is discussed in Chapter 8.

Toxicity. Hypersensitivity is a possible adverse reaction to iodine and should be considered whenever iodine or iodides are given, especially when preparations containing iodides are given intravenously for diagnostic studies.

Iodism may occur in a patient receiving preparations containing iodine. Symptoms include brassy taste of iodine, sore gums, a burning sensation in the mouth, Coryza and swelling of the eyelids, excessive salivation and tenderness of the salivary glands and skin eruptions.

Commercial preparations for oral use:

STRONG IODINE SOLUTION, U.S.P. (LUGOL'S SOLUTION). Along with 5% iodine, this solution contains 10% potassium iodide to enhance the solubility of free iodine.

IODINE SOLUTION, N.F. This aqueous solution is composed of 2% iodine along with 2.4% sodium iodide. It is used for the same therapeutic purposes as strong iodine solution.

Trace Minerals

COPPER. The synthesis of hemoglobin in the bone marrow, the formation and maintenance of compounds having enzymatic activity, central nervous system physiology and pigment metabolism are all concerned in some way with copper. A deficiency in man is unlikely, because of the wide distribution in food and the extremely small amounts required in the daily diet.

COBALT. Although cobalt is required in extremely small amounts, its deficiency may lead to pernicious anemia since it must be incorporated into the vitamin B_{12} molecule by microorganism synthesis.

FLUORINE. The fluoride ion is recognized as a constituent of the skeletal system. Small amounts are often added to drinking water as this has been found to significantly lower the rate of dental caries in children. Increased or excessive amounts, however, will cause mottling of the dental enamel.

MANGANESE. The exact function of manganese is not known. It is a growth factor, important in maintaining normal reproductive functions, related at least indirectly to the metabolism of calcium and phosphorus, and is an activator of certain enzymes.

ZINC. A deficiency of zinc brings about disturbance of growth and alopecia. It appears that the physiologic functions served by zinc are associated with the action of enzymes.

GUIDE FOR THE ASSESSMENT OF A PATIENT RECEIVING VITAMIN SUPPLEMENTS

I.   What vitamin(s) is the patient receiving? Why? For therapeutic reasons, physical or psychologic? For a deficiency? What are the indications of the deficiency? Why does the deficiency exist? Because of a physiologic dysfunction that impedes the production and/or absorption of the vitamin? Because of a diet deficient in the vitamin? Physical inability to eat? Socioeconomic reason? Improper methods of food preparation?

II.   Is the therapy effective? Are the signs and symptoms of the deficiency diminishing? What is the patient's attitude toward the therapy?

III.   Has the patient experienced any side effects? Can these be reduced by nursing measures?

IV.   What are the patient's and family's learning needs? Nutrition and food preparation? Directions for administration and storage? Side effects to be reported?

QUESTIONS FOR DISCUSSION AND REVIEW

1.   Note the advertisements for vitamin preparations in magazines, on television, and elsewhere. On the basis of what you now know, are the claims made for these preparations always justified? Give specific examples.

2.   Give five examples in which additional vitamin therapy would be advantageous.

3.   What effect does the preparation and storage of foods containing vitamins C, B_1 and B_2 have on their vitamin content? Would it be theoretically possible for a "balanced diet" to be vitamin deficient?

4. Why are oral vitamin B_{12} preparations usually unsatisfactory in deficiency states?

5. Give the general treatment which would be indicated in:
   a. scurvy
   b. pellagra
   c. beriberi
   d. rickets
   e. night blindness
   f. hemorrhagic disorders
   g. osteoporosis

6. What are the reasons why a patient would need a parenteral form of vitamin K rather than an oral preparation?

7. What are the symptoms of hypokalemia? What are the reasons or conditions in which hypokalemia occurs?

8. What are the symptoms of hyperkalemia? What are common conditions causing it? What means can be used to reduce a high potassium level?

9. What are the nursing observations and responsibilities related to the intravenous administration of potassium chloride?

10. Outline a teaching plan for a patient whose diet is deficient in iron.

BIBLIOGRAPHY

Cooley, D. G.: What is a vitamin? *Today's Health, 41*:20, 1963.

Gordon, E. S. and Sevringhaus, E. L.: *Vitamin Therapy in General Practice.* Chicago, Year Book Publishers, Inc., 1940.

Govoni, L. E. and Hayes, J. E.: *Drugs and Nursing Implications.* 2nd Ed. New York, Appleton-Century-Crofts, 1971.

Hass, R. L.: The case of fluoridation. *Amer. J. Nurs., 66*:328, (February) 1966.

Human Nutrition. (Reprint of Part I of the Yearbook of Agriculture, 1939.) Washington, D.C., U.S. Government Printing Office, 1940.

Joliffe, N., Tisdall, F. F. and Cannon, P. (ed.): *Clinical Nutrition.* New York, Paul B. Hoeber, Inc., 1950.

Manning, M. L.: The psychodynamics of dietetics. *Nurs. Outlook, 13*:57, (April) 1965.

Morris, E.: How does a nurse teach nutrition to patients? *Amer. J. Nurs., 60*:67, (January) 1960.

Potassium Imbalance (Programmed Instruction). *Amer. J. Nurs., 67*:343, (February) 1967.

Pratt, F.: Vitamins. *Canad. J. Psychiat. Nurses, 9*:12, (November) 1968.

Prichard, J. A. and Mason, R. A.: Iron stores of normal adults and replenishment with oral iron therapy. *J.A.M.A., 190*:897, 1964.

Sherman, H. C.: *The Science of Nutrition.* New York, Columbia University Press, 1943.

Sisk, S. A.: Pernicious Anemia. *Nurs. Times, 66*:531, (April 23) 1970.

Snively, W.: Potassium salts and intestinal ulcer. *J.A.M.A., 195*:977, 1966.

Stare, F. J.: Good nutrition from food not pills. *Amer. J. Nurs., 65*:86, (February) 1965.

Vitamin Manual. Kalamazoo, Michigan, The Upjohn Company, 1965.

Westerman, R. and Snively, W.: Potassium deficit: clinical aspects. *G.P., 33*:85, (June) 1966.

Chapter 7 Antihistamines and Immunizing Agents

Important Concepts Discussed

1. *Antigens, when introduced into the body, induce formation of counteracting antibodies.*
2. *Histamine, which is liberated in the course of antigen-antibody reactions, appears to be the immediate cause of allergic symptoms.*
3. *Immunity to disease is brought about by the same mechanism that produces antibodies to allergens.*
4. *Immunity may be attained by natural or acquired, active or passive, methods.*
5. *The nurse must be constantly alert in preventing and detecting allergic responses.*
6. *The nurse has an important role in the prevention of disease by encouraging adequate immunization of the public.*

THE NATURE OF ALLERGY

Observations of phenomena that are now recognized as allergic have been recorded in clinical medical literature from the earliest years. Hippocrates must have seen certain evidence that prompted his sixty-fourth aphorism: "It is a bad thing to give milk to persons having headache." For untold generations mothers have recognized that certain infants were "poisoned" by cows' milk or eggs and that an occasional child had an attack of coryza or asthma after contact with animals.

Practically all human beings are capable of becoming sensitized to certain large-molecular substances—usually proteins—which on gaining entrance to the body induce a response against themselves. Such a substance is called an *antigen*. The production of a specific antibody that combines with the antigen is the principal feature of the body's response to an antigen (the *antigen-antibody reaction*).

The animal body does not acquire the ability to distinguish between its own and other kinds of macromolecules until around the time of birth (the precise time varies in different species and with regard to different antigens). Until this time it accepts all the macromolecules that develop normally in it or are injected into it as its own, and it remembers and recognizes them all thereafter as its own, and so does not react against them. In order for a macromolecule to act as an antigen in a given body, it must not only be foreign to that body, it must also be *recognized* as being foreign.

An allergic reaction is a specific kind of antigen-antibody reaction. The most common kinds of antigens (or *allergens*) producing an allergic reaction include plant pollens, animal dander, certain foodstuffs such as eggs and milk, and numerous drugs and other chemicals. The nature of the response may vary widely, and may involve the respiratory tract, the gastrointestinal tract, the skin or other body organs. Among the human ills now generally recognized as allergic diseases may be numbered asthma, allergic rhinitis (hay fever), urticaria (hives), angioneurotic edema, allergic dermatitis, serum sickness and anaphylactic shock.

The principal characteristics of an allergic reaction may be summarized as follows:

1. It is highly specific to a particular causative agent.

2. The reaction may be transferred passively by a blood transfusion into a normal individual.

3. There is an incubation period (varying in length).

4. The reaction occurs only after prolonged contact with, or the second introduction of, an antigen.

5. The antigen enters the body via the respiratory tract, the gastrointestinal tract, the skin or by parenteral injection.

TERMINOLOGY. Because there are many types of allergic reactions, immunologists over the years have developed their own professional language by coining words to designate the special phases and types of the allergic response:

Allergy. The term applied to a state which is qualitatively altered from normal and which occurs following an antigen-antibody reaction.

Hypersensitivity reaction. A marked physiologic response to an agent which is ordinarily not troublesome to an average individual.

Idiosyncrasy. An abnormal susceptibility to a drug resulting in symptoms not related to its usual pharmacologic action.

Anaphylaxis. A severe allergic reaction which may cause death unless emergency measures are taken. It is characterized by a drop in blood pressure and body temperature, cardiac abnormalities and leukopenia (due to a fall in the circulating blood volume).

Allergen. A substance capable of producing an allergic reaction; the term may be used interchangeably with antigen.

Serum sickness. A condition occurring in man usually following the parenteral injection of a sufficient amount of antigen. The reaction appears 8 to 10 days after the introduction of the antigen and is characterized by high fever, joint pains and swelling, enlarged glands and widespread hives.

HISTAMINE IN ALLERGIC REACTIONS. The possibility that histamine plays a part in allergic reactions was first mentioned by Dale and Laidlaw in 1910 when the similarity between the immediate symptoms of anaphylactic shock and those elicited by large doses of histamine was first noted.

Histamine is a natural constituent of many tissues, both plant and animal, and apparently exists in combination with some constituent of the cell. There have been many demonstrations that histamine can be released from cells by noxious stimuli of either a chemical or physical nature. And it has been shown that antigens cause the release of histamine from the tissues of sensitized animals. The signs and symptoms produced by the injection of an antigen and those evoked by simple chemicals that release histamine are very similar. Therefore the thesis has been developed that the intracellular reaction between antigen and antibody results in the activation of a proteolytic enzyme which releases histamine bound to intracellular protein.

It is the histamine, then, that causes the typical symptoms of an allergic response—red, watery eyes, sneezing, coryza, rash, bronchiolar constriction, etc.

DETERMINING THE SOURCE OF THE ALLERGEN. If a food allergy is suspected, the person may be requested to make a record of all food he has ingested for a period of a week or more. Foods that are suspected of causing the allergy are then removed from the diet until allergic symptoms subside. Implicated foods are then added to the diet one at a time in an attempt to determine the exact food causing the allergy. The allergy is then controlled by eliminating this food from the diet.

Sensitivity testing may also determine the

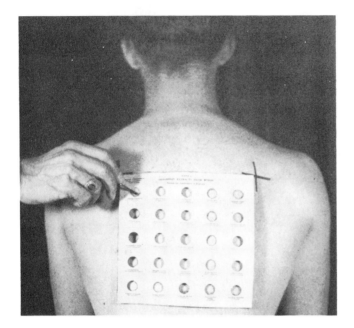

FIGURE 26. Method of conducting multiple skin sensitivity tests. (Claus, E. P.: *Pharmacognosy.* 4th ed. Lea & Febiger, Philadelphia, 1961, p. 492.)

allergen involved. This is done by placing a drop of a test extract into the eye. Tearing and redness of the conjunctiva will occur if the person is allergic to the extract used.

Test extracts may be injected intradermally at spaced intervals in the scapular region (see Figure 26) or on the forearm or lateral aspect of the upper arm. Sensitivity tests may also be done by sealing suspected allergens against the skin for several days, or by placing test extracts on the skin and then scratching the skin lightly. Positive reactions indicating that the person is allergic to the particular allergen used is based on the development of pronounced redness or the formation of a wheal. After the allergen has been isolated, attempts may be made to desensitize the person by injecting increasing amounts of the allergen at intervals over an extended period of time.

NURSING IMPLICATIONS

In administering medications and caring for patients, the nurse must be constantly alert for indications of an allergic response. Although some drugs are more likely to cause allergies, hypersensitivity reactions can occur when any drug or substance is administered. Allergic responses may de-velop even when patients have taken a drug previously with no indication of hypersensitivity. A person with a history of allergies is more prone to develop additional allergic responses to other drugs or allergens.

During admission, the patient should be questioned about any allergies he is known to have. It may be necessary to ask the patient this in other terminology since he may not know what an allergy is, but will indicate foods he "can't take" or may indicate allergic symptoms such as rashes he has experienced with a drug or food. Allergies should be reported and recorded prominently, usually on the doctor's order sheet, the front of the patient's chart and on the nursing Kardex. Patients should carry identification cards or Medic Alert tags indicating their allergies.

Nurses should be familiar with the purpose of Medic Alert, its tags and its symbols in order to teach the patients about this service, and to insure appropriate action when the tags are seen on a patient. See Chapter Two for additional information.

The nurse should observe patients for symptoms of allergic response in general. Such symptoms may include rash, urticaria, coryza, rhinitis, wheezing, gastrointestinal disturbances, severe symptoms of serum sickness or anaphylaxis. Certain drugs produce characteristic rashes when they cause an allergic response.

Serum sickness can be prevented by sensitivity tests performed before an antitoxin or other serum is given to a person. Usually antitoxins and sera are administered only by the physician because of the danger of immediate anaphylaxis.

Anaphylaxis is an acute emergency which requires immediate treatment to prevent death. The nurse should be alert for early symptoms such as redness and edema formation at the site where a drug has been injected. She should also watch for sneezing, itching and a tingling sensation in the throat. This is soon followed by edema of the face, hands and other areas of the body, wheezing respirations, cyanosis, dilated pupils, drop in blood pressure and rapid weak pulse. Death may follow within a short period of time.

Emergency drugs, particularly epinephrine, antihistamines, adrenocorticosteroids and aminophylline, should be immediately available. Oxygen and suction equipment may be needed, and a tracheostomy kit may be indicated in certain cases. If the allergic response occurs after a drug is injected into an extremity, a tourniquet can be applied above the site of injection to prevent further absorption of the drug into the systemic circulation until emergency measures have been instituted.

THE ANTIHISTAMINIC DRUGS

After the role of histamine in the allergic reaction was discovered, it was evident that an agent blocking the effect of histamine would be a useful therapeutic tool. However, in spite of efforts on the part of numerous chemists and pharmacologists, a quarter of a century elapsed before an agent was discovered which had significant histamine-blocking activity. This first agent was too weak and too toxic for clinical use, and the first clinically useful antihistaminic agent, Antergan, was not introduced until 1942. Soon afterward pyrilamine (Neo-Antergan), a more effective and less toxic agent, was introduced.

Following the successful use of these agents, a host of newer variants were developed and there are now in existence approximately 50 antihistaminic drugs. Most of these have approximately the same mechanism of action, that is, they apparently combine with the body's receptor sites for histamine and thus prevent histamine from acting with the receptors and causing a reaction.

ANTIHISTAMINES IN THERAPY. Antihistaminic drugs exert their greatest beneficial effect on nasal allergies. Seasonal hay fever is benefited more than vasomotor rhinitis. The drugs do not, however, prevent or effectively relieve asthma, which frequently complicates hay fever. The place of the antihistaminic drugs in the treatment of the symptoms of the common cold remains in question.

Urticaria, angioneurotic edema, serum sickness and drug reactions are usually relieved by administration of an antihistaminic drug, as is itching accompanying atopic dermatitis, contact dermatitis, pruritus ani and vulvae and insect bites.

The addition of certain parenteral antihistamines (e.g., chlorpheniramine maleate) to blood diminishes the incidence of unfavorable reactions due to blood transfusions and aids in the symptomatic treatment of non-hemolytic, nonpyrogenic transfusion reactions.

For reasons that are not entirely clear, certain of the antihistamines are effective in preventing or relieving the symptoms of motion sickness, and these same agents have also been used as antiemetics in postoperative vomiting and the nausea and vomiting of pregnancy.

ADMINISTRATION. Because they are rapidly absorbed from the intestinal tract, the antihistamines are usually given by mouth. The optimum effect is obtained in from 30 to 60 minutes after administration. Inactivation and excretion are fairly rapid, and the dose must be repeated every three to six hours unless a delayed-release dosage form is administered. Some antihistamines may be given intravenously or intramuscularly, but most of them cannot be so administered because of their irritating nature. Many may be used in the form of ointments or creams for topical application and have been found useful to allay itching in skin conditions. A few may be instilled into the eye. It should be noted, however, that the rate of occurrence of dermatologic complications resulting from allergic responses to antihistamines has been reported to be as high as 2 to 4%, and therefore their topical use has not been as widespread as might be expected.

TOXIC EFFECTS. The only notable side effect when antihistamines are administered orally is drowsiness, which may become hazardous if the individual is working with machinery or driving. Patients should also be cautioned about the possibility of an increased sedative effect if alcohol or other depressants are taken with antihistamines. Safety measures, such as the use of side rails and assistance in ambulating, may be needed with some patients.

SOME TYPICAL ANTIHISTAMINES

DIPHENHYDRAMINE HYDROCHLORIDE, U.S.P., B.P. (BENADRYL).

Moderate antispasmodic activity renders diphenhydramine useful in relieving bronchial spasm as well as serum reactions, urticaria, drug reactions, etc. It has also been found useful in controlling symptoms of Parkinson's disease, especially when combined with belladonna alkaloids, whose activity it potentiates.

Diphenhydramine may be used as a mild sedative or hypnotic, and is particularly useful in the elderly when barbiturates and other hypnotics are inadvisable. It may be employed as a mild sedative for children as well.

diphenhydramine hydrochloride*

---

* Note that in most cases the structural formulas do not show the salt or ester form of the drug.

DOSE. Oral—50 mg. three or four times daily. I.M.—10–50 mg. three times daily.

CHLORPHENIRAMINE MALEATE, U.S.P., B.P. (CHLOR-TRIMETON MALEATE, TELDRIN).

This compound exists also in the form of a dextro-rotatory isomer, dexchlorpheniramine maleate (Polaramine), which is approximately twice as potent as chlorpheniramine itself. Both forms are commonly used in the form of delayed-release preparations which provide antihistaminic activity for 8 to 12 hours. They are used for conditions such as hay fever, urticaria, rhinitis, and contact dermatitis.

chlorpheniramine maleate

DOSE. Chlorpheniramine—4 mg. orally three or four times daily. Dexchlorpheniramine—2 mg. orally three or four times daily.

DIMENHYDRINATE, U.S.P., B.P. (DRAMAMINE).

Originally introduced for the prevention or control of motion sickness, dimenhydrinate has subsequently found use in many conditions characterized by nausea, vertigo or vomiting and has proved to be remarkably effective. The very nature of nausea or vomiting, however, frequently prohibits oral medications; therefore, the drug is also used parenterally. It should not be mixed in the same syringe with other medications because of the likelihood of incompatibilities.

DOSE. 50 mg. orally or I.M. two to four times daily.

METHAPYRILENE HYDROCHLORIDE, N.F. (HISTADYL, THENYLENE).

In addition to the antihistaminic and local anesthetic properties of this compound, it exerts a relatively strong sedative effect in many individuals. For this reason methapyriline is a popular ingredient in several nonprescription sedative preparations (e.g., Dormin, Nytol), intended for the treatment of insomnia. It has also been used to treat the nausea and vomiting of pregnancy.

TOXICITY. The chief side effect is drowsiness; however, anorexia, vertigo and excitement may also occur. Ingestion of large doses may produce nausea, vomiting, tremors, convulsions, anuria, cyanosis, unconsciousness and cardiorespiratory depression. Topical application may cause cutaneous hypersensitivity reactions.

DOSE. 50 mg. orally four times daily.

TRIPELENNAMINE HYDROCHLORIDE, U.S.P., B.P. (PYRIBENZAMINE HYDROCHLORIDE). An antihistamine with a fairly low incidence of side effects, tripelennamine is used orally, parenterally and topically for the relief of urticaria, serum sickness, allergic rhinitis, dermatitis venenata and other pruritic dermatoses.

tripelennamine

DOSE. 50 mg. orally four times daily, then reduced.

BROMPHENIRAMINE MALEATE, N.F. (DIMETANE). Differing from chlorpheniramine only in the substitution of bromine for chlorine, brompheniramine exhibits good antihistaminic action with a low incidence of side effects. It is used for much the same purposes as chlorpheniramine.

DOSE. 4 mg. orally three to six times daily.

METHDILAZINE HYDROCHLORIDE (TACARYL). Structurally related to the tranquilizers, this agent acts in overcoming bronchoconstriction in experimental animals. It appears to

have more antipruritic activity in humans than most other drugs and thus is especially useful in treating pruritus, both allergic and nonallergic in origin.

DOSE. 8 mg. orally twice daily.

PROMETHAZINE HYDROCHLORIDE, U.S.P., B.P. (PHENERGAN HYDROCHLORIDE). Promethazine probably is the most potent of all histamine antagonists, and its action lasts two to three times as long as that of most other antihistamines. It causes a high incidence of drowsiness. It is often combined with narcotics as preoperative medication for both its sedative and secretion-drying effects, and will potentiate the effects of the narcotic agent.

Only clear parenteral solutions should be used and open vials should be refrigerated.

DOSE. Oral—25 mg. three to four times daily. I.M.—25 to 50 mg. as necessary.

COMBINATIONS OF DRUGS

Antihistamines are often used in combined form, either with other antihistamines or with drugs having other effects, for example nasal decongestants and aspirin-like drugs. Some of these combinations are listed in Tables 3 and 4, and a few are discussed in more detail below.

PYRROBUTAMINE COMPOUND (CO-PYRONIL). The compound form is used much more often than plain pyrrobutamine. Pyronil consists of:

Methapyrilene	25 mg.
Pyrrobutamine	15 mg.
Cyclopentamine HCl	12.5 mg.

Methapyrilene has a prompt onset of action but a short duration of effect, whereas pyrrobutamine requires 40 to 60 minutes for onset, but lasts for several hours. Cyclopentamine has an action similar to that of the sympathomimetic amines, enabling it to produce a local vasoconstrictor effect and a systemic pressor effect, but with only slight cerebral excitation. It makes a very effective combination for allergic disorders.

DOSE. One capsule orally every eight hours.

TABLE 3 Some Commonly Used Sympathomimetic-Antihistamine Combinations†

PRODUCT	SYMPATHOMIMETIC	ANTIHISTAMINE	OTHER INGREDIENTS
Allerest tablets	phenylpropanolamine HCl 25 mg.	chlorpheniramine maleate 2 mg. methapyrilene fumarate 5 mg.	—
Allerest time capsules	phenylpropanolamine HCl 50 mg.	pyrilamine maleate 15 mg. methapyrilene fumarate 10 mg.	—
Contac spansules	phenylpropanolamine HCl 50 mg.	chlorpheniramine maleate 4 mg.	belladonna alkaloids 0.2 mg.
Coricidin "D" Tablets	phenylephrine*	chlorpheniramine maleate*	aspirin* caffeine*
Coryban-D	phenylpropanolamine HCl 25 mg.	chlorpheniramine maleate 2 mg.	ascorbic acid 25 mg. caffeine 30 mg. phenacetin 160 mg. salicylamide 230 mg.
Dristan tablets	phenylephrine HCl 5 mg.	phenindamine tartrate 10 mg.	aspirin* caffeine* aluminum hydroxide* magnesium carbonate*
Dristan (12-hour) capsules	phenylephrine HCl 20 mg.	chlorpheniramine maleate 4 mg.	—
Novahistine elixir and tablets	phenylephrine HCl 5 mg., 5 cc. or tab	chlorpheniramine maleate 1 mg.	elixir includes chloroform 13.5 mg.; menthol 1 mg./5 cc. alcohol 5%
Sinutab	phenylpropanolamine HCl 25 mg.	phenyltoloxamine citrate 22 mg.	acetyl-p-aminophenol 150 mg. phenacetin 150 mg.
Vicks Tri-Span Time core tablets	ephedrine sulfate* phenylpropanolamine HCl*	pyrilamine maleate*	N-acetyl-p-aminophenol 3 gr. caffeine*

* Quantitative statement not included on label of product.
† From Zupko, A. G. and Stempel, E.: J.A.Ph.A., NS6:544, 1966.

TABLE 4 Sympathomimetic Constituents of Nasal Decongestants*

SYMPATHOMIMETIC DRUG	PROPRIETARY COMPOUND
cyclopentamine hydrochloride	constituent of Clopane Hydrochloride solution, 0.5%
1-desoxyephedrine	constituent of Vicks Inhaler
ephedrine (as the lactate)	constituent of Gluco-Fedrin
ephedrine (with gluconic acid)	constituent of I-Sedrin plain and I-Sedrin compound
methylhexaneamine	constituent of Forthane inhaler
naphazoline hydrochloride	constituent of Privine Hydrochloride solution, spray, jelly
phenylephrine hydrochloride	constituent of Isophrin Hydrochloride solution
phenylephrine hydrochloride	constituent of Neo-Synephrine Hydrochloride solution, spray, jelly
propylhexedrine	constituent of Benzedrex inhaler
tuaminoheptane equivalent	constituent of Tuamine inhaler
tuaminoheptane sulfate	constituent of Tuamine Sulfate solution, 1%

*From Zupko, A. G. and Stempel, E.: J.A.Ph.A, NS6:544, 1966.

ORNADE. This also is a combination consisting of:

Chlorpheniramine maleate	8 mg.
Phenylpropanolamine HCl	50 mg.
Isopropamide	2.5 mg.

Ornade is often used in common cold therapy since it combines an antihistamine (chlorpheniramine) with a decongestant (phenylpropanolamine) and an anticholinergic (isopropamide) to reduce nasal and lacrimal secretions. It is to be used with caution in patients with severe hypertension, and is contraindicated in those with glaucoma or prostatic hypertrophy.

DOSE. One capsule every 12 hours.

ACTIFED. Actifed is a combination of:
Triprolidine 2.5 mg. (antihistamine)
Pseudoephedrine 60 mg. (decongestant)
Like Ornade, this is employed chiefly for the common cold and similar conditions.

DOSE. One tablet orally two or three times daily.

CORICIDIN. A combination of:

Chlorpheniramine maleate	2 mg.
Aspirin	0.39 Gm.
Caffeine	0.03 Gm.

This combines an antihistamine with aspirin and caffeine to relieve the secondary symptoms of colds as well as allergic reactions.

DOSE. One tablet orally three or four times daily.

DIMETAPP. This compound is produced in a form that permits delayed release of action and gives continuous therapeutic effects for 10 to 12 hours.

Each "extentab" contains:

Brompheniramine maleate	12 mg.
Phenylephrine	15 mg.
Phenylpropanolamine	15 mg.

DOSE. One tablet orally twice daily.

TUSS-ORNADE. Each "spansule" (delayed-release capsule) contains:

Caramiphen ethandisulfonate	20 mg.
Chlorpheniramine maleate	8 mg.
Phcnylpropanolamine	50 mg.
Isopropamide	2.5 mg.

Here a cough depressant (Caramiphen) has been added to help make this drug effective in treating the common cold.

DOSE. One capsule orally twice daily.

NALDECON. Each sustained action tablet contains:

Phenylpropanolamine HCl	40 mg.
Phenylephrine HCl	10 mg.
Phenyltoloxamine citrate	15 mg.
Chlorpheniramine maleate	5 mg.

This is a combination of sympathomimetic and antihistaminic drugs for use in symptomatic relief of hay fever and other allergic disorders. The delayed action tablet provides relief for six to eight hours.

DOSE. One tablet orally three times daily.

EMPRAZIL. Each tablet contains:

Pseudoephedrine HCl	20 mg.
Chlorcyclizine HCl	15 mg.
Acetophenetidin	150 mg.
Aspirin	200 mg.
Caffeine	30 mg.

The decongestant (pseudoephedrine) and the antihistamine (chlorcyclizine) with APC help to provide symptomatic relief of the common cold, grippe and influenza.

DOSE. One or two tablets orally three times daily.

TRIAMINIC

Phenylpropanolamine HCl	50 mg.
Pyrilamine maleate	50 mg.
Pheniramine maleate	25 mg.

DOSE. One tablet orally three times daily.

TRIAMINICIN

Pyrilamine maleate	12.5 mg.
Pheniramine maleate	12.5 mg.
Phenylpropanolamine	25 mg.
Aspirin	225 mg.
Acetophenetidin	150 mg.
Caffeine	30 mg.
Vitamin C	50 mg.
Dried aluminum hydroxide	180 mg.

The new additions are the vitamin C to aid in the maintenance of normal epithelial tissue and the antacid aluminum hydroxide.

DOSE. One tablet orally three times daily.

IMMUNITY

Immunity to infectious disease or invasion of a microorganism is brought about by the same mechanism that produces antibodies in response to invading foreign nonliving proteins.

Immunity is said to exist when the level of circulating antibodies against specific infection is high enough so that the individual is not susceptible to that infection. There are various types of immunity:

I. Natural immunity—that with which a person is born.

A. *Individual*—occurs when circulating antibodies are present at birth; it is extremely rare. More common is the occurrence of antibodies to various blood groups.

B. *Species.* Certain animal species are immune to the diseases of other species, e.g., humans are not susceptible to hog cholera.

C. *Racial.* E.g., civilized races seem less susceptible to tuberculosis than are primitive races; Mongolians are immune to scarlet fever.

II. Acquired immunity—obtained after birth.

A. *Active*—acquired through contact with the antigen itself. The body manufactures antibodies in response to the antigen.

1. *Natural*—occurs after exposure to the disease itself. May develop whether or not clinical symptoms of the disease have appeared.

2. *Artificial*—obtained by immunization, that is, the artificial introduction of an antigen into the body. This is more desirable in most cases than permitting the disease to run its course with the concurrent possibility of secondary harmful effects.

It is possible to utilize cross reactions in antibody production, i.e., the antibody to antigen of similar properties. In such a case it is possible to immunize by introduction of the less virulent antigen. In some instances *heterophile* antigens (also known as heterogenetic antigens) may be employed for immunization. These are antigens common to more than one species of animal, and capable of reacting with tissues from other animals, or even from plants.

Immunization may be accomplished in several ways:

a. Introduction of living, virulent organisms just as they occur in nature (ordinarily not done, however, as it is obviously dangerous).

b. Introduction of attenuated organisms that are alive but no longer capable of producing disease.

c. The use of dead organisms; antibody production will occur as usual.

d. Secretions such as exotoxins and/or cellular components of organisms are used relatively often.

e. In certain cases heterophile antigens, or other cross-reacting antigens, may be administered. For example, it has been learned that the use of antibodies that are formed by reaction with the nontoxic *Bacterium prodigiosum* will protect against infection by the virulent anthrax bacillus.

B. *Passive*. In passive immunity the individual is the receptor of already-formed anti-bodies, manufactured in the blood of some other human or animal. Passive immunization is provided when immediate, temporary protection against a disease is needed. Passive immunity may also be acquired naturally, but in these instances is effective only briefly and only during early infancy.

1. *Natural:*
a. Passed from mother to unborn child through placental membrane.
b. Secreted in colostrum (first milk) to provide protection until the infant is able to manufacture its own antibodies. For a short time after birth infants are apparently able to absorb antibodies through the gastrointestinal tract. This ability is lost in a relatively short time.

2. *Artificial.* The serum of animals (usually horses) serves as the vehicle for most antibody administration; occasionally human serum is also used. These sera are used both for prophylaxis and for treatment of disease. Serum therapy must be administered early in the course of a disease, however, since when the organisms have multiplied sufficiently, an adequate amount of serum cannot be administered to resist the disease effectively.

The chief disadvantage of passive immunity, besides the danger of serum sensitivity, is its short duration. The peak of activity is at two to three weeks, and immunity decreases to virtually no protection after six weeks. This ordinarily allows sufficient time to begin building an active immunity to the disease, since a vaccine may be administered concurrently if the disease threat is expected to continue.

Serious and even fatal allergic reactions may occur with the animal sera. Optimally, skin testing should be performed before administration. Animal sera are contraindicated in patients with a history of rash, febrile reaction, etc., upon previous injections. Human serum forms may then be used as a substitute.

AGENTS THAT PROVIDE ACTIVE IMMUNITY

Active immunity, as previously described, is achieved only when the antigen or some form of it is injected. The term vaccination, now broadened to include all such antigen administration, was originally coined to describe immunization against vaccinia (cowpox), a procedure first attempted by Jenner to build smallpox immunity. Vaccines are usually administered subcutaneously or intramuscularly, but a few may be taken orally. They may never be administered intravenously.

The nurse has an important role in teaching patients and families as well as the general public the necessity of adequate immunizations to prevent disease. Because of the success of immunizations in preventing or greatly reducing the incidence of once rampant communicable diseases, the need for continued surveillance and immunizations is no longer of great public concern. Young children should be under the medical supervision of private physicians or well-child clinics. Adults should continue to receive booster doses if and when indicated; initial immunizations for adults may also be indicated as vaccines are developed.

DIPHTHERIA TOXOID, U.S.P.   Diphtheria toxoid is a sterile solution of the formaldehyde-treated toxic products of the diphtheria bacillus, *Corynebacterium diphtheriae*. The specific toxicity of the toxin has been reduced to a low level or completely removed. The antigenic property, however, remains unchanged, so that antibody production is stimulated as usual. Ehrlich theorized that the toxin molecule consisted of two portions: the toxophore group which is easily destroyed by chemicals and is the carrier of the toxic qualities, and the much more stable haptophore group which is nontoxic but can neutralize antitoxin and acts as an antigen to incite body cells to produce specific antitoxins.

Four forms of anti-diphtheria prophylactic agents are recognized:

1. *Formol toxoid or anatoxin.*   The formol toxoid is composed of diphtheria toxin treated with a solution of formaldehyde until the specific toxicity has been completely removed. The active immunity produced may last for several years.

DOSE.   Three doses of 0.5 cc. intra-

muscularly at intervals of three to four weeks.

2. *Alum-precipitated toxoid.*   This preparation is a sterile suspension of diphtheria toxoid precipitated by alum from a formaldehyde-treated solution of the products of growth of the bacillus. It has been observed that addition of alum to diphtheria toxoid results in precipitation of the toxoid while leaving in solution many of the culture medium components occurring in plain diphtheria toxoid, thus reducing the chances of untoward secondary reactions. Furthermore, the alum-precipitated toxoid is somewhat more active as an immunizing agent than is the regular diphtheria toxoid.

Because of the comparative insolubility of the alum-precipitated form, however, it is more likely to produce local reactions than are other preparations of the antigen. A local reaction is almost always caused by the injection, but in children this consists of nothing more than the formation of a small subcutaneous nodule which after a few days is painless and slowly absorbed. Occasionally erythema is seen at the site of the injection, and the arm may be painful for several days after administration of the toxoid. Very rarely the subcutaneous nodule will open through the skin and discharge pus. Bacteriological cultures of this pus are sterile, and these lesions are called "sterile abscesses" or "alum cysts."

Beyond 12 years of age, reactions are frequent and often severe. Adults seem to be allergic to the proteins contained in the diphtheria toxoid, and the immunization of adults should be undertaken with extreme care. Immunization should not be neglected because of this, however, because recent studies have shown the incidence of diphtheria to be increasing in adults while it is decreasing in children.

DOSE.   Two doses of 1 cc. each intramuscularly at intervals of four to six weeks.

3. *Aluminum hydroxide–absorbed diphtheria toxoid, U.S.P.*   Alum-precipitated toxoid, although considerably more powerful than the formol toxoid as an immunizing

agent, is variable in its purity, and antigenic properties. In order to overcome these deficiencies, the toxoid may first be refined by ammonium sulfate or alcohol precipitation, then adsorbed on pure alumium hydroxide by addition of the toxoid to an aluminum hydroxide gel.

> DOSE. Two doses of 1 cc. each intramuscularly at intervals of four to six weeks.

4. *Toxoid-antitoxin floccules.* This preparation is made by adding to diphtheria toxin (which has been treated to reduce or remove the specific toxicity) a quantity of diphtheria antitoxin equivalent of about 80 per cent of the toxoid. These toxin-antitoxin mixtures were introduced some years ago, in an attempt to render diphtheria toxin safer for immunization. They are not ordinarily employed at the present time as the attenuated forms produce more satisfactory results in immunization procedures.

TETANUS TOXOID, U.S.P.; TETANUS VACCINE, B.P. Two preparations of the toxoid are commonly used:

1. *Tetanus toxoid, fluid.* Tetanus toxoid is a sterile solution of the formaldehyde-treated products of the growth of the tetanus bacillus *Clostridium tetani.* It is used for active immunization against tetanus. By two weeks after the third injection most individuals will have developed an antibody titer sufficient to protect against tetanus. A maximum immunity is reached in three to five months. Booster injections given subsequently at the time of injury cause an appreciable rise in antibody titer within four days.

> DOSE. Three doses of 0.5 cc. subcutaneously at three-week intervals.

2. *Alum-precipitated tetanus toxoid.* Alum precipitation from a formaldehyde-treated solution of the products of growth of the tetanus bacillus results in a product that is more purified and less likely to cause untoward reactions. It may be used for the same general purposes as tetanus toxoid, but has the advantage of requiring administration of only two doses instead of three.

> DOSE. Two doses of 0.5 cc. intramuscularly at four- to six-week intervals.

TETANUS AND DIPHTHERIA TOXOIDS COMBINED, ALUM-PRECIPITATED, U.S.P. The combined product is intended for simultaneous active immunization against tetanus and diphtheria.

> DOSE. Three doses of 0.5 cc. intramuscularly at three- to four-week intervals.

DIPHTHERIA AND TETANUS TOXOIDS AND PERTUSSIS VACCINE, COMBINED, ALUM-PRECIPITATED, U.S.P.; DIPHTHERIA, TETANUS AND PERTUSSIS VACCINE, B.P. Use of the pertussis (whooping cough) vaccine with the two toxoids is approved and accepted prophylactic practice. Such a combination reduces the number of necessary injections and does not impair the resultant immunity.

Immunization should be postponed in the presence of acute infection. A history of central nervous system damage or convulsions is an indication to postpone primary immunization until the second year of life, and in this instance, the use of single, rather than combined, antigens is preferred.

In older individuals the reactions due to sensitivity to the proteins of the pertussis and diphtheria organisms are more frequent and more severe. The effect is more evident with combined antigens, and in these cases also the single forms are preferred.

Febrile reactions occurring in young children following immunization appear within 8 to 12 hours and subside in 24 to 36 hours. They are generally controlled with oral salicylates.

> DOSE. Three doses of 0.5 cc. intramuscularly at four- to six-week intervals.

POLIOMYELITIS VACCINE, U.S.P., B.P. One of the newest additions to the immunization field, poliomyelitis vaccine provided a long-awaited solution to the problem of the crippling and often fatal poliomyelitis. In addition to the original Salk vaccine, the newer oral forms of the Sabin vaccine now are in use in many parts of the world.

1. *Salk vaccine.* The Salk vaccine is an aqueous preparation of killed poliomyelitis viruses containing three types of virus strains. The three strains are grown separately under aseptic conditions in a medium containing viable cells from monkey kidneys and a nutrient fluid.

The color of the vaccine is from amber to cherry red, varying because of slight changes in pH shown by the indicator, phenol red, which is present in the vaccine. The more air space there is in the vial, the deeper the color is likely to be, because of the escape of carbon dioxide from the liquid to the air above. For this reason, the color of the remaining vaccine in bulk vials tends to deepen after withdrawal of individual doses. These color changes do not affect the efficacy or safety of the vaccine, however. Occasionally after use the vial may become cloudy or contain a precipitate. This may be due to bacterial contamination and in this case the vial should *not* be used.

Local and systemic reactions are mild and infrequent. There may be some erythema and tenderness at the site of injection with moderate soreness of the extremity for 24 to 36 hours. General malaise and low-grade fever of short duration are observed occasionally. Allergic symptoms following administration are very rare.

Whenever possible, immunization should be completed before the seasonal increase in the incidence of poliomyelitis occurs. However, the presence of the acute infection in a community is not considered to be a contraindication to the administration of the vaccine.

Very small amounts of penicillin may be present in the vaccine, and persons highly sensitive to penicillin should be tested intradermally before the vaccine is administered.

> **DOSE.** Three doses of 1 cc. intramuscularly or subcutaneously each at four- to six-week intervals. A booster injection is recommended annually.

2. *Sabin vaccine.* The oral form of polio vaccine is a suspension of the live, attenuated organisms of either type 1, 2 or 3 (monovalent forms) or a combination of all three types (trivalent form). The organisms are propagated on monkey kidney tissue under controlled conditions.

The vaccine requires particular care to preserve its potency, and must be stored continuously below 0° C. After thawing, it may be kept for a maximum of seven days at 2 to 10° C. Color changes may occur on storage or thawing, but have no significance.

The efficacy of poliovirus vaccine when given orally is dependent on the multiplication of the virus within the gastrointestinal tract. Other enteroviruses may interfere with this multiplication; therefore it is preferable that vaccination be carried out at a time when interference from enteroviruses is at a minimum (November through May). Vaccination should be postponed in the presence of persistent vomiting and diarrhea. There are no known contraindications to the use of the oral form.

> **DOSE.** Monovalent—each type is administered individually by mouth at minimum intervals of six weeks. Type 1 is given first, then 3 and lastly 2. Trivalent—two doses at 8-week intervals.

INFLUENZA VIRUS VACCINE, U.S.P., B.P. The vaccine is prepared from extraembryonic fluids of virus-infected chick embryos (Fig. 27). Formaldehyde is used as an inactivating agent. The vaccine is polyvalent, containing virus material from several different strains of both type A and type B viruses. Because of the prevalence of influenza during the winter, the first dose is usually given as soon as practicable after September 1 and the course of immunization should be completed by mid-December. Routine annual injection is recommended for certain high-risk groups such as patients with cardiovascular disease, pulmonary, renal or metabolic disorders, pregnant women and persons in older age groups.

Since the vaccine is prepared in hens' eggs, it should not be administered to individuals who have a history of hypersensitivity to eggs, chicken or chicken feathers. Skin testing with vaccines prepared from eggs is also contraindicated in such individuals.

> **DOSE.** Two doses of 1 cc. each subcutaneously at two-month intervals.

TYPHUS VACCINE, U.S.P., B.P. The vaccine consists of a suspension of the rickettsiae that cause louse-borne epidemic typhus, prepared by a yolk-sac culture method. The organisms are killed by formaldehyde. The indications for vaccine prophylaxis against typhus fever in the United States are rather limited because of the infrequency of the disease. The chief use is during epidemics or for the vaccination of contacts or those in attendance on typhus cases. In addition, it is recommended for those who travel through areas where danger from epidemic typhus exists.

Since the vaccine is prepared from eggs, it should not be administered to sensitive individuals.

DOSE. Two doses of 0.5 cc. subcutaneously at intervals of 7–28 days.

TYPHOID VACCINE, U.S.P. Prepared from a suspension of killed typhoid bacilli, the vaccine is used chiefly as a prophylactic against typhoid fever. It is not claimed that it produces such an absolute resistance to infection that one may neglect all sanitary precautions without any danger of infection, but it does produce such a high degree of immunity that under ordinary circumstances

it is improbable that the patient will develop typhoid fever. Also, if the disease does develop, as a result of unusual exposure, it runs a much milder course than it does in the unprotected person. Immunity lasts roughly one to two years.

DOSE. Three doses of 0.5 cc. subcutaneously with intervals of 7 to 28 days.

TYPHOID AND PARATYPHOID VACCINE, U.S.P., B.P. The vaccine contains killed typhoid and paratyphoid A and B bacilli. Combined immunization is recommended in combating epidemics and in emergencies (such as floods) which may interrupt water and milk supplies. It is recommended also in rural areas where enteric fevers are prevalent and for those who live or travel outside the United States.

Typhoid and paratyphoid vaccine may be used to produce artificial fevers. In chorea and certain inflammatory conditions, notably arthritis, thromboangiitis obliterans and ocular inflammation, fever therapy has been found helpful. Recent evidence sug-

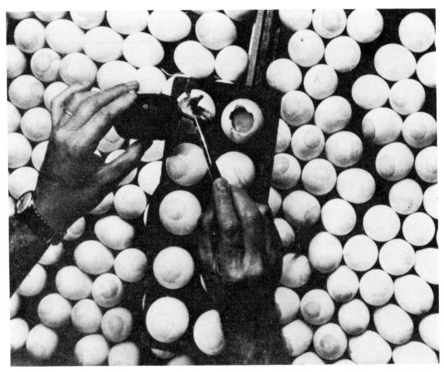

FIGURE 27. Preparation of influenza vaccine from virus-infected chick embryo. (Claus, E. P.: *Pharmacognosy.* 4th Ed., Lea & Febiger, Philadelphia, 1961.)

gests that this type of foreign-protein therapy may act by stimulating the adrenal cortices.

Like other immunizing biologicals, this vaccine should not be given during an acute illness. Infants with histories of febrile convulsions or cerebral damage should be given a small initial dose to test their tolerance. Use of the vaccine for fever therapy is contraindicated in elderly, asthenic, cachectic, arteriosclerotic or anemic patients, and in those with cardiac disease or obvious subacute or latent infections other than that being treated.

DOSE. Three doses of 0.5 cc. subcutaneously from one to four weeks apart.

MEASLES VACCINE (LIRUGEN). Composed of a lyophilized suspension of the live, attenuated rubeola virus, the vaccine is prepared by growing the virus in chick embryo tissue culture maintained in a nutrient fluid. It is recommended for immunization of individuals susceptible to rubeola (hard measles, ten-day measles, red measles). It will not protect against rubella (German measles).

Administration of the vaccine produces a noncommunicable measles infection. The reaction is manifested by fever beginning on the sixth to tenth day after injection and lasting two to five days. About half of those injected develop a mild measles-like rash. The illness is usually not accompanied by the coryza, cough and conjunctivitis that are so prominent with the natural disease. Encephalitis, a well recognized complication of natural measles, has not been reported following administration of measles vaccine.

The vaccine is contraindicated in pregnancy and in patients with leukemia, lymphoma and other generalized neoplasms. It should not be administered to persons receiving therapeutic agents that depress resistance, such as steroids, alkylating agents, antimetabolites and irradiation, or to patients with febrile illnesses. If gamma globulin has been administered within the preceding six weeks, immunization should be deferred since the globulin may inhibit a vaccine take. In addition, a recent blood transfusion, because of the probable immune globulin content, may temporarily inhibit the response to vaccinations.

Since the vaccine is prepared in chick embryo tissue, it may cause allergy.

DOSE. One dose of 0.5 cc. injected subcutaneously.

RUBELLA VIRUS VACCINE, LIVE (CENDEVAX, MERUVAX, RUBELOGEN). Live rubella virus vaccine produces active immunity to rubella (German measles) within 28 days of inoculation. The duration of immunity to the vaccine is not as yet established, but antibody levels are known to persist at least four years.

The vaccine is recommended for use in children from 12 months to puberty, and is often given as a part of mass immunization programs. Children are most susceptible to the communicable diseases, thus they are the greatest source of infection to pregnant women. The vaccine is not recommended for use in women of childbearing age since there is a danger of administration during an early, unrecognized pregnancy with possible deleterious effects to the fetus. If it is administered to adult women, there should be no chance of pregnancy occurring for at least three months after inoculation.

TOXICITY. Severe reactions are rare in children. Transient arthralgia has been reported occasionally in children but in 20 to 40 per cent of adults receiving the vaccination, skin rash, lymphadenopathy, mild febrile reactions symptoms of upper respiratory infections and rarely anaphylactoid reactions have been reported. It should not be administered in the presence of infection or when the patient has a severe underlying disease such as leukemia, lymphoma or other malignancy, since these may be potentiated by the vaccine. It should not be administered to patients whose resistance has been lowered by therapy with corticosteroids, alkylating agents, antimetabolites or irradiation.

DOSE. 0.5 cc. Subcutaneously or I.M., once.

MUMPS VACCINE. This suspension of killed mumps virus is prepared for extra-embryonic fluid of the virus-infected chick embryo. The virus is killed with formaldehyde.

Epidemics of mumps are apt to occur in segregated populations, such as in the armed forces, schools, and orphanages and among medical students and nurses. Epidemics may be prevented by routine administration of vaccine to all susceptible individuals. Administration of the vaccine prevents complications, such as orchitis, which sometimes occur when the natural disease is contracted.

The duration of the immunity is not known, but it is probably not safe to assume it lasts more than six to twelve months. Routine administration before adolescence is not recommended, as immunity may wane and permit infection to occur at an older age when there is a greater danger from complications.

Local and systemic reactions to the vaccine are usually mild. Slight erythema and some tenderness may appear at the site of injection; fever and malaise are uncommon. Immune individuals may have serious reactions, however. Immunity to mumps is found in many who have never had clinical symptoms of parotitis. Before the vaccine is administered to adults, a skin test should be performed; if it is positive, vaccination should be omitted.

DOSE. Two doses of 1 cc. subcutaneously at four- to six-week intervals.

CHOLERA VACCINE, U.S.P., B.P. The vaccine, a suspension of killed vibrio organisms used to produce active immunity to cholera, is prepared from two types of *Vibrio comma*. The organisms are killed with phenol solution. Although the vaccine provides a definite protective effect, it is impossible to immunize an individual so that he is unable to contract the disease in the face of massive exposure to cholera organisms. Booster injections may be required as often as every six months to maintain an effective immunity.

Local and systemic reactions may occur. There may be erythema, swelling and ten-derness at the site of injection. Malaise and low-grade fever are also seen. The symptoms may begin immediately or may be delayed from three to ten days. They usually subside in 20 to 48 hours.

DOSE. 0.5 cc. intramuscularly followed in 7 to 10 days by 1 cc. Booster of 1 cc. every six months.

ROCKY MOUNTAIN SPOTTED FEVER VACCINE. Embryonic chick tissues are used to prepare the vaccine to this acute infectious disease, which is found in many parts of the United States, but chiefly in the Rocky Mountain states and in those lying east of the Appalachian Mountains from New York to Georgia. The disease vector is the common tick; the infecting organism is *dermacentroxenus*. The usual precautions should be taken for vaccines grown in chick embryo.

DOSE. 3 doses of 1 cc. each subcutaneously at 7 to 10-day intervals.

SMALLPOX VACCINE, U.S.P., B.P. Smallpox is a highly contagious disease, and is one of the most fatal of acute diseases. At one time it was more common than measles and was the most common cause of blindness. It is caused by the variola virus. Domestic animals are afflicted by a closely related virus, but the infection is far milder among them. It was Edward Jenner who proved that cowpox is readily transferred to man and produces a mild infection which subsequently protects against smallpox.

The living virus of vaccinia (cowpox) is obtained under aseptic conditions from healthy, vaccinated calves and consists of a smooth, aqueous suspension of the vesicular tissue. Primary vaccination is recommended between the sixth and twelfth months of age, with repeat vaccinations every five years thereafter.

After vaccination, neither pads nor shields of any kind should be used, as they retain heat and moisture and thus encourage bacterial infections. Tight sleeves should be avoided and the arm protected from injury.

"Autovaccination" is the result of scratching the site with the fingers and transferring the virus to the mucous membranes of the

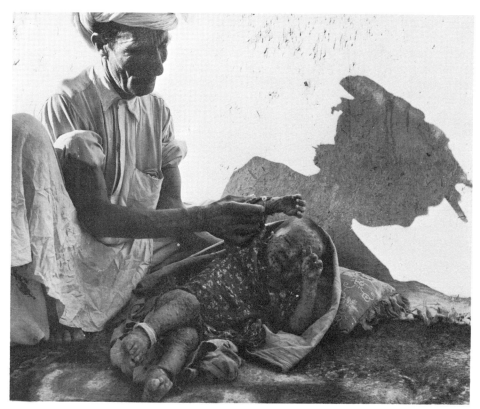

FIGURE 28. Smallpox, an extremely rare disease because of the effective vaccine. (Courtesy World Health Organization; photo by W. Wilkie.)

nose, mouth, vagina or any part of the skin. Vesicles may appear at these distant places. If the material is introduced into the eye, blindness may result.

> **DOSE.** A small amount of the vaccine is introduced by incision or linear abrasion or multiple puncture of the skin. The excess is wiped off.

YELLOW FEVER VACCINE, U.S.P., B.P. The vaccine is composed of the living virus of an attenuated strain of yellow fever virus selected for high antigenic activity and safety.

Yellow fever is transmitted from one person to another only by the bite of an infected mosquito. The places of its occurrence are confined to the limits of the zone in which its chief vector *Aedes aegypti* is found.

Immunity to the disease develops in seven days and usually lasts for many years. Revaccination should be performed every six to nine years.

> **DOSE.** 0.5 cc. subcutaneously.

RABIES VACCINE. Rabies vaccine is a preparation of killed, fixed virus which has been grown in duck embryo tissue. It provides active immunity to rabies if it is administered before the rabies virus attacks the nervous system of the patient. If symptoms of active rabies have occurred, the vaccine is of no benefit. Ideally, the attacking animal should be observed and examined, and if shown to be rabid, immunizations should be started as soon as possible. If the bite has been the result of a wild animal such as a squirrel, bat, etc. which has subsequently escaped, and it is known that there is a reservoir of rabies in the wild animal population in the area, vaccination is usually begun prophylactically. The side effects of this vaccine prohibit its routine use, however, unless there is a definite indication.

Immediate and thorough local treatment of all bite wounds and scratches remains of paramount importance. All wounds should be treated with copious flushing with soap and water, followed by thorough rinsing, then application of one of the quaternary ammonium compounds such as a 1:1000 solution of benzalkonium chloride. As previously discussed, all soap must be removed from the area before benzalkonium chloride is applied or its activity is neutralized.

Antirabies serum may be given concurrently with the vaccine to provide earlier protection, but they should not be given in the same syringe nor in the same injection site as neutralization of the vaccine can occur.

TOXICITY. Severe neurologic reactions may occur following administration of the vaccine including peripheral neuritis, encephalomyelitis, polyneuritis and anaphylactic shock. Fatalities have occasionally be reported. Less severe symptoms such as lethargy, weakness, stiff neck, fever and local reactions at the administration site occur more frequently. Regional lymphadenopathy near the site of injection has been reported.

The vaccine should be administered with caution to patients with a history of allergy to chicken or duck eggs or proteins and the patient should be tested for hypersensitivity to the vaccine. If necessary, antihistamines may be administered concurrently with the vaccine to minimize allergic reactions, and epinephrine should be available to treat possible anaphylactic reactions.

DOSE. 1 cc. subcutaneously daily for 21 days, or 1 cc. subcutaneously twice daily for 14 days, then daily for 7 days.

Injection sites should be rotated to include abdomen, lower back or lateral thigh.

BCG VACCINE, U.S.P., B.P. Bacillus Calmette-Guérin vaccine is a vaccine against tuberculosis. It consists of a suspension of living cells of a strain of the bacillus of Calmette and Guérin. This strain is maintained so as to preserve its power of sensitizing man to tuberculin, and also to preserve its relative nonpathogenicity to man and laboratory animals.

Calmette and Guérin transplanted cultures of a highly virulent bovine strain of tuberculosis bacillus to a potato medium in 1902. After thirteen years and 230 transplantations, the organism no longer produced progressive tuberculosis in susceptible animals, but produced instead nodular lesions with no evidence of progression. Despite the loss of virulence, the culture retained its antigenic characteristics and the animals were resistant to the progressive infection. All strains used for the production of this vaccine are traceable to the original culture.

BCG vaccine is used to produce an active immunization against tuberculosis, especially in persons likely to be exposed to the infection. Despite the extensive use of the vaccine, there is a diversity of opinion regarding its value. This is largely due to a lack of adequately controlled investigations and to the difficulty of dissociating the specific protective role of BCG from the almost universal decline in the morbidity and mortality of tuberculosis, which began before the use of the vaccine.

BCG vaccine is not recommended for those who present evidence of tuberculous infections as indicated by a positive skin test. It is recommended for those tuberculin-negative persons whose professional duties may expose them to tuberculous patients, or to material that may contain virulent tubercle bacilli. It is also recommended for those population groups, including newborn children, in whom the morbidity and mortality from tuberculosis are high and conditions favor the spread of the disease.

DOSE. 0.1 cc. intradermally.

POISON IVY EXTRACT (Ivyol). The extract is a 1:1000 solution of the active principles derived from poison ivy in sterile olive oil. Probably because of wide variation in susceptibility, clinical reports have not always been unanimous with respect to the value of these extracts. A number of clinical reports have indicated, however, that the use of poison ivy extract renders individuals immune or definitely less susceptible to casual contact with the plants *Rhus toxicodendron* (poison ivy), *Rhus diversiloba* (poison oak), and *Toxicodendron vernix* (poison sumac). The use of poison ivy extract is not recommended for treatment of persons already suffering from *Rhus* dermatitis.

> **DOSE.** Four doses of 0.5 cc. orally at weekly intervals beginning in the early spring.

AGENTS THAT PROVIDE PASSIVE IMMUNITY

A passive immunity, as previously discussed, is a short-lived immunity obtained by injecting already-formed antibodies. The high degree of resistance that the preparations bestow within a relatively short time makes them the agents of choice when temporary protection is desired, as in the case of an epidemic, or when an individual is exposed to a disease at a time when it would be inadvisable or dangerous to let the disease run its course.

These agents are given by the physician because of the danger of anaphylactic reactions. Patients should be questioned carefully about allergies, and sensitivity tests should be made before the agent is administered. Epinephrine 1:1000 should be immediately available along with other emergency drugs and equipment.

DIPHTHERIA ANTITOXIN, U.S.P., B.P. This is a sterile, concentrated, isotonic solution of antitoxin-bearing globulins obtained from the plasma of horses immunized with diphtheria toxoid and diphtheria toxin.

Following exposure to diphtheria, susceptible persons can be provided with temporary passive immunity by the administration of antitoxin. The duration of protection afforded by prophylactic doses is variable, but usually it lasts from 10 to 21 days. Exposed persons who have been immunized previously may be given a booster injection of diphtheria toxoid rather than the antitoxin.

Nearly all reactions to the antitoxin are allergic in nature. The highly sensitized individual may have an immediate, dangerous anaphylactic reaction, even to a skin test dose. If there is reason to fear such a reaction, epinephrine may be injected at the time the antitoxin is administered. A delayed reaction (serum sickness) may occur 8 to 10 days after the serum administration. The antihistaminic drugs are useful in this condition. If there are asthmatic symptoms, ephedrine or epinephrine may be given. The corticosteroids have also been found to be helpful.

A skin or eye test for sensitivity to equine serum may be performed to determine whether sensitivity exists. A skin test involves the intradermal injection of 0.05 to 0.1 cc. of a 1:10 dilution of serum. The appearance of a wheal in 10 to 30 minutes is a positive reaction. The eye test is done by instilling one drop of a 1:10 dilution of serum in the lower conjunctival sac. In sensitive individuals, lacrimation and conjunctivitis will be apparent in 10 to 30 minutes. The conjunctival reaction may be terminated with one or two drops of epinephrine 1:1000.

It is important to note, however, that negative sensitivity tests do not rule out a delayed reaction. The sensitivity tests are of value in determining the possibility of an immediate reaction.

> **DOSE.** Prophylactic—10,000 units intramuscularly.
> Therapeutic—10,000 to 200,000 units intramuscularly or intravenously.

TETANUS ANTITOXIN, U.S.P., B.P. Although a horse serum preparation is usually employed, in the event of sensitization both bovine and human serum products are available. The human serum would be preferable in all cases, but the extremely high cost of preparing it prohibits its routine use.

The antitoxin will neutralize circulating tetanus toxin and thus is indicated both in therapy and in prophylaxis of tetanus.

> **EQUINE ANTITOXIN:**
> **DOSE.** Prophylactic—5,000 to 10,000 units intramuscularly.
> Therapeutic—40,000 to 60,000 units intramuscularly.

HUMAN ANTITOXIN (HYPER-TET):

DOSE Prophylactic—250 units intramuscularly.

Therapeutic—3,000 to 6,000 units intramuscularly.

GAS GANGRENE ANTITOXIN, B.P. Horse serum normally is employed in this antitoxin also. The bivalent form is most commonly used, containing antibodies to *Clostridium perfringens* (*Cl. welchii*) and to *Cl. septicum.* It is indicated for the treatment of gas gangrene infections due to these causative organisms. They gain entry through contaminated wounds and cause infection chiefly in traumatized muscle. *Cl. perfringens* may be found in gangrenous appendices and in puerperal infection as well.

Two other types of antitoxin are available: the trivalent, which contains antibodies to the three most prevalent strains of the organism, and the pentavalent, which contains antibodies against all five of the gas gangrene causative organisms. The pentavalent type is used only when necessary, since it is impossible to attain as high an antibody titer when five different antibodies are present. In addition, as the number of specific antibodies increases, the number of sensitivity reactions may increase also.

DOSE. Prophylactic—5,000 to 10,000 units intramuscularly.

Therapeutic—20,000 to 60,000 units or more intramuscularly.

TETANUS—GAS GANGRENE ANTITOXIN, N.F. Each vial contains 1500 units tetanus antitoxin, and 2000 units each of *Cl. perfringens* and *Cl. septicum* antitoxins. The combination form is usually desirable for wounds requiring gas gangrene prophylaxis as there is usually a concurrent threat of tetanus.

DOSE. One to three vials intramuscularly.

BIVALENT BOTULISM ANTITOXIN, U.S.P. Botulism antitoxin, bivalent, types A and B, is indicated in the treatment of all cases of toxemia in which the toxin is known or suspected to be produced by *Clostridium botulinum* types A or B. The antitoxin is prepared from horse serum. The combination of the antitoxins is necessary because the best re-

sults will be obtained if the antitoxin is administered as soon as possible, without waiting for determination of the type causing the toxemia.

DOSE. The antitoxin is diluted 1:10, preferably with 10 per cent glucose. Ten cc. of this mixture (containing 1 cc. or 1000 units of antitoxin) is injected very slowly intravenously over five minutes. After 15 minutes the remaining 90 cc. may be injected more rapidly. A syringe containing epinephrine 1:1000 (1 cc.) should be available whenever this antitoxin is administered and should be injected at once if respiratory difficulty or other signs of allergic reaction occur. This dose may be repeated every four hours until the toxic condition is alleviated.

SCARLET FEVER ANTITOXIN (STREPTOCOCCUS ANTITOXIN). A vial of this preparation contains a sterile solution of antitoxic substances obtained from the serum or plasma of healthy animals immunized against the toxin formed by *Streptococcus pyogenes,* the causative agent of scarlet fever.

The advent of sulfonamides and antibiotics has made it possible to treat the streptococcal infection specifically rather than merely treating the toxemia and rash by administration of the antitoxin. Therefore the antitoxin is rarely used at the present time.

DOSE. Prophylactic—2000 units intramuscularly.

Therapeutic—5,000 to 10,000 units intramuscularly.

PERTUSSIS IMMUNE GLOBULIN, U.S.P. This preparation consists of the gamma globulin fraction of the serum of human adults who have been hyperimmunized with pertussis (whooping cough) vaccine. Pertussis is still a very serious disease in nonimmunized infants less than one year old. The maximum therapeutic effect is obtained when this hyperimmune gamma globulin preparation is administered within the first seven days of illness. It appears to shorten the course, lessen the severity, and reduce the frequency of complications of the disease.

DOSE. Prophylactic—1.25 to 2.5 cc. intramuscularly (infants).
Therapeutic—1.25 cc. intramuscularly every 24 to 48 hours (infants).

MUMPS IMMUNE GLOBULIN (HYPAROTIN). Like the pertussis immune globulin, this product is prepared from the gamma globulin fraction of humans, in this case hyperimmunized with mumps virus vaccine. Treatment with the immune globulin after the onset of symptoms can be expected to have little or no therapeutic effect. Used as early as possible before the onset of other symptoms than parotitis, the globulin may, if used in large doses, prevent complications such as orchitis. The therapeutic dose should not be less than five times the minimum prophylactic dose and preferably more.

DOSE. Prophylactic—3 to 4.5 cc. intramuscularly.
Therapeutic—15 to 20 cc. intramuscularly.

IMMUNE SERUM GLOBULIN, U.S.P. Immune serum (or gamma) globulin is prepared by pooling extracts of human placentas. The globulin can be used to prevent or modify various virus diseases such as measles, poliomyelitis, infectious hepatitis, German measles (rubella), chickenpox (varicella), herpetiform lesions and herpes zoster, and as replacement therapy in dysgammaglobulinemia syndromes (e.g., agammaglobulinemia and hypogammaglobulinemia). It is used occasionally to modify the symptoms of measles vaccination, and as adjuvant treatment in refractory infections which do not respond to antibiotic therapy alone.

DOSE. Wide variation due to various uses. Ranges from 0.01 cc./lb. to 20 to 50 cc. monthly in dysgammaglobulinemia therapy. All doses are administered intramuscularly.

RH$_o$(D), IMMUNE GLOBULIN (HUMAN), (RHOGAM). This fractional concentrate of human immune globulin is standardized to contain a high concentration of the antibody to the Rh(D) antigen, the antigen most commonly involved in Rh incompatibilities of the newborn.

Following extensive research into the problem of Rh incompatibilities, it was found that the sensitization of the Rh negative mother occurred to the greatest extent at or just following parturition, when large amounts of the Rh+ blood cells of the infant could be transferred to the mother via numerous open blood vessels remaining from detachment of the placenta. The mother's immune system then formed antibodies, often in high concentration which subsequently were on hand to cause incompatibility reactions should later pregnancies also be Rh+ babies. Erythroblastosis fetalis (hemolytic disease of the newborn) is then produced by antigen-antibody reactions with the blood cells of an Rh+ baby in a previously sensitized Rh− mother. The condition increases in severity with each pregnancy involving an Rh+ fetus and often results in serious damage or death to the fetus.

Rh$_o$(D), if administered within 72 hours after delivery, has been shown to diminish antibody formation in the mother presumably by neutralizing antigenic cells which have escaped into the mother's bloodstream before the immune system of the mother can react to them. It is administered under the following conditions:

a. The mother is Rh(D) negative
b. The mother is not sensitized to Rh(D) by a previous pregnancy
c. The baby is Rh(D) positive and has a negative direct Coombs test (The Coombs test in this case detects previous sensitization of the mother by demonstrating the presence of antibodies in the baby's red cells).

The preparation may be administered after each subsequent pregnancy involving an Rh+ child.

TOXICITY. Slight temperature elevations may occur, as well as mild local reactions at the site of injection. Systemic reactions are rare. A cross reaction of the patient's blood and the serum must be performed before administration.

DOSE. 2 cc. I.M.

ANTIRABIES SERUM, U.S.P. Antirabies serum is a concentrated antiserum for passive immunization against rabies. It is obtained from horses hyperimmunized by repeated injections of rabies virus. The antiserum delays virus propagation in the body, thus allowing more time for rabies vaccine to induce antibodies to the virus.

In cases in which the biting animal cannot be located, or if there is a high index of suspicion that is may be rabid, the antiserum is administered immediately and the series of vaccination injections are begun. There is no established time limit for the administration of antirabies serum, but it is preferable that it be administered within 24 hours. If the interval between exposure and treatment is greater than 24 hours, or if there are severe wounds about the head or neck, two or three times the recommended amount of antirabies serum should be administered.

> **DOSE.** 1000 to 6000 units administered by multiple infiltration at the site of the wound.

ANTIVENINS

Antisera containing antibodies against snake venoms or against the poison produced by the black widow spider are called antivenins. Most of these are made from horse serum.

ANTIVENIN CROTALIDAE POLYVALENT, U.S.P. (North and South American antisnakebite serum.) This equine antivenin contains protective substances against the venoms of the pit vipers of North and South America including the rattlesnakes, water moccasin (cottonmouth) and highland moccasin (copperhead) as well as other relatively common species.

Antivenin should be administered as soon as possible after the bite. It is essential to inject a large enough initial dose to overwhelm the poison. The *smaller* the body of the patient, the *larger* the initial dose that is required. Although this is in direct contrast to most therapeutic procedures, it is necessary in this case because children have less resistance and less body fluid with which to dilute the poison. They may require twice the dose of serum that suffices for adults.

> **DOSE.** 1 to 5 vials intramuscularly or intravenously.

ANTIVENIN LATRODECTUS MACTANS (LYOVAC; BLACK WIDOW SPIDER ANTIVENIN). The venom of the black widow spider acts on the myoneural junctions or on the nerve endings, causing an ascending motor paralysis or destruction of the peripheral nerve endings. The groups of muscles most frequently affected first are those of the thigh, shoulder and back. After a varying length of time, the pain spreads to the abdomen and becomes more severe, and weakness and tremor usually develop. The abdominal muscles assume a boardlike rigidity. The symptoms increase in severity for several hours, perhaps a day, and then very slowly become less severe, gradually passing off in the course of two or three days, except in fatal cases.

As soon as a diagnosis of arachnidism due to the black widow spider is made, the patient should receive the antivenin, made from horse serum. Symptoms usually subside in one to three hours. Although one dose of antivenin is usually sufficient, in some cases it has been found necessary to administer two doses over a period of time.

> **DOSE.** 6000 units intramuscularly.

IMMUNOSUPPRESSIVES

AZATHIOPRINE (IMURAN). Azathioprine has been shown to suppress the immune mechanism, but the precise mechanism of action is as yet unknown. It is a known antagonist to purine metabolism and may inhibit RNA and/or DNA synthesis.

The immune suppressive response has been shown to be useful in the treatment of patients with organ transplants, as rejection reactions are suppressed or at least delayed by the drug. It may be used in conjunction with other immunosuppressive therapy such as irradiation, corticosteroids or other cytotoxic drugs. The maximum effectiveness occurs when this drug is administered during the induction period of the immune response, thus it is usually started within two days of an organ transplant operation.

TOXICITY. Bone marrow depression, nausea, vomiting, diarrhea, anorexia, ulceration of oral mucosa, dermatoses, serum sickness, alopecia, arthralgia, retinitis, Raynaud's disease, jaundice and pulmonary edema have been reported. The immunosuppressive reaction will also make the patient more susceptible to infections by depleting the body's natural immune reactions.

DOSE. 3 to 5 mg./kg. orally daily.

CORTICOSTEROIDS AND IMMUNIZATION

Concurrent therapy with oral or parenteral (not topical or intra-articular) corticosteroids is considered by many to be a contraindication to the administration of vaccines. This contraindication is mentioned in some instructions for the use of live and killed vaccines, and is intended to apply to booster doses as well as to primary inoculations. The steroids are known to suppress antibody production and other immune responses and thus decrease the effectiveness of the vaccines.

Exceptions to this contraindication must be made, however, where the steroids are necessary for survival, as in systemic lupus erythematosus or for relief of acute allergic reactions. If immunization is essential, as in persons likely to contract diseases such as poliomyelitis and measles, it should be carried out notwithstanding concurrent administration of corticosteroids. The contraindication also does not apply to persons who require continuous corticosteroid therapy, such as patients with adrenal insufficiency or congenital adrenal hyperplasia. Such individuals are especially susceptible to measles and other infectious diseases and immunization should be carried out.

When corticosteroid therapy can be safely withdrawn or when other effective drugs are available, as in rheumatoid arthritis, it is advised that the corticosteroid therapy be discontinued for at least 72 hours before a vaccine is administered. The time required for the development of optimum immune responses varies with different vaccines. When possible, corticosteroid therapy should not be resumed until about two weeks after the vaccine has been given.

GUIDE FOR THE NURSING ASSESSMENT OF A PATIENT RECEIVING AN ANTIHISTAMINE

I. Why does this patient need an antihistamine? What is he allergic to? Has the allergy, if known, been reported and recorded appropriately? Has the source of the antigen been removed if possible?

II. Has the antihistamine produced the intended effect? Are the symptoms of allergy receding? Is there a decrease in urticaria, skin eruptions, wheezing, sneezing, coryza, etc.? Is the dosage scheduled so that antihistamine action is in effect over a 24 hour period whenever possible?

III. Has the patient experienced any side effects? Has he experienced drowsiness or sedation? Did this occur initially or has it decreased with continued administration? Has the patient experienced dryness of the mouth, incoordination, nausea and vomiting, insomnia? Is the patient receiving barbiturates or ingesting alcohol which may produce an increased sedative effect?

IV. What are the patient's (and family's) learning needs? Does the patient understand the purpose of the antihistamine? Does he understand the cause of the allergy, if known? Does he know the measures he can take to avoid contact with the allergen?

If he is allergic to a drug: Is he aware of drug combinations which may contain the drug (e.g., aspirin in A.P.C. and Darvon Compound)? Is he aware of a possible need to carry information concerning the allergy on his person (e.g., identification card, Medic Alert)? Does he know that he should avoid the use of dangerous machinery or automobiles when drowsiness and sedation occur? Does he understand the potential effect of alcohol or barbiturates when taken with antihistamines?

QUESTIONS FOR DISCUSSION AND REVIEW

1. Trace an allergic reaction from the time the pollen dust is inhaled until the symptoms of asthma develop.

2. May antihistamines be taken routinely without apparent ill effects? What untoward effects may be experienced by certain individuals?

3. Is it always a good idea to take antihistamines at the first sign of a cold? What should be kept in mind if such a practice is routinely followed?

4. Give an example of a natural active acquired immunity.

5. What immunities do you have? What types are they, i.e., active or passive, natural or acquired?

6. What are the advantages and disadvantages of a passive immunity? of an active immunity?

7. If a new mother asks you what immunizations her baby should have and when, how should you respond?

8. What drugs and emergency equipment should be available in the event of an anaphylactic reaction? Are these on the emergency cart in your hospital?

BIBLIOGRAPHY

Ager, E. A.: Current concepts in immunization. *Amer. J. Nurs., 66*:2004, (September) 1966.

Allergy and Hypersensitivity: A Programmed Review for Physicians. 2nd Ed. New York, Pfizer Laboratories, 1964.

AMA Drug Evaluations. Chicago, American Medical Association, 1971.

Anderson, R.: Smallpox immunization. *Practitioner, 195*:281, 1965.

Boyd, W. C.: *Fundamentals of Immunology.* 2nd Ed. New York, Inter-Science Publishers, Inc., 1947.

Brand, J. J. and Perry, W. L. M. Drugs used in motion sickness. *Pharmacol. Rev., 18*:895, 1966.

Browne, C. M.: Pertussis immunization. *Practitioner, 195*:292, 1965.

Brunner, L. S., et al.: *Textbook of Medical-Surgical Nursing.* 2nd Ed. Philadelphia, J. B. Lippincott Co., 1970.

Bruton, M. R.: When tetanus struck. *Amer. J. Nurs., 65*:107, (October) 1965.

Cannon, D. A.: Poliomyelitis immunization. *Practitioner, 195*:302, 1965.

Carpenter, P. L.: *Immunology and Serology.* 2nd Ed. Philadelphia, W. B. Saunders Co., 1965.

Cirksena, W. J.: Tetanus. *Amer. J. Nurs., 62*:65, (April) 1965.

Cole, L.: Tetanus immunization. *Practitioner, 195*:296, 1965.

Cooke, R. A.: *Allergy in Theory and Practice.* Philadelphia, W. B. Saunders Co., 1947.

Council on Drugs: A new agent for prophylaxis of tetanus: tetanus immune globulin (Hyper-Tet). *J.A.M.A., 192*:471, 1965.

Davenport, F. M.: Prospects for control of influenza. *Amer. J. Nurs., 69*:1908, (September) 1969.

Editorial: Cholera immunization. *J.A.M.A., 192*:995, 1965.

Fish, S. A.: Medic Alert. *Nurs. Forum, 8*:428, 1969.

Frazier, C. C.: Those deadly insects. *R.N., 34*:49, (April) 1971.

Friend, D. G.: The antihistamines. *Clin. Pharmacol. Ther., 1*:5, 1960.

Govoni, L. E. and Hayes, J. E.: *Drugs and Nursing Implications.* 2nd Ed. New York, Appleton-Century-Crofts, 1971.

Henderson, L. L.: A special article: anaphylaxis. *Ann. Allergy, 23*:525, 1965.

Johnson, K. J.: Allergic injections. *Amer. J. Nurs., 65*:121, (July) 1965.

Keele, C. A. and Neil, E.: Samson Wright's Applied Physiology. 11th Ed. London, Oxford University Press, 1965.

Main, R. J. and Richardson, A. W.: *Physiology.* 2nd Ed. St. Louis, C. V. Mosby Co., 1953.

Mostow, S. R.: Why influenza vaccine does not do the job. *Amer. J. Nurs., 70*:2126, (October) 1970.

Peebles, T. C., et al.: Tetanus-toxoid emergency boosters — A reappraisal. *New Eng. J. Med., 280*:575, 1969.

Pruzansky, J. J., et al.: Immunologic changes during hyposensitization therapy. *J.A.M.A., 203*:805, 1968.

Rodman, M. J.: Drugs for allergic disorders. *R.N., 34*:63, (June) 1971.

Rodman, M. J.: Drugs for the relief of asthma. *R.N., 30*:35, (March) 1967.

Rodman, M. J.: Drugs for treating coughs and colds. *R.N., 27*:85, (March) 1964.

Rosenthal, S. R.: The tuberculine tine test. *G.P., 34*:116, (November) 1966.

Sabin, A. B.: Oral poliovirus vaccine. History of its development and prospects for eradication of poliomyelitis. *J.A.M.A., 194*:872, 1965.

Shafer, K. N., et al.: *Medical-Surgical Nursing.* 4th Ed. St. Louis, C. V. Mosby Co., 1967.

Shaffer, J. and Sweet, L.: Allergic reactions to drugs. *Amer. J. Nurs., 65*:100, (October) 1965.

Swartz, H.: *Allergy: What It Is and What To Do About It.* New Brunswick, N.J., Rutgers University Press, 1949.

Von Magnus, H.: Measles vaccine present status. *Med. Clin. N. Amer., 51*:599, 1967.

Voorhorst, R.: *Basic Facts of Allergy.* Leiden, Holland, H. E. Stenfert Kroese N.V., 1962.

Chapter 8 Topical Anti-infectives

Important Concepts Discussed

1. *Topical anti-infectives may be applied orally, rectally, vaginally or to any body surface under specific conditions.*
2. *The effectiveness of a topical anti-infective must be balanced against its tissue destructiveness.*
3. *Anti-infectives may act either to inhibit, kill or retard the growth of microorganisms.*
4. *The phenol coefficient of an anti-infective is a measurement of its ability to kill microorganisms as compared to the effect of phenol.*
5. *The effectiveness of an anti-infective is dependent to a great extent on its correct use by the nurse and other health personnel.*

The antimicrobial drugs occupy a unique niche in the history of medicine. The development of the germ theory of disease was the starting point of a dramatic revolution in medicine, bringing about a long-overdue awareness of the importance of aseptic procedures and anti-infective drugs.

Drugs in this category are applied locally, that is, topically, although a few may also be administered systemically. Hundreds of chemical compounds having germicidal activity are available, but, unfortunately, many of these have a very limited effectiveness in the presence of serum or other organic matter, or else are excessively damaging to the tissues. Tissue damage, of course, is not of concern when such agents are employed for use in the disinfection of inanimate objects. On the other hand, corrosiveness, staining and other effects then become important considerations.

There are four chief classes of agents that will kill or inhibit microorganisms by topical action. We may classify them as follows:

Disinfectant or germicide. An agent that kills microorganisms capable of producing infection.

Bactericide. An agent that kills bacteria.

Bacteriostatic. A substance that inhibits or prevents growth of bacteria.

Antiseptic. A substance that either inhibits or kills microorganisms.

FACTORS INFLUENCING THE ACTION OF ANTI-INFECTIVES

Various factors may influence the effectiveness of disinfecting agents:

1. *The nature and concentration of the disinfectant.* While some agents are effective in relatively low concentrations, others require very high concentrations to affect the rate of growth and kill the microorganism. If such an agent is used in low concentrations, it may actually stimulate the growth of the microorganism instead of inhibiting it.

2. *The duration of treatment.* All the organisms are not killed at the same time, but rather there is a gradual decrease in the number of organisms in the medium.

3. *pH.* The acidity or alkalinity of the medium affects both the microorganism and the disinfectant. The optimum pH varies with the disinfectant.

4. *Temperature.* Disinfection is enhanced by an increase in temperature. In many cases heat alone is sufficient to produce disinfection.

5. *The nature of the organism.* The presence or absence of capsules or spores, the chemical composition, species, etc. all influence the effectiveness of the disinfectant.

6. *The presence of foreign matter.* Organic matter such as blood, pus and cell debris as well as other foreign materials can greatly decrease the effectiveness of certain chemical agents.

In using anti-infectives the nurse employs her knowledge of these factors and her knowledge about the particular agent in order to promote the desired antibacterial action. She uses the appropriate strength and length of time, based on the type of microorganism involved or suspected.

Articles to be disinfected should be thoroughly washed with soap and mechanical friction to remove foreign matter and reduce the bacterial flora. They should be rinsed and dried completely before being disinfected in order to remove soap and avoid dilution of the disinfectant.

Before applying a topical anti-infective to the skin or wound, the nurse should be sure that blood, pus and drainage are removed. Careful observations for signs of local irritation or hypersensitivity at the site of application should be made in addition to observations for effectiveness.

COMPARING ANTI-INFECTIVES

As more and more topical anti-infectives came into use, a practical method of comparing them was needed. The method used at the present time compares the anti-infective with phenol (see p. 133), which is used as a standard, and thus classifies these agents according to a known value.

The *phenol coefficient* is a term which expresses the bactericidal efficiency of a disinfectant as compared with that of phenol tested under identical conditions. To obtain the phenol coefficient figure, the dilution of the disinfectant that kills the organism in 10 minutes, but not in 5 minutes, is divided by the dilution of phenol that does likewise. A phenol coefficient greater than 1.0 indicates that the tested anti-infective is more effective than phenol under similar conditions. For example, a sample anti-infective may kill the organism in a 1:300 dilution, whereas phenol accomplishes the same in a 1:90 dilution. The phenol coefficient would then be:

$$\frac{sample}{phenol} = \frac{300}{90} = 3.3$$

The phenol coefficient is of only limited value because conditions of comparison may vary greatly in respect to some or all of the factors mentioned previously.

OXIDIZING AGENTS

Oxidizing agents are substances that undergo decomposition and liberate oxygen when in contact with organic material. The oxygen has a harmful effect on living matter, especially anaerobic bacteria. These agents are quite useful as antiseptics, deodorants and cleansing agents.

POTASSIUM PERMANGANATE, U.S.P., B.P. Potassium permanganate is commercially available as dark purple crystals that are readily soluble in water. It is a powerful oxidizing agent, and in the absence of organic matter it is superior in disinfectant power to phenol. When in contact with body fluids, however, it is rapidly reduced, thus losing some of its beneficial effects. The reduced compound, manganese dioxide (MnO_2), has a dark brown appearance in contrast to the purple color of the fresh solution. Any preparation in which this muddy brown precipitate is noted should not be employed for disinfectant purposes since it is practically useless.

Potassium permanganate has three therapeutic properties: it is bactericidal, oxidizing and astringent. The solution is used to cleanse suppurating wounds such as cancerous ulcerations, and for vaginal or bladder irrigations. It may be employed in the form of compresses, wet dressings or soaks in skin conditions and is especially useful in instances where there is secondary infection. For extensive dermatoses the entire body may be bathed in the solution. Dilute acids, such as lemon juice, may be used to remove brown stains on clothing and linens.

CONCENTRATION. 1 : 10,000–1 : 4000.

HYDROGEN PEROXIDE SOLUTION, U.S.P., B.P. Hydrogen peroxide solution is a colorless liquid with a slight odor. Its most important use is as an antibacterial agent, and it owes its activity to the release of oxygen.

The germicidal action of hydrogen peroxide is often greatly overestimated. Its action is quite short-lived and it must be in fairly concentrated solution to have any appreciable effect. The solution is used therapeutically to cleanse wounds, suppurating ulcers and similar conditions. Its actual value probably lies more in its ability to remove organic debris through its effervescent action than in its direct antibacterial effect. Because of its lack of toxicity, hydrogen peroxide is often the agent of choice for application to the oral mucous membranes. Prolonged use will cause some irritation of the mouth surfaces, however.

Hydrogen peroxide has been employed as a vaginal douche in the treatment of *Trichomonas* infections, but more effective therapeutic agents have largely replaced it at the present time.

Solutions of hydrogen peroxide decompose rapidly upon standing, and they should be stored in tight, light-resistant containers and kept in a cool place.

CONCENTRATION. 1.5–3%.

SODIUM PERBORATE, N.F. Sodium perborate occurs as a white powder which is stable in dry, cool air but rapidly decomposes with the liberation of oxygen in warm or moist air. It is likewise unstable in solution, decomposing to form sodium metaborate and hydrogen peroxide. The liberation of oxygen from solution, however, makes the solution useful in the treatment of lesions of the oral mucous membranes such as glossitis, gingivitis and stomatitis. In addition, the solution may be used as a wet wound dressing because of its antiseptic and deodorizing properties.

Occasionally the dry powder is applied to oral lesions as this form has some hemostatic properties.

MEDICINAL ZINC PEROXIDE, U.S.P. Medicinal zinc peroxide contains a mixture of zinc peroxide, zinc carbonate and zinc hydroxide. It is used as a disinfectant, astringent and deodorant for topical application to wounds, and is of especial benefit in wounds infected with anaerobic bacteria.

Upon application, medicinal zinc peroxide is slowly decomposed to liberate oxygen. The reduced compound, largely consisting of zinc oxide, remains at the site of application and exerts mild protective and astringent action.

Zinc peroxide dressings have been used for postoperative anorectal wounds and in addition have been placed in opened pleural cavities for the treatment of empyema. Zinc peroxide may be used in the form of a paste or suspension and applied to the gums for the treatment of gingivitis. Pastes of this compound have been used experimentally upon exposed, infected cancer sites with some benefit in the treatment of the secondary infection.

PHENOL AND RELATED COMPOUNDS

PHENOL, U.S.P., B.P. (CARBOLIC ACID). Depending upon the concentration used, phenol may have topical anesthetic, disinfectant or caustic properties when applied to the skin. Although phenol formerly was the most widely used disinfectant and it is the standard by which the effectiveness of other agents is measured, its use as a topical disinfectant is somewhat limited at the present time because of the availability of less caustic and equally effective agents.

phenol

Phenol and the compounds related to it are rapidly absorbed by bacteria and firmly bound to them. As a result, amino acids and other essential nutrients are lost from the microorganisms. This effect may be due to an alteration of the permeability of the cell wall, to a disturbance of intracellular metabolism, or to a combination of both effects. In high concentrations, phenols have a denaturing effect on all proteins.

Phenol is often incorporated into topical preparations for its local anesthetic effect. It exerts both antipruritic and antiseptic action.

Since a toxic effect may be obtained if phenol is absorbed systemically from topical preparations, it should not be applied to large, denuded areas. It is highly toxic if taken internally as a result of caustic erosion of the oral and gastric mucous membranes and the subsequent loss of tissue fluids. Shock and death may ensue if treatment is not begun immediately.

CONCENTRATION. 0.5–1%.

SAPONATED CRESOL SOLUTION, N.F., B.P. Cresol is a mixture of several forms of phenol. It is applied topically in the form of a soap solution or emulsion (well known under the trade name Lysol) because it is relatively insoluble in water.

When organic material is not present, saponated cresol solution has a phenol coefficient of 3.0. With organic material the phenol coefficient is decreased to 1.87, but cresol is still significantly more effective than phenol under similar circumstances.

Although cresol is less caustic than phenol, the general belief that it is less toxic has proved to be false. Many deaths have been reported from cresol poisoning.

The solution is employed for sterilizing instruments and skin. Occasionally it is still used as a vaginal douche; however, it has largely been replaced by less toxic agents.

CONCENTRATION. 1–5%.

RESORCINOL, U.S.P., B.P. Resorcinol is used almost exclusively in the treatment of skin diseases such as eczema, seborrhea of the scalp, ringworm and psoriasis. In addition to its antiseptic properties, resorcinol is useful for its keratolytic, exfoliating and antifungal effects when applied topically.

resorcinol

This compound is a primary irritant and in addition can produce a sensitization reaction, and severe allergic reactions have been noted upon its continued use. It may be absorbed systemically if used over large denuded areas, and exerts toxic effects especially in the case of infants and young children.

Resorcinol should be stored in a dark, tightly capped container.

CONCENTRATION. 1%.

HEXYLRESORCINOL, N.F. (S. T. 37). Hexylresorcinol is reported to have the highest bactericidal effect and the lowest toxicity of any of the substituted phenolic compounds. Its phenol coefficient has been given variously, ranging from 42 to 108.

This compound has a low surface tension and consequently is able to wet substances easily. These soaplike properties are in large part responsible for its effectiveness as a disinfectant. It should be stored in light-resistant containers.

Hexylresorcinol may be incorporated in soaps and disinfectants and may be taken orally to treat roundworm, hookworm and whipworm infestations (see p. 194).

CONCENTRATION. 1 : 1000 (topical use).

THYMOL, N.F., B.P. Thymol is employed topically as a disinfectant for the same purposes as phenol. It is more effective than phenol as a disinfectant when there is no organic material present; however, its efficiency is greatly reduced in the presence of large amounts of proteinaceous material.

It is incorporated into many topical preparations and mouthwashes for its antiseptic action. Its more agreeable odor and taste make it more acceptable than phenol in these preparations.

CONCENTRATION. 1-2%.

HEXACHLOROPHENE, U.S.P. Hexachlorophene is employed as a disinfectant in many soaps and other dermatologic formulations. It has a phenol coefficient of approximately 125.0.

hexachlorophene

Even when the compound is used daily over a prolonged period of time, no tissue reaction is seen on wounds and burned surfaces from the action of this agent. Preparations containing it are very useful as adjunctive treatment in the management of acne, furuncles, diaper rash, eczema, pyogenic dermatoses and similar conditions. When it is used over a period of time the residual bacterial count on the skin is significantly reduced.

Preparations should be applied to previously moistened skin which has been cleansed of blood and other organic matter.

Hexachlorophene is the active germicidal ingredient in Gamophen, Hex-o-san, Dial, Septisol and pHisoHex, among other preparations.

TOXICITY. In recent publications the FDA has warned against indiscriminate or prolonged use of the higher concentrations of hexachlorophene. It has been shown that this substance is absorbed through the skin, particularly in newborn infants. Animal studies have shown that pathologic changes i.e., nervous system cystic lesions, will occur if high blood levels are sustained. It is currently felt that cleansing agents containing the 3 per cent concentration of hexachlorophene i.e., pHisoHex, should not be routinely used for total body bathing of infants.

CONCENTRATION. 3%.

SALTS OF HEAVY METALS

Heavy metals are able to exert their antiseptic or antibacterial activity by combining with the protein components of microorganism cells, resulting in the precipitation of cellular protein. Although their effectiveness in this regard is certainly undisputed, they nevertheless have limited application in medicine because of their toxicity when in contact with human cells. If these agents are absorbed following application to large, denuded areas of skin, serious and even fatal heavy metal poisoning may result.

MERCURY PREPARATIONS

MERCURY BICHLORIDE, N.F., MERCURIC CHLORIDE, B.P. (CORROSIVE SUBLIMATE). Mercury bichloride has long been classed among the most potent and reliable disinfectants. Its highly toxic properties have greatly limited its use on the skin, although relatively weak solutions are still occasionally employed as a preoperative vaginal douche.

The chief use of mercury bichloride at present is in the disinfecting of inanimate objects such as dishes, bedpans and utensils. Its antiseptic action is greatly decreased by the presence of protein, sulfides, carbonates and many other substances both organic and inorganic.

Because of the availability of the tablets for use in the preparation of solutions, mercury bichloride has been used with suicidal and homicidal intent. If it is taken internally the symptoms may range from a mild gastritis with prompt recovery to severe necrosis of the gastrointestinal mucosa with resultant pain, vomiting and blood in the feces. The likelihood of death following ingestion of this drug depends upon the dose ingested, the form in which it was taken, the promptness with which vomiting is induced and subsequent therapy.

Less toxic mercury salts are administered as diuretics because of their effect on the proximal tubule cell enzymes (Chapter 19), and it may be expected that mercury bichloride will have similar effects on the kidney cells. Severe, irreversible kidney damage may result from the systemic absorption of this compound.

CONCENTRATION. 1:2000–1:1000.

PHENYLMERCURIC NITRATE, N.F., B.P. Phenylmercuric nitrate, an organic mercurial compound, may be employed both in solution and in ointment form for application to the skin and mucous membranes for its antiseptic properties.

When mercury is combined with an organic compound the toxicity is sufficiently decreased to permit its use on the skin. The same combination reduces the germicidal properties, however, so that this agent is not used as extensively as mercury bichloride for the disinfection of inanimate objects.

CONCENTRATION. 1:500.

MERBROMIN SOLUTION, N.F. (MERCURO-CHROME). Although the nonirritating and relatively nontoxic properties of merbromin make it a popular antiseptic solution for application to minor cuts and abrasions, its antiseptic activity is open to question. Some studies have reported that the efficacy of tinctures of merbromin is due chiefly to the alcohol content and that the aqueous solution cannot be counted upon to reduce the bacterial population of the skin by more than one-half.

CONCENTRATION. 1–2%.

THIMEROSAL, N.F. (MERTHIOLATE). Although the reports concerning the antibac-terial properties of thimerosal are somewhat varied, it is quite useful as a nonirritating bacteriostatic and fungistatic agent. Spore-forming bacteria are resistant to its action, however, as is true of most of the organic mercurials.

Solutions of thimerosal are applied to intact skin and mucous membranes and to wounds and abrasions, and are used for irrigating the mucous membranes of the nose, throat, eye and urethra.

CONCENTRATION. 1:1000.

NITROMERSOL, N.F. (METAPHEN). Since nitromersol has only slight protein-precipitating and astringent properties, it is nonirritating and relatively nontoxic. The combination of mercury with an organic chemical makes this compound safe for use on rubber and metallic instruments, and it is often used as a bacteriostatic agent for surgical instruments. Like thimerosal, this compound is not effective against spore-forming bacteria.

CONCENTRATION. 0.2–0.5%.

SILVER PREPARATIONS

SILVER NITRATE, U.S.P., B.P. Silver nitrate is an effective protein precipitant, and forms an eschar or crust upon the skin following topical application. The formation of this crust prevents any activity beyond the top surface layers, however. The precipitated albumin is at first white, but soon becomes darkened from the reduction of silver upon its surface.

Silver nitrate solutions are employed in several concentrations as genitourinary tract irrigants for the treatment of gonococcal infections and are instilled into the eyes of newborn infants for prophylactic therapy against gonococcal ophthalmia neonatorum. Many states require by law the application of silver nitrate in the eyes of all newborn infants; however, it is being replaced more and more by antibiotic ointments which are less irritating to the conjunctiva. After instillation in the eyes, physiologic saline is used to irrigate the eyes. Physiologic saline may also be used if healthy skin is accidentally affected.

Solutions of silver nitrate are also applied as wet dressings to aid in the healing of skin ulcers and to check the formation of excessive granulation tissue in wounds.

Stains on clothing or linens resulting from silver nitrate may be removed by first applying an iodine solution or tincture followed by a 5% solution of sodium thiosulfate to the stain.

Silver nitrate sticks may be used as a local hemostatic agent.

CONCENTRATION. 1%—ophthalmia neonatorum. 1:10,000–1:1000—bladder irrigation. 1:1000–1:750—wet dressings.

MILD SILVER PROTEIN, N.F. (ARGYROL, LUNARGEN, SILVOL). Mild silver protein is a colloidal solution that contains from 19 to 23 percent silver. When in combination with protein, the silver ions are released very slowly, so that this preparation is much less irritating than silver nitrate solution when applied to the skin. The slower liberation of the silver makes this combination much less effective as a disinfectant, however, and it has been largely replaced by more effective agents.

Silver salts do not produce severe toxicity symptoms upon oral ingestion since they are readily precipitated by the chloride ions in the stomach. Some gastrointestinal irritation is produced, however, which may be relieved by the subsequent administration of albumin or salt solution.

Upon prolonged application of silver salts to the skin or mucous membranes the silver is absorbed in sufficient quantities to produce argyria, that is, deposition of the silver salts in the tissues of the body giving the skin a permanent grayish or cyanotic hue. This can be distinguished from cyanosis by inspection of the fingernails, however.

CONCENTRATION. 19–23% silver.

STRONG SILVER PROTEIN (PROTARGIN). The strong silver protein preparation actually has a lower silver content (7.5–8.5%) than the mild solution; however, this preparation delivers more silver to the skin surface per unit time and thus produces an antiseptic effect somewhere between that of the mild

silver protein and silver nitrate solution. Strong silver protein is more irritating, however, and is no longer listed as an official preparation.

CONCENTRATION. 7.5–8.5% silver.

ZINC PREPARATIONS

ZINC SULFATE, U.S.P., B.P. Zinc sulfate solutions are used externally for their astringent activity. They have only mild antiseptic activity, however. They may be used as an astringent wash for the mucous membranes of the eye, nose, throat and genital tract or as a wet dressing for skin conditions.

Solutions of zinc sulfate must be buffered carefully, since in neutral or alkaline solutions the basic salt zinc hydroxide precipitates from solution. The solution should be discarded immediately if a precipitate appears.

CONCENTRATION. 0.1–1%—ophthalmic solution.
4% topical application to the skin.

ZINC OXIDE, U.S.P., B.P. Zinc oxide is used topically as a mild antiseptic and astringent in a wide variety of skin disorders. It may be incorporated into ointments, pastes, lotions or powders for application to the skin. A paste prepared from zinc oxide, gelatin, glycerin and water is used as a supportive and protective plaster for eczema and varicose ulcers.

CONCENTRATION. 8–20%.

HALOGENS

The halogens are fluorine, chlorine, bromine and iodine. All the halogens are potentially bacteriostatic agents, only chlorine and iodine are sufficiently nonirritating to be applied to the skin.

IODINE PREPARATIONS

IODINE TINCTURE, U.S.P. Elemental iodine is one of the most potent and useful of the available germicides, and one of the oldest in current use. Tincture of iodine was first used as an antiseptic in France in 1839, and was used in the American Civil War.

Tincture of iodine contains 2 per cent iodine and 2.4 per cent sodium iodide diluted in alcohol. The alcohol, which is necessary to dissolve the iodine, contributes somewhat to the irritating nature of this compound when applied to abraded tissues. Strong solutions may produce some tissue necrosis. The tincture may be used as a disinfectant for inanimate objects or applied to the skin. It also may be used to disinfect water. One drop of iodine tincture in one quart of water kills amebae and bacteria in 15 minutes. The phenol coefficient has been estimated at around 200.

The action of iodine tincture is not strictly limited to the skin surface since it is able to penetrate skin to some degree and reach subsurface abscesses.

CONCENTRATION. 2–7%.

STRONG IODINE SOLUTION, U.S.P. (LUGOL'S SOLUTION). Strong iodine solution is composed of 5 per cent iodine and 10 per cent potassium iodide in an aqueous solution. It is not as effective as the alcoholic tincture when applied to the skin surface, and its chief application in medicine is that of an iodine supplement to the diet. The solution may also be administered in higher doses to suppress the thyroid gland in the treatment of hyperthyroidism.

CONCENTRATION. 5% iodine.

IODOCHLORHYDROXYQUIN,   U.S.P. (VIOFORM). Although the chief use of iodochlorhydroxyquin is in the treatment of amebic dysentery (p. 183), it may be applied topically to treat various skin conditions. It exhibits antibacterial, antifungal and antipruritic properties when applied to the skin and may be used in the treatment of virtually every kind of eczema. Both water-soluble creams and ointments of iodochlorhydroxyquin are available commercially.

CONCENTRATION. 3%.

POVIDONE-IODINE SOLUTION, N.F. (BETADINE). Produced by the interaction of polyvinylpyrrolidone (PVP) and iodine, this compound is assumed to form a fine membrane on the skin when exposed to air. It is thought to act as a lethal curtain for the pathogens beneath it and for those deposited on its outer surface from the air above.

This preparation produces no appreciable pain or irritation when poured upon denuded surfaces and does not cause skin reactions. It has a long duration of action and maintains its germicidal activity in the presence of blood, pus, serum and proteinaceous materials.

The commercial surgical soap compound of povidone-iodine is frequently used as a surgical scrub, and the solution is used in bacterial and mycotic skin infections, thrush, stomatitis, tonsillitis, pharyngitis, vaginal moniliasis and *Trichomonas vaginalis* infections.

CONCENTRATION. 1–1.5%.

CHLORINE PREPARATIONS

Chlorine is a very potent germicide, and is widely used for the purification of water supplies. Because the element exists as a gas, and because in solution it is unstable, it is not often used in elemental form as an antiseptic. However, many chlorine compounds are available that slowly give off hypochlorous acid, which has a strong bactericidal effect, and these compounds can be used in the disinfection of certain inanimate objects, and in surgery.

SODIUM   HYPOCHLORITE SOLUTION, N.F., (DAKIN'S SOLUTION). Although it is inactivated in the presence of large amounts of organic material, sodium hypochlorite solution is of some value as an oxidizing and antiseptic agent. It may be used for the disinfection of inanimate objects such as thermometers or glassware which are not affected by the bleaching action of the solution.

The oxidizing properties of the solution render it quite effective as a deodorizing wash. It may be used as a foot-bath for the prophylaxis of athlete's foot, and is effective against amebae, gram-negative bacteria and spore-forming bacteria. Solutions are unstable and should be freshly prepared.

CONCENTRATION. 5% solution diluted with 4–10 parts water.

DILUTED SODIUM HYPOCHLORITE SOLUTION, N.F., B.P. (MODIFIED DAKIN'S SOLUTION). The diluted solution of sodium hypochlorite has generally the same uses as the stronger solution. It is less irritating to the skin, however, and is preferred when the solution is to come in contact with living tissue. When used in wet dressings on wounds, care should be taken to avoid contact of the solution with healthy skin. It is inactivated in the presence of pus or tissue fluids.

A small amount of sodium bicarbonate is added to the solution to neutralize the acidity. The sodium bicarbonate must be added shortly prior to use since the neutralized solution deteriorates much more rapidly than does the original solution. Solutions should be freshly prepared before use.

CONCENTRATION. Full strength or diluted 1:4 with water.

CHLORAMINE-T. This organic compound retains the oxidizing properties of chlorine but is less irritating to the skin than sodium hypochlorite solution. In addition, it has the advantages of a longer duration of action, and a relative resistance to inactivation by organic material.

Chloramine-T has been employed as an oxidizing and antiseptic mouth wash, and for irrigation of the bladder, uterus and other internal body cavities. It has also been used to purify water, in which case the unpleasant taste can be masked by the addition of a little citric acid.

CONCENTRATION. 0.1–0.2%.

HALAZONE, N.F. Like chloramine-T, halazone is composed of chloride bound to an organic molecule. It is primarily used for the sterilization of drinking water. Since the antibacterial activity of halazone is greatly enhanced by the presence of alkali, the commercial tablets contain, in addition to halazone, sodium chloride with either sodium carbonate or sodium borate. The tablets should be allowed to stand in the water 30 minutes before drinking.

CONCENTRATION. 4–9 mg. (1–2 tablets) per liter.

DYES

Many dyes are quite useful in medicine as antiseptic and antifungal agents and in addition some have wound-healing properties.

In using dyes, staining of the skin is inevitable, but the patient should be assured that the discoloration will eventually disappear. The nurse should be especially observant, since some dyes and staining may obscure signs of irritation and inflammation. The nurse should take precautionary measures to prevent staining of linen and clothing.

Based on their chemical structures, the medicinal dyes may be classified into three groups: triphenylmethane, acridine and azo dyes.

TRIPHENYLMETHANE (ROSANILINE) DYES

METHYLROSANILINE CHLORIDE, U.S.P., CRYSTAL VIOLET, B.P. (GENTIAN VIOLET, METHYL VIOLET). Methylrosaniline chloride is quite useful as a bactericidal agent, and is particularly effective against the gram-positive organisms. It has little or no effect against gram-negative organisms or the tubercle bacilli, however.

When the dye is in contact with necrotic tissue a precipitate is formed, so that it is of value in the treatment of necrotic wounds. It is used to treat burns, otitis, cystitis, urethritis, superficial ulcers, decubiti, pruritus ani, thrush and similar disorders.

Aqueous solutions will stain clothing and linens; the stains may be removed by washing or in some cases by the application of dilute ammonia solution.

CONCENTRATION. 1%.

CARBOL-FUCHSIN SOLUTION, N.F. (CASTELLANI'S PAINT, CARFUSIN). Although this preparation has largely been replaced, it is still occasionally employed in the treatment of superficial fungus infections, especially athlete's foot. The solution is a mixture of fuchsin, phenol, resorcinol and boric acid in an acetone-alcohol-water solution.

ACRIDINE (FLAVINE) DYES

PROFLAVINE HEMISULPHATE, B.P. Solutions of proflavine hemisulphate are relatively nontoxic and nonirritating when applied to the skin and mucous membranes. They are often used as antiseptic washes on open wounds. Upon prolonged use, proflavine may cause tissue damage and necrosis, thus reversing the healing process in wounds.

These solutions deteriorate rapidly in sunlight, so they should be stored in dark, tight containers and should be discarded when turbidity develops.

CONCENTRATION. 0.1%.

ACRIFLAVINE. Although acriflavine is not a potent bactericide, it is quite effective as a bacteriostatic agent and is applied to open wounds for this purpose. It is somewhat more irritating than proflavine, however, and is more toxic if absorbed. Rarely, acriflavine may be employed as a bladder irrigation, or for the treatment of impetigo.

CONCENTRATION. 0.1% (topical).
1:5000 (bladder irrigation).

AZO DYES

SCARLET RED OINTMENT. Unlike the acridine dyes, the azo dyes have a stimulating effect on the growth of epithelium. Scarlet red ointment is used to aid in the healing of clean, dry ulcerations. It loses its activity rapidly in the presence of pus or tissue fluid. The ointment should be applied to the edges of the ulceration rather than over the entire denuded area since the healing effect is most efficient in this area.

The use of scarlet red ointment is somewhat limited at present, in part because of its extensive staining properties.

CONCENTRATION. 5%.

PHENAZOPYRIDINE HYDROCHLORIDE (PYRIDIUM). Pyridium is administered orally for its topical anesthetic and antiseptic effect on the mucosa of the urinary tract. Urinary frequency and discomfort are relieved following administration of the drug. Patients should be informed that the dye will cause a reddish brown discoloration of the urine. The nurse should also be aware of this since the reddish discoloration of urine may cause her to suspect hematuria. Pyridium may be administered alone or in combination with other urinary antiseptics.

DOSE. 100 mg. orally three or four times daily.

SURFACE-ACTIVE AGENTS

The surface-active agents, or detergents, are considerably more effective than soaps in their wetting and emulsifying properties. The reduction in surface tension that they cause enables these agents to penetrate surface films and aid in the mechanical removal of debris.

Some surface-active agents also have bactericidal or bacteriostatic potency in addition to their mechanical effects, and are effective as irrigants or antiseptic washes. Their antiseptic properties are not sufficient to render them effective if their ability to partially remove harmful substances by surface action is not employed, however. The presence of organic material inhibits the effectiveness of these agents.

CATIONIC DETERGENTS

The cationic, or positively charged, detergents generally have greater antiseptic power than the anionic agents. Although they are not effective as germicides, they are bacteriostatic for both gram-positive and gram-negative microorganisms. The best known of these agents are the quaternary ammonium compounds.

These agents may be used as antiseptic storage solutions, although alone they are not effective for instruments that must be "cold sterilized"; a more potent germicide is generally employed for this purpose.

The surface-active properties of the cationic detergents render them useful as antiseptic washes, as bladder irrigants, to moisten catheters prior to insertion, and to aid in the liquefaction of mucus when administered along with other inhaled medications.

The cationic detergents are rapidly inactivated by the anionic detergents and soaps, so that these must be completely removed prior to application of these agents.

These preparations should be stored in light-resistant containers.

BENZALKONIUM CHLORIDE, U.S.P., B.P. (ZEPHIRAN CHLORIDE). Benzalkonium chloride is a mixture of alkyldimethylbenzylammonium chlorides of the general structure shown herewith. The R represents a mixture of the alkyls from C_8H_{17} to $C_{18}H_{37}$.

$$C_8H_{17} \text{ to } C_{18}H_{37} - \overset{+}{N} \overset{CH_3}{\underset{CH_3}{\overbrace{}}} CH_2 - \bigcirc \quad \cdot Cl^-$$

benzalkonium chloride

This compound is nonirritating to the skin and has found many uses as a topical antiseptic agent. It may be applied to the skin, mucous membranes or open wounds. It is used to treat superficial injuries or fungal infections, for preoperative disinfection of the skin, for instillation into the eye, vagina, bladder or urethra, and for irrigation of deep, infected wounds. It is often used as a storage solution for instruments.

CONCENTRATION.   1 : 5000–1 : 750.

BENZETHONIUM CHLORIDE, N.F. (PHEMEROL CHLORIDE). Although the properties of benzethonium chloride closely resemble those of benzalkonium chloride, its primary use has been as an antiseptic agent applied to the mucous membranes of the eye and nose, and as a local antiseptic for intact skin. It is prepared commercially as a solution and a tincture.

CONCENTRATION.   1 : 100–1 : 500   (skin) 1 : 4000–1 : 2500 (ophthalmic and nasal).

CETYLPYRIDINIUM CHLORIDE, N.F. (CEEPRYN CHLORIDE, INCORPORATED IN CEPACOL LIQUID AND LOZENGES). Cetylpyridinium chloride is used chiefly as a topical antiseptic for small skin abrasions. Occasionally it has been employed as a preoperative antiseptic or for irrigation of body cavities. Although it would be effective as an antiseptic storage solution, it is usually not used for this purpose.

CONCENTRATION.   1 : 10,000–1 : 1000.

METHYLBENZETHONIUM CHLORIDE, N.F. (DIAPARENE CHLORIDE).   As its commercial name suggests, methylbenzethonium chloride is used primarily in the disinfection of diapers. It is also applied topically in the form of an ointment for the prevention of diaper rash.

Tablets are available which may be added to a pail of water for disinfection of diapers. All soap should be removed carefully prior to placing the diapers in this solution, however, since like the other cationic detergents Diaparene is readily inactivated in solutions containing soap.

CONCENTRATION.   1 : 250.

ANIONIC DETERGENTS

The anionic detergents are salts of high molecular weight acids. Unlike soaps, which also come under the heading of anionic surface-active agents, these agents are not precipitated in hard water or by other inorganic cations. The anionic detergents are inactivated by high molecular weight cations such as the cationic detergents, and the two types must never be applied simultaneously. The anionic detergents generally are inferior to the cationic agents in their antiseptic properties, but they are effective nevertheless in the mechanical removal of bacteria and debris from the skin and mucous membranes.

SODIUM TETRADECYL SULFATE (SOTRADECOL). Sodium tetradecyl sulfate has been incorporated in various external preparations for its surface-active properties in order to enhance the penetrability of medications. It has been used as a sclerosing agent for the treatment of varicose veins although it may be quite painful when used in this way. Sensitization has occurred only rarely with this drug.

CONCENTRATION.   1–5%.

PHISODERM.   This commercial preparation has the primary advantage of being adjusted to correspond to the pH of normal skin. It is nonirritating, and in emulsion form it is somewhat effective as a topical antiseptic. It may be used to replace soap entirely on sensitive or dry skin.

PHISOHEX.   Like pHisoderm, this preparation contains an anionic detergent in a buffered emulsion, but in addition pHisoHex contains 3% hexachlorophene. It may be used as a preoperative scrub, as a surgeons' scrub, as an antiseptic wash for abraded skin, in infants' baths, and as prophylactic therapy for acne or other skin conditions.

When used as an antiseptic wash, a few drops are rubbed on previously moistened hands or arms, or one teaspoonful to one tablespoonful may be added to the bath water. For irrigations, 5 to 15 cc. is added to one pint of water.

The questions raised concerning the potential toxicity of this cleansing agent are noted previously in the chapter under Hexachlorophene.

MISCELLANEOUS AGENTS

Ethyl alcohol, U.S.P., B.P. (alcohol, ethanol, grain alcohol). In addition to its oral uses, ethyl alcohol is quite an effective agent when applied topically. It is most effective as an antiseptic in 70% concentration. Unlike most topical agents, solutions of higher concentrations lose some effect as antiseptic preparations.

Because of its ability to precipitate cellular protein, alcohol has some value as an astringent. It is quite useful in the skin care of bedridden patients and the prevention of decubitus ulcers. Because of its drying effect on the skin, its use should be avoided if the skin is already dry, since cracking of the skin may occur; an emollient should be used on dry skin. Since alcohol evaporates readily it is usually the agent of choice for the sponging of febrile patients.

Although there has been much controversy concerning the effectiveness of alcohol as an antiseptic on rubber stoppers of multiple dose vials and on the skin prior to injection, it continues to be the practical agent of choice for this purpose. Some studies have shown it to be grossly ineffective unless it remains in contact with microorganisms for at least one-half hour, so that its benefits—if any—on rubber stoppers is that of flushing away dirt or debris. Its effect on the skin is likewise negligible. It is believed by some authorities that alcohol may remove skin lipids that are bactericidal to

pathogens on the skin; alcohol, therefore, may promote rather than combat bacterial growth.

> **CONCENTRATION.** 25–30% (sponging of febrile patients).
> 70% (antiseptic).

Isopropyl alcohol, N.F. Because isopropyl alcohol does not have to be recorded as taxable alcohol and is not denatured for external use, it is used by many institutions instead of ethyl alcohol. In contrast to ethyl alcohol, solutions of isopropyl alcohol of increasing strength are increasingly antiseptic. It is less corrosive to surgical instruments than is ethyl alcohol, thus is preferred for storage. It is considerably more toxic if accidentally ingested, however.

> **CONCENTRATION.** 75–100%.

Formaldehyde solution, U.S.P., B.P. (formalin). Formaldehyde solution contains not less than 37% formaldehyde with a small amount of methanol added to prevent polymerization. Formaldehyde is approximately equivalent to phenol in germicidal properties; however, it is irritating to the skin, and is rarely used as a topical antiseptic. It is used as a deodorant, to disinfect bedpans and surgical equipment, as a cold sterilizer solution, and as a fumigant. It may be used as a fixing agent for tissue specimens.

The Bard-Parker solution for cold sterilization contains formaldehyde, isopropyl alcohol and antirust tablets. If instruments are allowed to remain in the solution for 12 hours all organisms, including spores, may be presumed to be killed.

> **CONCENTRATION.** 0.5–40%.

Boric acid, U.S.P., B.P. Boric acid may be used in the form of solutions, ointments or dusting powders for application to the skin and mucous membranes. Toxic reactions may result due to the absorption of this drug if it is applied repeatedly to large, denuded areas. It has largely been replaced for this purpose by equally effective and less toxic agents.

> **CONCENTRATION.** 2% (eye).
> 4% (skin and mucous membranes).

NITROFURAZONE, N.F. (FURACIN). Nitrofurazone has been shown to have bacteriostatic and bactericidal activity and is effective both in vitro and in vivo against a variety of gram-negative and gram-positive microorganisms. It appears to interfere with essential enzyme systems within bacterial cells, and is effective even where the invading microorganisms have acquired resistance to the sulfonamides or antibiotics.

nitrofurazone

It may be applied to superficial mixed infections, in the treatment of burns, to promote healing by encouraging the growth of healthy granulation tissue, for the treatment of nonspecific urethritis, for acute or chronic otitis media and for ophthalmic infections.

Continued application of nitrofurazone is often complicated by the development of drug sensitivity.

Discoloration from exposure to light may occur, but this does not affect its effectiveness.

CONCENTRATION. 0.2%.

FURAZOLIDONE, N.F. (FUROXONE). Furazolidone is used in the treatment of vaginal and intestinal infections. It is reported to be effective against *Shigella* and *Salmonella* infections of the gastrointestinal tract. For this purpose it is given orally in the form of a liquid or tablets in a dose of 100 mg. four times daily.

For use in *Trichomonas* vaginitis or in mixed trichomonal and monilial vaginitis, furazolidine is often combined with nifuroxime under the brand name of Tricofuron. This agent is available as a vaginal powder and as suppositories. Sensitization may occur to this drug, in which case treatment should be discontinued and a cleansing douche administered.

Furazolidone may cause flushing, fever and a sensation of chest constriction if the patient ingests alcohol during or within four days of administration. It may also act as a MAO-inhibitor when used in large, prolonged doses.

CONCENTRATION (TRICOFURON).
0.1% (powder).
0.25% (suppositories).

TRICLOBISONIUM CHLORIDE. Triclobisonium is an organic compound with antimicrobial activity against a wide variety of microorganisms, including *Trichomonas* and *Candida albicans*. It is the active ingredient in Trib vaginal suppositories and cream and in the topical ointment and cream, which are sold under the trade name Triburon.

The vaginal preparations are indicated for use in infections produced by the previously mentioned microorganisms and *Haemophilus vaginalis,* staphylococci and streptococci. They are particularly effective when used preoperatively, post partum and following such procedures as cauterization, conization and irradiation.

Triburon topical ointment and cream may be used against many microorganisms commonly found in wound infections and may be applied prophylactically to burns, wounds and skin grafts.

Sensitization phenomena, although rare, do occur. If urticaria or rashes appear, the drug should be withdrawn.

CONCENTRATION. Trib Vaginal Cream—0.1%.
Trib Vaginal Suppositories—0.1% (one suppository vaginally morning and night).
Triburon Ointment—0.1%.
Triburon Hydrocortisone Cream (triclobisonium 0.1%, hydrocortisone 1%).

ANTIFUNGAL AGENTS

Fungal infections are difficult to correct because of the tendency of fungi to spore formation. Patients need much support and encouragement during the prolonged course of treatment. It is important that the nurse instruct the patient and his family in measures to prevent the further spread of the infection.

TRIACETIN (ENZACTIN). Triacetin, or glyceryl triacetate, is frequently employed in the treatment of superficial fungal infections of the skin, hair and nails. Although most fungi are quite sensitive to the drug and do not appear to become resistant to it, *Candida albicans* is sensitive only to high concentrations and requires a longer period of treatment. The action of triacetin is dependent upon the release of acetic acid by the action of esterases, enzymes present in the organisms and in human tissue fluids.

Sensitivity reactions have been noted following prolonged therapy. Triacetin is available in the form of aerosols, ointments, powders and liquids.

CONCENTRATION. 25–33%.

CHLORQUINALDOL (STEROSAN). Chlorquinaldol, like triacetin, is applied to the skin in the treatment of various fungal infections. It is especially effective when combined with oral antifungal therapy in the form of griseofulvin. It is available as a cream and an ointment.

CONCENTRATION. 3%.

CHLORDANTOIN (SPOROSTACIN). Chlordantoin is applied in the form of a lotion or cream to treat fungal infections of the skin or vagina. Sensitivity reactions have been observed with therapy.

CONCENTRATION. 1%.

TOLNAFTATE (TINACTIN). Tolnaftate is a new topical drug claimed to eliminate a wide variety of common pathogenic fungi from the skin. It appears to be useful, especially in superficial fungal infections resistant to other topical agents. Patients treated unsuccessfully with keratolytic agents, undecylenic acid preparations and with oral griseofulvin frequently will respond to tolnaftate solution.

Tolnaftate is inactive systemically, does not produce sensitivity and does not ordinarily cause local irritation upon application to intact or broken skin. It is indicated in the treatment of tinea infections of all parts of the body. It is not effective against *Candida albicans* infections.

As yet it is not known whether susceptible fungi can acquire a resistance to tolnaftate.

CONCENTRATION. 1% solution in a propylene glycol base.

UNDECYLENIC ACID, N.F. This unsaturated fatty acid has considerable antifungal and antibacterial activity when applied topically, and for this reason has been employed quite extensively in powders and ointments to treat conditions such as athlete's foot and various other topical fungal infections.

Its main advantage is that it is not irritating to skin or mucous membranes when applied in the suggested concentrations. Reports of its effectiveness vary greatly, however, and some cases of athletes' foot can persist for a long time despite intensive treatment with preparations containing undecylenic acid.

CONCENTRATION. Mucous membranes —1%.
Skin—5 to 10%.

OTHER ANTIFUNGAL AGENTS

GENERIC NAME	TRADE NAME	CONTENTS
Caprylic compound	Naprylate	10% sodium caprylate 5% zinc caprylate
Zinc undecylenate ointment	Desenex, Undesol, Undex	20% zinc undecylenate 5% undecylenic acid
Propionate compound	Propion Gel	10% calcium propionate 10% sodium propionate
Propionate-caprylate mixture	Sopronol	Mixture of the zinc, calcium, sodium salts of propionic and caprylic acids

SCABICIDES

Scabicides are a class of topical anti-infectives employed for the treatment of scabies, a skin disease caused by the mite *Sarcoptes scabiei*, usually under poor hygienic conditions. The main symptom is pruritus, which may result in secondary infection due to skin breakdown from scratching.

Application of the drugs will relieve the present infection, but hygienic measures must be taken to prevent subsequent invasion by the parasites. All articles of clothing should be sterilized before reuse following an infection. The source of the infestation should be determined and possible contacts should be located and treated, if necessary.

BENZYL BENZOATE LOTION, U.S.P., B.P. (BENYLATE, ALBACIDE). This mixture of benzyl benzoate with soap and isopropyl alcohol is widely used as a treatment for scabies. The lotion is applied vigorously for five minutes with a shaving brush after a thorough scrubbing of the entire body with soap and a ten-minute soaking in a bath at 100° F. After the first application dries, a second one is put on and a bath taken in 24 hours. The treatment kills larvae as well as mature forms, but the eggs are somewhat more resistant, and at times an additional treatment may be necessary.

Calamine lotion may be used as an adjunct to therapy if areas of the skin are irritated.

CONCENTRATION.   25%.

GAMMA BENZENE HEXACHLORIDE, U.S.P., B.P. (LINDANE, HEXACHLOROCYCLOHEXANE, KWELL). This drug is used topically as a lotion or ointment to treat scabies and louse infestation. For body infestation, a single liberal application left in place for 24 hours and then washed off thoroughly is usually sufficient to control the infestation. If necessary, the treatment may be repeated in four days. Prolonged treatment is unnecessary and undesirable because of the toxicity and absorbability of this compound.

CONCENTRATION.   1%.

CROTAMITON (EURAX).   Crotamiton is quite effective as a topical scabicide and in addition possesses antipruritic action which is useful in the treatment of a wide variety of skin diseases. The ointment or lotion is applied to the entire body, excluding the head, then reapplied 24 hours later to insure removal of all the mites.

CONCENTRATION.   10%.

CHLOROPHENOTHANE, U.S.P. (DDT, DICOPHANE).   Chlorophenothane, in addition to its household use as an insecticide, finds some clinical application in the treatment of mite infestations and pediculosis. For the treatment of head or pubic lice, the powder is rubbed into the hair and allowed to remain for several days. For the treatment of body lice, the underclothes are thoroughly dusted with the powdered preparations. One application is usually sufficient, although the treatment may be repeated in a week if necessary. Oily preparations are readily absorbed and are too toxic for medicinal use.

CONCENTRATION.   5–10%.

QUESTIONS FOR DISCUSSION AND REVIEW

1. Which topical anti-infectives are useful for:
   a. vaginal irrigations?
   b. ophthalmic infections?
   c. fungal infections?
2. What anti-infectives are used in your hospital for:
   a. disinfecting bedpans?

    b. disinfecting and storing thermometers?
    c. cleaning units?
    d. surgical scrubs?
    e. disinfecting operating rooms?
    f. cold sterilization of instruments?
    g. storage of instruments?

3. In what strength and in what length of time should the anti-infectives indicated in the previous question be used?

4. What would be the significance of a phenol coefficient of 6.0? What possible uses would there be for such an anti-infective? What special properties must be considered before it may be used on the skin, mucous membranes or in the eye?

5. What topical anti-infectives would be useful for cleaning a badly infected wound? Which would have little or no usefulness?

6. What precautions must be taken before using Zephiran as a topical anti-infective? Why?

7. What hygienic measures should you teach a patient who has:

    a. monilial vaginitis?
    b. athlete's foot?
    c. scabies?
    d. pediculosis?

BIBLIOGRAPHY

AMA Drug Evaluations. Chicago, American Medical Association, 1971.

Bettley, F. R.: Some effects of soap on the skin. *Brit. Med. J., 1*:1675, 1960.

Brunner, L. S., et al.: *Textbook of Medical-Surgical Nursing*. 2nd Ed. Philadelphia, J. B. Lippincott Co., 1970.

Carney, R. G.: Topical use of antibiotics. *J.A.M.A., 186*:646, 1963.

Claudia, M., Sr.: TLC and sulfamylon for burned children. *Amer. J. Nurs., 69*:755, (April) 1969.

Done, A. K.: Boric acid in hospitals. *J.A.M.A., 189*:336, 1964.

Edgeworth, D.: Nursing and asepsis in the modern hospital. *Nurs. Outlook, 13*:54, (June) 1963.

Fox, C. L., Jr.: Silver sulfadiazine—a new topical therapy for pseudomonas in burns. *Arch. Surg., 96*:184, 1968.

Govoni, L. E. and Hayes, J. E.: *Drugs and Nursing Implications*. 2nd Ed. New York, Appleton-Century-Crofts, 1971.

Henley, N. L.: Sulfamylon for burns. *Amer. J. Nurs., 69*:2122, (October) 1969.

Hugo, W. B.: The mode of action of antiseptics. *J. Pharm. Pharmacol., 9*:145, 1957.

Kretzer, M. P., et al.: Effective use of antiseptics and disinfectants. *R.N., 32*:48, (May) 1969.

Kundsin, R. B.: Antiseptics and disinfectants. *Practitioner, 200*:15, 1968.

Lentx, M., Seaton, R. and Macmillan, B.: Silver Nitrate treatment of thermal burns. *J. Trauma, 6*:399, 1966.

Pories, W. J., et al.: Acceleration of healing with zine sulfate. *Ann. Surg., 165*:432, (March) 1967.

Reddish, G. F. (ed.): *Antiseptics, Disinfectant, Fungicides and Chemical and Physical Sterilization.* 2nd Ed. Philadelphia, Lea and Febiger, 1957.

Richards, R. C.: Some practical aspects of surgical skin preparation. *Amer. J. Surg., 100*:575, 1963.

Rodman, M. J.: Drugs for treating skin infections. *R.N., 28*:77, (February) 1965.

Shafer, K. N., et al.: *Medical-Surgical Nursing.* 5th Ed. St. Louis, C. V. Mosby Co., 1971.

Shaw, B. L.: Current therapy for burns. *R.N., 34*:33, (March) 1971.

Smith, D. T., Conant, N. F. and Willett, H. P. (eds.): *Zinsser Microbiology.* 14th Ed. New York, Appleton-Century-Crofts, 1968.

Spaulding, E. H. and Emmons, E. K.: Chemical disinfection. *Amer. J. Nurs., 58*:1238, 1958.

Thompson, L. R.: Evaluating disinfectants. *Amer. J. Nurs., 62*:82, (January) 1962.

Thompson, L. R.: Thermometer disinfection. *Amer. J. Nurs., 63*:113, (February) 1963.

Taylor, J. W. et al.: For effective thermometer disinfection. *Nurs. Outlook, 14*:56, (February) 1966.

Wexler, L.: Gamma Benzene Hexachloride in treatment of pediculosis and scabies. *Amer. J. Nurs., 69*:565, (March) 1969.

White, A. W., Handler, P. and Smith, E. L.: *Principles of Biochemistry.* 3rd Ed. New York, McGraw-Hill Book Co., 1964.

Wood, M., Kenny, H. A. and Price, W. R.: Silver nitrate treatment of burns. Technique and controlling principles. *Amer. J. Nurs., 66*:518, 1966.

Chapter 9 Systemic Anti-infectives

Important Concepts Discussed

1. *Microorganisms often have the ability to destroy or inhibit each other. Antibiotics are products of living microorganisms that exert a deleterious effect on other microorganisms.*

2. *Slight alterations in the chemical structure of an antibiotic can have notable effects upon the incidence of side effects and sensitivity reactions experienced by the recipient of the drug.*

3. *A broad-spectrum antibiotic is effective against many strains of microorganisms; a narrow-spectrum antibiotic is effective against a limited number of microorganisms.*

4. *Sulfonamides owe their antibacterial effectiveness to their chemical resemblance to para-aminobenzoic acid (PABA), a substance needed for microorganism metabolism. Normal utilization of PABA is inhibited when sulfonamides are present.*

5. *Nursing action is directed toward promotion of optimum effectiveness and prevention of side effects.*

Several classes of therapeutic agents fall into the group of systemic anti-infectives. We will consider the classes separately.

ANTIBIOTICS

An antibiotic is a substance produced by living cells that is detrimental to the life activities of other organisms. The term, although originally restricted to the metabolic products of microorganisms, now includes certain synthetic and semisynthetic variants of these products.

HISTORY

Since World War II an extraordinary amount of basic research has been directed toward the search for microbial products that are of primary importance as antibiotics. These investigations have resulted in the introduction of many new types of antibiotics—and the end is nowhere in sight.

The relatively recent interest and research in antibiotic therapy has developed from the discovery by Sir Alexander Fleming in 1928 that an obscure mold, *Penicillium*, produces a potent substance (which he named penicillin) that is naturally destructive to many disease-producing microorganisms. Penicillin still ranks as one of the most widely used antibiotics in the control of infectious diseases, but many other antibiotics discovered since penicillin have attained a high rank in medicine.

CLASSIFICATION

Antibiotics can be classified according to their activity against the various classes of microorganisms—gram-positive and gram-negative bacteria, rickettsiae, viruses, spirochetes, fungi and protozoans. Antibiotics that have shown in vitro effectiveness against many strains or classes of organisms are referred to as "broad-spectrum" antibiotics, while those effective against only one or two classes are referred to as having a "narrow spectrum." This general classification, however, should not be used as a guide to the therapeutic application of antibiotics without taking cognizance of many other factors such as the disease being treated, the condition of the patient and individual sensitivity problems.

In addition, antibiotics may be only inhibitory (*bacteriostatic*), or they may have lethal (*bactericidal*) effects on the microorganisms, depending on the susceptibility of the invading microorganism and the concentration of the antibiotics at the site of infection.

RESISTANCE

The susceptibility of microorganisms to antibiotics may vary considerably from strain to strain, and variations in resistance may occur within an individual strain. The development of resistant strains has been given much study; the phenomenon may be explained merely by the survival of resistant strains which at first were not very apparent among the other nonresistant varieties, or, less probably, by the ability of organisms to form resistant strains by spontaneous mutation or adaptation.

The susceptibility or resistance of a specific invading organism can be determined by noting inhibition of bacterial growth around an antibiotic-containing disc on a culture medium, whereas a more accurate comparison of microorganism susceptibility to the antibiotic can be determined by serial dilution tests. In the serial dilution test the concentration of antibiotic relative to the number of microorganisms is varied to determine the concentration necessary to inhibit the growth of the organism. These in vitro tests are generally valid and are helpful guides to the choice of the right antibiotic. The only disadvantage is the time it takes to culture the organism on plates, since very often it may be dangerous to delay therapy until the culture can be read. In most cases treatment is instituted using a broad-spectrum antibiotic; then a change is made subsequently if the results of the in vitro tests make it seem advisable.

CHOOSING AN ANTIBIOTIC

Before deciding to treat a patient with an antibiotic, certain considerations need to be taken into account. Among these, the susceptibility of the responsible organisms is in the forefront. Other points to be considered are: the increasing incidence of resistant bacteria, the possibility of complication arising from each antibiotic and the manner of dealing with them, and the history of the patient with regard to allergic manifestations. Obviously the lowest dose compatible with effective treatment is desirable when administering antibiotics.

The concentration of an antibiotic that is attainable in body fluids may be useful in judging the relative merits of different preparations of the same drug (i.e., oral route vs. parenteral, various salts, etc.), but blood level is not synonymous with antibacterial activity. Indeed, a low blood level may well be more effective against a susceptible organism in one case than a relatively high blood level in another infection where the organism is only moderately susceptible. Then, too, blood levels may be misleading because bacterial infections are often localized in tissues other than blood, or in organized abscesses or areas of necrotic tissue with a poor blood supply. Blood levels in themselves do not necessarily provide adequate information about the effectiveness of the antibiotic at the site of infection.

Some anti-infectives will pass the blood-brain barrier, while others will not; some are excreted rapidly and thus attain high concentrations in the urine, but inadequate levels in the blood or tissues; some are almost completely absorbed from the gastrointestinal tract and others are not absorbed at all. Prior to choosing an antibiotic, the physician must become familiar not only with the effectiveness of the drug against the causative organism, but with the pharmacodynamics of drug absorption, utilization and excretion.

COMBINATIONS

There are very few clearly substantiated cases for combination therapy with antibiotics. One of the few well-documented indications is the concurrent administration of penicillin and streptomycin. In many cases antagonism may develop between two active agents so that the combination would be less effective than either drug given alone. Antagonism of this sort occurs in the concurrent use of penicillin and chloramphenicol, whereas in other cases such as the combination of erythromycin, lincomycin and/or chloramphenicol the second antibiotic employed adds nothing to the effect, yet the patient is exposed to the side effects of two drugs.

PROBLEMS IN ANTIBIOTIC THERAPY

A number of lines of action have been tried to prevent the gastrointestinal disturbances that often follow oral antibiotic therapy. Substances such as sodium hexametaphosphate and citric acid have been used to enhance the absorption of some antibiotics, e.g., the tetracyclines, and to enable the prescribing of a lower dose. Clinical trials have not fully substantiated the theoretically enhanced absorption, however.

Another problem in therapy has been the discomfort and diarrhea caused by second-ary infections due to antibiotic-resistant bacteria or fungi often present in the intestines. These microorganisms are ordinarily kept in check by the normal flora of the intestinal tract, but when the normal flora is inhibited by the antibiotics, a free field is left for the resistant pathogens. Once firmly established, such resistant microorganisms are difficult to eradicate. In the event of overgrowth of fungi, notably *Candida albicans,* therapy with nystatin (Chapter 18) is effective, and has been recommended for prophylactic purposes as a concomitant of all oral therapy with the tetracyclines, chloramphenicol or neomycin.

NURSING IMPLICATIONS

ALLERGIC REACTIONS. The possibility that a patient may have an allergic reaction to an antibiotic, or to some other drug, is a major concern of the nurse. The nurse is often the first to detect the signs of allergy, and she should know the more subtle signs as well as the more dramatic signs and symptoms of anaphylactic shock. Allergy may be indicated by formation of a wheal at the site of injection. She should know what emergency drugs and equipment may be indicated and where they are located. If an allergy to a drug is suspected for any reason, the drug should be withheld and the physician notified.

Several measures may be taken to reduce the possibility of administering a drug to which a patient is sensitive. On admission the patient should be asked if he has any allergies or has ever had hives. All known allergies should be recorded on the patient's chart, the doctor's order sheet, and the nursing Kardex. Some hospitals provide special tags for this purpose.

With the growing use of Medic Alert tags, nurses should remember to check routinely for these, especially on patients who are admitted unconscious or are for any reason unable to communicate.

Before actually administering a drug that is likely to produce an allergic reaction, such as penicillin, the nurse should ask the patient if he has any allergies or is allergic to penicillin. Patients receiving injections of any type on an outpatient basis, as in clinics or doctors' offices, should remain near the medical facility for 20 to 30 minutes after the injection lest an allergic reaction occur.

The fact that the patient does not have a history of sensitivity to a particular drug that he has received in the past does not eliminate the possibility of allergic reaction. Having received the drug in the past may actually increase the likelihood of the patient's developing an allergic reaction when he receives it at a later time.

Patients who have a history of any kind of allergy tend to be more easily sensitized to antibiotics. Those who have a history of asthma, hay fever or urticaria should be given antibiotics with caution and should be observed carefully for manifestations of allergy. Sensitivity testing may be done by the physician if an allergy to a particular drug is suspected.

There are several measures that the nurse can use to help prevent the development of resistant strains of bacteria. Careless handling of antibiotics can allow normally harmless bacteria in the environment to become selectively killed, thus promoting the emergence of a resistant population. Any antibiotic that is spilled should be removed thoroughly and promptly. Nurses should avoid "squirting" parenteral preparations from the needle when preparing an antibiotic injection.

Strict observance of the principles of medical and surgical asepsis is essential to reduce the number of pathogens in the hospital environment. Carelessness and relaxation of technique often occurs because of a false sense of assurance or a belief by personnel that antibiotics will correct any infection. It is essential to realize that many infections are becoming more difficult to counteract because of the problem of resistance.

This problem of resistance has helped to prompt the search for new drugs to deal with resistant microorganisms. Some hospitals maintain a reserve supply of certain types of antibiotics that are not allowed to be used routinely. These drugs are reserved for emergencies when an organism is found to be resistant to most other antibiotics. Some hospitals may have a special committee or department which is concerned with the problem of hospital infections, and may regulate the use of antibiotics.

Certain hospitals limit the length of time that an order for an antibiotic is considered valid: the physician must then review the patient's condition and reorder the drug if he wishes the patient to continue on therapy. In this way unnecessarily prolonged antibiotic therapy is avoided, and the patient is not submitted to the relatively dangerous side effects of many of these drugs.

NURSING OBSERVATIONS. *Fever* is one of the most commonly used criteria to judge the degree of infection or the effectiveness of an antibiotic. The nurse should therefore check the patient's temperature frequently while he is receiving antibiotics or when an infectious process is suspected.

Other evidence should also be sought that the infection is being affected by therapy. This will depend on the location and type of infection, but may include observation of decreased purulent drainage, increased sense of well-being and increased appetite.

The nurse should know the possible *side effects* of the antibiotic and observe carefully for them. A great many antibiotics and other drugs affect the hematopoietic system. The nurse should therefore know the signs and symptoms of blood dyscrasias and be aware of the results of laboratory tests (see chart, pp. 40–41).

Expiration dates should be carefully checked and patients instructed to discard unused antibiotics, since deterioration of some drugs may cause adverse reactions. The manufacturer's directions for the reconstitution and storage of the drug should be carefully followed.

Secondary infection or superinfection by organisms or fungi that are unaffected by or resistant to the antibiotic is a fairly common complication of antibiotic therapy. The nurse must be alert for any evidence of a new infectious process anywhere in the body. Common sites involved are the mouth, the gastrointestinal tract and the vagina. Diarrhea, change in character of the stool, and vaginal discharge are signs to be noted.

Proper oral hygiene and inspection of the mouth should be performed routinely to check for signs of secondary infection or blood dyscrasias.

Other measures to promote the patient's health and ability to fight infection should be included in the care of the patient. Such measures include adequate nutrition, adequate hydration, rest and general cleanliness. A guide for the nursing assessment of a patient receiving an antibiotic, which appears at the end of this chapter, offers additional suggestions for proper and thorough nursing care.

Penicillin

The penicillins are produced by strains of the mold *Penicillium*, notably *P. notatum* and *P. chrysogenum*. By altering the contents of the culture media, different forms of penicillin may be produced, all having the same basic structure but differing in the side chain attached to the molecule. Penicillins F, G, K, O, V and X have been produced; however, only penicillins G, O and V are used therapeutically at the present time.

Laboratory synthesis of penicillin has been achieved. The process is very complicated, however, and the yields are too poor for the synthesis to be practical on a large scale. Interruption of the process at a specific time permits isolation of a reasonable yield of the basic building block of all penicillins, 6-aminopenicillanic acid. Synthetic methods have been used to attach hundreds of different side chains to this basic compound. Some of these so-called semisynthetic penicillins are currently used to a considerable

extent in therapy, and others have shown sufficient action to warrant further study.

MODE OF ACTION

Some of the properties of penicillin make it an almost ideal chemotherapeutic agent. Apart from its capacity to kill or inhibit the growth of certain pathogenic organisms, it is virtually nontoxic; it is soluble, diffusible and readily absorbed.

Penicillin may be bactericidal or bacteriostatic depending on the concentration obtained at the site of infection and the relative susceptibility of the organism. Its antibacterial activity is apparently due to its ability to interfere with bacterial cell wall synthesis by blocking cross-linkage of the cell wall precursors. Without adequate cell walls, the microorganisms are easily killed.

Although a certain amount of penicillin is inactivated in the body, for example by being reversibly bound to serum proteins, the greater part of a dose administered parenterally remains active as it circulates in the blood and is excreted in the urine still in an active form. Some microorganisms, however, secrete penicillinase, an enzyme that destroys the penicillin molecule, and in these instances penicillin is rapidly inactivated. At best the half life of penicillin (that is, the period during which the blood level is at its peak) is very short—only about 60 to 90 minutes; therefore the dose must be repeated frequently, and the drug should be administered promptly at the time intervals ordered by the physician.

Penicillin maintains its activity in the body by its wide distribution, not only in the circulating blood and in many normal secretions and tissues, but in some inflammatory

penicillinic acid
6-aminopenicillanic acid
penicillanic acid

and traumatic exudates as well. It is excreted chiefly by the kidneys, and as indicated above, excretion takes place quite rapidly.

ADVANTAGES OF PENICILLIN

A successful anti-infective agent not only must be able to eliminate infection, but must be able to do so without producing toxic effects on the patient. This characteristic is displayed by penicillin to such a degree that it has had some confusing consequences in the matter of working out dosages. Doses of penicillin are expressed in units, a unit being the antibiotic activity of a standard sample of penicillin against a test organism. Recommended doses vary according to the type of penicillin (see below) and the method of administration. For instance, adult doses of penicillin G range from 250,000 to 20,000,000 units or more, depending upon the route of administration and the antibiotic blood level desired. In contrast to many other antibiotics, high circulating levels of penicillin are quite safe, even in the presence of kidney damage. This has proved to be of great advantage since penicillin may be employed in instances when other antibiotics may be contraindicated. Possible allergic manifestations must be borne in mind, however, especially when administering extremely high doses.

Even when kidney damage is present, there is no reason to suppose that circulating penicillin adds to a patient's serious condition. In a severe infection the advantage of absence of toxicity outweighs all the inconveniences in administration that are imposed by the chemical and pharmacological properties of penicillin. The clinician is able to give as large a dose as may be required and yet to watch the progress of the disease without confusion from signs and symptoms due to any toxic action of the drug.

DISADVANTAGES

Allergic reactions remain the chief disadvantage in penicillin. They have caused death in some instances. The usual mechanism is hypersensitization, induced by a second or later exposure to the drug. It is thought that about 15 per cent of Americans at present are sensitized to some type of penicillin. Some of the forms of allergic reactions caused by these agents are skin rashes, oral lesions, fever, and the type of illness usually known as serum sickness. The possibility of causing allergic reactions has made it less and less safe to give penicillin topically, that is, locally, and this mode of administration is seldom used now.

In respect to its stability, penicillin has some undesirable characteristics, i.e., its gradual decomposition in solution unless refrigerated, its destruction by bacterial enzymes (penicillinases) if exposed to contamination, and the impracticality of sterilizing a solution by boiling.

Oral administration of penicillin was thought to be impractical in the early days of its use, because of the destruction of this agent by gastric hydrochloric acid and because of its limited absorption through the intestinal wall. However, the use of newer forms of penicillin, and the realization that high doses could be given safely, have now made oral administration more common. It must be remembered, however, that oral administration is considerably less reliable than parenteral administration and serious infections should always be treated with intramuscular or intravenous therapy.

INDICATIONS FOR PENICILLIN

Penicillin is used in infections caused by most cocci, both gram-positive and gram-negative. In some cases the use of penicillin has resulted in the selective killing of susceptible strains with the resultant overgrowth of resistant strains. It is now thought that from 15 to 20 per cent of staphylococci isolated outside of hospitals are resistant to penicillin G. (In strains isolated within hospitals the incidence may be as high as 90 to 95 per cent.)

The meningococcus is somewhat less sensitive to penicillin than other cocci. Meningitis due to this organism is usually treated with a combination of sulfonamides and penicillin.

Penicillin also is effective against most

other gram-positive organisms. In general the gram-negative bacilli, such as the colon-typhoid-dysentery group, are not very susceptible to penicillin. The agent is generally ineffective against protozoal, rickettsial, viral and fungal infections, and against the tubercle bacillus. Penicillin may be described as a narrow-spectrum antibiotic.

TYPES OF PENICILLIN

PENICILLIN G

POTASSIUM PENICILLIN G, U.S.P. (SODIUM PENICILLIN G, N.F.; BENZYLPENICILLIN, B.P.). Benzyl penicillin, or penicillin G, is the form most commonly used in parenteral therapy and is employed as either the potassium or sodium salt. This crystalline, soluble form may be used for subcutaneous, intramuscular, intravenous or intrathecal injection. Intramuscular injection of penicillin G provides a maximal blood concentration within 30 to 60 minutes. Peak concentrations are attained in about five minutes following intravenous injection, and in about 60 minutes following subcutaneous injection. The duration of action is relatively short, requiring injection every three to four hours to maintain a satisfactory blood level. Because of the frequency of injection and the pain produced by the medication, the injection should be given deeply into the muscle and the sites of injection should be carefully rotated.

potassium penicillin

This drug must be refrigerated once it is prepared in solution form by adding sterile water or sterile saline. Contact with penicillin may cause a local dermatitis. If large numbers of penicillin injections are to be administered, the nurse should wear gloves to protect her hands.

Although penicillin G can be used orally, it is largely inactivated by gastric acidity, absorption is poor and unsatisfactory blood levels are attained. When administered orally, penicillin G should be given between meals to reduce its destruction by gastric secretions.

USES. Streptococcal and pneumococcal infections, bacterial endocarditis, meningitis; gonorrhea, syphilis and miscellaneous infections caused by penicillin-susceptible organisms.

DOSE. 1 to 50 million units every 3 to 4 hours intravenously or intramuscularly. 250,000 to 800,000 units every 4 hours orally.

LONG-ACTING FORMS OF PENICILLIN G

Since the duration of action of penicillin G in the crystalline form is so short, efforts were made to create an insoluble form of penicillin which would remain in the tissues forming a "depot" from which the penicillin could be slowly leached away, thus maintaining the effective blood level for a longer time. The first really successful method of prolonging penicillin blood levels for a clinically significant period of time following intramuscular injection was a preparation of the soluble penicillin G in a vehicle of vegetable oil and beeswax. This method had several disadvantages, and more acceptable forms have largely replaced the oil and wax mixture at the present time.

A method that involves the preparation of sparingly soluble salts of penicillin G which can be suspended in appropriate vehicles and injected as suspensions has been the most satisfactory technique for prolonging the duration of penicillin action. Several of these forms are in current use. All are given intramuscularly.

PROCAINE PENICILLIN G, U.S.P., B.P. (ABBOCILLIN, CRYSTICILLIN, DURACILLIN, WYCILLIN). Incorporation of procaine into the penicillin molecule results in a slightly soluble salt with more prolonged duration of action than the crystalline form of penicillin. However, prolonged action is attained at the expense of blood concentrations, for the peak blood level of procaine penicillin G is only a fraction of that of soluble penicillin salts following injection. This preparation should not

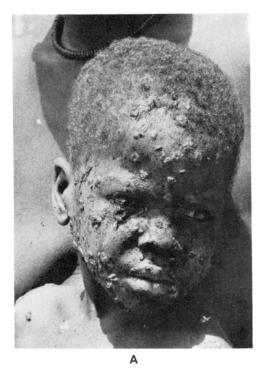 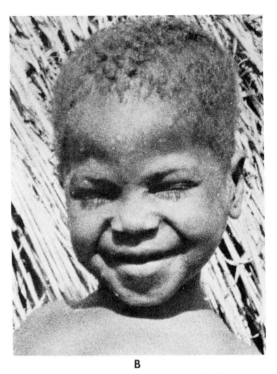

A   B

FIGURE 29. A, Yaws, a widespread, disfiguring treponemal disease causing deep-seated infirmity if untreated. B. The same child 10 days after receiving a single injection of long-acting penicillin. (Courtesy World Health Organization; photo by Eric Schwab.)

be given to a patient who is allergic to procaine.

When immediate as well as prolonged action is desired, injectable mixtures of the soluble penicillin with procaine penicillin may be used.

Procaine penicillin G has actions and uses similar to those of the crystalline form.

Procaine penicillin, like other repository forms, is a thick suspension that may pose problems when it is injected. Before injecting it, care must be taken in aspirating to be sure the needle is not in a blood vessel.

Because of the thickness of the preparation, the plunger on the syringe may actually move, but suction may not be transferred to the patient's tissue, and aspiration will not take place. The nurse should look carefully to be sure that the fluid moves when she pulls back on the plunger. Before inserting the needle, she should be certain that it is not clogged.

Procaine penicillin should be given deep in a large muscle and the sites of administration should be rotated if frequent injections are necessary.

procaine penicillin

DOSE. 600,000 units every 8 to 12 hours.

BENZATHINE PENICILLIN G, U.S.P., B.P. (BICILLIN). Benzathine penicillin is a repository (that is, long-acting) form of penicillin which is very slightly soluble in water. Following intramuscular injection the duration of action is much more prolonged than with either crystalline or procaine penicillin. Blood levels sufficient for the inhibition of very susceptible organisms persist for 14 to 21 days following injection.

The actions and uses are similar to those for the other forms of penicillin.

> **DOSE.** 600,000 to 1,200,000 units every 4 or 5 days; may be given every other day for severe infections. For prophylaxis of rheumatic fever 1,200,000 units is given every four weeks; in treatment of primary and secondary syphilis a single dose of 2,400,000 units is recommended.

COMBINATION FORMS OF PENICILLIN

PEN S-R, DURACILLIN FORTIFIED. This combination of 300,000 units procaine penicillin with 100,000 units crystalline provides immediate availability of penicillin along with a moderately long-acting form.

> **DOSE.** One vial every 8 to 12 hours.

BICILLIN C-R. Equal parts of procaine and benzathine penicillin provide a faster onset of action than would be obtained using the benzathine alone.

> **DOSE.** 600,000 units every 2 to 3 days.

BICILLIN A-P. Each vial contains:
  Benzathine penicillin G   600,000 U.
  Procaine penicillin G   300,000 U.
  Potassium penicillin G   300,000 U.
The combination of the three forms make this a suitable preparation for many instances in which penicillin therapy is indicated.

PENICILLIN V

PHENOXYMETHYL PENICILLIN, N.F., B.P. (PENICILLIN V, PEN-VEE, V-CILLIN, COMPOCILLIN-V). POTASSIUM PHENOXYMETHYL PENICILLIN, U.S.P. (PEN-VEE-K, V-CILLIN K, COMPOCILLIN-VK). Pencillin V, also known as phenoxymethyl penicillin, exhibits a high degree of stability in the presence of gastric acidity. Because of this unique characteristic, significant antibiotic loss does not occur in the stomach, and effective blood levels may be attained using the oral route. The potassium salt of penicillin V is used in the same way.

For optimum absorption and decreased possibility of unfavorable effects of gastric secretions, oral penicillin preparations should be given between meals.

> **USES.** Has been shown to be effective in the treatment of streptococcus, pneumococcus and gonococcus infections and in those caused by sensitive strains of staphylococcus. Especially recommended for prophylaxis of rheumatic fever in patients with a previous history of the disease.
>
> Oral penicillin is not indicated in the treatment of meningitis, peritonitis or syphilis; neither can the oral form be recommended for treatment of all forms of bacterial endocarditis.
>
> **DOSE.** 125 to 250 mg. orally every 4 hours.

PENICILLIN O

SODIUM PENICILLIN O (CER-O-CILLIN SODIUM). Penicillin O, or allylmercaptomethyl penicillin, has been demonstrated clinically to be less likely to give rise to sensitivity or allergic reactions than penicillin G. Some patients sensitive to penicillin G may receive penicillin O without developing allergic reactions; however, others may be sensitive to both forms. It is recommended that appropriate sensitivity testing be carried out before administering a therapeutic dose of penicillin O to patients who are known to be sensitive to penicillin G. The action and effects of penicillin O are the same as those of penicillin G.

USES. Same as for penicillin G.

DOSE. 1 to 5 million units every 3 or 4 hours intramuscularly or intravenously.

SEMISYNTHETIC PENICILLINS

POTASSIUM PHENETHICILLIN, N.F. (ALPEN, DARCIL, MAXIPEN, SYNCILLIN). Like phenoxymethyl penicillin, phenethicillin is able to resist inactivation in acid media, and is quite effective when taken orally. Phenethicillin, however, produces higher peak blood levels than does an equal dose of phenoxymethyl penicillin. The antibacterial activity is about comparable, nevertheless, for phenethicillin is less active than either potassium penicillin G or phenoxymethyl penicillin.

DOSE. 125 to 250 mg. orally three times daily.

SODIUM METHICILLIN, U.S.P. (DIMOCILLIN, STAPHCILLIN). Methicillin is available only for injection since it is unstable in acid solution. By virtue of its unusual stability in the presence of staphylococcal penicillinase, methicillin is clinically effective against many strains of staphylococcus that are resistant to other penicillins. It has about the same order of toxicity as penicillin G.

This drug should not be mixed in the same syringe with other drugs. Solutions stored at room temperature should be discarded after 24 hours. Refrigerated solutions may be kept for four days.

USES. Only in the treatment of infections caused by penicillinase-producing staphylococcus that are resistant to other forms of penicillin.

DOSE. 1 to 1.5 Gm. I.M., 1 to 2 Gm. I.V. every 4 to 6 hours.

NAFCILLIN SODIUM (UNIPEN). Like methicillin, nafcillin is resistant to inactivation by staphylococcus penicillinase. It has the advantage of being stable in acid and so may be given orally. The serum levels attained following oral administration vary considerably from one individual to another; often they are low and in some patients not

sufficient even at peak levels to inhibit staphylococcus. The parenteral preparation for I.M. use should be refrigerated and discarded after 24 hours.

USES. Primarily reserved for severe infections caused by penicillin G–resistant staphylococcus. Has a narrow spectrum of activity and no particular advantage over other forms of penicillin for parenteral therapy.

SIDE EFFECTS. Mild to moderate pain at the site of intramuscular injection is a frequent side effect. Development of sterile abscesses at the site of injection has been reported. Thrombophlebitis has occurred occasionally following intravenous administration.

DOSE. 250 to 500 mg. every 6 hours. orally, I.M. or I.V.

SODIUM OXACILLIN, U.S.P. (PROSTAPHLIN, RESISTOPEN). Like the aforementioned semisynthetic penicillins, oxacillin possesses the property of resistance to inactivation by staphylococcus penicillinase. In addition, it is acid-resistant, and therefore can be conveniently administered in oral form.

Diffusion of oxacillin into various body fluids differs from that of other penicillins. Therapeutic levels are achieved in bile and pleural fluids, and activity may be detected in spinal fluid, placental cord serum, amniotic fluid and human milk. Diffusion into synovial fluid appears to be poor and diffusion into peritoneal and pericardial fluids is little or absent.

USES. Only in the treatment of infections caused by penicillinase-producing staphylococcus that are resistant to other forms of penicillin.

DOSE. 500 mg. orally every 4 to 6 hours.

AMPICILLIN, B.P. (POLYCILLIN, PENBRITIN, OMNIPEN). Ampicillin is a broad-spectrum antibiotic which is active in clinically attainable concentrations against a number of gram-negative bacilli as well as against the gram-positive cocci and the other organisms generally susceptible to penicillin.

ampicillin

Ampicillin is destroyed by penicillinase, and therefore is inactivated by strains of staphylococcus and gram-negative bacilli that produce this enzyme. It is generally well absorbed following oral administration, although absorption is somewhat slow and serum levels decrease rather slowly as well. Low concentrations of the antibiotic are usually present in the serum six hours after the drug is given.

Reconstituted solutions for parenteral use must be used within one hour.

USES. Primarily in the treatment of infections caused by gram-negative bacteria. Good results have been obtained in urinary tract and soft tissue infections.

DOSE. 500 mg. every 6 hours orally, I.M. or I.V.

DISODIUM CARBENICILLIN (GEOPEN). This semisynthetic penicillin is effective when administered parenterally in the treatment of *Pseudomonas, Proteus* and some *E. coli* infections. It has been shown to be relatively free of untoward side effects when used in patients with preexisting renal damage.

USES. Urinary tract infections, septicemia and severe systemic infections, infected burns and other soft tissue infections and acute and chronic respiratory infections.

TOXICITY. Skin rashes, nausea, anemia, neuromuscular irritability. Occasionally disturbances in clotting mechanisms have been noted.

DOSE. 1 to 2 Gm. I.M. or I.V. every 4 to 6 hours. In severe systemic infections doses to 40 Gm. daily have been administered.

CLOXACILLIN SODIUM (TEGOPEN). This semisynthetic penicillin derivative is resistant to inactivation by penicillinase, thus has a broader spectrum of activity than penicillin.

It is effective when administered orally, but food interferes with absorption, thus it should be given to patients between meals, at least one hour before and not sooner than three hours after the last meal.

It is used primarily for infections caused by staphylococcal, pneumococcal and streptococcal infections, particularly in the respiratory tract, soft tissues and skin.

TOXICITY. Cross sensitivity to penicillin has been noted, thus it is not administered to patients with a history of penicillin sensitivity. GI disturbances, mild leukopenia and dermatoses have occurred with therapy.

DOSE. 0.25 to 1 Gm. orally four to six times daily.

TREATMENT OF ALLERGIC REACTIONS TO PENICILLIN

PENICILLINASE (NEUTRAPEN). This preparation of a highly purified injectable penicillinase was introduced for intramuscular or intravenous use in the management and treatment of allergic reactions to penicillin. Penicillinase destroys only the antigen (penicillin), and thus halts the progress of the allergic reaction. Although good results were obtained with this preparation at first, it has now been found that severe hypersensitivity reactions to the enzyme may develop, and it must be used with great caution.

Other drugs, such as corticosteroids and antihistamines, may also be used as discussed in Chapter 7.

DOSE. 800,000 U. in sodium chloride solution I.M. or I.V.

Other Antibiotics

STREPTOMYCIN SULFATE, U.S.P., B.P. Streptomycin is a sugar-containing antibiotic that was first isolated from *Streptomyces griseus* and has proved highly effective as an antibacterial agent. Although considerable research has been performed in order to determine the basis of its antibiotic action, this has not been completely established at the present time. Streptomycin is presumed to act by interfering with microbial protein synthesis, theoretically by binding soluble RNA with the wrong specificity, thus inducing the manufacture of faulty and ineffective bacterial proteins.

streptomycin sulfate

It is not absorbed following oral administration, and for systemic therapy it is administered only by the intramuscular route. Following injection, peak blood levels are obtained in one to two hours, and only trace amounts are found in the blood after four hours.

Since resistance to streptomycin develops rapidly during therapy, this antibiotic is rarely used alone. It is often combined with penicillin in the treatment of meningitis, bacteremia and urinary tract infections caused by strains of *Proteus, Pseudomonas, Klebsiella* and *Aerobacter.*

Probably the most important single use of streptomycin is in the treatment of tuberculosis. Here again, it is not used alone, but in combination with other antitubercular drugs such as para-amino salicylic acid (PAS) (p. 180) and isoniazid (INH) (p. 180). It is useful for all forms of tuberculosis, including miliary tuberculosis and lesions of the meninges and genitourinary tract, as well as the pulmonary form of the disease.

Limitations. The most prevalent side effect of streptomycin therapy is the progressive and permanent hearing loss that occurs with prolonged treatment. Since prolonged therapy is always necessary in tuberculosis,

this toxic effect is commonly observed. Cases of auditory damage have even been recorded in infants following treatment of pregnant women with streptomycin. This drug should be administered with extreme caution to patients with preexisting renal disease, in whom excretion would be delayed, allowing high blood levels for several days with the obvious sequelae of ototoxicity. It is recommended that auditory testing should be done frequently during streptomycin therapy. Other toxic reactions observed include urticaria, stomatitis and paresthesias. These usually subside when therapy is discontinued.

The nurse should wear gloves during the preparation of streptomycin since frequent exposure to this drug may cause contact dermatitis.

TOXICITY.   As above.

DOSE.   0.5 to 1 Gm. daily intramuscularly. After tuberculosis is somewhat controlled, the dosage is often reduced to 1 Gm. I.M. two or three times weekly.

TETRACYCLINE HYDROCHLORIDE, U.S.P., B.P. (ACHROMYCIN, PANMYCIN, STECLIN, TETRACYN, POLYCYCLINE).   Tetracycline is the parent compound of a group of antibiotics known jointly as the tetracyclines. Three others of this group are discussed below. All members of the group have essentially the same actions and properties. They are broad-spectrum compounds active against a variety of both gram-negative and gram-positive bacteria. Although in vitro they are primarily bacteriostatic, in high concentrations they may have bactericidal activity.

Citrates, phosphates, glucosamine and other agents have been added to tetracycline preparations in an effort to increase their absorption from the gastrointestinal tract. Such buffering or the use of the tetracycline phosphate complex may produce somewhat higher blood levels but well controlled studies have not confirmed these claims, and any increased absorption is probably clinically insignificant. Preparations containing ascorbic acid may cause false-negative results of certain tests for glycosuria.

tetracycline

Tetracycline hydrochloride may be administered orally or by the intramuscular or intravenous route. Intramuscular injection should be given deeply, although tissue irritation may still occur.

Cautions. Irritation of the gastrointestinal tract by tetracycline frequently causes nausea and vomiting. This can be relieved somewhat by giving the medication with meals. However, foods or drugs high in calcium, such as milk, should not be given before or with tetracycline since calcium impedes the absorption of tetracycline.

Photosensitization of the skin may occur from exposure to the sun, the patient should be instructed to avoid exposure to sun and to report any signs of skin discomfort.

Diarrhea may become a problem because of irritation of the gastrointestinal tract and possible superinfection by resistant or unaffected organisms such as yeast. For this reason antifungal drugs are often used concurrently with oral tetracyclines. The most common antifungal agent used is Mycostatin. Pruritus ani may result from contamination with breakdown products of tetracycline and can be relieved by carefully cleansing the anal area after each bowel movement.

The expiration date on tetracycline products should be checked carefully before administering since products of degradation may cause adverse effects on kidney function. Degradation may also occur as a result of exposure to heat, extreme humidity and light.

USES. Indicated in a wide variety of infections caused by susceptible bacteria including: respiratory tract infections, genitourinary infections, infections of the nervous system, surgical infections, infections in obstetrics and gynecology and other miscellaneous conditions caused by susceptible organisms.

TOXICITY. In addition to the problems mentioned above, glossitis, dermatitis and allergic reactions may occur, but are rare. Use during tooth development (last trimester of pregnancy, neonatal period and early childhood) may cause discoloration of the teeth to a yellow-brown shade. This occurs mostly during long-term use but has also been observed in short treatment courses.

DOSE. Oral—250 mg. every 6 hours. Intravenous—500 mg. every 12 hours. Intramuscular—100 mg. two to three times a day.

CHLORTETRACYCLINE HYDROCHLORIDE, N.F., B.P. (AUREOMYCIN). Chlortetracycline hydrochloride, a product of *Streptomyces aureofaciens*, is closely related to tetracycline in its action and uses. Aqueous solutions of this drug, however, are less stable than aqueous solutions of tetracycline or oxytetracycline hydrochloride, and some decomposition may be expected during extended intravenous infusions.

DOSE. Oral—250 mg. every 6 hours. Intravenous—500 mg. every 12 hours. Intramuscular—100 mg. two to three times a day.

OXTETRACYCLINE HYDROCHLORIDE, N.F., B.P. (TERRAMYCIN). The actions and uses of this agent are closely related to those of tetracycline. It is manufactured by *Streptomyces rimosus.*

DOSE. Oral—250 mg. every 6 hours. Intravenous—500 mg. every 12 hours. Intramuscular—100 mg. two to three times a day.

DEMETHYLCHLORTETRACYCLINE HYDROCHLORIDE, N.F. (DECLOMYCIN). Differing slightly from the structures of the other tetracyclines, this agent produced by *Streptomyces aureofaciens* is more stable in acid or basic aqueous solutions than the other forms. The clinical applications are the same; however, the dose is reduced to about three-fifths that of the

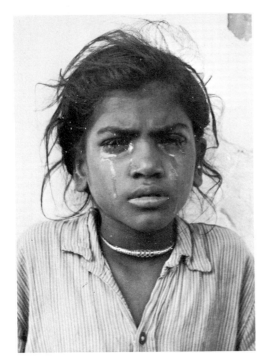 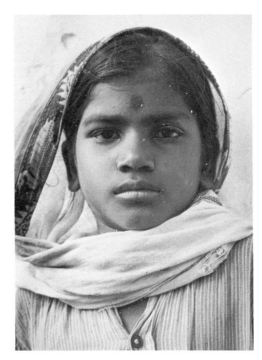

FIGURE 30. A, Trachoma, a common cause of blindness among the people of India. B, The same girl after 10 days of therapy with chlortetracycline ophthalmic ointment. (Courtesy World Health Organization; photo by Homer Page.)

other tetracyclines since this form is better absorbed and maintains higher blood levels.

DOSE.   150 mg. orally every 6 hours.

CHLORAMPHENICOL, U.S.P., B.P. (CHLOROMY-CETIN).   Following its recovery from *Streptomyces venezuelae* the first noted effect of chloramphenicol was on the rickettsiae of typhus. This action was the first example of a rickettsial disease showing susceptibility to an antibiotic. Subsequent studies of its antibacterial action showed that chloramphenicol was active against a wide range of organisms with varying biological characteristics.

Chloramphenicol diffuses rapidly following oral or parenteral administration, but its distribution is not uniform. Highest concentrations are found in the liver and kidney, and lowest are in the brain and cerebrospinal fluid. Chloramphenicol enters cerebrospinal fluid even in the absence of meningeal inflammation, appearing in concentrations about half that found in the blood. This antibiotic has also been reported to occur in pleural and ascitic fluids, in saliva and in milk, and it readily diffuses to all parts of the eye. Transport occurs across the placental barrier, with somewhat lower concentrations in cord blood of newborn infants than in maternal blood.

Untoward reactions.   Mucous membrane lesions such as stomatitis are the most common complications of chloramphenicol treatment. It appears also that changes similar to those occurring in the mouth may take place in other parts of the gastrointestinal tract. The changes make themselves known by the symptoms of flatulence, nausea, and, rarely, vomiting. Intestinal bleeding occasionally occurs; this effect may be due to disturbance in the gastrointestinal flora that normally manufactures vitamin K for the body.

Allergic reactions occur, but are not nearly so common as following penicillin therapy.

The most serious side effect, and the one which has caused the most difficulty during and subsequent to chloramphenicol therapy, is the deleterious effect on the bone marrow and thence on the production of the blood cells. Reports of purpura, reduced platelet counts and deficient production of various blood cells began to appear in considerable numbers. Soon an alarming incidence of blood disorders with a relatively high incidence of fatal aplastic anemia brought a generalized warning from the U.S. Food and Drug Administration suggesting restriction of the use of the drug to cases in which it was definitely indicated. In infections due to susceptible organisms, the advantages of the excellent antibiotic activity by far outweigh the dangerous side effects if its use is properly controlled by the physician.

The nurse should be particularly alert for any signs or symptoms of blood dyscrasias (see chart on common drug side effects in Chapter 2) and should report her observations to the physician immediately.

USES. In acute infections caused by Salmonella typhi, i.e., typhoid fever. It is not recommended for the carrier state. Serious infections caused by microorganisms not susceptible to other antibiotics, i.e., rickettsiae and gram-negative organisms, and as a cystic fibrosis regimen.

TOXICITY. As above.

DOSE. Oral—250 to 500 mg. as often as every 3 hours. Parenteral—1 Gm. every 8 to 12 hours.

ERYTHROMYCIN, U.S.P., B.P. (ILOTYCIN, ERYTHROCIN). An antibiotic produced from a strain of *Streptomyces erythreus*, erythromycin has an antimicrobial spectrum similar to that of penicillin. It diffuses rapidly into body tissues, as well as into the peritoneal, pleural, ascitic and amniotic fluids, into the placental circulation, and across the lining membranes of pulmonary tissue. Under ordinary circumstances it diffuses poorly into the spinal fluid; however, diffusion across the meninges is somewhat improved if the

meningeal membranes are inflamed. Erythromycin is excreted in the bile, as well as in human milk, feces and urine.

Because this drug may be affected by gastric juices and enzymes when given orally, it should ideally be given between meals.

After the dry form of erythromycin has been made into a solution, it must be refrigerated and discarded after seven days.

USES. Effective against beta-hemolytic streptococci, pneumococci and some strains of staphylococci. Inhibits the growth of diphtheria bacilli and may be used in conjunction with diphtheria antitoxin in the treatment of diphtheria.

Since its spectrum of activity is so close to that of penicillin, this is often the drug of choice in the treatment of patients who are allergic to penicillin.

TOXICITY. Nausea, vomiting, abdominal distress and diarrhea are the chief side effects, but occur infrequently at adult dosages not exceeding 1 gram daily. Changes in the bacterial flora leading to overgrowth of yeast and fungi occur less frequently than with other antibiotics, but the possibility should be borne in mind when it is administered orally. Skin reactions have been reported, as well as fatal anaphylactic shock, due possibly to injection of large amounts of erythromycin. Contact dermatitis is possible.

DOSE. 250 to 500 mg. every 6 hours orally. 0.5 to 1 Gm. every 6 hours I.M. or I.V.

ERYTHROMYCIN ESTOLATE (ILOSONE). This lauryl sulfate salt of the propionic acid ester of erythromycin gives higher, more predictable and more prolonged antibiotic blood levels than erythromycin base. It has the same uses.

TOXICITY. Jaundice has been reported following use of this salt, in contrast to other forms of erythromycin. Contraindicated in patients known to have liver disorders.

DOSE. 250 to 500 mg. orally every 6 hours.

ERYTHROMYCIN ETHYLCARBONATE, U.S.P. ILOTYCIN ETHYL CARBONATE). The ethylcarbonate ester of erythromycin is used to prepare oral suspensions. These preparations are stable for two weeks at room temperature.

DOSE. 250 mg. orally every 6 hours.

ERYTHROMYCIN ETHYLSUCCINATE. Because it is less irritating to tissue than other forms when it is injected intramuscularly, this form is ordinarily employed for the intramuscular injection. This preparation must not be mixed with other aqueous solutions. Consult a pharmacist or the manufacturer's instructions before mixing with other drugs.

DOSE. 100 mg. every 8 to 12 hours intramuscularly.

ERYTHROMYCIN GLUCOHEPTONATE, U.S.P. (ILOTYCIN GLUCOHEPTONATE). This salt is administered by intravenous infusion because of its solubility and relative stability. The powder should be dissolved in sterile water only to provide complete solubility. Once dissolved in water, it can then be added to an isotonic solution for infusion.

DOSE. 250 mg. every 6 hours I.V.

ERYTHROMYCIN LACTOBIONATE, U.S.P. (ERYTHROCIN LACTOBIONATE). Although intramuscular injection of this salt does not produce tissue damage, it does produce pain at the site of injection. It is generally reserved for intravenous therapy. Powdered preparations should be dissolved with sterile water.

DOSE. 250 mg. every 6 hours I.V.

NEOMYCIN SULFATE, U.S.P., B.P. (MYCIFRADIN). Neomycin sulfate is the soluble salt of an antibiotic obtained commercially from cultures of *Streptomyces fradiae*. The antibiotic is active over a pH range of 2 to 9 and is not inactivated by tissue exudates, bacterial enzymes, or by-products of bacterial growth. Its mechanism of action is similar to that of streptomycin in that it interrupts bacterial protein synthesis.

It is not useful orally for systemic infections since absorption from the gastrointestinal tract is minimal, but it may be given by mouth to sterilize the bowel prior to surgery. It is quite effective as a topical antibiotic, but its use in systemic therapy is quite limited owing to serious toxic reactions.

Toxic reactions. When a total dose of neomycin exceeding 15 mg. per kg. of body weight (more than 1 gram of neomycin per day) is continued for more than 10 days, signs of toxicity affecting renal, central nervous system and auditory functions are likely to develop. In the presence of preexisting renal disease, neomycin excretion is impaired with resulting increase in serum concentrations and concomitant increase in toxic reactions. The eighth nerve damage appears to be additive to that produced by streptomycin, dihydrostreptomycin, and other ototoxic antibiotics so that these antibiotics should not be used concurrently. Signs of kidney damage, including mild albuminuria, presence of granular casts and depression of urinary output with elevation of blood urea nitrogen, are reversible, usually disappearing upon discontinuance of the drug. The auditory effects, however, may progress even after administration of the neomycin is discontinued and the changes are irreversible.

USES. Intramuscular injections should be restricted to individuals with serious systemic infections caused by susceptible organisms that are resistant to other less toxic antibiotics. Particularly useful in treatment of infections caused by *Klebsiella pneumoniae, Hemophilus influenzae, Proteus vulgaris,* and *Pseudomonas aeruginosa* and in urinary tract infections caused by strains of *Ps. aeruginosa, Escherichia coli, P. vulgaris* or *Aerobacter aerogenes.* Topically it is used in solution form for wound or bladder irrigation or in the form of an antibacterial ointment. Sensitivity reactions and systemic absorption are possible if applied topically to large denuded areas.

TOXICITY. As above.

DOSE. Systemic therapy—10 to 15 mg.

per kg. body weight. The maximum daily dose should not exceed 1 Gm.

Preoperative—0.5 to 1 Gm. orally every hour for 4 hours, then every 4 hours for 24 to 72 hours.

TRIACETYLOLEANDOMYCIN, N.F. (TAO). Triacetyloleandomycin is an antibiotic obtained from a species of *Streptomyces antibioticus.* It is quite effective orally due to its stability in acid solution. Because of the toxic reactions seen with prolonged use of this antibiotic, it should not be given unless the causative organism has demonstrated susceptibility to this antibiotic and resistance to other less toxic agents.

USES. Acute infections caused by staphylococci, streptococci, pneumococci and gonococci. Has been used less frequently in severe infections of the respiratory tract, connective tissue, genitourinary tract and gastrointestinal tract caused by other susceptible organisms.

TOXICITY. May cause liver damage, and when therapy is expected to last beyond ten days, other agents should be used when possible. Contraindicated in preexisting liver disease. Allergic reactions are infrequent and seldom severe, but those of the anaphylactoid type have occurred on rare occasions.

DOSE. 250 mg. orally every 4 to 6 hours.

BACITRACIN, U.S.P., B.P. (BACIGUENT). Bacitracin is an antibiotic derived from *Bacillus subtilis.* It is therefore a bacterial product rather than the product of a mold, in contrast to most other antibiotics. It is active against a broad spectrum of gram-positive organisms, including streptococci, staphylococci, pneumococci, clostridia, corynebacteria, spirochetes, as well as certain gram-negative cocci, including gonococci and meningococci. It is ineffective against most gram-negative bacilli.

USES. Employed by topical application in ointment form or in aqueous or saline solution for local wound irrigation. Use may result in systemic absorption if area to which it is applied is large and denuded. Solutions should be refrigerated since deterioration takes place rapidly at room temperature.

TOXICITY. Rather severe kidney damage may be produced by systemic therapy with bacitracin. For this reason it is primarily useful in local or topical antibiotic therapy where absorption is not sufficient to produce serious systemic reactions. Other side effects include nausea, vomiting, low-grade fever and urticaria. It is rarely, if ever, used systemically except for experimental purposes.

DOSE. 500 units per gram or cc. for topical application.

KANAMYCIN SULFATE, U.S.P. (KANTREX). Kanamycin is an antibiotic isolated from *Streptomyces kanamyceticus.* The drug is rapidly absorbed after intramuscular injection, with peak levels reached within approximately one hour after administration. Levels are within the active range for sensitive organisms for only two or three hours, then decline quite rapidly.

This antibiotic diffuses readily and rapidly into most body fluids but does not cross the blood-brain barrier nor the blood-amnion barrier following intramuscular injection. It is excreted almost entirely through the kidney by glomerular filtration and is not reabsorbed by the renal tubules. Patients with impaired renal function excrete kanamycin much more slowly—roughly in proportion to the extent of renal damage. In such cases excessive serum levels are obtained which greatly increase the risk of hearing loss.

Toxic reactions. The most important toxic effect of systemic kanamycin is injury to both the auditory and vestibular portions of the eighth cranial nerve. Hearing loss is often preceded by tinnitus or dizziness, is progressive, and usually has been irreversible. Renal injury is the other major toxic effect. This may be manifest initially by casts, albuminuria and microscopic hematuria, but occasionally acute renal tubular necrosis has resulted. Adequate fluid intake is necessary in order to reduce these toxic effects on renal function. Other side effects include skin rash, nausea, vomiting, diarrhea, fever, headache, malaise and aberrant skin sensations.

Orally administered kanamycin produces few serious side effects because it is poorly absorbed from the gastrointestinal tract. Continued oral administration may result in overgrowth of nonsusceptible organisms and may necessitate treatment with antifungal agents later. It obviously should not be given orally in the face of possible bowel obstruction.

> **USES.** Parenteral use restricted to the treatment of serious infections caused by organisms resistant to other antibacterial agents. It should not be mixed in the same syringe with other drugs. Useful in the short term treatment of gram-negative or staphylococcal urinary tract, respiratory tract and soft tissue infections and occasionally in osteomyelitis and septicemia caused by susceptible strains. Orally, because of its limited absorption, kanamycin is used for preoperative intestinal antisepsis and for inhibition of the bowel flora in patients with hepatic coma and cirrhosis in order to decrease the amount of nitrogenous by-products released to the blood stream.
>
> **TOXICITY.** As above.
>
> **DOSE.** 1.5 Gm. daily, orally or I.M.; for bowel antisepsis – 1 Gm. every hour for 4 hours, then 1 Gm. every 6 hours for 36 to 72 hours.

SODIUM NOVOBIOCIN, N.F., B.P. (ALBAMYCIN, CATHOMYCIN).

A product of *Streptomyces niveus,* this antibiotic should be used only in the treatment of susceptible staphylococcus and *Proteus* infections that are resistant to the more commonly used antibiotics and sulfonamides. The antibiotic is readily absorbed from the gastrointestinal tract; it diffuses readily into the pleural and ascitic fluids but does not diffuse into the spinal fluid unless the meninges are inflamed. Novobiocin is excreted in the bile, urine and feces.

> **USES.** As above.
>
> **TOXICITY.** Blood dyscrasias, jaundice have been reported.
>
> **DOSE.** 250 mg. orally every 6 hours. 500 mg. every 12 hours I.V. or I.M.

POLYMYXIN B SULFATE, U.S.P., B.P. (AEROSPORIN).

A polypeptide antibiotic from the spore-forming soil bacterium *Bacillus polymyxa,* this agent is bactericidal in vitro against most gram-negative organisms. Bacteria initially susceptible to the antibiotic rarely acquire a resistance to it. Given intramuscularly, peak blood levels are attained in 30 minutes and are maintained for 4 to 6 hours. It does not enter cells or pass into the spinal fluid, however. Approximately 60 per cent is excreted in the urine, but only a small amount is in a biologically active form. Preparations of this drug should be protected from exposure to air and light.

> **USES.** Intramuscularly or intravenously in the treatment of infections caused by *Pseudomonas, E. coli, Aerobacter* or *Haemophilus.* Since only small amounts pass from the blood stream into the spinal fluid, it is of little value in the treatment of meningitis even when caused by these susceptible organisms unless it is injected intrathecally. Intrathecal injection has been performed for the treatment of *Pseudomonas* meningitis and may be used for other types of meningitis if the organism is not susceptible to the less toxic drugs.
>
> **TOXICITY.** Neurologic disturbances and kidney damage occur, along with dizziness, weakness, blurring of vision and paresthesias. An intake of fluids to maintain a minimum of 1500 cc. output is important in reducing toxicity.
>
> **DOSE.** Oral – 75 to 100 mg. four times daily. I.M. – 1.5 to 2.5 mg/kg/24 hours in 3 divided doses. I.V. – 2.5 mg./kg./ 24 hours in one or two divided doses.

VANCOMYCIN, U.S.P., B.P. (VANCOCIN). Vancomycin is a bactericidal antibiotic obtained from strains of *Streptomyces orientalis* which is active against staphylococci, hemolytic streptococci, enterococci, pneumococci, corynebacteria and clostridia. Bactericidal concentrations can be readily maintained by intravenous administration and can be demonstrated in pleural, pericardial, ascitic and synovial fluids and in the urine. The drug does not readily diffuse across normal meninges into the spinal fluid unless the meninges are inflamed.

> **USES.** Intravenously in the treatment of severe septicemia or meningitis caused by organisms not susceptible to other antibiotics.

> **TOXICITY.** Thrombophlebitis may be produced by multiple intravenous injections of vancomycin. Care should be taken to avoid extravasation, since sloughing of the skin may occur. Chills, drug fever, eosinophilia and various skin reactions occur in varying degrees in many patients. Too rapid administration intravenously may cause nausea.

> **DOSE.** 1 Gm. every 12 hours I.V.

CEPHALOTHIN (KEFLIN). Cephalothin is a semisynthetic derivative of the cephalosporins, a group of compounds with antibiotic activity derived from the fungus *Cephalosporium acremonium.* Cephalothin is a broad-spectrum bactericidal compound active against streptococci, pneumococci and staphylococci, as well as a majority of the strains of *H. influenzae, Proteus, E. coli* and *Aerobacter. Pseudomonas* organisms and many strains of enterococci are resistant to the drug.

It should be noted that the administration of cephalothin affects the activity of certain agents used for testing the urine for sugar in diabetes. In persons taking the drug, urine specimens tested with copper-reducing agents such as Clinitest or Benedict's solution show a black-brown color that interferes with the interpretation of the test. This difficulty is not encountered with glucose oxidase testing material such as Testape and Combistix.

Because of the rather poor solubility of cephalothin in aqueous solutions, relatively large volumes must be injected. Warming the vial may be necessary to redissolve the solute if a precipitate has formed. When diluted according to the manufacturer's recommendation, a 1 Gm. dose makes an injection of 4 ml. Because of this large volume, and also because cephalothin may cause pain, the sites of injection should be carefully rotated. The doctor may order lidocaine (Xylocaine) or some other local anesthetic to be injected along with cephalothin.

Reconstituted solutions may be kept at room temperature for 6 hours, or for 48 hours if refrigerated.

> **USE.** In respiratory tract, urinary tract, soft tissue and skin infections as well as osteomyelitis and septicemia caused by susceptible microorganisms. Since its spectrum of activity includes penicillin-susceptible organisms, it is often the drug of choice in patients allergic to penicillin.

> **TOXICITY.** Neutropenia, allergies and injection site discomfort have been reported. Cross sensitivity to this drug has been noted in patients allergic to penicillin.

> **DOSE.** 0.5 to 2 Gm. I.M. or I.V. every 4 to 6 hours.

CEPHALOGLYCIN DIHYDRATE (KAFOCIN). Cephaloglycin is a member of the cephalosporin family of pharmacologic agents, but has the advantage of absorption after oral administration. It may be taken with food, since absorption does not appear to be affected significantly. It is readily concentrated and excreted in the urine after oral administration.

> **USES.** In the treatment of acute and chronic genitourinary tract infections, including pyelonephritis, cystitis and asymptomatic bacteruria. It is particularly effective against *E. coli, Klebsiella, Proteus,* staphylococci and enterococci.

TOXICITY. Nausea, vomiting, diarrhea, dermatitis, fever, chills, headache, dizziness and malaise. Prolonged use may be accompanied by overgrowth of yeast or fungi.

DOSE. 250 mg. four times daily orally for 10 days.

CEPHALEXIN MONOHYDRATE (KEFLEX).

Also a semisynthetic derivative of cephalosporin, this agent is effective against a variety of microorganisms; excellent blood levels may be obtained upon oral administration.

USES. In respiratory infections, particularly caused by pneumococci or streptococci. It may be useful in the treatment of urinary tract infections or skin and soft tissue infections.

TOXICITY. Nausea, vomiting, diarrhea, genital pruritus, neutropenia and skin reactions.

DOSE. 250 to 1000 mg. orally four times daily.

CLINDAMYCIN HYDROCHLORIDE HYDRATE (CLEOCIN).

Clindamycin is an orally effective inhibitor of protein synthesis in the bacterial cell, permanently affecting bacteria so that protein synthesis cannot be resumed. This latter fact has been interpreted to indicate death of the microorganism, thus bactericidal activity has been ascribed to this antibiotic, in contrast to the bacteriostatic effect of many antibiotics.

USES. Infections of the upper respiratory tract, skin and soft tissue infections and dental infections. It is indicated in the treatment of conditions caused by gram-positive organisms, particularly streptococci, pneumococci, and staphylococci.

TOXICITY. Nausea, vomiting, diarrhea, skin rash, transient leukopenia and various allergic reactions have been noted.

DOSE. 150 to 300 mg. orally every 6 hours.

LINCOMYCIN (LINCOCIN).

This new antibiotic produced by *Streptomyces lincolnensis* is different chemically from all other clinically available antibiotics. It has been shown to be effective against most of the common gram-positive organisms. It is well absorbed orally or by intramuscular or intravenous injection and is excreted in the bile and by the kidneys.

USES. May be administered orally in mild infections, and parenterally in more severe infections of the soft tissue, bone and respiratory system. Has been employed to treat otitis media, septic arthritis, meningitis, empyema, urinary tract infections and pustular acne. Useful in the treatment of patients allergic to penicillin.

TOXICITY. Diarrhea, nausea, vomiting, rash, vaginitis, urticaria. Its use is not recommended in patients with pre-existing liver, kidney, endocrine or metabolic disorders. Until further studies are completed, it is not recommended for use in the newborn.

DOSE. Oral—500 mg. three times daily. Parenteral—600 mg. every 12 hours.

CEPHALORIDINE (LORIDINE).

This agent is a broad-spectrum antibiotic which is effective when administered parenterally against a wide variety of microorganisms. It is bound to plasma protein, thus is found in high concentrations in the kidney. It does not pass the blood-brain barrier and is not used for meningeal infections.

USES. Intramuscularly or intravenously in the treatment of severe respiratory tract infections, genitourinary tract infections, osteomyelitis, syphilis (when penicillin is contraindicated) and gonorrhea.

TOXICITY. May cause kidney damage, thus renal function should be monitored closely during therapy. Skin rashes, nausea, vomiting and leukopenia have been reported, but are rare.

DOSE. 500 to 1000 mg. I.M. or I.V. three times daily.

GENTAMICIN SULFATE (GARAMYCIN). Gentamycin sulfate is a member of the aminoglycoside group of antibiotics. It is ineffective upon oral administration, but excellent blood levels are obtained after intramuscular injection, thus this is the method of choice. Very high renal levels of this drug may be obtained since it is almost entirely excreted by the kidneys.

USES. The use of this drug should be limited to serious infections caused by susceptible organisms, particularly *Pseudomonas, Proteus, E. coli,* and *Klebsiella.* It is effective in bacteremia, infected surgical wounds, soft tissue infections, respiratory tract infections and urinary tract infections caused by these microorganisms.

TOXICITY. May cause kidney damage or ototoxicity. Auditory loss is particularly noted in patients who have pre-existing renal damage, since in these cases the drug is excreted more slowly. When administering this drug to patients with impaired renal function, the dosage should be reduced approximately in half. Rash, purpura, anemia, drug fever, hypotension, convulsions, vomiting and liver damage have been reported as well.

DOSE. 60 to 100 mg. I.M. twice daily.

ANTIBIOTICS ACTIVE AGAINST FUNGI

AMPHOTERICIN B, U.S.P. (FUNGIZONE). Amphotericin B is a fungistatic antibiotic derived from strains of *Streptomyces nodosus.* Clinical evidence indicates that it is very active against a wide variety of deep-seated fungi and yeasts; it is ineffective against bacteria and viruses. Demonstrable blood levels persist for 18 hours after intravenous infusion, since kidney excretion is quite slow. Although poorly absorbed from the gastrointestinal tract, amphotericin B is active against species of *Candida* in the intestine, and small doses may be given orally to treat monilial overgrowth resulting from oral antibiotic therapy.

The drug is available in powder form. Both the powder and solutions made from it should be refrigerated and protected from light. Unused material should be discarded after 24 hours. Any precipitated solution should not be used. I.V. infusion should be freshly prepared and protected from light.

USES. Specifically for the treatment of disseminated mycotic infections including coccidioidomycosis, cryptococcosis, disseminated moniliasis, histoplasmosis, South American leishmaniasis and North and South American blastomycosis.

TOXICITY. Transient anorexia, chills and fever. Headache, nausea and vomiting are early toxic manifestations requiring a reduction of the total daily dosage. Increase in blood urea nitrogen (BUN) and nonprotein nitrogen (NPN) levels is the main dosage limiting factor. If these levels exceed 20 mg. and 40 mg. per 100 ml. respectively, it may be advisable to interrupt therapy until the values return to normal. Elevated blood creatinine level may also require interruption of therapy or a temporary decrease in dosage. Decreases in hemoglobin and drop in hematocrit have occurred. Hematologic, bone marrow and kidney and liver function tests as well as BUN and NPN level determinations should be conducted prior to therapy and at least once weekly during treatment. Inflammation or thrombophlebitis may occur at the site of infusion.

DOSE. 50 mg. in I.V. infusion over a period of 6 hours. Total daily dose should not exceed 250 mg./kg. of body weight. Recommended concentration for intravenous infusion is 0.1 mg. of amphotericin for each milliliter of 5% dextrose in water.

GRISEOFULVIN, U.S.P., B.P. (FULVICIN, GRIFULVIN, GRISACTIN). A major advance was made in antifungal therapy with the introduction of griseofulvin, a product of *Penicillin griseofulvum,* and the first agent that could be administered orally for the treatment of topical fungal infections. The exact mechanism of the fungistatic activity has not yet been determined.

Following systemic absorption, it is incorporated into all areas of skin and dermal appendages such as hair and nails. These infected tissues are then gradually replaced by healthy new growth. The response to therapy varies individually with the rate of keratinization of new tissue. The patient should be taught the importance of cleanliness to prevent reinfection, and the necessity of continuing with the prescribed therapy. The patient should be advised to use alcohol cautiously since griseofulvin may potentiate the action of alcohol.

USES.   Effective orally in the superficial mycoses, that is, ringworm of the scalp, body, feet and nails, produced by species of *Trichophyton, Microsporum* and *Epidermophyton.* Limited effectiveness in infections caused by *Sporotrichum schencki* and *Nocardia brasiliensis.* Griseofulvin is no more effective topically than other fungistatic compounds.

TOXICITY.   Side effects may include headache, vertigo, angioneurotic edema, skin disorders, monilial overgrowth, heartburn, epigastric discomfort, nausea and diarrhea, and, rarely, photosensitization and transient hearing loss. Large doses have produced mental confusion and transient psychologic disorders. A tendency toward leukopenia, which disappears when the drug is discontinued, has been observed on occasion.

DOSE.   500 mg. to 1 Gm. orally per day.

NYSTATIN, U.S.P., B.P. (MYCOSTATIN).   Nystatin is an antifungal antibiotic obtained from *Streptomyces noursei.* It is active against many species of yeasts and molds but is ineffective against bacteria. The drug is poorly absorbed following oral administration and detectable serum levels can be achieved only by massive oral doses. Following oral administration the drug is excreted unchanged in the feces.

USES.   Orally for the treatment of monilial infections of the oral cavity, for intestinal moniliasis and for treatment of monilial superinfection sustained during antibiotic or corticosteroid therapy. Topically, in the form of ointment for the treatment of monilial infections of the mouth (thrush), vagina and labia, and for monilial infections of the skin and nails. For oral infections, give between meals. No value in the treatment of systemic monilial infections.

TOXICITY.   Side effects occur infrequently and are mild and transitory. High dosage may produce nausea, vomiting and diarrhea. Hypersensitivity reactions occur very rarely.

DOSE.   Oral—500,000 to 1,000,000 units three times daily. Suppositories—100,-000 units three times daily. Topical—solutions containing 100,000 units per cc.

SULFONAMIDES

During the decade before penicillin became generally available the sulfonamides were the principal chemotherapeutic agents in use. They were widely employed during World War II. Although the introduction of antibiotics has caused the sulfonamides to be used less commonly today, they are still widely employed and have a number of advantages, such as low cost and ease of administration.

The discovery, in Germany in 1935, that mice with streptococcal and other infections could be protected by prontosil, an azo dye, led to clinical trial and the development of other similar agents. Splitting the prontosil molecule yielded para-aminobenzenesulfonamide (sulfanilamide), which was demonstrated to be as effective as prontosil in curing experimental infections. Numerous derivatives of sulfanilamide were soon synthesized and given clinical trials.

MECHANISM OF ACTION

Many theories have been proposed as to the mechanism of action of sulfonamides. The most generally accepted of these suggests that there is a competitive antagonism between para-aminobenzoic acid (PABA) and sulfonamide. The normal utilization of

NH_2

$COOH$

PABA

PABA by bacteria is thereby prevented. Sulfonamides prevent PABA from being incorporated into the folic acid molecule. Sulfonamide-sensitive organisms therefore are those that require folic acid and must synthesize this compound themselves. Those that do not require folic acid or that can utilize preformed folic acid are not affected by sulfonamides.

NH_2

SO_2NH_2

sulfanilamide

ABSORPTION, DISTRIBUTION AND EXCRETION

Certain sulfonamides are readily absorbed from the gastrointestinal tract and are distributed throughout all tissues of the body. Other sulfonamides are absorbed very poorly and are used as local anti-infectives on organisms in the gastrointestinal tract. If large enough doses are given systemically, enough of the drug will reach the cerebrospinal fluid to be effective in meningitis. Therefore use of the intrathecal route is unnecessary in sulfonamide therapy.

Both acetylation and oxidation of the sulfonamides occur in the liver and other tissues, and the drug is largely excreted in the urine. Small amounts are found in the feces and in some body secretions.

TOXICITY

The newer sulfonamides exhibit a much lower rate of toxic reactions than did those that were formerly used. Kidney damage and urinary complications such as urolithiasis, oliguria, hematuria, renal colic, obstruction anuria and nitrogen retention occur after sulfapyridine, sulfathiazole and sulfamerazine administration, but occur more rarely with sulfadiazine, sulfamethoxypyridazine, sulfisoxazole, sulfisomidine and sulfacetamide therapy.

Kidney damage and resulting complications may be due to the precipitation of sulfonamide crystals or their detoxification product, acetylsulfonamide, in the kidney tubule, or to a direct toxic action of the drug on the renal epithelium. Such damage may be prevented or reduced in severity by maintaining a fluid intake of approximately 2500 cc. a day in order to insure a urinary output of not less than 1000 cc. a day, and by the concurrent administration of sodium or potassium bicarbonate to alkalinize the urine. An accurate record of intake and output should be kept and the pH of the urine tested. Increasing acidity of the urine should be reported. Any decrease in output, hematuria or other symptoms of kidney damage should be reported immediately.

Fever, dermatoses and blood dyscrasias occur occasionally. These and other side effects of sulfonamide therapy are discussed in a nursing assessment guide, which appears at the end of this chapter.

Severe hypoglycemia may result when sulfonamides are administered with the antidiabetic sulfonylurea drugs such as tolbutamide. These similar agents potentiate each other's action.

COMBINATIONS OF SULFONAMIDES

Administration of two or more sulfonamides concurrently will usually lower the incidence of renal complications, since each sulfonamide is independently soluble. That is, even though 0.5 Gm. of each of three sulfonamides will give the therapeutic benefits of 1.5 Gm. of sulfonamide, each behaves in solution as if the others were not present. This results in a lower incidence of renal complications caused by precipitation of the drugs from solution.

The incidence of fever, rash and conjunctivitis is greater when combination therapy is used, however.

Sulfonamide Preparations

PHTHALYLSULFATHIAZOLE, U.S.P., B.P. (SULFATHALIDINE). Because phthalylsulfathiazole is only slightly absorbed from the gastrointestinal tract following oral administration, it is used preoperatively and postoperatively to reduce the bacterial flora in the intestinal tract when surgery is performed. Large doses may cause cramping in the abdomen, increased liquid consistency of the stool and frequent bowel movements.

DOSE.   3 to 7 Gm. daily orally.

SUCCINYLSULFATHIAZOLE, U.S.P., B.P. (SULFASUXIDINE). Succinylsulfathiazole is employed orally in the treatment of ulcerative colitis and ileitis and for bowel sterilization prior to surgery. Like phthalysulfathiazole, this agent is not absorbed from the gastrointestinal tract.

DOSE.   17 Gm. initially followed by 4 Gm. every 4 hours.

SULFACETAMIDE, N.F. (SULAMYD). Sulfacetamide is used primarily in the treatment of urinary tract infections such as pyelitis, cystitis and pyelonephritis. Unlike many other sulfonamides, it is soluble in acid as well as alkaline urine so that there is less danger of precipitation in the kidney tubules when high doses are employed. It is also used topically in the treatment of eye infections. Aqueous solutions must be refrigerated and prevented from exposure to light.

DOSE.   1 Gm. orally three or four times daily. 10 to 30 per cent solutions employed topically.

SULFADIAZINE, U.S.P., B.P. Sulfadiazine readily penetrates cerebrospinal fluid and when given intravenously is the sulfonamide of choice in treatment of meningococcal meningitis. If kidney function is impaired, sulfadiazine will accumulate in the blood and tissues; it is less toxic than many of the other sulfonamides, but will precipitate in acid urine.

DOSE.   2 to 4 Gm. orally initially, then 1 Gm. every 4 hours. 50 to 100 mg./kg. body weight every 6 to 8 hours I.V.

SULFAMETHIZOLE, N.F., B.P. (THIOSULFIL, UROLUCOSIL). Sulfamethizole is rapidly absorbed from the gastrointestinal tract and excreted. Crystalluria is rare but the usual precautions of sulfonamide therapy should be observed. It is used primarily in the treatment of urinary tract infections.

DOSE.   75 to 100 mg./kg. body weight daily orally.

SULFISOXAZOLE, U.S.P. (GANTRISIN). Probably the most commonly used of all the sulfonamides, this drug is characterized by a high degree of solubility even in neutral and slightly acid body fluids with a resultant decrease in the likelihood of renal blocking or crystalluria. It is used orally in the treatment of urinary infections due to gram-positive staphylococci and streptococci and to some gram-negative organisms. The drug should be protected from light.

Sulfisoxazole is also available for parenteral and ophthalmic use in the form of the soluble diethanolamine salt.

DOSE.   4 to 6 Gm. initially, then 1 or 2 Gm. every hour, intravenously. 500 mg. to 1 Gm. every 6 to 8 hours orally. 4% solution in ophthalmic preparations.

SULFAMETHOXAZOLE (GANTANOL). Although this drug is closely related to sulfisoxazole, its rate of excretion is somewhat slower, and a lower dosage may therefore be used.

DOSE.   2 Gm. initially, then 1 Gm. twice daily.

SULFAMETHOXYPYRIDAZINE,   U.S.P.,   B.P. (KYNEX, MIDICEL). Because of its slow excretion and long-lasting blood levels, this agent is recommended for use in urinary tract infections, upper respiratory tract infections, bacillary dysenteries and surgical and soft tissue infections. Crystalluria and hematuria due to its use are exceptionally rare. Administration of Kynex after meals may help to decrease gastrointestinal irritation.

DOSE. 1 Gm. orally the first day, then 500 mg. daily orally.

SULFADIMETHOXINE, N.F. (MADRIBON). Another low dosage sulfonamide, this is useful in a wide range of infectious disorders as well as in prophylactic therapy.

DOSE. 2 Gm. initially, then 0.5 Gm. daily orally.

SALICYLAZOSULFAPYRIDINE (AZULFIDINE). This compound, a derivative of sulfapyridine, is metabolized in the body to aminosalicylic acid and sulfapyridine. The salicylate derivative is intended to add an analgesic action to the action of the sulfonamide. If the urine is alkaline, this drug causes it to become orange-yellow in color.

DOSE. I Gm. four to six times daily orally.

Other sulfonamide preparations are:

SULFAPYRIDINE, U.S.P., B.P.

DOSE. I Gm. three times daily.

SULFISOMIDINE, SULPHADIMIDINE, B.P. (ELKO-SIN)

DOSE. 1 Gm. three times daily.

p-NITROSULFATHIAZOLE (NISULFAZOLE)

DOSE. Rectally in the form of a 10% suspension for the treatment of ulcerative colitis.

COMBINATIONS OF SULFONAMIDES

TRISULFAPYRIMIDINES ORAL SUSPENSION, U.S.P. Sulfadiazine, sulfamerazine and sulfamethazine are combined in equal parts in this suspension to provide 10 Gm. of sulfonamide per 100 cc. suspension.

DOSE. Initially 40 cc. (4 Gm.), then 10 cc. (1 Gm.) every 4 hours.

TRISULFAPYRIMIDINES TABLETS, U.S.P. (SULFOSE, TERFONYL TRUOZINE). Each tablet contains 0.167 Gm. each sulfadiazine, sulfamerazine and sulfamethazine for a total of 500 mg. mixed sulfonamides per tablet.

DOSE. Initially 4 Gm. then 1 Gm. every 4 hours.

ALDIAZOL-M TABLETS. Each tablet contains 0.125 Gm. each of sulfadiazine and sulfamerazine with 0.25 Gm. sodium citrate. The sodium citrate aids in maintaining an alkaline medium to enhance the solubility of the sulfonamides.

DOSE. The dosage schedule of this and the following mixed sulfonamides closely parallels that of the trisulfapyrimidine preparations.

DUOZINE DULCET TABLETS. Each tablet contains 0.15 Gm. each of sulfadiazine and sulfamerazine.

CITRASULFAS M. This oral suspension contains 0.216 Gm. each of sulfadiazine and sulfamerazine with 1 Gm. sodium citrate per 5 cc.

PANSULFA TABLETS, TRICOMBISUL TABLETS. These similar preparations each contain sulfacetamide, sulfadiazine and sulfamerazine in equal parts to make 500 mg. tablets.

URINARY ANTISEPTICS

In order to be effective as a urinary antiseptic, a drug must be excreted in the urine and concentrated in sufficient amounts to have an antiseptic effect in the urinary tract.

Some of the sulfonamides and antibiotics are currently used as urinary antiseptics, but a number of other agents are employed almost exclusively for their effect on the urinary tract. The choice of the specific antiseptic agent depends largely on the pathogen involved in the infection.

MANDELIC ACID; AMMONIUM, CALCIUM AND SODIUM MANDELATE. Although any of these four agents may be used, calcium mandelate has certain advantages over the other three forms. It causes less gastric irritation than does mandelic acid, it does not interfere with the acidification of urine as does sodium mandelate, and being relatively tasteless, it is more acceptable to the patient than the ammonium salt.

In an acid urine (pH 5.5 or less) mandelic acid and its salts are bacteriostatic or bactericidal against *E. coli, A. aerogenes* and *S. faecalis;* they are effective against some strains of *Proteus, Pseudomonas, Alcaligenes, Salmonella* and *Shigella.*

Fluid intake during therapy should not exceed 1200 cc. daily in order to concentrate the drug effectively in the urine. If a noticeable improvement in the infection is not obtained in 12 to 14 days, additional therapy should be instituted.

> **TOXICITY.** Contraindicated in the presence of preexisting kidney damage because the drug cannot be effectively concentrated or excreted in the urine. Systemic acidosis may result from elevated retention of this drug. Nausea, diarrhea, dysuria and hematuria occur but rarely become serious problems.

> **DOSE.** 3 Gm. four times a day orally.

METHENAMINE MANDELATE, U.S.P. (MANDELAMINE). Methenamine mandelate is used in the management of urinary tract infections, including pyelitis, pyelonephritis, cystitis, and infections accompanying neurogenic bladder and urine retention. It is effective against most of the causative agents of urinary tract infection such as *E. coli, Staphylococcus aureus, Staph. albus, Streptococcus faecalis,* and some other strains. It has antiseptic action only, and has limited efficacy when used alone in the treatment of severe or chronic urinary tract infections.

The action of methenamine mandelate is due both to the properties of mandelic acid, which is excreted in the urine, and the production of formaldehyde, which is formed in an acid urine from methenamine. An acid urine is essential for the optimal action of this drug and the pH may go no higher than 6.0. Intermittent testing of the urinary pH should be carried on during therapy. Ammonium chloride or sodium acid phosphate in doses of 0.5 to 1 Gm. should be administered concurrently to ensure proper acidity of the urine.

> **TOXICITY.** Side effects are few and relatively uncommon. Gastrointestinal upsets occur occasionally. The drug is contraindicated in renal insufficiency since metabolic acidosis may result.

> **DOSE.** 1 Gm. three to four times daily orally.

METHYLENE BLUE, U.S.P. This agent is a synthetic dye which also has antiseptic properties and is used to treat cystitis and urethritis both by oral administration and by local irrigation of the bladder. Internal administration imparts a greenish yellow or blue color to the urine and patients should be forewarned of this fact when they are placed on oral therapy.

An additional property of this drug—that of changing hemoglobin to methemoglobin—makes it of some use intravenously as an antidote in cyanide poisoning, for the cyanide combines with methemoglobin to form a nontoxic compound, cyanmethemoglobin. In this way the enzyme systems of the body are protected against the effects of the cyanide molecules.

> **TOXICITY.** Irritation of the bladder occurs occasionally.

> **DOSE.** Irrigation—0.1 to 0.2% solution. Oral—120 to 300 mg. every 4 hours. Intravenous—1% aqueous solution.

NALIDIXIC ACID (NEGGRAM). Nalidixic acid is rapidly absorbed from the gastrointestinal tract and readily excreted in the urine in active form. Effective levels of the drug appear in the urine even after a single dose of 500 mg. Although antibacterial serum levels may be obtained following oral administration, considerably higher doses are required for systemic therapy than are needed for antibacterial urine concentration, and the use of the drug in the treatment of systemic infections is still under investigation.

The drug is used in the treatment of infections of the urinary tract, and is the drug of choice in *Proteus* infections, although it is quite active against the other common organisms producing urinary infections as well. There has been no evidence that the effectiveness of nalidixic acid is dependent on urinary pH. Combination therapy with other urinary antiseptics is often desirable as resistance to therapy is a problem if nalidixic acid is used alone.

TOXICITY. The most common side effects are nausea and vomiting, although weakness, dizziness, headache and drowsiness occur as well. Sensitivity reactions and mild eosinophilia have occurred. Periodic blood counts during therapy are advisable to check for possible bone marrow suppression.

DOSE. 1 Gm. four times a day, orally.

nalidixic acid

NITROFURANTOIN, U.S.P., B.P. (FURADANTIN). A genitourinary agent that is bactericidal to many gram-negative and gram-positive organisms, this drug is also characterized by a low incidence of bacterial resistance. It is effective against most strains of *E. coli, Proteus, Micrococcus pyogenes albus, M. pyogenes aureus, Streptococcus pyogenes, Aerobacter aerogenes* and *Paracolobactrum*. Although it is usually administered orally for infections of the urinary tract, it may occasionally be administered intravenously for refractory bacterial infections caused by susceptible organisms when oral therapy is not feasible. Nitrofurantoin may cause the urine to have a brownish tint.

TOXICITY. Oral administration may produce peripheral neuritis, nausea, vomiting, hemolytic anemia or allergic reactions; in many cases these effects may be controlled simply by a reduction in dosage or by giving the drug with food or milk. The drug is contraindicated in the presence of preexisting renal damage. It should not be used in infants under one month of age.

DOSE. 100 mg. four times a day orally. 180 mg. twice daily I.V.

PHENAZOPYRIDINE HYDROCHLORIDE (PYRIDIUM). Although phenazopyridine, an azo dye, inhibits various microorganisms in vitro, it has little or no antibacterial effect in vivo. Its chief value in urinary tract infections lies in its local anesthetic effect on the urinary tract mucosa, thus diminishing the constant urgency that often accompanies infections.

The drug is used orally as an adjunct to the treatment of cystitis, prostatitis, urethritis and pyelonephritis. Patients should be forewarned about the orange or red color the drug will impart to the urine, when the drug is taken orally, and the nurse should not be led to confuse this with hematuria.

Phenazopyridine is often combined with the sulfonamides to treat urinary infections.

TOXICITY. Some allergic reactions have been noted as well as infrequent cases of methemoglobinemia. Severe hepatitis and uremia are contraindications to the use of this drug.

DOSE. 100 to 200 mg. three times a day orally.

ETHOXAZENE HYDROCHLORIDE (SERENIUM). Like phenazopyridine, ethoxazene exhibits antibacterial activity in vitro, but has little or no effect in vivo after oral administration. Its chief value lies in its anesthetic effect on the urinary mucosa. It is often used as an adjunct to sulfonamides or antibiotics in the treatment of acute urinary infections.

TOXICITY. Should be used with caution in patients with pyelonephritis or pregnancy or gastrointestinal disorders. It is contraindicated in the presence of uremia, severe hepatitis and chronic glomerular nephritis.

DOSE. 100 mg. three times a day orally.

FURAZOLIDONE, N.F. (FUROXONE). Furazolidone is a nitrofuran derivative which is believed to exert its antibacterial action through interference with carbohydrate metabolism in the bacterial cell. When administered orally, it is useful in the treatment of gastrointestinal infections caused by susceptible bacteria such as *Salmonella, Shigella, Staphylococcus, Aerobacter* and *Escherichia.* It is excreted via the urine and may impart a brown color to it. Testing of the urine for sugar may be invalid while the drug is being taken.

Furazolidone is also applied as a powder insufflate and in suppository form for the treatment of *Trichomonas vaginalis* vaginitis.

The drug should be protected from exposure to light.

Toxicity. Nausea, vomiting, headache and dermatoses may occur upon oral use of furazolidone. Blood dyscrasias have been noted upon prolonged administration. This drug has been shown to inhibit monoamine oxidase in experimental animals. When administered to a number of patients, an increase in urinary tryptamine excretion was observed, together with a 5- to 25-fold enhancement of sensitivity to the pressor effect of tyramine. These changes are characteristic of monoamine oxidase inhibitors (Chapter 11). Because of these experimental reports, a warning has been given that oral treatment with furazolidone may induce hypersensitivity to ingested amines such as those found in sharp cheeses, wine—especially Chianti—and beer. These foods and beverages should be avoided during furazolidone administration and for four days after the drug has been discontinued.

DOSE. Oral—100 mg. four times daily. Insufflation—0.1% concentration. Suppositories—0.25% furazolidone.

GUIDE FOR THE NURSING ASSESSMENT OF A PATIENT RECEIVING AN ANTIBIOTIC

I. Why is the patient receiving an antibiotic? Where is the locus of the infection? What are the results of the culture and sensitivity test, if done? What organism(s) is (are) involved? Are the organisms sensitive to the prescribed antibiotic?

II. Does this patient have any condition for which the antibiotic is contraindicated? Any renal impairment? Any allergies?

III. Is the drug being administered correctly? Is the physician's order still valid or should it be questioned? Is it being given on time in order to maintain blood levels? If given orally, is it given at a time which promotes maximum systemic absorption? If given intramuscularly, is recommended technique used (e.g., deep I.M.) and are sites rotated? Are there signs of tissue irritation? If given intravenously, is the correct preparation of the drug used? Is this antibiotic compatible with the I.V. solution used? Is the rate of flow correct? Are there signs of thrombophlebitis?

IV. Is the antibiotic effective? Is there a decrease in fever, white blood cell count, signs of inflammation, purulent drainage, cough and sputum production, malaise and other subjective symptoms? Do repeated cultures indicate a decrease in the number of pathogens?

V. Are there any drug-food interactions with this antibiotic? Are there any drug interactions likely to occur with other drugs the patient is receiving?

VI.   Has the patient experienced any side effects of this antibiotic? Any rashes or other signs and symptoms of allergy? Any signs or symptoms of secondary infection? Any signs or symptoms of blood dyscrasias (see chart in Chapter 2)? Do any of the laboratory tests indicate damage to kidney, liver, or hemopoietic system? Any signs of toxicity to the eighth cranial nerve such as tinnitus, dizziness, loss of hearing? Is there adequate urinary output? Are nursing measures being initiated to decrease side effects whenever possible?

VII.   What are patient's (and family's) learning needs? Does he know the purpose of the antibiotic? Does he understand clearly directions for taking the antibiotic, if at home? Does he understand the advisability of discarding unused antibiotics when no longer needed? Does he understand the dangers of self-prescribing of antibiotics, as well as other drugs?

GUIDE FOR THE NURSING ASSESSMENT OF A PATIENT RECEIVING A SYSTEMICALLY ABSORBED SULFONAMIDE

I.   Why is the patient receiving the sulfonamide? For systemic infection? For urinary tract infection?

II.   Does this patient have any condition for which this drug is contraindicated? Is he hypersensitive to sulfa drugs? Does he have a history of renal calculi?

III.   Is the drug producing the desired effect? Is the blood level of the drug being maintained by administering the drug on time? Is there a decrease in signs of infection, such as decreased fever, decreased white blood cell count? Are signs of urinary tract infection decreased? Is there a decrease in urgency, frequency and dysuria? Do cultures of urine show a decrease in bacteria?

IV.   Has the patient experienced any side effects? Any signs or symptoms of hypersensitivity to sulfa drugs? Is crystal formation avoided by measures to prevent acidity of the urine? Is fluid intake sufficient to maintain a urinary output of at least 1000 cc.? Is sodium bicarbonate ordered to be given with this drug? Is there any decrease in urinary output? Hematuria? Are there any indications of blood dyscrasias? Is the patient a diabetic who is receiving a sulfonylurea as an oral hypoglycemic agent? If so, has the patient experienced signs and symptoms of hypoglycemia?

V.   What are the patient's (and family's) learning needs? Does the patient understand why he is receiving the drug? Does he understand the directions for administering the drug? Does he understand the need for an adequate fluid intake? Is he aware of signs and symptoms which he should report immediately?

QUESTIONS FOR DISCUSSION AND REVIEW

1.   Explain the mechanism by which it is possible for a patient to have severe dermatitis following repeated doses of penicillin.

2.   When are the long-acting forms of penicillin used? When is it necessary to use the short-acting forms?

3.   What symptoms would be indicative of an allergic reaction to penicillin? What drugs and equipment should be on hand?

4.   Which sulfonamides are useful for systemic infections? Which are not absorbed after oral administration?

5.   What are the primary advantages in using long-acting sulfonamides? What would be the disadvantages?

6.   What are the toxic symptoms of griseofulvin? Which would necessitate withdrawal of the drug?

7.   What is the primary value of phenazopyridine in urinary tract infections? Is it of value if given alone in serious infections?

8.   What nursing measures can be taken when a drug causes gastrointestinal distress by irritating the mucosa?

9.   Explain how secondary infection or superinfection occurs.

10.   Why should the patient have an adequate urinary output when he is receiving a systemic sulfonamide?

11.   What are the signs and symptoms of blood dyscrasias that commonly occur with antibiotics?

BIBLIOGRAPHY

Abraham, E. P.: The cephalosporins. *Pharmacol. Rev.*, *14*:473, 1962.

Abraham, E. P.: The chemistry of new antibiotics. *Amer. J. Med.*, *39*:692, 1965.

AMA Drug Evaluations. Chicago, American Medical Association, 1971.

Bercovitz, Z. T. (ed.): *Clinical Tropical Medicine.* New York, Paul B. Hoeber, Inc., 1944.

Best, W. R.: Chloramphenicol-associated blood dyscrasias. *J.A.M.A.*, *201*:181, 1967.

Block, B.: Site of injection of penicillin, (Questions and Answers). *J.A.M.A., 188*:95, 1964.

Council on Drugs: A new antibacterial agent for infections of the genitourinary tract—Nalidixic acid (NegGram). *J.A.M.A.*, *192*:628, 1965.

Council on Drugs: A new oral penicillin—Ampicillin. *J.A.M.A.*, *191*: 1071, 1965.

Council on Drugs: A new semisynthetic penicillin—Sodium Nafcillin. *J.A.M.A., 191*:930, 1965.

DiPalma, J. R.: The antibiotics and their use. *R.N., 32*:57, (October) 1969.

DiPalma, J. R. (ed.): *Drill's Pharmacology in Medicine.* 4th Ed. New York, McGraw-Hill Book Co., 1971.

Eggers, H. J., and Tanim, I.: Antiviral chemotherapy. *Ann. Rev. Pharmacol., 6*:231, 1966.

Florey, M. E.: *The Clinical Application of Antibiotics*. London, Oxford University Press, 1961.

Friend, D.: Penicillin G. *Clin. Pharmacol. Ther., 7*:421, 1966.

Friend, D.: Penicillin therapy—newer semisynthetic penicillins. *Clin. Pharmacol. Ther., 7*:706, 1966.

Gause, G. F.: *The Search for New Antibiotics*. New Haven, Yale University Press, 1960.

Goodman, L. S., and Gilman, A.: *Pharmacological Basis of Therapeutics*. 4th Ed. New York, Macmillan Co., 1970.

Gorini, L.: Antibiotics and the genetic code. *Sci. American, 214*:102, (April) 1966.

Goth, A.: *Medical Pharmacology*. 3rd Ed. St. Louis, C. V. Mosby Co., 1968.

Govoni, L. E., and Hayes, J. E.: *Drugs and Nursing Implications*. 2nd Ed. New York, Appleton-Century-Crofts, 1971.

Griffiths, R. S., and Black, H. R.: Cephalothin—a new antibiotic. *J.A.M.A., 189*:823, 1964.

Hall, J. W.: Drug therapy in infectious diseases. *Amer. J. Nurs., 61*:56, 1961.

Jager, B. V.: Untoward reactions to antibiotics. *Amer. J. Nurs., 54*:966, 1954.

Kunin, C. M.: Effects of antibiotics on the gastrointestinal tract. *Clin. Pharmacol. Ther., 8*:495, 1967.

Martin, W. I.: Newer penicillins. *Med. Clin. N. Amer., 51*:1107, 1967.

Moulton, F. R. (ed.): *A Symposium on Human Malaria*. No. 15. Washington, D.C., Am. Assn. for the Adv. of Sci., 1941.

Murdock, J. McC.: Toxicity of the sulfonamides. *Practitioner, 194*:26, 1965.

Richardson, I., et al.: The meaning of antibiotic resistance in bacteria 2. Genetic mechanisms of bacteria. *Nurs. Times, 65*:884, (July 10) 1969.

Ridley, M.: The age of antibacterial chemotherapy. *Nurs. Times, 66*:77, (January 15) 1970.

Ridley, M.: The semisynthetic penicillins and other antibacterial agents. *Nurs. Times, 66*:103, (January 22) 1970.

Ridley, M.: The clinical use of antibacterial agents. *Nurs. Times, 66*:146, (January 29) 1970.

Rodman, M. J.: Combating urinary tract infection. *R.N., 31*:59 (November) 1968.

Rodman, M. J.: New drugs for fighting infection. *R.N., 30*:55, (June) 1967.

Schaffer, L., et al.: Lincomycin—a new antibiotic. *Clin. Pediat., 2*:642, 1963.

Smith, D. T., Conant, N. F. and Willett, H. P. (eds.): *Zinsser Microbiology*. 14th Ed. New York, Appleton-Century-Crofts, 1968.

Smith, L. H. and Martin, W. J.: Infections of the urinary tract. *Med. Clin. N. Amer., 50*:1127, 1966.

Toxicity of tetracyclines. *Lancet, 2*:283, 1963.

VanArsdel, P. P., Jr.: Allergic reactions to penicillin. *J.A.M.A., 191*:238, 1965.

Weinstein, Z., Kaplan, K. and Chang, T.: Treatment of infections in man with Cephalothin. *J.A.M.A., 189*:929, 1964.

White, A. W., Handler, P. and Smith, E. L.: *Principles of Biochemistry*. 3rd Ed. New York, McGraw-Hill Book Co., 1964.

Wolfe, A. D. and Hohn, F. E.: Erythromycin: mode of action. *Science, 143*:1445, 1964.

Yaffe, S. J.: Antibiotic dosage in newborn and premature infants. *J.A.M.A., 193*:818, 1965.

er 10 Systemic Anti-infectives in Specific Infections

Important Concepts Discussed

1. *Antitubercular drugs, although quite effective in many cases of tuberculosis, have a high incidence of serious side effects and microorganisms acquire resistance to them very quickly.*
2. *Sulfones, drugs used in the treatment of Hansen's disease, bear a chemical resemblance to the sulfonamides, but have a different mechanism of action.*
3. *Most antimalarial drugs are effective only against a particular phase in the life cycle of the parasite.*
4. *Although worm infestation can be effectively treated by specific pharmacologic agents, patient teaching in hygiene must accompany drug therapy to prevent reinfection.*
5. *The nurse has an important role in the prevention and treatment of disease by insuring the correct administration of drugs and promoting health through teaching and case-finding.*

ANTITUBERCULOSIS DRUGS

Pulmonary tuberculosis is a persistent infection caused by the acid-fast microorganism *Mycobacterium tuberculosis.* Although infections by this organism are largely centered in the lungs, they are also found in other body tissues and organs such as the bone, kidneys, spleen and meninges.

The tuberculosis bacillus is difficult to treat by drug therapy primarily because of the frequency with which resistance to therapy occurs, but also because there is an allergic response at the site of infection with an inflammatory reaction resulting in encapsulation of the lesion.

Because of the inflammatory reaction at the site of the lesion, the invasion of the area by numerous inflammatory cells and subsequent fibrous tissue deposition around the area, the blood supply becomes poor. Eventually caseation necrosis occurs. The area of necrosis is likely to liquefy and involve a branch of the bronchial tree in the process. The liquefied necrotic material then drains out and is expectorated, leaving a cavity in the lung parenchymal tissue. When this occurs, efficient and effective drug therapy becomes an even greater problem.

Consequently, if x-ray examinations do not show reduction in size of the cavity after four to six months of treatment, surgery is usually indicated.

In order to delay the appearance of resistant organisms, combinations of drugs are used in the treatment of tuberculosis. The use of streptomycin in this disease has already been discussed in Chapter 9. Streptomycin is combined primarily with para-aminosalicylic acid (PAS) and isoniazid (INH) to delay the development of resistance, but even this therapy is not always effective in healing the lesions before resistance occurs. In this event additional anti-tuberculosis agents are employed. These agents are generally withheld until treatment with the standard drugs has proved ineffective, however, because almost without exception serious drug toxicity reactions occur with them.

The antituberculosis drugs act by inhibiting multiplication of the tubercle bacilli, thus enabling the body's own resources to cope with the disease and develop an immunity to it. These agents are thus bacteriostatic rather than bactericidal in effect, and are often referred to as tuberculostatic drugs.

The patient receiving anti-infectives for tuberculosis should be observed for the effectiveness of the drug. Signs and symptoms of improvement include a decrease in fever, decreased malaise and a feeling of well-being, increased appetite and weight gain and decreased coughing and production of sputum. A negative sputum culture and regression in size of the lesion on x-ray are particularly significant as indications of drug effectiveness. Patients sometimes need encouragement and supervision in continuing drug therapy when the symptoms of tuberculosis have disappeared in their view.

Teaching the patient hygiene measures, the need for good nutrition and adequate rest and exercise is an important aspect of the plan of care. Follow-up on the patient's personal contacts is needed to curb the spread of tuberculosis and to diagnose and treat, in the early stage, any cases found.

Further suggestions for patient care are offered in the nurse's assessment guide at the end of this chapter.

AMINOSALICYLIC ACID, U.S.P. (PARA-AMINOSALICYLIC ACID, PAS, PAMISYL, PARAPAS, PARASAL).

Aminosalicylic acid is rapidly absorbed from the gastrointestinal tract when taken orally and diffuses throughout the body with the highest concentration being found in the kidney, lungs and liver. The presence of the drug in the urine may interfere with the results of Benedict's test for glycosuria. When used singly, this drug has a low level of antituberculosis activity, but it is quite useful in delaying the emergence of resistant strains of the microorganism when used in conjunction with streptomycin and/or isoniazid.

p-aminosalicylic acid

Early symptomatic improvement occurs when PAS is used, however, and the patient experiences less coughing and sputum production, increased appetite, slowing of the pulse and respiration, and reduction of the accompanying fever. It is important for the nurse to note and chart these beneficial effects. This drug should be given with food or after meals, and an antacid may be needed to counteract the gastric discomfort sometimes experienced.

The expiration date of the drug should be checked before it is administered, and it should be stored away from heat and humidity in a tightly sealed container.

TOXICITY. Gastrointestinal disturbances consisting of nausea, vomiting and diarrhea. These effects are usually overcome by using a different preparation, such as the calcium salt of PAS, or by stopping the drug for a few days. Hepatitis, dermatitis and drug fever occur occasionally as do more serious goitrogenic effects resulting from inhibition of iodine accumulation in the thyroid gland. Electrolyte disturbances are occasionally noted. Other salicylates should be avoided in order to prevent salicylate poisoning.

DOSE. 4 to 5 Gm. orally three times daily. This dosage requires the patient to take a relatively large number of tablets each day.

$$CO-NH-NH_2$$

isoniazid

ISONIAZID, U.S.P., B.P. (INH, ISONICOTINIC ACID HYDRAZIDE, NICONYL, NYDRAZID, RIMIFORN, TYVID). Although isoniazid is quite effective when used singly, it is active for only a short time because of the rapid development of resistance. When this drug is used alone, resistance develops almost a thousand times as fast as it does when streptomycin is used singly. Accordingly INH is only used in combination therapy. A highly specific drug, INH is totally inactive against any organism except *Mycobacterium tuberculosis.*

Like PAS, this drug is rapidly absorbed from the gastrointestinal tract and is distributed throughout all body tissues including the brain and spinal fluid.

It is rapidly inactivated, however, and 90 per cent of the hydroxylation and acetylation products appear in the urine within 24 hours. The remainder is excreted in the feces, milk, saliva and other exocrine secretions.

INH alone is used as prophylactic therapy for one year after a previously nonreactive individual converts to a positive tuberculin skin test, when no active tubercular disease can be detected.

TOXICITY. At recommended dosage levels, toxic reactions are not usually a problem with this drug. Toxic doses produce symptoms of anorexia, weight loss, liver damage, febrile reactions, vertigo, constipation, dryness of the mouth and delayed micturition. Since this drug is related to pyridoxine, symptoms of pyridoxine deficiency occasion-

ally occur in the form of peripheral neuritis. This can be corrected by administering pyridoxine in doses of 25 to 50 mg./day. Rarely symptoms of central nervous system irritability occur. Should be used with caution in patients with a history of convulsions or epileptic seizures, since these are occasionally precipitated by this drug.

DOSE. 100 mg. orally twice daily.

PYRAZINAMIDE (PZA). Pyrazinamide is indicated in the treatment of tuberculosis only when bacterial resistance has developed to the primary drugs (streptomycin, PAS, INH) and other drugs cannot be used because of intolerance or allergic manifestations.

Because of its limited usefulness and the possibility of liver damage, pyrazinamide is not considered a suitable drug for initial treatment. When used, it may be given alone or in combination with INH for one to three months. Intolerance or resistance usually preclude its use for longer periods.

TOXICITY. Liver damage may be progressive and irreversible and may result in death upon prolonged use of this drug. In mild to moderate cases of impaired liver function, the symptoms may be reversible upon discontinuation of therapy. Blood uric acid levels should be performed routinely during therapy since uric acid is often increased sufficiently to precipitate attacks of gout during therapy.

DOSE. 0.75 Gm. orally twice daily.

VIOMYCIN SULFATE, B.P. (VINACTANE, VIOCIN). This antibiotic produced by *Streptomyces puniceus* has been shown to be less effective and more toxic than many of the drugs used in the treatment of tuberculosis. It does seem capable of potentiating the bacteriostatic ability of other drugs, and is always used in combination with other agents.

Since absorption following oral administration is poor, viomycin is administered intramuscularly. Only small amounts diffuse into the spinal fluid, so that it is of limited use in tuberculous meningitis. Excretion occurs largely via the kidneys.

TOXICITY. Auditory nerve damage occurs, and precautions must be taken when this drug is combined with other ototoxic agents such as streptomycin. Patients with impaired kidney function should be followed closely since high levels of the drug may accumulate if excretion is impaired. Albuminuria and cylindruria are observed frequently, and microscopic hematuria occurs, but rarely. The renal toxicity caused by this drug appears to be reversible, but patients with preexisting renal disease should be given it only with closely regulated testing of kidney function.

DOSE. 2 Gm. I.M. every third day, given in divided doses at 12 hour intervals for up to six weeks.

CYCLOSERINE, B.P. (SEROMYCIN). Cycloserine, an antibiotic produced by *Streptomyces orchidaceus,* is active in vitro against a wide variety of gram-positive and gram-negative organisms including the tubercle bacillus. Because of toxic reactions, its use is limited almost exclusively to the treatment of tuberculosis, and it is used in this disease only when treatment with the standard drugs has decreased in effectiveness. Cycloserine is more effective in combination with INH; however, it may be used alone.

$$H_2C \text{------} CH\text{-}NH_2$$

cycloserine

TOXICITY. When the individual dose does not exceed 250 mg. few toxic reactions are observed. Administration of 1 Gm. or more daily may cause drowsiness, dizziness, allergic reactions, hyperreflexia and convulsions. Central nervous system effects may be minimized or controlled by the concurrent administration of pyridoxine, anticonvulsants, tranquilizers or sedatives. Contraindicated in patients with a history of epilepsy and should be used with caution in patients with renal insufficiency since

delayed excretion enhances the appearance of side effects.

DOSE. 250 mg. orally every 12 hours.

ETHIONAMIDE (TRECATOR). This analogue of nicotinamide is one of the newer agents effective against *M. tuberculosis.* When administered orally it is readily distributed to all body tissues including the brain and meninges. The organism becomes resistant rapidly, however, and it should be used only in combination therapy.

TOXICITY. Gastrointestinal symptoms, postural hypotension, depression, drowsiness, peripheral neuropathy, dermatoses and hepatitis have been noted. Should not be administered to patients with diabetes mellitus since management may become a problem when this drug is given.

DOSE. Initially 250 mg. twice daily, gradually increased to 500 mg. twice daily. Only administered orally at the present time.

ETHAMBUTOL (MYAMBUTOL). This agent appears to be effective orally in the treatment of tuberculosis. It has proved effective in cases when most other agents had become relatively useless.

TOXICITY. Studies are incomplete, but there are possible reversible effects on the vision following prolonged use. Muscular incoordination and labored respiration have been noted in animal experiments.

DOSE. 25 to 50 mg./kg. daily orally.

AMEBICIDES

Amebiasis, or infection by organisms of the ameba group, is very common throughout the world. A large proportion of the cases are due to nonpathogenic organisms, and even among those caused by pathogenic organisms, symptoms are often mild. The term amebiasis, however, is usually limited to severe infection caused by the *Entamoeba histolytica.* The primary site of infection is the large intestine, and the usual symptom is diarrhea (amebic dysentery). However, motile (trophozoite) forms of the parasite may invade the body tissues and travel to other parts of the body, where metastatic abscesses occur. The most common sites of abscesses are the liver and the mucosa of the duodenum and colon. Abscesses of the brain and other organs occur rarely.

The incidence of amebiasis in any population is determined by the level of sanitation. Originally the disease was thought of as tropical in distribution, but it is now found throughout the world. It occurs particularly where human excreta is used as the chief fertilizer for vegetables, and wherever fecal contamination of drinking water occurs. Carriers of the parasite excrete it in the feces in a cyst form, which reverts to the motile form after ingestion by a new host.

Drug therapy of amebiasis may have several different aims, including treatment of the asymptomatic carrier of cysts, and treatment of the various manifestations of amebic infection within the body. Amebicidal drugs may vary in their effectiveness for these different purposes. A complete cure of amebiasis denotes complete eradication of the parasites from the body, and may require many months or even years.

In caring for a patient with amebiasis, the nurse should remember that the portal of entry for the parasite is the gastrointestinal tract, usually through food and water contaminated by feces. The number of stools as well as their characteristics should be noted, with particular observation for the presence of cysts, mucus and blood. The nurse should use careful handwashing technique, and the necessity of handwashing to prevent reinfection and spreading to others should be explained to the patient.

Persons who are carriers, i.e., those who have only mild gastrointestinal distress but unknowingly pass cysts, must be located and restricted from any food handling.

Sanitary facilities and procedures in the home may need to be evaluated and corrected. Fecal material should be flushed immediately. Bedpans should be disinfected by boiling at least once a day.

If amebiasis results in severe or persistent diarrhea, electrolyte imbalance may occur and correction will be needed. The diet should be high in caloric value, low in residue and should contain plenty of fluids.

EMETINE HYDROCHLORIDE, U.S.P., B.P. Emetine, an alkaloid obtained from ipecac, is of little value in the cure of intestinal amebiasis, but is most valuable for controlling the symptoms. It is of no value in the treatment of asymptomatic cyst passers.

Contrary to its ineffectiveness in the intestinal form of the disease, emetine is of value in the treatment of amebic hepatitis and abscess of the liver, lungs, brain and skin.

This drug is a general protoplasmic poison that is slowly eliminated from the body following parenteral administration. It continues to be eliminated in the urine for 40 to 60 days after a single dose is administered. Preexisting kidney damage increases the time necessary for excretion, so that dangerously high blood levels may be accumulated within a relatively short period.

The pulse and blood pressure should be followed closely during therapy. A decrease in blood pressure and an elevated pulse may indicate toxicity to cardiac muscle. The drug should never be administered for more than 10 days at a time with a 30 day rest period intervening between courses of therapy. Bed rest is recommended during the course of therapy; the activity of the patient should be regulated after therapy is stopped.

> **TOXICITY.** Nausea, vomiting, diarrhea, dizziness, tachycardia and sudden cardiac failure may occur. In addition, there may be cellular degeneration of the liver, heart, intestinal tract, kidney and skeletal muscles. Contraindicated in patients with heart disease, liver or kidney disorders, in aged or debilitated persons, and in pregnancy. Should be used with caution in children.

Local edema and necrosis may occur at the site of injection. Sites of injection should be carefully rotated. Care should be taken when aspirating before injection, since intravenous administration of this drug is dangerous.

DOSE. 60 mg. subcutaneously or intramuscularly daily for four to six days.

CHLOROQUINE PHOSPHATE, U.S.P., B.P. (ARALEN). Although this drug is used primarily as an antimalarial (p. 192), it is used with considerable success in the treatment of extraintestinal forms of amebiasis. Its absorption in the upper gastrointestinal tract precludes its usefulness in the intestinal form of the disease.

The actions and side effects of this drug will be discussed more thoroughly in the antimalarial section.

DOSE. 2 Gm. orally daily for two days, then 250 mg. twice daily.

BIALAMICOL (CAMOFORM). Bialamicol is employed to relieve the symptoms of acute amebiasis and is quite effective in this regard. It is of little effect in the treatment of asymptomatic cyst passers, however, and it is found that cysts persist in the stools of many patients treated with this drug.

It is quite readily absorbed following oral administration and is accumulated rapidly in most body tissues with high concentrations of the liver, kidney, spleen, lungs and lymphoid tissues of the intestinal wall and mesentery.

The drug should be protected from exposure to light.

TOXICITY. Usually well tolerated. Reversible enlargement of the liver occurs occasionally with high doses or prolonged treatment. Gastrointestinal symptoms and skin reactions have been reported in some cases. The latter may be aggravated by exposure to the sun or to ultraviolet rays.

DOSE. 250 to 500 mg. orally three times daily.

CARBARSONE, U.S.P. This organic arsenical is quite useful in the treatment of the amebic cysts as well as the trophozoite forms of the parasite. Since arsenic is only slowly excreted in the urine, it is necessary to give

interrupted therapy with this drug in order to avoid possible cumulative toxic effects.

TOXICITY. The drug should be discontinued immediately if symptoms of nausea, vomiting, diarrhea, pulmonary congestion, neuritis, skin reactions, albuminuria or liver and spleen enlargement occur. Contraindicated in patients with preexisting liver and kidney disorders (including abscess or inflammation of the liver of amebic origin.)

DOSE. 250 mg. orally twice daily for 10 days for carriers without diarrhea. For deep colon ulceration 2 Gm. rectally as a retention enema in 200 cc. of 2% sodium bicarbonate solution every other night for a maximum of five doses.

GLYCOBIARSOL, N.F. (MILIBIS). This organic compound contains both arsenic and bismuth and is widely used in the treatment of the intestinal form of amebiasis. Because of its limited water solubility, it is poorly absorbed from the gastrointestinal tract, and therefore is ineffective against the extraintestinal forms of the disease.

TOXICITY. This drug causes reduced peristalsis owing to the bismuth component. Should not be used in patients sensitive to arsenic or bismuth and is contraindicated in the presence of liver and kidney disorders. Because of the poor solubility, gastrointestinal symptoms and hepatitis occur only rarely.

DOSE. 500 mg. orally three times daily for 7 to 10 days.

iodochlorhydroxyquin

IODOCHLORHYDROXYQUIN, N.F. (ENTERO-VIO-FORM, VIOFORM). This iodine-containing organic compound is effective against both the trophozoite and cyst forms of amebae. The greater part of the oral dose remains in the gastrointestinal tract; hence the drug is of little value in the treatment of extraintestinal forms of the disease.

The drug will stain clothing and linens yellow.

TOXICITY. Generally low. Infrequent, mild gastrointestinal symptoms occur along with skin disorders. Contraindicated in patients with iodine intolerance or thyroid, hepatic or renal disorders.

DOSE. 250 mg. orally 3 times daily for 10 days followed by a rest period of 8 to 10 days.

CHINIOFON, N.F. (YATREN). Although this drug has little effect on the ameba in vitro, it is quite effective in vivo; it is probably changed into an active form within the body. Very little of an orally administered dose is absorbed, and its usefulness is confined to the intestinal form of the disease. Chiniofon is often combined with other drugs for total therapy of amebiasis.

TOXICITY. Serious symptoms are rare, although diarrhea has occasionally been noted. To be used with caution in patients with liver damage and contraindicated in individuals sensitive to iodine or with thyroid disorders.

DOSE. 0.75–1.0 Gm. orally three times daily for 7 to 10 days. Rectally, as a retention enema, 6 Gm. is dissolved in 200 cc. of lukewarm water and is administered for ten days.

DIIODOHYDROXYQUIN, U.S.P., DI-IODOHYDROXYQUINOLINE, B.P. (DIODOQUIN, MOEBIQUIN, YODOXIN). This compound is effective against both the cyst and trophozoite forms of amebae. Since it is well absorbed following oral administration, it is of definite value in the treatment of the extraintestinal forms of the disease. It may be taken prophylactically for the prevention of amebiasis when in endemic areas.

TOXICITY. The greater part of the toxic effects of this drug are due to the iodine it contains. Symptoms of iodism occur with prolonged use, including

furunculosis, dermatitis, sore throat, rhinitis, chills, fever and headache. Occasionally gastrointestinal symptoms have been reported. The same precautions and contraindications as for chiniofon apply.

DOSE. 650 mg. orally three times daily, preferably between meals.

DRUGS USED IN LEPROSY

Leprosy, or Hansen's disease, is an infectious disease caused by *Mycobacterium leprae*. It is a systemic infection characterized by a prolonged incubation period and a chronic course in which skin changes predominate in some cases and nerve changes in others. The average healthy person is resistant to the disease, and when contracted it takes many years to run its course. Death usually results due to some other condition.

Leprosy lesions are due to the actual presence of large numbers of the causative organisms in the affected tissues, and do not become evident for some time. The areas most often affected are the skin of the face and extremities, the nasal mucous membranes, the nerve trunks, the lymph nodes and the testes. During febrile episodes, the bacilli are often demonstrable in the blood.

Two main types of lesions are recognized:

1. The lepromatous or nodular type, in which exaggerated tissue response to the organisms results in the nodules containing enormous numbers of the Mycobacterium. Eventually large nerve trunks are affected and there is anesthesia of the extremities and other nerve damage.

2. The tuberculoid type, in which there is a more intense cellular reaction that begins in the papillary and subpapillary layers. Nodules containing epithelioid cells and lymphocytes are seen about the capillaries, but bacilli are usually not present in the lesions. As the masses expand, scaling and hypopigmentation develop.

Two other less distinct types of leprosy are recognized, the indeterminate and borderline forms.

There are two cardinal symptoms of

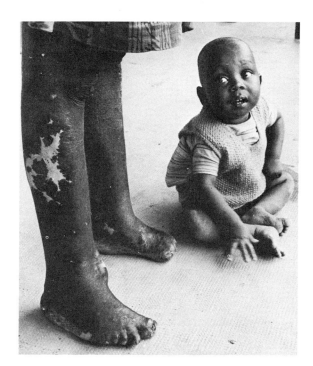

FIGURE 31. Lesions of leprosy. (Courtesy World Health Organization; photo by Pierre Pittet.)

leprosy in its early stages: anesthesia and skin lesions. Anesthesia may be the only symptom for many years. The first noticeable symptom is the loss of discrimination between heat and cold; then this is followed by loss of pain and finally touch in the affected areas.

The drugs that have proven most valuable in the treatment of leprosy are the sulfones. Streptomycin is also used, however. These agents are bacteriostatic, not bactericidal, and a long period of treatment is required for clinical cure. The average duration of therapy is about 18 months.

An important aspect of caring for a patient with leprosy is that of dispelling the fears and misconceptions of the patient and family about the disease. Isolation of the patient is indicated only if lesions demonstrate the presence of the organism, and should be avoided whenever possible because ot the psychologic effect of isolation on patients who may already feel rejected and outcast by society.

The optimal health of the patient should be promoted by providing good nutrition, rest and exercise and a clean environment. Precautionary measures may be needed if the patient has areas of numbness which are likely to sustain injury from heat, cold or pressure without his realizing it.

Rehabilitation measures are usually initiated when the acute phase of the disease is controlled.

SULFONES

The sulfones are synthetic drugs derived from a parent compound, diaminodiphenylsulfone. They are used in the treatment of both lepromatous and tuberculoid forms of leprosy and are generally the drugs of choice. In the lepromatous form, the inflammatory and ulcerative lesions are usually noticeably improved within the first three to six months of therapy, along with relief of nasal obstruction, epistaxis, dyspnea and hoarseness. The lepromatous lesions occurring on the skin do not respond as quickly to treatment as do the mucosal lesions.

If sensation has not been impaired to an extreme extent, therapy usually improves it somewhat. Extensive areas of anesthesia are generally not improved by treatment, however.

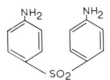

diaminodiphenyl sulfone

All sulfones are readily absorbed following oral administration and are distributed rapidly in most tissues and organs of the body.

Toxicity. Although these drugs have a high margin of safety, some toxic effects occur after prolonged periods of treatment. Hemoglobin levels usually fall during the first few weeks of therapy, but then stabilize or gradually increase toward normal levels. Leukopenia occurs less often, but periodic blood counts should be performed during treatment. Other reactions include skin reactions, drug fever, hepatitis and allergic rhinitis. In larger doses liver damage, psychotic episodes, gastrointestinal disorders, paresthesias and neuralgias have occurred.

. Extreme caution should be used if the drug is administered to individuals with pre-existing kidney, liver or cardiovascular disease or blood dyscrasias.

Sodium acetosulfone (Promacetin)

DOSE. 0.5 to 1.5 Gm. orally daily. Treatment schedules should be interrupted every four months for rest periods of 10 to 15 days.

Sodium sulfoxone, U.S.P. (Diasone)

DOSE. 330 mg. daily orally for the first week, then increased to 660 mg. daily for one to three weeks, then to the maximum dosage of 990 mg. daily.

Dapsone, U.S.P. (Avlosulfon)

DOSE. 100 mg. twice weekly orally for the first four weeks, then 200 mg. twice weekly for three weeks, then 300 mg. for three weeks followed by 400 mg. twice weekly thereafter.

Glucosulfone sodium, U.S.P. (Promin).
Although this sulfone may be absorbed orally, the toxic reactions that follow this mode of administration generally require the drug to be given parenterally.

DOSE. 2 to 5 Gm. intravenously for 6 days out of 7. Therapy should be interrupted for one week at the conclusion of each two week treatment period.

ANTISYPHILITIC DRUGS

Syphilis is an infectious disease caused by the spirochete, *Treponema pallidum.* Under natural conditions, syphilis occurs only in man and the infection must be transmitted from one human being to another by direct contact since the spirochete is extremely fragile and is destroyed rapidly when exposed to air or drying. A former method of treatment for syphilis was to expose the individual to malaria, since the high fever experienced with this disease destroyed the spirochete. It is also easily killed by chemical agents or by storing donor blood in the refrigerator for three days.

There are three stages of syphilis:

1. *Primary.* The primary lesion, or chancre, is a circumscribed, painless lesion that occurs two to six weeks after exposure and usually appears on the genitalia.

2. *Secondary.* Following the spontaneous healing of the primary lesion the patient is usually asymptomatic for a period of two to six months before the appearance of multiple secondary lesions of secondary syphilis on the skin and mucous membranes. These lesions are quite infectious, but may involute and may or may not recur after a latent period of three to twelve months.

3. *Tertiary.* Following a latent period of 20 to 30 years, an allergic reaction to the by-products of the spirochete causes the formation of gummatous lesions. These often occur in the nose, producing a "saddle nose," or in the heart, brain and other organs. Tabes dorsalis appears about this time and is characterized by a loss of balance and syphilitic gait. Often the joints are swollen, and there is a loss of sensation from the waist down due to involvement of the spinal cord ganglia.

Congenital syphilis occurs in the infants born of infected mothers. The severity of infection varies: the child may be born apparently normal but with a positive serologic reaction and may have extensive tissue involvement, or may die in utero.

Penicillin is the treatment of choice in syphilis. The treponemata are extremely sensitive to penicillin and a single injection of benzathine penicillin 2,400,000 units is usually sufficient to eliminate the infection in the primary or secondary stages. The tertiary stage is more difficult to treat, however, and serious allergic reactions may be precipitated by therapy with antibiotics owing to the release of large numbers of organisms along with proteinaceous by-products into the blood stream. Such a reaction is known as the Jarisch-Herxheimer reaction.

If the patient is hypersensitive to penicillin, oxytetracycline, chlortetracycline and chloramphenicol are also effective. (See Chapter 9 for dosages of these antibiotics.)

Certain other systemic agents, particularly bismuth preparations, are still used occasionally in the treatment of syphilis.

Case-finding and education of the public are vital roles for the nurse and other health personnel in the prevention and treatment of venereal disease, the incidence of which has been rapidly increasing. The general public, especially adolescents, need a great deal of information about this disease — the seriousness and necessity of early treatment, where medical help is available in the community, the means of transmission of the disease and its signs and symptoms.

Misconceptions and lack of knowledge contribute to the problem. Veneral disease is considered an indication of masculinity by some. Natural immunity is not induced by infection; therefore, reinfection may occur.

Although case-finding for syphilis is helped somewhat by serology examinations required for marriage licenses, Armed Forces screening and routine screening of hospitalized patients, many cases are not detected and contacts are usually difficult to locate.

The nurse should take special precautions to protect herself when giving an injection to a patient who has syphilis. Syphilis may be transmitted via the blood, and she should avoid contact with the needle after it has been removed from the patient's tissue. In addition, the surface skin lesions of secondary syphilis are very infectious. The nurse should avoid contact with them if possible, and should wear gloves if it is necessary to touch skin lesions of primary or secondary syphilis.

BISMUTH SODIUM TRIGLYCOLLAMATE (BISTRI-MATE). Since this preparation is not as effective in the treatment of syphilis as the antibiotics, it is primarily reserved for use in individuals intolerant to other agents. It is well absorbed from the gastrointestinal tract and may be administered orally; its administration after meals may reduce gastrointestinal irritation. The patient and the nurse should be aware that bismuth causes the stool to become black.

This drug is also useful in controlling dermatologic conditions such as lupus erythematosus, lichen planus and scleroderma.

TOXICITY. The chief toxic effect is directed toward the kidney. Adequate fluid intake should be insured and urinalysis should be performed frequently during therapy; the drug should be discontinued at the first appearance of albuminuria. Other toxic symptoms include gastrointestinal disorders, myalgias, peripheral neuritis, leukopenia and dermatologic reactions.

DOSE. 400 mg. three times daily orally, after meals.

BISMUTH SUBSALICYLATE. In contrast to the sodium triglycollamate salt, this bismuth preparation is not absorbed orally, and must be administered intramuscularly. It is used occasionally in combination therapy with penicillin, but is usually reserved for cases in which penicillin therapy is inadvisable.

TOXICITY. Same toxic effects as with bismuth sodium triglycollamate.

DOSE. 100 mg. intramuscularly at weekly intervals.

TREATMENT OF GONORRHEA

Gonorrhea is an inflammation of the genitourinary tract mucous membranes caused by *Neisseria gonorrhoeae*. Infection is almost always the result of sexual contact but, following the initial invasion, the gonococci may spread to extragenital sites producing arthritis, tenosynovitis, endocarditis and meningitis.

The incidence of gonorrhea is unknown, but conservative estimates state that there are at least 1.5 million new cases per year.

In the female the symptoms of the disease may begin with dysuria, urgency and frequency after an incubation period of two to eight days. Cervicitis often follows, accompanied by a mucopurulent discharge. Abscesses of Skene's ducts or Bartholin's glands are common. The duration of symptoms from an untreated infection that remains localized in the lower genital tract is usually no longer than one or two months; however, the female may be a carrier of the disease for many months after this. Inflammation of the fallopian tubes occurs not infrequently and may be manifest by acute abdominal pain and abscess formation which may or may not require surgical intervention. More often there is a subacute infection in the tubes resulting in adhesions and partial or complete blockage. It is a leading cause of tubal pregnancies and sterility in women.

In the male the onset of dysuria, urgency and frequency is associated with mucoid urethral discharge that becomes purulent. Ascending infections produce prostatitis, seminal vesiculitis or epididymitis. As in the female, although acute symptoms subside, the gonococci are able to survive in the prostate for many months during which time the male is a carrier. Urethral strictures, acute urinary retention and sterility are common side effects of gonorrhea in the male.

In caring for a patient with gonorrhea, the nurse should use careful handwashing technique and avoid touching her hands to her face or eyes. In treatments or care involving the perineal area, such as catheterizations or douches, the nurse should wear gloves and glasses to protect her eyes from the possibility of contamination by splashing of liquid containing the gonococcus which, if untreated, can lead to blindness.

As in syphilitic infections, penicillin remains the drug of choice in the treatment. Usually a single injection of 2.4 million to 4.8 million units is given intramuscularly using procaine penicillin. A culture is usually taken one week after treatment, and if relapse occurs the patient should be treated with double the original dose over a period of one to two days.

Patients allergic to penicillin, or in cases where the organism is resistant to penicillin, may be treated with tetracycline or erythromycin in doses of 500 mg. orally every 4 hours to a total dose of 3 Gm.

TRICHOMONACIDES

Of the many trichomonads that infect man, only one strain, *Trichomonas vaginalis,* is pathogenic. This organism may be detected in the urine, vaginal and urethal secretions and prostatic fluid. Vaginal infections are characterized by localized itching, burning and pruritus accompanied by a white, viscous discharge.

Trichomonal infections are contracted by direct or indirect contact with an infected individual, e.g., through coitus or by fomite contact as in the common use of towels. Occasionally the disease may be acquired congenitally from an infected mother.

Various anti-infectives are used to destroy the pathogen.

In addition to hygienic measures to prevent the spread of this infection, the patient may need to be instructed in the use of vaginal treatments, such as douches, vaginal suppositories and applicators to apply vaginal creams.

CARBARSONE, U.S.P.   Previously discussed under amebicides, this drug may also be used in trichomonal infections in the form of oral tablets or vaginal suppositories.

DOSE.   Orally—0.25 Gm. two or three times daily for 10 days. Additional courses should be undertaken only after a 10 to 14 day rest period. Suppository —130 mg. nightly for two weeks.

DIIODOHYDROXYQUIN, U.S.P., DI-IODOHY-DROXYQUINOLINE, B.P. (DIODOQUIN, MOEBIQUIN, YODOXIN). This drug is primarily employed in the treatment of amebiasis, but it may be given orally in the treatment of trichomonal infections as well.

> **DOSE.** 650 mg. orally three times daily for 20 days.

IODOCHLORHYDROXYQUIN, U.S.P. (VIOFORM). Vaginal suppositories of this drug are prepared commercially with small amounts of lactic and boric acids in order to aid in the restoration of the normal vaginal pH. Vaginal creams may be prepared with the addition of carbohydrates to replenish the depleted glycogen of the vaginal mucosa. Because of the staining of clothing by this drug, the patient should be advised to wear a sanitary pad during the course of treatment.

> **DOSE.** 250 mg. vaginal suppositories; one inserted nightly for 7 to 10 days. Ointment or cream in 3% concentration.

METRONIDAZOLE (FLAGYL). The advantage of this agent over those previously discussed in the treatment of trichomonal infections is that it is extremely effective when taken orally. It is perhaps the most effective agent now used for therapy in these conditions. Side effects, when they occur, are few and minor.

> **TOXICITY.** The most frequent side effects are associated with the gastrointestinal tract and include nausea, anorexia, cramping and occasionally vomiting and diarrhea. There is sometimes a metallic taste in the mouth. Psychic disturbances and skin reactions occur but infrequently. On prolonged administration drug fungus overgrowths do occur, but they may be treated by concurrent administration of an antifungal drug.

> **DOSE.** 250 mg. orally three times daily for 10 days.

ANTIMALARIALS

Malaria is endemic in a number of countries in the world and is still a major cause of ill health in many areas. The name itself means "bad air" and the disease was so called because people who resided in damp, foul areas contracted it readily.

Malaria is a systemic and severe, often chronic disease. Attacks of the disease commonly begin with a brief illness followed by a shaking chill and rapidly rising temperatures, usually accompanied by headache and nausea and ending with profuse sweating. The patient needs rest and supportive nursing measures during this period. After a symptom-free interval the cycle is repeated. If untreated an attack may be fatal.

Cerebral malaria and blackwater fever are dangerous complications of *Plasmodium falciparum* invasion. Blackwater fever is characterized by extensive hemolysis of red blood cells and consequent hemoglobinuria with the production of dark red or black urine. In cerebral malaria, sludging of blood vessels by the malarial organism occurs, producing severe brain damage.

Malaria is ordinarily transmitted by the bite of an *Anopheles* mosquito (Fig. 32), but may also be transmitted by blood transfusions from infected individuals or by the use of contaminated syringes. Isolation of the patient is usually not indicated unless Anopheles mosquitos are present. The life cycle of the malarial micoorganisms may be divided into two stages: the sporogenous or sexual cycle, which takes place in the mosquito, and the schizogonous or asexual, which occurs in man (Fig. 33).

There are four types of malaria as distinguished by the causative organisms:

1. *Plasmodium vivax.* Benign or tertian malaria is caused by the *P. vivax.* The sporozoite is injected into man by the mosquito and invades the red blood cells. The blood cell gradually enlarges and the sporozoite becomes a motile trophozoite with a bizarre outline. This proceeds to the *schizont* stage where nuclear division occurs in the trophozoite, forming 12 to 24 nuclei. The red blood cell is now $1\frac{1}{2}$ times normal size.

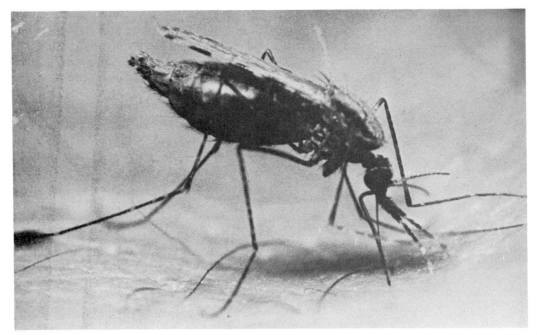

FIGURE 32. The *Anopheles* mosquito, vector responsible for the transmission of malaria. (Courtesy World Health Organization; photo by Schweizerisches Tropeninstitut Bâle.)

Following directly upon nuclear division is the segmenter stage in which cellular division of the trophozoite occurs with cytoplasm surrounding each of the nuclei. These daughter cells are now called *merozoites.* The red blood cell soon ruptures with the release of the merozoites, along with pigment or altered hemoglobin that accumulates within the red blood cell as the microorganism feeds. This pigment when released acts as a foreign protein to cause the typical febrile reaction of malaria.

Sometimes the ameboidal forms, instead of becoming schizonts, develop into large uninucleate parasites with scattered pigment granules called *gametocytes.* These undergo no further change in man and either disintegrate or are picked up by a mosquito where they undergo the sexual phase of the cycle and become the spindle-shaped sporozoites. Sixteen to 35 days later they may reinfect man through the bite of the mosquito.

2. *P. falciparum.* Red blood cell enlargement is not notable in this type of malaria, which is also known as malignant tertian or estivoautumnal malaria. This is the most severe form of malaria, and attacks may prove rapidly fatal if not treated. Early and complete treatment will eradicate the infection, however, and if reinfections do not occur, there is no relapse. In recent years some strains of *P. falciparum* have shown resistance to chemotherapeutic agents, and therapy has become more difficult.

3. *P. malariae.* This type is known as quartan malaria. There is no red blood cell enlargement; however there may be "band forms" in the blood cells caused by the parasite extending as a band across the cell. There may or may not be brain involvement. This type of malaria may last 17 to 21 years and transfusion from an infected person may transmit infection even though the disease has been latent.

4. *P. ovale.* This relatively uncommon form of malaria resembles *P. vivax* infections in many respects. Without reinfection the disease persists for one year.

OBJECTIVES OF TREATMENT OF MALARIA

Drug therapy may be given in order to prevent, suppress or treat the active manifestations of malaria. The drugs of choice

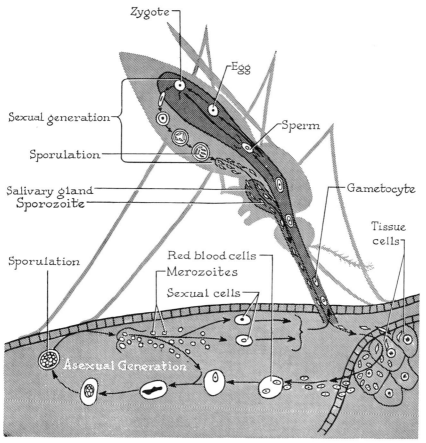

FIGURE 33. A diagram of the life cycle of the malaria parasite. (From Villee, Walker, and Smith: *General Zoology.* Ed. 3. W. B. Saunders Co., Philadelphia, 1968.)

vary according to which phase of the disease is being treated. The drugs will be listed below under the different modes of therapy, then discussion of each drug will follow in more detail.

Prophylaxis. In order to prevent the active manifestations of malaria during travel through an endemic area, drug therapy is directed toward destruction of the malaria parasites in the blood before they enter the red blood cells. Transmission of the disease is also decreased with this therapy since fewer gametocytes develop to be transmitted to another susceptible individual by the mosquito.

Drugs used: primaquine (falciparum and vivax), chloroguanide (falciparum) and pyrimethamine (falciparum).

Suppression. Although infection of the red blood cells by the parasite is not pre-

vented with drugs used for suppressive therapy, these agents do inhibit or slow the progression of the disease in the erythrocytic stage, thus decreasing the clinical manifestations of the disease.

Drugs used: chloroquine, chloroguanide and pyrimethamine.

Treatment of clinical attacks. Agents used during full-blown attacks of malaria act by interfering with the multiplication of the parasite within the red blood cell, and subsequently halt the rupture of the erythrocyte and release of the proteinaceous material into the blood stream.

Drugs used: chloroquine, amodiaquine.

Clinical cure. Following the suppression of the clinical attack of malaria, treatment must be instituted to remove the parasite from the body.

For falciparum malaria prolonged suppression of the disease effects a clinical cure. Chloroquine, chloroguanide or pyrimethamine is given, with treatment continuing for four weeks beyond the last exposure to mosquitos in the endemic area.

Vivax malaria is treated with pyrimethamine for ten weeks after leaving the area.

QUININE SULFATE, N.F. This alkaloid from the bark of the cinchona tree was the first curative agent known for malaria. It is incapable of preventing attacks of the disease, but it is quite effective in killing the parasite in the schizont stage. It has no effect on the sporozoites or pre-erythrocytic forms. It is less effective and produces more side effects than the newer antimalarials; it has largely been replaced by them.

Following the discovery that quinine had

quinine

an antipyretic effect in malaria, it was used for this purpose in other infectious diseases, but with little benefit. It does have analgesic effects that are similar to those of aspirin, however, and is occasionally prescribed for various conditions accompanied by muscle and joint pain.

TOXICITY. Tinnitus, headache, nausea, visual disturbances, skin flushing, confusion, renal damage and hemolytic anemia.

DOSE. 300 to 600 mg. orally three times daily.

AMODIAQUINE HYDROCHLORIDE, N.F. (CAMO-QUIN). Amodiaquine is rapidly absorbed after oral administration and soon reaches a concentration in the red blood cells that is double that in the plasma. It is used to treat clinical attacks of vivax and falciparum malaria and may be used as a suppressive for either type.

TOXICITY. Nausea, vomiting, diarrhea, fatigue, excessive salivation and hyperpigmentation of the skin have been noted.

DOSE. 0.4 Gm. orally three times daily for 5 days, then 0.4 Gm. once weekly.

CHLOROQUINE PHOSPHATE, U.S.P., B.P. (ARALEN PHOSPHATE). Chloroquine provides rapid symptomatic relief during clinical attacks of malaria. While the true mechanism of action is not known, it has been observed to react strongly with nucleoproteins, this effect perhaps explaining its lethality on the rapidly dividing schizonts within the red blood cell. This agent has little effect against the exo-erythrocytic forms of the disease even when given in massive doses and is of limited value in suppression of the disease.

In addition to its usefulness as an antimalarial, chloroquine is used in the treatment of amebiasis and various other diseases such as rheumatoid arthritis and discoid lupus erythematosus. It is quite effective as an anti-inflammatory agent and is useful in the treatment of photoallergic reactions.

TOXICITY. Gastrointestinal symptoms, dermatoses, headache, dizziness, lethargy and visual disturbances have occurred. The drug should be used with caution in the presence of liver disease and severe gastrointestinal, neurological and blood disorders.

DOSE. Therapeutic—1 Gm., then 500 mg. in 6 to 8 hours, and 500 mg. on each of two consecutive days, orally. Give before or after meals.
Suppressive—500 mg. orally on same day each week.

HYDROXYCHLOROQUINE SULFATE, U.S.P. (PLAQUENIL). Like chloroquine, hydroxychloroquine provides suppressive prophylaxis and termination of clinical attacks of both falciparum and vivax malaria. When used according to the dosage schedule it brings about a radical cure of the falciparum type.

In addition, this agent is a moderately effective anti-inflammatory agent and may be used alone or in conjunction with salicylates or corticosteroids.

TOXICITY. Gastrointestinal, visual and skin disturbances and anemia have been reported.

DOSE. 800 mg. initially followed by 400 mg. in 6 to 8 hours. An additional 400 mg. is given on each of two successive days.

PRIMAQUINE PHOSPHATE, U.S.P., B.P. Unlike chloroquine, this agent does not exert antipyretic or analgesic activity. Its primary use at present is in the prophylaxis and clinical treatment of vivax malaria. For the treatment of acute attacks, however, it should be combined with other agents.

TOXICITY. Usually tolerated well when given orally in the suggested doses. Occasionally abdominal cramping, mild anemia and dermatologic reactions have occurred. Negroes and some Caucasians seem more susceptible to hemolytic reactions due to this drug, which may be explained by the congenital absence or deficiency of an enzyme needed to withstand the oxidative effects of the drug on the red blood cells. In the event that this enzyme is missing, rather severe hemolytic crises may occur following therapy. Frequent blood counts and observations of the urine for darkening or reddening should be done to check on this.

DOSE. 15 mg. orally daily for 14 days for treatment of relapsing vivax malaria.

pyrimethamine

PYRIMETHAMINE, U.S.P., B.P. (DARAPRIM). Pyrimethamine is a folic acid antagonist which owes its efficacy in the treatment of malaria to the parasite's requirement for folic acid as a nucleic acid precursor. Because of its ability to arrest cell division, it is most effective in the schizont and segmenter stages of the disease.

It has a slow onset of administration when administered orally, and it has been used primarily in the prophylaxis of falciparum and vivax malaria.

TOXICITY. Few side effects are noted with recommended doses. High doses or prolonged therapy interfere with formation of red blood cells, causing mild to moderate anemia. Dermatoses have been noted.

DOSE. 25 mg. orally once weekly for suppressive therapy.

QUINACRINE HYDROCHLORIDE, U.S.P. (MEPACRINE HYDROCHLORIDE, B.P., ATABRINE). Quinacrine is effective in the management of all forms of malaria. It is used to destroy the erythrocytic asexual forms of vivax, falciparum and quartan malaria and the sexual forms of vivax and quartan malaria.

In addition, this drug has been used in the treatment of giardiasis.

TOXICITY. Yellow discoloration of the urine, sclerae and skin may occur with therapy. Patients should be assured that the skin discoloration will disappear in about two weeks. Mild intestinal disturbances, anorexia, dermatoses and generalized cramping may occur.

DOSE. Prophylactic—100 mg. orally daily for 6 days a week or 400 mg. two times a week, given after meals and with a full glass of water.
Acute infection—200 mg. every 6 hours for five doses, then 100 mg. three times daily for 6 days.

ANTHELMINTICS

Although worm infestations may be found throughout the world, they are especially abundant in the warmer climates. This is due in part to the favorable climatic conditions that facilitate survival of the larvae, but, perhaps more important, it is also due to the primitive sanitary practices of the individuals living in these areas. Many cultures of the world have no organized method of disposing of human excreta, so that it is allowed to pollute streams, soil, water supplies and food. In some areas human excreta is used for fertilization and the larvae or eggs, which survive well in the warm, moist soil, are consumed with the raw or partially cooked food, thus continuing the cycle.

Most human worm infestations are quite amenable to drug therapy. In order to be effective, these agents must obviously be differentially toxic to the worms and their hosts. The various agents employed accomplish this by different means. Some, when taken orally, act to selectively paralyze the worms in the gastrointestinal tract so that they are no longer able to contract against the peristalsis of the intestine and are carried out with the feces. Other agents may act by interfering with the energy production, glycogen storage or enzyme activity of the parasite. In other cases, however, there may be only a slight margin of safety between the dose of the drug that is effective in removing the parasite and that which begins to bring about toxic symptoms in the human host.

Nursing responsibilities involve the teaching of the patient and his family in order to prevent the transmission and further spread of the infestation. The need for careful handwashing should be particularly emphasized. The family must be included in the plan of care since they are often infected also.

Stools should be examined daily for the presence of worms. Separate toilet facilities should be provided if this is possible. If not, the affected persons should be instructed to wash the toilet seat with soap and water after each use. In the United States, disposal through the sewer systems is usually sufficient. Patients who use bedpans should have one for their own individual use; handwashing should be carried out by patient and staff after each use.

Nursing interventions should also be directed toward alleviating the symptoms caused by the infestation. Adequate nutritional and fluid intake, and plenty of rest are needed by most patients.

Following is a brief outline describing the more common worms that infest humans along with the drugs of choice for their treatment. The various anthelmintic agents will

be discussed in more detail following the outline.

I. ROUNDWORMS OR NEMATODES

A. *Roundworm.* The *Ascaris lumbricoides* are large round worms very similar to the earthworm and measuring 15 to 35 cm. in length. They are found all over the world and infect mud-eating children. In order to cause an infection, the eggs must have embryonated in the soil prior to ingestion, a process that takes two to three weeks. After ingestion, the eggs hatch in the intestine liberating small larvae that penetrate blood or lymph vessels, eventually reaching the lungs from which they migrate up the trachea and down the esophagus to reach the intestine once more. A heavy infestation is often accompanied by symptoms of lobar pneumonia with fever, coughing and hemoptysis. The adult worm often migrates within the body and may come out the mouth, nose or anal sphincter at night.

Drug of choice: Piperazine.

B. *Hookworm.* Infestations are caused by *Necator americanus*, *Ancylostoma braziliense* and *Ancylostoma caninum*. The eggs of these worms hatch in the soil and form filariform larvae that are able to penetrate intact skin. The larvae reach the lungs via the blood, then migrate up the trachea and down the esophagus to the intestine where they mature into adults measuring 5 to 14 mm. A secondary hemorrhagic anemia is very common in hookworm infestations because the adult worms attach to the intestinal wall, causing constant bleeding from these sites.

Drug of choice: Bephenium hydroxynaphthoate.

C. *Whipworm.* The *Trichuris trichiura*, which closely resembles a whip, causes infections when embryonated eggs are ingested. The adult worms, which measure 40 to 50 mm. in length, ordinarily do not produce severe symptoms, but occasionally will cause appendicitis or prolapse of the rectum if present in large numbers.

Drug of choice: Dithiazanine iodide.

D. *Dwarf threadworm.* *Strongyloides ster-*

coralis, like the hookworm, buries itself in the duodenal mucosa to suck blood and from there liberates eggs that are excreted in the feces. In the soil the eggs mature into filariform larvae that continue the cycle by penetrating intact skin and migrating to the lungs and intestine.

Drugs of choice: Pyrvinium pamoate, thiabendazole.

E. *Pinworm.* The *Enterobius vermicularis* is commonly called the pinworm because it measures only 2 to 13 mm. in length. The eggs, after ingestion, hatch in the intestine. When maturation has occurred the adults migrate to the anal area where they lay their eggs. The pruritus this produces induces scratching of the area, and the eggs are transferred via the fingernails to inanimate objects or to the mouth where reinfection occurs. Whole families are readily infected from one individual.

Drugs of choice: Piperazine or pyrvinium pamoate.

F. *Pork roundworm.* *Trichinella spiralis* infection, or trichinosis, is widespread throughout all regions of the world where pork is eaten. (There is a 17% incidence in some areas of the United States.) The worms gain entrance to the human gastrointestinal tract when poorly cooked pork containing encysted larvae is eaten. The larvae mature in the intestine, mate and produce additional larvae which burrow through the intestinal wall and eventually are encysted in skeletal muscle where they become calcified and remain viable for approximately 30 years. In severe infestations, allergic reactions to the larvae may cause death. Once encysted, there is no way to remove larvae from the muscle; treatment consists of drugs that attack the intestinal forms along with anti-inflammatory agents to minimize the allergic reaction.

Drugs of choice: Cortisone or ACTH to alleviate the allergic response; thiabendazole or piperazine for the intestinal forms.

G. *Filariae.* Members of the Filarioidea family, notably *Wuchereria bancrofti,* produce extraintestinal infections. The parasite is spread from one human to another by an insect bite and the organism, similar to the malarial parasite, must undergo a matura-tion cycle in the insect before it is again infective for man. In man the filariae produce inflammatory reactions in the lymph channels and progressive obstruction of these channels by scar tissue, leading to an edematous elephantoid appearance of the affected part (elephantiasis). Obstructions occur most frequently in the extremities, external genitalia and breast tissue. Drug therapy cannot reverse the process once obstruction has taken place, but is aimed toward destruction of the circulating parasite.

Drug of choice: Diethylcarbamazine.

II. Tapeworms or Cestodes

A. *Beef tapeworm.* *Taenia saginata* infestations in man result from ingestion of poorly cooked beef. The worm attaches to the intestinal wall, but the patient is often asymptomatic and the infection unnoticed until segments are passed with the feces.

Drug of choice: Quinacrine.

B. *Pork tapeworm.* *Taenia solium* infects man following ingestion of poorly cooked pork. The larvae hatch in the intestine and migrate to various tissues in the body where they become encapsulated. Treatment is directed toward eliminating the worms remaining in the gastrointestinal tract.

Drug of choice: Quinacrine.

C. *Fish tapeworm.* The larvae of *Diphyllobothrium latum,* often called the broad tapeworm, are ingested by eating poorly cooked fish that harbor the larvae. This worm competes with man for vitamin B_{12}, so that it often produces concomitant symptoms of pernicious anemia. Vitamin B_{12} and folic acid are often given as supportive therapy.

Drug of choice: Quinacrine.

III. Flukes or Trematodes

A. *Blood flukes.* Like all of the flukes to be discussed in this section, *Schistosoma japonicum, S. haematobium* and *S. mansoni* are infective for man only following a maturation cycle in the snail. Drinking infested water or even wading in it may cause infection with the flukes. In human beings the blood flukes act as a foreign protein in the blood, producing an allergic response with a daily afternoon temperature rise that falls to normal the next morning. Abscesses may occur in the liver or lungs in severe infections.

Drugs of choice: *S. mansoni* and *haematobium*—potassium antimony tartrate; *S. japonicum*—stibophen.

B. *Lung fluke.* The *Paragonimus westermani,* when they reach the lung, produce tubercle-like lesions that may be suppurative and even ulcerate. Treatment with available drugs is not entirely satisfactory.

Drugs of choice: Concurrent use of emetine and sulfadiazine.

C. *Liver fluke.* The *Clonorchis sinensis* and *Fasciola hepatica,* or liver flukes, invade the biliary passages causing hyperplasia of the connective tissue and cirrhosis of the liver. Drug therapy is palliative only and cannot cause reversal of the inflammatory reaction or cirrhosis.

Drugs of choice: *C. sinensis*—chloroquine; *F. hepatica*—emetine.

D. *Intestinal fluke.* The giant fluke, or *Fasciolopsis buski,* produces intestinal infestation only. Drug therapy is generally quite satisfactory.

Drugs of choice: Tetrachloroethylene or hexylresorcinol.

ANTHELMINTIC AGENTS

PIPERAZINE CITRATE, U.S.P. (ANTEPAR). Piperazine citrate is useful in both pinworm and *Ascaris* infestations. It acts as an anthelmintic because of its peculiar property of rendering the parasite's neuromuscular junctions insensitive to acetylcholine. Flaccid paralysis of the worms ensues, they are no longer able to maintain their position in the intestine by antiperistaltic contractions, and they are excreted in the feces.

TOXICITY. Toxicity is low; however, nausea, vomiting, headache and skin reactions occur occasionally. It is contraindicated in patients with preexisting kidney damage in whom excretion is impaired, allowing toxic levels to accumulate in the blood.

DOSE. 50 mg./kg. body weight orally daily for seven days.

BEPHENIUM HYDROXYNAPHTHOATE (ALCOPARA). This drug, although only recently discovered to be effective against hookworms, is now the drug of choice for the treatment of these conditions. It is quite effective when administered orally, and since it is poorly absorbed from the gastrointestinal tract, few systemic side effects occur. It is packaged in granules to enable more rapid dispersal in the stomach; these are quite bitter, and the drug is more palatable if the granules are administered in chocolate milk, orange juice or a carbonated beverage.

TOXICITY. No serious side effects have been reported. A small percentage of patients have experienced nausea, vomiting and diarrhea. In seriously debilitated patients electrolyte balance should be monitored carefully. Safety for use in pregnancy has not been established.

DOSE. One 5 Gm. packet (2.5 Gm. bephonium ion) orally twice in one day. The dose may be repeated in a few days if necessary.

PYRVINIUM PAMOATE, U.S.P. (POVAN). This drug decreases glucose uptake by the worm and depletes glycogen stores. It is the drug of choice for the treatment of dwarf threadworm and is also quite effective in pinworm infestations. Patients should be informed that this drug will color the stool a bright red, and that the liquid preparation will stain clothing if spilled on it. Patients should be instructed not to chew the tablet form since this staining may occur on the teeth.

TOXICITY. Few toxic effects are noted following oral administration of this drug, because of its failure to be absorbed from the gastrointestinal tract. It is contraindicated in any condition in which gastrointestinal absorption might take place, e.g., denuded intestinal epithelium. It is also contraindicated in suspected intestinal obstruction or acute abdominal disease, and must be used with caution in patients with liver or kidney disorders.

DOSE. Orally in a single dose of 5 mg./kg. body weight, either in a suspension or tablets.

THIABENDAZOLE (MINTEZOL). Thiabendazole is a broad-spectrum anthelmintic, which is the drug of choice in the treatment of threadworm and trichinosis, but is also effective in pinworm, hookworm, whipworm and *Ascaris* infection. In trichinosis it relieves allergic manifestations, fever and eosinophilia; however, its effect on the viability of the encysted larvae is not well defined as yet. Some animal studies have shown that the encysted population may be somewhat decreased in overwhelming infestations, but human studies have been inconclusive.

TOXICITY. Causes drowsiness similar to that produced by antihistamines, so patients should be warned against engaging in hazardous occupations or driving. Other side effects include nausea, vomiting, diarrhea, pruritus and headache. Transient leukopenia has been noted.

DOSE. 10 mg./kg. body weight orally twice daily for one day, to be repeated in 7 days. The recommended maximal daily dose is 3 Gm.

DIETHYLCARBAMAZINE CITRATE, U.S.P., B.P. (HETRAZAN). The drug of choice in filariasis, diethylcarbamazine is also effective in hookworm and *Ascaris* infestations. It has little or no effect on tapeworms. Following oral administration it is rapidly absorbed from the gastrointestinal tract and is excreted chiefly in the urine.

TOXICITY. Side effects are usually transient and mild, but they occur frequently. They include: nausea, vomiting, headache, lethargy, dermatoses and weakness. These effects occur more frequently in the debilitated or malnourished, but regress when the drug is discontinued. Severe febrile and allergic-type reactions occasionally occur, probably due to the absorption of the foreign protein from dying microfilaria or adult worms. These symptom may appear within a few hours after the initial

dose and induce hyperpyrexia, tachycardia, arthralgia, papular rash, pruritus and G-I distress.

DOSE. 2 mg./kg. body weight orally three times daily after meals for 7 to 21 days.

QUINACRINE HYDROCHLORIDE. Quinacrine is more thoroughly discussed in the section on antimalarial drugs, and will be mentioned in this section only briefly as the drug of choice in all tapeworm infestations.

DOSE. 0.2 Gm. orally every 5 minutes on an empty stomach immediately following a saline enema, to make a total dose of 1 Gm. A cathartic is given 24 hours after the medication is given. Treatment may be repeated in one week if the scolex or head of the worm is not passed in the stool. The stool should be carefully strained in order to detect the scolex.

ANTIMONY POTASSIUM TARTRATE, U.S.P., B.P. (TARTAR EMETIC). This agent is the drug of choice for the blood flukes *S. mansoni* and *S. haematobium,* but is somewhat less effective against *S. japonicum.* It acts as an anthelmintic because of its ability to inhibit an enzyme (phosphofructokinase) which is necessary for the anaerobic metabolism of glucose to lactic acid. The intermediary product, fructose-6-phosphate, accumulates and the flukes die. Antimony salts are also toxic to humans, however, and should never be used in higher doses or for periods of time longer than those recommended.

Intravenous injection should be given by a physician, and the vital signs should be checked before, during and after administration. Emergency drugs and equipment should be available. The patient should be kept in a recumbent position for at least one hour after the injection.

TOXICITY. Coughing immediately on injection is a frequent symptom. More serious effects include hypotension, decreased cardiac output and respiratory depression. Occasionally nausea, vomiting and joint and muscle stiffness will occur. Contraindicated in the presence of severe heart, liver or kidney disease.

DOSE. First dose 8 cc. of 0.5% solution intravenously; on alternate days the dose is increased by 4 cc. each time until a maximum dose of 28 cc. is reached. This regimen may be repeated 15 times.

STIBOPHEN, U.S.P., B.P. (FUADIN). Stibophen is the drug of choice for *S. japonicum* infection. It also is an antimony-containing compound and generally has the same mode of action as antimony potassium tartrate. In this case antimony is present in the trivalent form in a cyclic structure, so that it attaches more slowly to circulating erythrocytes and is somewhat less toxic than the tartrate salt.

TOXICITY. Similar to that for antimony potassium tartrate, but less severe.

DOSE. Intramuscularly as a 6.3% solution. 1.5 cc. is given the first day; 3.5 cc. the second day; then 5 cc. on alternate days until a total of 40 cc. has been administered. If necessary, the course of therapy may be repeated after two to three weeks.

EMETINE HYDROCHLORIDE, U.S.P. Emetine is the drug of choice in the treatment of lung flukes and the liver fluke *Fasciola hepatica.* The actions and side effects are discussed more thoroughly in the section on amebicides.

DOSE. 1 mg./kg. body weight per day subcutaneously or intramuscularly for 10 days. The daily dose should not exceed 60 mg.

CHLOROQUINE PHOSPHATE, U.S.P., B.P. (ARALEN). Chloroquine is the drug of choice in the treatment of infestations by the liver fluke *Clonorchis sinensis.* The actions and side effects are discussed in the section on antimalarials.

DOSE. 0.5 Gm. twice daily for 3 days, then 0.5 Gm. daily for 20 days.

TETRACHLOROETHYLENE, U.S.P., B.P. The drug of choice in the treatment of intestinal fluke infestations, tetrachloroethylene also has long been used with success in the treatment of hookworm. It acts by paralyzing the worms sufficiently to cause them to release their attachment to the intestinal wall. They are then eliminated from the intestine by peristaltic contractions. Theoretically, very little absorption from the intestine should occur upon oral administration, but when the drug is absorbed, relatively serious toxic effects ensue.

Tetrachloroethylene should be stored in a cool place to prevent poisonous phosgene from being formed. Fats, oils and alcohol should not be ingested during therapy with this drug since these substances seem to promote absorption of tetrachloroethylene from the gastrointestinal tract.

TOXICITY. The most common side effects consist of burning in the stomach, cramps, nausea and vomiting. Headache, dizziness and unconsciousness occur less frequently.

DOSE. 3 cc. orally in the morning on an empty stomach. Two or more treatments at four day intervals may be necessary.

HEXYLRESORCINOL, N.F., B.P. (CRYSTOIDS). Hexylresorcinol is one of the drugs of choice in intestinal fluke infestations and has also been used with success in the treatment of hookworm, *Ascaris,* and beef, pork, fish and dwarf tapeworms. Because of its broad spectrum of activity, it is particularly useful in mixed infestations.

Although it is usually administered orally, it may be employed in a retention enema and mixed with a radiopaque substance such as barium sulfate which can be guided to the infested area under fluoroscopy.

TOXICITY. Systemic reactions are rare owing to the poor absorption from the gastrointestinal tract; however, repeated doses may cause severe gastrointestinal irritation and necrosis of the small bowel. When this occurs, systemic absorption is likely, with the most serious effects on the heart and liver. The drug is contraindicated in patients with gastroenteritis or peptic ulcer. Alcohol is contraindicated during treatment with this drug as it increases absorption.

DOSE. 1 Gram orally in the morning on an empty stomach; no food for 4 hours thereafter. The medication is supplied in the form of soft gelatin capsules which must be swallowed whole. Irritation of the mouth may occur if a capsule is broken in swallowing. A saline cathartic is given 24 hours after the drug is taken in order to remove the worms from the bowel.

GUIDE FOR THE NURSING ASSESSMENT OF A PATIENT RECEIVING AN ANTITUBERCULOSIS DRUG

I.   What is the patient's understanding of tuberculosis and the therapeutic plan? What misconceptions does he or his family have? What socioeconomic factors may affect the therapeutic plan for this patient?

II.   Is the drug producing the intended effect? Is there an increase in weight? Is there a lessening of coughing and sputum production? Has the degree of fever, pulse and respiratory rate decreased? Does the patient have less fatigue and a sense of well-being? Do the result of cultures of sputum and gastric washings indicate a reduction or absence of the tubercle bacillus? Do x-ray examinations indicate regression, stabilization in size, or healing? Are other essential measures, such as good nutrition and adequate rest, being carried out?

III.   Has the patient experienced any side effects common to the particular drug or drugs? Are any side effects interfering with the patient's continuing with drug or other therapy? Can any side effects be alleviated by nursing measures?

IV.   What are the patient's and family's learning needs? What is his understanding of his condition? Does he understand the necessity of continuing drug therapy even when he feels subjective improvement? Does he know what signs and symptoms should be reported? Does he understand the rationale behind other therapeutic measures, such as good nutrition and adequate rest? Is he carrying them out? Does he understand the need and know the procedures for preventing the spread of tuberculosis to others? Have family members and other close contacts been screened for tuberculosis? Have steps been taken to provide for follow-up care of this patient?

QUESTIONS FOR DISCUSSION AND REVIEW

1.   Is tuberculosis still a threat in this country? Why?

2.   What can a public health nurse do to decrease the social stigma still existing regarding persons with Hansen's disease?

3.   Why is syphilis a disease to be carefully watched and controlled? What are the early signs and symptoms? What special precautions should be taken when caring for a person with syphilis? What drugs are most useful in combating this condition?

4.   What are the signs and symptoms of gonorrhea? What precautions should the nurse take in caring for a patient with gonorrhea?

5.   Can malaria be completely cured? Explain.

6.   What are the symptoms of worm infestation?

7.   What types of worm infestations are of most importance in the United States? Give the drugs used for each.

8.   Explain the mechanism of action of the sulfones in Hansen's disease.

9.   What actions and precautions should the nurse take in caring for a patient with worm infestation? What observations should be made for the effectiveness of drug therapy in these patients?

10.   What hygienic measures should be taught to a patient with a worm infestation, who is going to be treated at home?

BIBLIOGRAPHY

AMA Drug Evaluations. Chicàgo, American Medical Association, 1971.

Bercovitz, Z. T. (ed.): *Clinical Tropical Medicine.* New York, Paul B. Hoeber, Inc., 1944.

Brown, W. J.: Acquired syphilis—drugs and blood tests. *Amer. J. Nurs., 71*:713, (April) 1971.

Bruce-Chwatt, L. J.: Changing tides of chemotherapy of malaria. *Brit. Med. J., 1*:581, 1964.

Brunner, L. S., et al.: *Textbook of Medical-Surgical Nursing.* 2nd Ed. Philadelphia, J. B. Lippincott Co., 1970.

Cohen, A. C.: *The Drug Treatment of Tuberculosis.* Springfield, Ill., Charles C Thomas, 1966.

Daniel, T. M.: Rifampin—a major new chemotherapeutic agent for the treatment of tuberculosis. *New Eng. J. Med., 280*:615, 1969.

Davis, J. H.: Newer drugs in therapy of pinworm infestation. *Med. Clin. N. Amer., 51*:1208, 1967.

DiPalma, J. R.: The antifungal drugs and their use. *R.N., 30*:35, (June) 1967.

DiPalma, J. R.: Drugs for malaria. *R.N., 30*:77, (April) 1967.

DiPalma, J. R.: Drugs for tuberculosis. *R.N., 29*:53 (July) 1966.

Finmara, N. J.: The treatment of syphilis. *New Eng. J. Med., 270*:1185, 1964.

Florey, M. E.: *The Clinical Application of Antibiotics.* London, Oxford University Press, 1961.

Frenay, M. A. C., Sr.: Drugs in tuberculosis control. *Amer. J. Nurs., 61*:82, 1961.

Gabriel, H. S.: Beware those jet-borne diseases. *R.N., 30*:37, (April) 1967.

Govoni, L. E. and Hayes, J. E.: *Drugs and Nursing Implications.* 2nd Ed. New York, Appleton-Century-Crofts, 1971.

Herban, N. L.: Nursing care of patients with tropical diseases. *Nurs. Clin. N. Amer.,* 5:157 (March) 1970.

Hopewell, P. C.: Chemoprophylaxis for the prevention of tuberculosis. *Amer. Rev. Resp. Dis.,* 97:721, (April) 1968.

Huff, C. G.: Man against malaria. *Am. J. Trop. Med.,* 14:339, 1965.

Juniper, K.: Treatment of amebiasis. *Mod. Treatm.,* 3:1016, (September) 1966.

Koonz, F. P.: Nursing in tuberculosis. *Nurs. Clin. N. Amer.,* 3:403, (September) 1968.

Manson-Bahr, P. E. C.: Treatment of parasitic infections (excluding amebiasis) *Mod Treatm.,* 3:1031, 1966.

McInnes, J. K.: Do patients take antituberculous drugs? *Amer. J. Nurs.,* 70:2152, (October) 1970.

Modell, W.: Malaria and victory in Vietnam. *Science, 162*:1346, 1968.

Most, H.: Treatment of the more common worm infections. *J.A.M.A., 185*:874, 1963.

Moulton, F. R. (ed.): *A Symposium on Human Malaria.* No. 15. Washington, D.C., Am. Assn. for Adv. of Sci., 1941.

Powell, R. D.: The chemotherapy of malaria. *Clin. Pharmacol. Ther.,* 7:48, 1966.

Shafer, K. N., et al.: *Medical-Surgical Nursing.* 5th Ed. St. Louis, C. V. Mosby Co., 1971.

Slatkin, M. H.: Trends in the diagnosis and treatment of syphilis. *Med. Clin. N. Amer.,* 49:823, 1965.

Smith, D. W., et al.: *Care of the Adult Patient.* 3rd Ed. Philadelphia, J. B. Lippincott Co., 1971.

Thompson, P. E.: Parasite chemotherapy. *Ann. Rev. Pharmacol.,* 7:77, 1967.

Trantman, L. P.: The management of leprosy and its complications. *New Eng. J. Med., 723*:756, 1965.

Weg, J. G.: Tuberculosis and the generation gap. *Amer. J. Nurs., 71*:495, 1971.

Weiss, M.: Chemotherapy and tuberculosis. *Amer. J. Nurs., 59*:1711, 1959.

Chapter 11 Drugs That Affect the Central Nervous System

Important Concepts Discussed

1. *All parts of the central nervous system may be either stimulated or depressed by appropriate pharmacologic agents.*

2. *Emotional factors play an important part in the evaluation of the effects of drugs affecting the central nervous system.*

3. *Psychotherapeutic drugs are not intended to be curative agents; they are administered to control the symptoms of the psychologic disorder until other therapy is effective.*

4. *Many psychotherapeutic drugs exert their effect upon the central nervous system by altering brain chemistry.*

5. *The attitude and approach of the nurse are important factors in the effectiveness of many drugs affecting the central nervous system.*

6. *Drugs should be used as an adjunct to, rather than a substitute for, nursing interventions to meet the needs of the patient.*

THE STRUCTURE OF THE CENTRAL NERVOUS SYSTEM

The central nervous system, a highly organized and intensely active complex of nerve cells, nerve fibers and their connections, provides the link between an individual and his environment.

The system is composed of the brain and spinal cord. In respect to function, however, the activities and effects of the various parts are much more varied than would be expected from their anatomic proximity. Centrally active pharmacologic agents do not affect each portion of the system in exactly the same manner, and the pharmacologic responses are varied as well.

CEREBRAL HEMISPHERES. The *cerebrum,* divided into two lateral hemispheres, is the largest portion of the brain. The *cortex,* or external covering of the cerebrum, is the origin of spontaneous activity, the link between some sensory organs and motor responses and the site of conditioned reflexes, intelligence, memory, consciousness and most sensations.

Drugs that depress the activity of the cerebral cortex may produce effects ranging from mild sedation to general anesthesia; extreme depression leads to death. Cortical stimulants at first increase awareness, responsiveness and activity. Overstimulation produces restlessness, agitation, incoherent speech and eventual convulsions as the motor centers are stimulated.

THALAMUS.   A bilateral mass of gray matter at the base of each hemisphere forms the thalamus. This nuclear mass relays afferent sensory impulses, integrates sensation and is believed to be a center of crude sensory awareness. Poorly defined sensations of pain, extreme temperature changes, pressure and skin contact may be "felt" in the thalamus. Fibers traveling through the thalamus to the higher centers in the cortex include those permitting a fine differentiation of such sensations as point localization, spatial discrimination, the position and movement of the limbs, light touch, barely noticeable differences in pain and the fine discrimination of temperatures. Thalamic activity seems to be associated with the concept of pleasant and disagreeable experiences and perhaps with conditioned responses related to these concepts.

Agents that depress the thalamus prevent transmission of many sensations to the cortex.

HYPOTHALAMUS.   This area, about and below the third ventricle, contains many nuclei and tracts and several physiologic centers. It is supplied by afferent fibers from the cerebral cortex, thalamus and brain stem and sends efferent fibers to the thalamus, brain stem, spinal cord and hypophysis. It controls vegetative functions rather than somatic movement.

Stimulation of this area may produce such vagal effects as bradycardia, hyperinsulinemia, increased motility and secretion of the gastrointestinal tract and micturition. Centers in this area control body temperature, carbohydrate and fat metabolism and water balance.

There is some evidence that a sleep center is located in the hypothalamus. Some hypnotic drugs are believed to act by depressing this area of the brain.

Midbrain, pons, medulla.   These areas, besides being composed of ascending and descending tracts and cranial nerve nuclei,

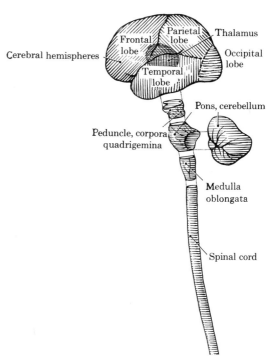

FIGURE 34.   Central nervous system. (Modified from *Dorland's Illustrated Medical Dictionary.* Ed. 24. W. B. Saunders Co., 1965.)

contain important physiologic centers. The micturition center lies between the posterior midbrain and the pons. The medulla contains the defecation, emetic, vasomotor and cardiac centers.   The primary respiratory center is in the medulla, but auxiliary respiratory centers are located in the pons.

RETICULAR FORMATION.   This area, which is composed of cells and nerve fibers, extends from the upper part of the spinal cord through the brain to the cerebrum. The reticular formation has been under considerable study during recent years, and all aspects of its activity are not yet understood. Its role appears to be that of integration of the functions of other parts of the nervous system. It is thought to be a very primitive part of the brain. Branches from cells in the sensory nuclei, in addition to synapsing with motor cells and ascending to higher centers, feed into this system. If the sensory input is the type the individual has learned is important, e.g., an unusual noise or the cry of a baby at night, the reticular formation is believed to send nonspecific impulses to the cerebral cortex. These fan out widely in the cortex and rouse the individual if asleep, or help to keep him alert if awake. Without this source of stimulation the cortex cannot interpret the specific sensory information brought to it.

Depression of the reticular formation produces a calming effect and eventual loss of consciousness. It is believed to be the site of action of many tranquilizers.

CEREBELLUM. The cerebellum is a center for balance and motor coordination. Impulses enter it from most sensory organs, but those from the proprioceptive organs in the muscles and the parts of the ear concerned with equilibrium play a particularly prominent role. The cerebellum keeps track of the orientation of the body in space and the degree of contraction of the muscles. "Copies," so to speak, of the motor directives sent out by the cerebrum to the muscles are also sent to the cerebellum. It in turn monitors the responses of the body and returns corrective signals to the cerebrum, or, in some cases, directly to the muscles.

Disturbances in the activity of the cerebellum may produce dizziness and loss of equilibrium.

SPINAL CORD. The cord consists mainly of motor and sensory tracts between muscles, viscera and sensory endings and the higher nervous centers. It also affords synaptic connections of the reflex arcs for purely spinal activity.

Stimulation of the spinal cord leads to hyperexcitability and convulsions.

CENTRAL NERVOUS SYSTEM STIMULANTS

Central nervous system stimulants are drugs that increase or enhance the cognitive and regulative functions of the central nervous system. Although many other drugs, such as some of the local anesthetics and anticholinergics, stimulate the central nervous system as a side effect, only agents that have this as their principal therapeutic action will be discussed in this chapter.

The central stimulants vary considerably in their effect on the brain and spinal cord, and they may thus be used rather specifically to obtain a desired therapeutic effect.

Some agents, such as caffeine, methylphenidate and the amphetamines, exert their principal effect on the higher centers of the cerebral cortex; thus they are useful for increasing alertness, wakefulness and, to some extent, mental activity.

Their effect is unfortunately not limited to the cerebrum, however, and in large doses or when taken for prolonged periods of time, the drugs produce side effects such as hypertension and tachycardia, which are due to stimulation of the medullary centers.

Other central nervous system stimulants may be used primarily for their effect on the medullary centers. These are used chiefly to stimulate the vomiting center (e.g., apomorphine) and the respiratory center (e.g., nikethamide). Agents used to stimulate the vasomotor center or the cardiac accelerator center (e.g., epinephrine) are generally not considered central stimulants, but exert their effects by other mechanisms of action.

Spinal cord stimulants, such as strychnine, are generally not used therapeutically because the side effects of such therapy far outweigh the therapeutic benefits.

When central nervous system stimulants are prescribed on a routine basis, the scheduling of the dosage should be arranged, if possible, so that the stimulating effect of the drug does not interfere with the patient's sleep. Generally, the last dose should be given at least six hours before bedtime. This will depend, however, on the particular drug, the intended purpose and the effect on the individual patient.

Many of the central nervous system stimulants, particularly the amphetamines, have been misused by the public. They have been used by truck drivers to maintain wakefulness on long driving trips. Students have used them to stay awake while studying for examinations; because of the excess fatigue which can result, it is doubtful whether learning is increased. Taking amphetamines for their appetite-suppressive effects has caused widespread abuse. Insomnia, which may occur with amphetamines, has led many people into a vicious cycle of hyponotics to induce sleep and amphetamines to maintain wakefulness.

A further discussion of the abuse of these drugs can be found in Chapter 25.

THE XANTHINE DERIVATIVES

Caffeine, theobromine and theophylline are closely related both pharmacologically and structurally in that they are all derivatives of the organic base molecule, xanthine.

All three drugs produce cerebral stimulation, diuresis and smooth muscle relaxation, but they vary somewhat in intensity of action. Caffeine is the most effective of the three as a central nervous system stimulant, theophylline is less effective and theobromine has little effect. Theophylline is the most effective both as a smooth muscle relaxant and as a diuretic. It is followed in activity by theobromine and last by caffeine. Caffeine, although it is the least potent of the three as a diuretic, has this effect following consumption of caffeine-containing beverages.

Theophylline ethylenediamine (aminophylline) is quite effective in overcoming spasms of the biliary tract because of its relaxant effect on smooth muscle; thus it is useful in the treatment of biliary colic. By the same mechanism of action it is quite useful either orally, parenterally or rectally for the treatment of acute asthma attacks.

Direct stimulation of the myocardium is produced particularly by theophylline and to a lesser extent by theobromine and caffeine. Theophylline ethylenediamine is used in cardiac conditions to increase cardiac output as well as to dilate coronary arteries and thus increase coronary flow. It is among the drugs of choice in the treatment of congestive heart failure and cardiac arrest.

caffeine

CAFFEINE, U.S.P., B.P.   Caffeine is an alkaloid that is contained in coffee, tea and cola.

Although its primary effect is exerted on the cerebral cortex, in larger doses it acts as a descending stimulant, progressively stimulating the medullary centers and finally the spinal cord. When taken orally in the form of beverages or when injected parenterally, caffeine relieves fatigue, allays drowsiness and increases the rapidity and accuracy of intellectual performance. There is increased perception of sensory stimuli, and reaction time to these stimuli is decreased.

Stimulation of the respiratory, vasomotor and vagal centers of the medulla is observed particularly when caffeine is administered parenterally. Similar effects may be noted when it is taken orally, but much larger doses are required.

The therapeutic rationale behind the incorporation of caffeine into headache formulae, e.g., APC capsules, is that a sharp decrease in cerebral blood inflow has been observed following parenteral administration of caffeine. The amounts of caffeine incorporated in these formulae would most probably not have a pronounced effect in this regard, but the central stimulation obtained from even this relatively small dose has proven of some benefit in combination with analgesic agents.

USES.   As a cerebral stimulant primarily. It is less often employed as a circulatory or respiratory stimulant or mild diuretic because of the availability of more potent and effective agents.

TOXICITY.   Since caffeine increases the flow of gastric hydrochloric acid, the use of caffeine-containing beverages is prohibited in patients with peptic ulcers. Overdoses of caffeine produce restlessness, insomnia, excitement, tinnitus, muscular tremor, tachycardia, cardiac irregularities and diuresis. Untoward reactions may be observed upon ingestion of 1 Gm. or more of caffeine, but this is highly variable since individual tolerance develops upon prolonged use of caffeine-containing beverages.

DOSE.   200 mg. orally three times daily. 500 mg. I.M. or subcutaneously in the form of caffeine sodium benzoate.

OTHER CENTRAL NERVOUS SYSTEM STIMULANTS

AMPHETAMINE SULFATE, N.F., B.P. (BENZEDRINE); DEXTROAMPHETAMINE SULFATE, U.S.P. (DEXEDRINE). These two commercial preparations will be discussed together because the only difference is that amphetamine is a racemic mixture of the dextro and levorotatory forms, whereas dextroamphetamine is a purified product containing the dextro form only. Most of the central nervous system stimulation is produced by this dextrorotatory form. This latter preparation is the form used primarily in therapy at present and may be administered in half the dose used in the racemic mixture.

Amphetamine is a sympathomimetic agent with pronounced cerebral stimulation, but it concurrently exerts its effect as a sympathetic agent, producing very undesirable side effects.

amphetamine sulfate

USES. Primarily in the treatment of mental depression, exhaustion, narcolepsy and catalepsy. They are used as adjuncts in the treatment of chronic alcoholism and orthostatic hypotension, as anorectic agents, and are quite effective in reducing body weight, probably because they cause an increased metabolic rate, due to increased activity, and a decreased appetite. The anorexia has been attributed to a stimulation of the prefrontal lobes, which in turn affects the satiety center of the hypothalamus. Some appetite loss has also been attributed to a singular depression of the sense of smell, which makes food less attractive to the dieter. When used as anorectic agents, they are often combined with a barbiturate to reduce the central stimulation and are administered in the form of a long-acting preparation that may be taken only once or twice daily to control the appetite. Its

use has been regulated by the Drug Abuse Control Amendments.

TOXICITY. Habit formation, tachycardia and hypertension leading to circulatory collapse have been noted upon prolonged use. Dosage should be withdrawn gradually. Hyperexcitability, gastrointestinal disturbances, headache, restlessness, insomnia and disturbances in bowel function have also been noted.

DOSE. Amphetamine: 10 mg. orally three times daily.
Dextroamphetamine: 5 mg. orally three times daily. The last dose should be administered at least six hours before bedtime. When given for obesity, the doses should be administered one hour before meals.

METHAMPHETAMINE HYDROCHLORIDE, U.S.P., METHYLAMPHETAMINE HYDROCHLORIDE, B.P. (DESOXYN, METHEDRINE, DESOXYEPHEDRINE). Methamphetamine is also a sympathomimetic amine, and its pharmacologic action on the central nervous system is between that of dextroamphetamine and amphetamine. The effect of this drug on the vasomotor system is less pronounced when administered orally, but is quite notable on parenteral administration, when a prompt and sustained increase in blood pressure and heart rate are noted. The duration of action is quite prolonged, and it is excreted slowly over a period of several days.

USES. Orally as an anorectic agent, in the treatment of chronic alcoholism, fatigue, enuresis and occasionally to overcome the effects of a mild overdose of barbiturates. It has been employed parenterally to prevent hypotension during spinal anesthesia and intravenous barbiturate administration. It is occasionally used intranasally to relieve congestion. This drug is commonly known as "speed" within the drug culture, where it is taken in extremely high doses.

TOXICITY. Insomnia, excitability irritability, hypertension, dizziness, headache, arrhythmias, muscular twitching, nausea, vomiting, abdominal cramps, constipation and dryness of the mouth. Delirium and hallucinations occur less frequently. It is contraindicated in cases of severe hypertension, hyperthyroidism, insomnia, arteriosclerosis, nephritis, coronary artery disease and myocardial damage.

DOSE. 5 mg. orally one to three times daily. It should be given one hour before meals when taken to suppress appetite, with the last dose given at least 6 hours before bedtime.

PENTYLENETETRAZOL INJECTION, N.F. (METRAZOL). Pentylenetetrazol is a central nervous system stimulant that acts on the higher centers of the cerebrum and produces violent convulsions in overdose. It also acts on the medulla, stimulating respiratory, vasomotor and vagal centers. Medullary stimulation is more prominent when this area is depressed than when it is functioning normally. Because the drug excites both sympathetic and parasympathetic nervous systems, the effect depends upon the status of the organism at the time of administration.

USES. Formerly used as a central nervous system stimulant to counteract the depressant action of overdoses of barbiturates, tribromoethanol, paraldehyde, opiates and chloral hydrate, but rarely employed for this purpose now, due to the harmful effects of overstimulation during the course of treatment. In the past pentylenetetrazol was used in the convulsive therapy of schizophrenia and other psychotic states, but it has now been generally replaced by electric shock therapy. Pentylenetetrazol is not a cardiovascular stimulant as was first thought and is not indicated in circulatory collapse or shock. Researchers believe that it is harmful in the resuscitation of the newborn.

Pentylenetetrazol is principally used now to enhance mental and physical activity in the elderly, and to treat the symptoms of chronic fatigue.

TOXICITY. Overdosage produces convulsions, which are the cause of a high incidence (43 per cent) of compression fractures of lumbar vertebrae, especially in patients under 21 and over 55. Osteoporosis is an absolute contraindication to the use of large doses of this drug; arthritis and other bone disorders are also contraindications. Disturbed cerebral function often follows its use in therapy and epileptoid changes in the electroencephalogram have been noted.

DOSE. 100 mg. I.V., I.M. or subcutaneously.

NIKETHAMIDE INJECTION, N.F., B.P. (CORAMINE). Nikethamide is a central nervous system stimulant that stimulates all levels of the spinal cord but is used therapeutically primarily for its effects on the medullary centers. It stimulates the respiratory center to increase the rate and depth of respiration and was formerly used for this effect to counteract the respiratory depression encountered in overdoses of narcotics and barbiturates. It is rarely used for this purpose at present because it is very difficult to administer the minimally effective dose, and rebound central stimulation may occur.

USES. Its stimulating effect on the vasomotor center increases the peripheral vascular tone and makes it useful in acute circulatory failure occurring during surgical procedures. The effects on peripheral circulation are inconsistent and somewhat unpredictable, and it has been largely replaced by more effective agents.

TOXICITY. Severe itching is often encountered during intravenous administration over a period of time. Intraocular pressure is increased; thus it must be administered with caution to patients with glaucoma. Overdosage may produce convulsions and may paradoxically cause death because of respiratory failure.

DOSE. 1 ml. of 25% solution intravenously as required by the patients condition.

ETHAMIVAN (EMIVAN).   Ethamivan acts on the respiratory center in the medulla to increase the depth and rate of respiration. Although it has no effect on cardiac rate or rhythm, it does induce mild vasopressor action.

The onset of action is within one minute of intravenous administration; the average duration of action is about 10 minutes. Although the drug is less active orally, a duration of action of about three to four hours is obtainable by this route.

USES.   As an adjunct in the emergency treatment of respiratory depression produced by barbiturates and tranquilizers as well as an adjunct in the treatment of chronic obstructive pulmonary emphysema and bronchial asthma.

TOXICITY.   Intravenous administration may produce sneezing, coughing, laryngospasm, excitement, muscular twitching, itching and flushing of the extremities. These side effects can usually be minimized by reducing the rate of administration. Overdosage may produce convulsions. It is contraindicated in patients with a history of epilepsy.

DOSE.   Oral—20 to 60 mg. two to four times daily. I.V.—1 Gm. infused at a rate of 10 mg./minute.

BEMEGRIDE, U.S.P., B.P. (MEGIMIDE)   Although the exact mode of action of bemegride has not been determined, it apparently stimulates the respiratory and circulatory centers and restores reflexes and consciousness. Overdosage may cause convulsions.

USE.   Bemegride is used chiefly as a respiratory stimulant in the treatment of barbiturate and glutethimide intoxication.

TOXICITY.   No chronic toxic reactions have been noted; the convulsions that are produced by overdosage are readily controlled with thiopental sodium. Suction equipment, airways and mouth gags should be on hand when the drug is used.

DOSE.   50 mg. I.V. every 3 to 5 minutes until response is noted.

ANORECTIC AGENTS.

The anorectic agents are synthetic drugs that have the appetite depressant effects of the amphetamines but are modified to minimize the undesirable sympathomimetic activity of the central nervous system stimulants.

Anorectic agents are usually ineffective in long-term weight reduction unless accompanied by changes in eating patterns and in the underlying psychological and emotional factors contributing to the obesity.

Patients should be instructed in the principles of nutrition and the importance of exercise. Emotional support and encouragement will also be needed. The importance of using the agents only as prescribed by a physician should be stressed.

BENZPHETAMINE HYDROCHLORIDE (DIDREX). Benzphetamine is an analog of amphetamine that is used as an anorectic agent. It causes loss of appetite and consequent loss of weight.

TOXICITY.   Side effects may include nervousness, dizziness, insomnia, dryness of the mouth, nausea, constipation, tachycardia and palpitation. The drug should be administered with caution to patients with hyperthyroidism, hypertension or other cardiovascular diseases since the sympathomimetic effects, although reduced, are still sufficient to produce undesirable effects in these patients.

DOSE.   25 mg. orally once or twice daily before meals.

The following agents are similar to benzphetamine in pharmacologic and toxic effects:

DIETHYLPROPION HYDROCHLORIDE (TENUATE, TEPANIL)

DOSE.   25 mg. orally three times daily before meals.

Phendimetrazine tartrate (Plegine)

DOSE. 35 mg. orally two or three times daily before meals.

Phenmetrazine (Preludin)

DOSE. 25 mg. orally two or three times daily before meals.

Phentermine hydrochloride (Ionamin)

DOSE. 8 mg. orally three times daily before meals.

Psychic Energizers

The psychic energizers, or mood elevators, are drugs that are used for the treatment of mental depression. The true psychic energizer often works indirectly through the body's enzyme system to produce an antidepressant effect. The true central nervous system stimulants, such as amphetamine, may also be used in psychotherapy, but these generally tend to have more untoward effects than the newer drugs; thus they have largely been replaced by this latter group of psychic energizers.

In observing for the effect of these drugs, the nurse should realize that there is often a greater chance that the patient will attempt suicide when depression lessens. The possibility of drug interactions with other drugs the patient is receiving should always be considered.

Methylphenidate hydrochloride, N.F. (Ritalin). Methylphenidate is a mild central nervous system stimulant with an action that falls between caffeine and amphetamine. It does not produce the anorectic effect of the amphetamines, nor does it produce significant changes in blood pressure, heart rate or respiratory functions.

USES. It is used orally to overcome various types of depression and intravenously to treat overdoses of tranquilizers, barbiturates and anticonvulsant drugs. In depressive conditions, methylphenidate brightens the mood and increases mental and motor activity. Its use is subject to the regulations of the Drug Abuse Control Act.

TOXICITY. Nervousness, insomnia, palpitation, dizziness, nausea and headache have been reported, but these side effects are usually minimal and may be controlled by decreasing the dosage. Its use concomitant with coumarin anticoagulants may require adjustment of the anticoagulant dose during and after Ritalin therapy. It should not be given with epinephrine or levarterenol since it potentiates their effects.

DOSE. 10 mg. orally two or three times daily. Last dose should be given at least six hours before bedtime. 50 to 100 mg. I.V., I.M. or subcutaneously or dosage as required to treat drug overdosage.

Imipramine hydrochloride, N.F., B.P. (Tofranil). Structurally this drug is closely related to another mild stimulant, amitriptyline. It is not a MAO inhibitor, nor does it directly stimulate the central cortex. Very little is known of its mode of action.

USES. Imipramine has been successfully used in the treatment of mild depression. It is not completely effective in the treatment of schizophrenia and other severe mental disorders. It is quite useful in small dosages for long-term treatment of senile depressive disorders. Unlike most stimulants, this agent has little or no effect on nondepressed individuals. The effect of this drug is usually not evident for at least two weeks. Dosage should be gradually decreased rather than discontinued abruptly to prevent reactive depression.

TOXICITY. Minor side effects, which disappear spontaneously or can be readily controlled by reduction of dosage, have been reported by many investigators. These are atropine-like and include dryness of the mouth, increased perspiration, tremor, constipation, dizziness, tachycardia, skin rash and blurred vision. Rarely obstructive jaundice has been associated with imipramine therapy; hypotensive reactions have been seen with some frequency.

When imipramine is administered during or shortly after treatment with MAO inhibitors, severe reactions, including markedly potentiated atropine-like effects, convulsions and muscular rigidity may occur. Barbiturates should not be used in treating such reactions because of potentiation of effects and the low margin of safety.

Patients with increased intraocular pressure should be treated with caution.

> **DOSE.**   100 to 200 mg. orally daily in divided doses.

AMITRIPTYLINE HYDROCHLORIDE (ELAVIL). Amitriptyline is a potent antidepressant with a low degree of toxicity. In addition, it is tranquilizing, which makes it particularly useful in depressed patients in whom anxiety or agitation is a predominant symptom. Patients usually do not show startling changes in behavior or attitude, but gradually develop more interest in their surroundings and show a slow elevation of mood. The drug is less effective if organic brain disease is present. Patients should be warned that their urine will be blue-green in color during administration of this drug.

> **USE.**   As a mild antidepressant for hospital and outpatient treatment.

> **TOXICITY.**   Side effects are usually mild. Drowsiness occurs occasionally, as well as dizziness, nausea, excitement, hypotension, tremor, headache, anorexia, increased perspiration and skin rash. Large doses may cause temporary confusion.

The combination of amitryptyline with other antidepressant drugs generally does not result in additional therapeutic effect and may cause untoward reactions.

> **DOSE.**   25 mg. orally three times daily.

NORTRIPTYLINE HYDROCHLORIDE (AVENTYL). This oral antidepressant drug is similar structurally to amitriptyline (Elavil), and similarly is used in the treatment of endogenous or reactive depression. It is less effective if organic brain damage is present.

> **TOXICITY.**   Serious reactions necessitating withdrawal of the drug are uncommon. Most frequently dryness of the mouth, drowsiness, blurred vision, tremor, fatigue, nausea and vomiting are observed. More rarely tachycardia, hypotension, confusion and hallucinations have been observed. It should be administered with caution to patients with a history of convulsive disorders, cardiovascular complaints or glaucoma. It is contraindicated for concurrent use with MAO inhibitors, since the combination leads to extreme agitation and hyperthermia. A lapse of 14 to 21 days should occur between discontinuance of the MAO inhibitor and institution of nortriptyline.

> **DOSE.**   10 to 25 mg. orally four times daily.

PROTRIPTYLINE HYDROCHLORIDE (VIVACTYL). This agent is a potent, rapidly acting antidepressant that is indicated for the treatment of mental depression in patients who are under close medical supervision.

Its mechanism of action is unknown, but it is not a monoamine oxidase inhibitor and, unlike amitriptyline, it does not have sedative or tranquilizing properties.

> **USES.**   In the treatment of anxiety, suicidal tendencies, fatigue, insomnia, agitation and anorexia.

> **TOXICITY.**   Because of its anticholinergic activity, this drug is contraindicated in the treatment of patients with glaucoma or urinary retention. It should not be given concomitantly with MAO inhibitors and should be used with caution in the elderly and in patients with cardiovascular or liver disorders. Monitoring of liver and bone marrow function is recommended during therapy. Dryness of the mouth, ataxia, tremor, blurring of vision, confusion, nausea, headache, dizziness, impotence, dermatoses, numbness and tingling of the extremities have been reported.

> **DOSE.**   15 to 40 mg. orally daily in divided doses.

DESIPRAMINE HYDROCHLORIDE (NORPRAMIN, PERTOFRANE). Desipramine is an effective antidepressant drug with a rapid onset of action. It is of benefit in endogenous depression, such as the manic-depressive reactions, psychotic depressive reactions and involutional depressive reactions, as well as in the less severe reactive depressions of neuroses. It is of little value in schizophrenia.

TOXICITY. Desipramine should not be given within two weeks of administratration of MAO inhibitors because adverse reactions occur. Because of its anticholinergic effects, the drug should not be given to patients with glaucoma, urethral or ureteral spasm or to those who have had a myocardial infarction within three weeks. The presence of a severe coronary disease with EKG abnormalities is a contraindication to the use of this drug.

Transient jaundice has been noted following therapy. The other side effects are similar to those of imipramine.

DOSE. 150 mg. orally daily in divided doses.

DOXEPIN HYDROCHLORIDE (SINEQUAN). This synthetic agent has been shown to have marked antidepressant and antianxiety effects on patients with psychoneuroses. It is recommended for the treatment of anxiety and/or depressive reactions, such as those that occur concurrently with alcoholism, as a result of organic disease or more severe mental illnesses such as involutional depression or manic-depressive reactions.

It has not been shown to be habit forming, patients do not have a euphoric reaction to the drug and withdrawal symptoms have not been observed.

TOXICITY. Drowsiness, potentiation to depression from alcoholic beverages, dry mouth, blurred vision, constipation, tachycardia and hypotension have been reported. This agent should never be administered sooner than two weeks after the discontinuing of MAO in-

hibitors in order to avoid extreme hypertensive effects and even death.

DOSE. 25 mg. orally three times daily.

MONOAMINE OXIDASE INHIBITORS

The introduction of monoamine oxidase (MAO) inhibitors into psychiatric medicine for the purpose of treating depression resulted from a search for improved antitubercular derivatives of isoniazid. One of the first derivatives, iproniazid, was found to have a persistent side effect of mood elevation. Because of the toxic reactions noted upon continued administration of this drug its therapeutic use was discontinued, but the search was continued for more useful and less dangerous MAO inhibitors after insight was gained into the changes in brain chemistry produced by this drug.

Monoamine oxidase (MAO) with catechol-O-methyl transferase (COMT) is responsible for the degradation of sympathetic amines, such as epinephrine, norepinephrine, serotonin and dopamine. When monoamine oxidase is inhibited, the amines are metabolized more slowly and thus accumulate in the brain and other tissues.

To absolutely attribute the pharmacologic effects of these drugs to the elevated amine level may be too much of an oversimplification. Much research is currently being directed to further clarification of the mode of action of these agents.

Because of the indirect action of these drugs, prompt relief of symptoms cannot be expected; it is ordinarily several weeks before a clinical response is observed in depressed patients.

TOXICITY

Unfortunately, the effects of the MAO inhibitors are not confined to endogenous serotonin and norepinephrine, but, because of the same metabolic interruption, they also enhance the toxic effects of exogenous amines, which are normally detoxified by MAO. Amines, especially tyramine, are found in high concentrations in aged cheeses, especially Swiss and cheddar. Some wines, especially Chianti, as well as beer and yogurt contain amines. Chicken liver, bananas and avocados have recently been added to the list of foods forbidden to patients taking MAO inhibitors. Although liver does not ordinarily contain tyramine, it seems likely that decarboxylase is activated during the preparation of the liver, thus converting the amino acid tyrosine, which is normally present, to tyramine. When a MAO inhibitor is taken concurrently with food containing amines, serious and even fatal hypertensive episodes may result. Patients should be taught to avoid these foods, and in the hospital, food selection should be carefully supervised.

Because of the numerous drug interactions with the MAO inhibitors, patients taking these drugs should be instructed not to take any medication that is not specifically prescribed by the physician. Numerous drugs are either contraindicated or should be administered with extreme caution to patients taking MAO inhibitors. These include drugs such as reserpine which, when given after pretreatment with MAO inhibitors, causes excitation rather than the usual sedation. This phenomenon is known as "reserpine reversal." The pharmacologic effect of reserpine, in simplified terms, is that of increasing the leakage of norepinephrine and serotonin from cellular storage sites. Under normal circumstances these amines are detoxified by MAO so that the net effect is a decrease in the level of circulating amines, resulting in a sedative and hypotensive effect. When MAO is inhibited, however, these amines are not detoxified, but leave the cell in active form and produce behavioral stimulation and pressor effects.

Other drugs that should be administered with extreme caution when MAO inhibitors are given are the ganglionic blocking agents, such as guanethidine (Ismelin), other mood elevators, such as imipramine (Tofranil) and amitryptyline (Elavil), as well as sympathomimetic drugs, such as epinephrine, neosynephrine, ephedrine and amphetamine.

In addition, the MAO inhibitors may potentiate the effects of morphine, meperidine (Demerol) and other narcotics, barbiturates, antihistamines and alcohol since they interfere with the detoxification of these drugs by the liver. These should be administered with caution to patients receiving the MAO inhibitors, and if given, symptoms of respiratory depression must be watched for.

It is now recognized that some MAO inhibitors potentiate the actions of insulin and the sulfonylureas (such as tolbutamide and chlorpropamide). Thus, their concurrent administration to a diabetic patient is dangerous unless the dose of the antidiabetic drug is reduced. The nurse must watch carefully for evidence of hypoglycemia in the diabetic patient who is receiving these drugs.

Optic damage, anemia, hepatic damage and renal difficulties have also been noted on prolonged administration of MAO inhibitors.

Since the risk of suicide is often greatest near the end of the depressive cycle, particular care should be exercised when patients with potential suicidal tendencies begin to respond to MAO inhibitors.

These drugs should always be withdrawn gradually, especially if large doses have been administered over a period of time, since a rebound effect may occur, which is characterized by headache, excitability and occasionally hallucinations.

NIALAMIDE (NIAMID). Nialamide may be given orally to treat neurotic and psychotic disorders characterized by depression. It has been recommended in the treatment of involutional melancholia, manic-depressive psychosis and schizophrenia; however, electroshock therapy is of more benefit than nialamide in severe depression and in patients with suicidal tendencies.

> **DOSE.** 75 to 100 mg. orally daily initially. The dose may be increased or decreased by 12.5 to 25 mg. at weekly intervals. As much as 200 mg. daily has been administered in the treatment of severe depression. Most patients may be maintained on 12.5 mg. every other day after a maximal effect has been reached.

PHENELZINE SULFATE (NARDIL). The uses and effects of phenelzine sulfate are similar to those of nialamide.

DOSE. 15 mg. orally three times daily initially. The average maintenance dose is 15 mg. every other day.

TRANYLCYPROMINE (PARNATE). Tranylcypromine is unrelated chemically to nialamide and phenelzine sulfate, but resembles them greatly in pharmacologic actions.

DOSE. 20 mg. orally daily for two or three weeks until a therapeutic response is noted. The dose is then gradually reduced to 10 to 20 mg. daily. In extreme cases as much as 60 mg. may be administered daily, but in doses of more than 30 mg. daily, postural hypotension is frequently observed.

CENTRAL NERVOUS SYSTEM DEPRESSANTS

The type of depression induced in the central nervous system by a pharmacologic agent depends to a large extent upon its site of action. An agent that depresses the motor areas of the brain, for instance, does not have the same effect as one that acts primarily upon the higher brain centers. In addition, the degree and type of depression may be varied by the dose and the mode of administration. In general, parenteral administration produces a much faster and more pronounced response than does oral administration.

General Anesthetics

Anesthesia may be loosely defined as a depression of the response to stimuli. Whereas local anesthesia implies depressed activity of certain peripheral nerves only, general anesthesia implies cortical depression with effects ranging from analgesia to loss of consciousness and severe depression of the medullary centers.

The stages of anesthesia were described by Guedel in 1920 as follows:

Stage I—stage of analgesia. In this stage the patient is still conscious and responds to commands and questions; analgesia is present, but is not of sufficient depth to allow surgery.

Stage II—stage of delirium. The patient loses consciousness; excitement and involuntary activity occur, but may vary greatly and may include laughing, shouting, thrashing about, irregularity of breathing, hypertension and tachycardia. Incontinence, nausea, vomiting and dilatation of the pupils may also occur. The use of combinations of anesthetic agents and the sophisticated techniques of anesthesiologists have reduced considerably the severity and duration of this stage.

Stage III—stage of surgical anesthesia. Within this stage there are several planes of anesthesia which the anesthesiologist monitors by observing the character of respirations, eyeball movement, pupil size and the presence or absence of certain reflexes. He must maintain the level of anesthesia within this stage.

Stage IV—stage of respiratory paralysis. This stage is characterized by respiratory arrest which may be followed by circulatory failure.

These stages may be observed and controlled by the anesthetist by observing muscle tone, pupil size, breathing patterns and EEG tracings. Each stage is passed through both in induction of the anesthetic and in reverse order during the recovery period.

Various theories have been proposed to explain the mechanism of action of the general anesthetics, ranging from dissolution of fatty substances from the brain to reversal of cell proteins and decreased electrical conductivity of nervous tissue, but perhaps no explanation has received as much credence as Pauling's hydrate monocrystal theory, formulated in 1961. This explains anesthesia by postulating interaction of molecules of the anesthetic agent with water molecules in the brain to form hydrate water crystals. These may interfere with the protein molecules and their electrically charged side chains and decrease the electrical energy in the brain, a process that is reversible upon

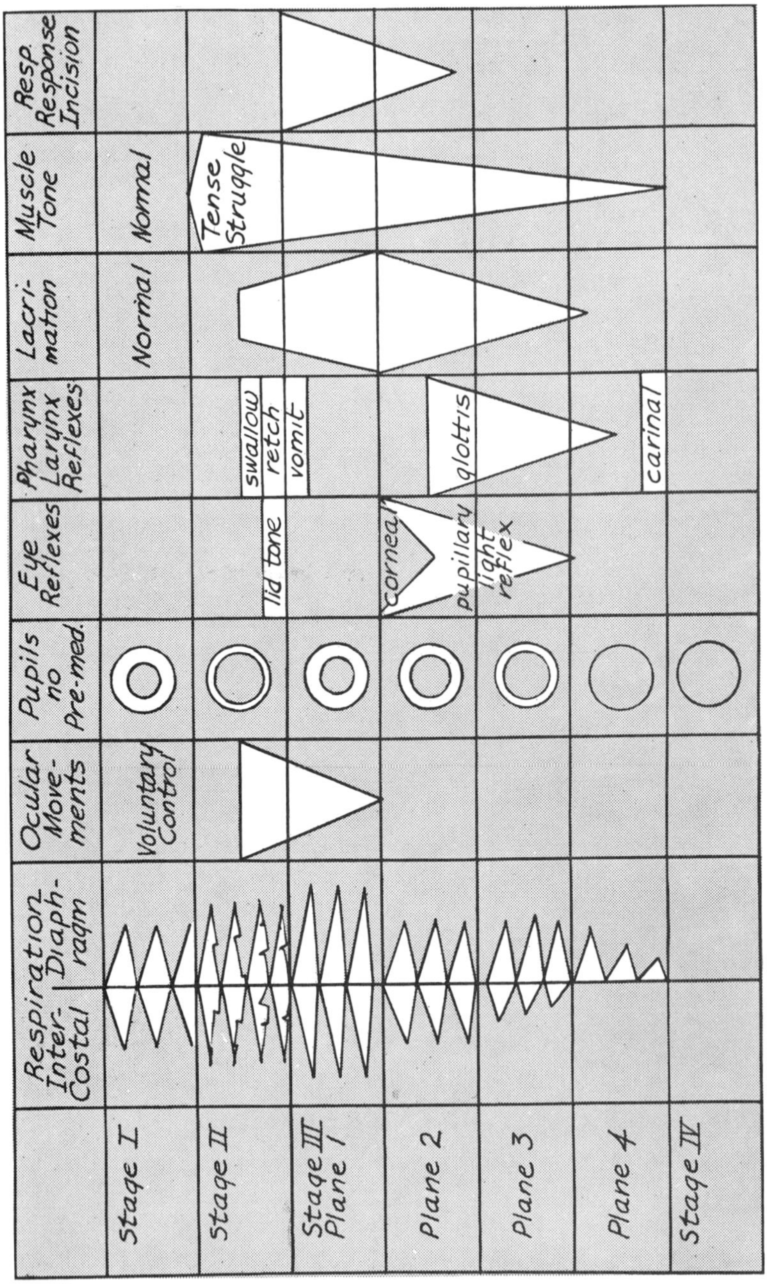

FIGURE 35. The signs and reflex actions of the stages of anesthesia. (After Gillespie, N. A.: *Anesth. and Analg.*, 22.)

elimination of the anesthetic from the body. It is possible that no one theory, but rather a combination of several, will be needed to explain anesthetic activity.

General anesthetics may be administered by inhalation, as is the case with the anesthetic gases, or intravenously in the form of short-acting barbiturates. The choice of anesthetic is dependent primarily on the estimated time of surgery and the degree of muscle relaxation or the depth of anesthesia desired during the procedure.

The nurse should be familiar with the common methods of administering anesthesia in order to carry out preoperative instruction of the patient. Her knowledge of anesthetic action and its common side effects should guide her observations and care of the patient during the postoperative period of recovery from anesthesia.

VOLATILE ANESTHETICS

ETHER, U.S.P. (ETHYL ETHER, DIETHYL ETHER). Ether was one of the first anesthetic gases employed for surgical procedures and is still one of the most popular agents. Almost any major surgical procedure may be performed under ether anesthesia since good skeletal muscle relaxation is readily attained. In addition, the stages of anesthesia are passed through slowly enough to permit close and accurate control. Deep surgical anesthesia may be maintained for relatively long periods without the danger of unpredictable respiratory depression.

Ether causes release of catecholamines in the body, providing an additional safety feature to counter-balance the depressant effect of the anesthetic on the myocardium. It is quite irritating to the respiratory mucosa, however, causing greatly increased salivation and bronchial secretion. Atropine is usually given as a preanesthetic medication to counteract this effect.

Ether is excreted, largely unchanged, via the lungs.

Since this agent is quite volatile it must be stored away from heat. When ether is exposed to air, peroxides are formed, which are highly explosive; thus it is packaged in sealed metal containers. It may not be used for anesthesia if the container has been opened for more than 24 hours.

USES. In any major surgery, it is especially useful in abdominal procedures because of the excellent skeletal muscle relaxation obtained. Its administration by inhalation produces remarkable bronchial dilation; thus it is often the drug of choice in the treatment of intractable status asthmaticus.

TOXICITY. Convulsions, dehydration, anoxia, fever, acidosis and depression of the respiratory center may occur with this agent. Vomiting occurs regularly upon recovery from the anesthesia; the patient should be positioned on his side to prevent aspiration of vomitus into the lungs.

CONCENTRATION. 10 to 15 volumes per cent by inhalation.

VINYL ETHER, N.F., B.P. (VINETHENE). Vinyl ether is an extremely rapidly acting anesthetic, giving smooth induction and producing surgical anesthesia two to three times as quickly as ethyl ether. The patient must be watched very carefully, however, because the fourth stage is easily and rapidly induced with this drug.

Excretion occurs via the lungs.

Vinyl ether is both flammable and explosive and may decompose if exposed to light and air.

USES. May be used for abdominal surgery, but muscle relaxation is not as complete as with diethyl ether. Recovery is more rapid and is accompanied by less vomiting than occurs with ethyl ether.

TOXICITY. Liver damage occurs, but it is not serious except in cases in which the anesthetic has been used over a prolonged period of time or an excessive dose has been administered. It is not safe for operations lasting longer than one hour.

CONCENTRATION. 2 to 4 volumes per cent by inhalation.

Chloroform, N.F., B.P. Chloroform may be used by inhalation to induce any desired stage of anesthesia. Induction is quicker than with ether; thus there is not the desirable safety feature of accurately determining each stage as it is being passed.

Upon exposure to heat, chloroform is converted to phosgene which, although irritating, is not dangerous. It is sensitive to light and highly volatile.

> **USES.** Chloroform is used in all forms of major surgery and in obstetrics to produce analgesia without loss of consciousness.
>
> **TOXICITY.** Liver damage in the form of central lobular necrosis is noted with administration of chloroform, but this can largely be prevented by adequate oxygenation and removal of carbon dioxide from the anesthetic mask. It is important to keep the anesthesia as light as possible to minimize the danger of circulatory depression. Chloroform depresses both the myocardium and the smooth muscles of the peripheral vascular system.
>
> **CONCENTRATION.** 1 volume per cent by inhalation.

Nitrous oxide, U.S.P., B.P. Nitrous oxide, or laughing gas, is widely used as an anesthetic agent. It is sweet-smelling and non-irritating and produces rapid induction when administered by inhalation. Although it is not inflammable or explosive, it supports combustion since it decomposes at high temperatures to form nitrogen and oxygen.

> **USES.** Useful only in short operations since, in order to induce deep anesthesia, extremely high concentrations must be used, and the patient readily becomes anoxic. It should not be used in concentrations greater than 80 per cent and must be accompanied by 20 per cent oxygen.
>
> **TOXICITY.** The chief disadvantage of nitrous oxide is that it produces anoxia when used in high concentrations. A few cases of sudden respiratory arrest

and death in healthy patients without anoxia have been reported, however.

> **CONCENTRATION.** 80 volumes per cent by inhalation.

Ethylene, N.F. This unsaturated hydrocarbon produces satisfactory anesthesia. It is not much more potent than nitrous oxide, however. It must be used in 80 per cent concentrations to be of value. Induction is rapid and pleasant, and there is no irritation of the respiratory mucosa. The incidence of nausea and vomiting upon recovery is somewhat higher than that noted with nitrous oxide, however.

Since there are practically no untoward effects on vital functions, it is one of the preferred anesthetics for poor risk patients.

Special precautions must be taken during the administration of ethylene because it is very explosive.

> **USES.** Used for short surgical procedures in which extensive abdominal relaxation is not required. Ethylene oxide is used in a 10 per cent concentration with 90 per cent carbon dioxide for gas sterilization.
>
> **TOXICITY.** Minimal.
>
> **CONCENTRATION.** 80 volumes per cent by inhalation.

Trichloroethylene, U.S.P. (Trilene). Trichloroethylene is a clear, colorless liquid with an odor resembling chloroform. It has the advantage of being nonexplosive in mixtures of the gas and oxygen or air normally used during anesthesia.

> **USES.** It is used by inhalation either as an analgesic or a general anesthetic for minor surgical procedures and obstetrics. In addition it has been found to be useful as an analgesic in the treatment of tic douloureux (trigeminal neuralgia), a painful neuritis of the fifth cranial nerve. It acts in this respect nonspecifically, however, merely functioning as a general central nervous system depressant, as it has no selective action on any of the cranial nerves.

TOXICITY. If trichloroethylene is used in a closed circuit with soda lime or one of the other carbon dioxide absorbers, toxic impurities are formed. One of these impurities, dichloroacetylene, is particularly toxic to the central nervous system, and it is also spontaneously explosive. This anesthetic, then, should always be administered by the open or semi-open technique.

DOSE. General anesthesia—0.25 to 0.75 volumes per cent in air. Trigeminal neuralgia—0.6 cc. by inhalation 3 to 4 times daily. No more than 4 cc. in 24 hours.

CYCLOPROPANE, U.S.P., B.P. Although cyclopropane is a very potent anesthetic, it has fallen into disuse recently chiefly because of its explosive properties. It may not be used with electrocautery or other electrical appliances during surgery. It may be used for patients in shock since it maintains a satisfactory blood pressure.

Like ether, this anesthetic causes release of epinephrine in the body. Epinephrine may not be administered concurrently because of the risk of ventricular tachycardia.

USES. Primarily in poor risk or hypotensive patients or when analgesia without loss of consciousness is desired.

TOXICITY. Arrhythmias, respiratory depression and decreased liver and kidney blood flow may occur. Excessive histamine release may occur and produce asthmatic symptoms in susceptible individuals.

CONCENTRATION. 3 to 5 volumes per cent for analgesia only, by inhalation. 13 to 23 volumes per cent for general anesthesia, by inhalation.

HALOTHANE, U.S.P., B.P. (FLUOTHANE). This chlorinated hydrocarbon is a modern equivalent of chloroform. It has some muscle relaxing properties but is only 25 to 50 per cent as effective as ether for this purpose. It is not a rapidly acting drug, and induction is often difficult and slow.

USES. Often used to provide a "bloodless" field for plastic surgery since it produces peripheral vasodilation. There is therefore less bleeding at incision sites. It has been used in obstetrics, but it inhibits uterine contraction during the period of anesthesia; it has largely been replaced by other agents for this purpose.

TOXICITY. In concentrations sufficient to produce general anesthesia, halothane is a respiratory depressant; therefore the patient's breathing must be assisted. It almost always produces blood pressure depression. This agent is a direct myocardial depressant; it must therefore be used with caution in patients with cardiovascular diseases.

It is contraindicated for use concurrently with Levarterenol (Levophed) or epinephrine.

CONCENTRATION. 1 to 3 volumes per cent by inhalation.

INTRAVENOUS ANESTHETICS

Intravenous anesthesia may be produced with a variety of substances ranging from opiates to the non-narcotic analgesics and barbiturates. Thiopental sodium is currently used almost exclusively for this purpose.

THIOPENTAL SODIUM, U.S.P. (PENTOTHAL). Thiopental, like the other barbiturates, produces cortical depression, but in addition is believed to produce unconsciousness by blocking the reticular activating center of the brain, which is responsible for wakefulness.

This agent is extremely rapidly acting when injected intravenously, and the patient falls asleep in a matter of seconds without passing through noticeable stages of analgesia and delirium. It is a poor analgesic, however, and when used alone it is not suitable for extensive surgical procedures.

USES. Used alone for short and nontraumatic surgical procedures, or prior to the administration of another general anesthetic to facilitate induction. It is administered alone for electroshock therapy and hypnosis.

TOXICITY. Respiratory depression, coughing, laryngospasm and allergic reactions.

CONCENTRATION. 2.5 per cent solution by intravenous drip.

LOCAL ANESTHETICS

Although local anesthetics are not central nervous system depressants, they will be covered with the general anesthetics in this section for the purpose of completeness.

Local anesthetics block or interfere with nerve conduction following application to a relatively small area. Depending upon the solubility and permeability of the individual agents, they may be applied locally to the skin or mucous membranes in solution or ointment form, or they may be ineffective unless injected subcutaneously.

Spinal anesthesia may be produced by introduction of a local anesthetic into the subarachnoid space of the spinal cord. These agents are often mixed with a few cc. of spinal fluid, which is first withdrawn from the subarachnoid space and then injected. The fluid remains in the lower areas of the cord by gravity, thus interfering with nerve conduction from all areas below the affected level of the cord.

COCAINE HYDROCHLORIDE, U.S.P., B.P. Cocaine is an alkaloid obtained from the leaves of *Erythroxylon coca.* When taken internally it is a potent central nervous system stimulant causing restlessness and excitement and an apparently increased capacity for muscular work because of loss of the sensation of fatigue. Central stimulation is soon followed by depression. In extreme cases the depression involves the vital medullary centers and death ensues.

Severe addiction to cocaine occurs readily, and its use in medicine has been outlawed except in preparations intended for topical use, because absorption from these sites is insignificant. It is covered by the Harrison Narcotic Act.

USES. The most important local action of cocaine is its ability to block nerve conduction when brought into direct contact with nerve tissue. It is frequently used in aqueous solutions for local anesthesia in the eyes, and in the mucous membranes of the nose and throat.

TOXICITY. Toxic effects are not noted from topical administration. Systemic poisoning is characterized by excitability, restlessness, confusion, rapid pulse, irregular respiration, nausea, vomiting, abdominal pain, convulsions, unconsciousness and even death.

CONCENTRATION. 1 to 20 per cent topically in solution or ointment form.

PROCAINE U.S.P., B.P. (NOVOCAIN). Procaine is probably the most widely used of all anesthetics. Unlike cocaine, it is not effective when applied topically to tissues, but must be injected subcutaneously. Procaine is read-

$$H_2N-\underset{}{\bigcirc}-\overset{O}{\underset{||}{C}}-O-CH_2CH_2-N\overset{C_2H_5}{\underset{C_2H_5}{}}$$

procaine

ily absorbed following injection and is excreted in the urine.

USES. Procaine solutions are infiltrated locally prior to minor surgical procedures. It is the local anesthetic of choice in dental practice and for spinal anesthesia.

TOXICITY. Occasionally systemic effects occur in unusually sensitive individuals and are akin to allergic reactions. Deaths following cardiovascular collapse have been reported from as little as 0.01 Gm. procaine. The central nervous system stimulation produced in sensitive individuals may be controlled by the use of barbiturates.

CONCENTRATION. 0.25 to 2 per cent subcutaneously for nerve block locally. Concentration used for spinal anesthesia varies greatly.

DIBUCAINE HYDROCHLORIDE, U.S.P. (NUPER-CAINE). Upon intravenous injection, dibucaine is six times as toxic as cocaine. However, it may be used for all types of procedures requiring a local anesthetic. It is the most potent and one of the more commonly employed local anesthetics.

CONCENTRATION. 0.05 to 0.1 per cent.

LIDOCAINE HYDROCHLORIDE, U.S.P. (XYLO-CAINE). A recently developed anesthetic, lidocaine is unique among local anesthetic agents in its chemical structure.

USES. When administered subcutaneously, it has approximately the same toxicity as procaine. It is nonirritating, has a longer duration of action than procaine, however, and is highly suitable for anesthetizing mucous membranes.

An oral form (Xylocaine Viscous) is prepared for application to areas within the oral cavity.

Lidocaine has recently become important in the control of cardiac arrhythmias. This use is discussed in Chapter 13.

CONCENTRATION. 2 per cent.

ETHYL CHLORIDE, U.S.P., B.P. Ethyl chloride is a liquid which, when sprayed on the skin or mucous membranes, evaporates rapidly, producing rapid cooling and surface anesthesia of the area. It has limited usefulness, however, since freezing may injure cells, lower resistance to infection and delay healing. Recovery from the anesthesia is painful.

USES. Ethyl chloride has been employed in the local treatment of burns, frostbite, bee stings and sprains and prior to minor surgical procedures.

TOXICITY. If ethyl chloride is used by inhalation, liver damage and cardiac irregularites may occur. Ventricular fibrillation and cardiac arrest have been noted as well. Ethyl chloride anesthesia, if used at all, should be limited to surgical processes lasting less than 15 minutes.

CONCENTRATION. Sprayed full strength locally on the skin or mucous membranes.

Other similarly acting local anesthetics:
PIPEROCAINE HYDROCHLORIDE, B.P. (METY-CAINE).

CONCENTRATON. 2 to 10 per cent ointment.

DIPERODON HYDROCHLORIDE (DIOTHANE).

CONCENTRATION. 0.5 to 1 per cent ointment.

PHENACAINE HYDROCHLORIDE, N.F. (HOLO-CAINE).

CONCENTRATION. 1 per cent ophthalmic solution.

Sedatives and hypnotics

The terms "sedative" and "hypnotic," although often used interchangeably, are actually quite distinct. A sedative is a drug used to calm and dispel anxiety or hyperactivity by mild depression of the higher brain centers. A hypnotic, on the other hand, is a drug used to induce sleep. The same drugs obviously may be used as either sedatives or hypnotics depending on the dose given and the response of the individual patient. One patient may become quite drowsy on a dose that will barely sedate another. Therefore, a patient receiving sedatives or other drugs capable of producing drowsiness should not drive an automobile or operate dangerous machinery.

NURSING IMPLICATIONS OF HYPNOTICS

Along with the administration of hypnotics, the nurse should use other measures to induce sleep. A soothing and relaxing back rub, a comfortable environment and a few moments spent with the patient promote sleep and reduce the need for hypnotics. Determining the patient's usual bedtime rituals and sleeping patterns helps in planning for adequate rest and sleep. Some patients may be sleeping in naps during the day; since this may be interfering with nighttime sleep, diversional activities and increase in physical activity should be considered.

Hospitalized patients may be somewhat reluctant to take a medication for sleep, possibly because of a fear of becoming addicted. Patients need to have these fears dispelled and may need to be encouraged to take a p.r.n. hypnotic. The nurse must remember that the hospital is a very noisy place, even at night. The patient is also in a strange setting, under many stresses and anxieties.

The patient should be observed to evaluate the effectiveness of the hypnotic. A patient who awakes a few hours after administration may need a longer-acting hypnotic. Some hypnotics may cause restlessness and confusion in certain patients, especially the elderly. The use of safety measures, such as bedside rails and availability of the call bell, should be considered.

If a patient is taking a hypnotic at home, it is a good idea for him to keep the medication away from the bedside in order to prevent accidental overdosage. The patient may wake up confused after taking one dose and think that he has not taken the hypnotic. The effort involved in getting out of bed to take another pill may awaken the patient enough to make him realize what he is doing.

THE BARBITURATES

The barbiturates are a much studied and much used class of central nervous system depressants that may be employed as either sedatives or hypnotics. The pharmacologic action of the various barbiturates is essentially the same; they merely differ in potency and duration of action.

Barbiturates differ from the narcotics in that, although they produce sedation or even sleep, they do not relieve pain. If they are given alone in the presence of pain, restlessness, confusion and delirium may occur. Thus, barbiturates would not be the drugs of choice if wakefulness is from discomfort due to pain. However, when they are com-

bined with analgesic agents, such as salicylates and codeine, the combination is more effective than the analgesic alone.

The basic formula for the barbiturates is shown below. An increase in length of one or both alkyl side chains on the basic barbiturate molecule results in enhanced potency and diminished duration of depression. If the potency of the compound as a hypnotic decreases, convulsant properties may appear.

Thiobarbiturates, derivatives of thiobarbituric acid (prepared by the substitution of sulfur in the molecule) are usually rapidly localized in the body fat depots and thus have a short duration of action. Thiopental, which is structurally similar to pentobarbital with the exception of the substitution of sulfur, is a very potent and rapidly acting drug. It is used solely as an intravenous general anesthetic and is not employed for daytime sedation or as a routine hypnotic.

Many of the barbiturates may be administered orally or parenterally as a preoperative sedative to calm the patient, allay his fears and thus indirectly facilitate induction with the general anesthesia.

The structure of the individual barbiturate determines how it is inactivated in the body. Barbital is largely excreted in the urine; amobarbital and pentobarbital are detoxified in the body, largely in the liver, and the metabolic products are excreted in the urine. The thiobarbiturates, as stated previously, are deposited in the body fat but eventually are also degraded by the liver and excreted by the kidney.

The barbiturates are used more commonly for the production of sleep than for any other purpose. With an adequate oral dose of a barbiturate, sleep occurs within 20 to 60 minutes and closely resembles normal sleep. There may be a morning "hangover," however, which seems rather distressing to some individuals.

In high doses all barbiturates are capable of inhibiting convulsions. Phenobarbital is the most effective as an anticonvulsant, however, since it seems to have a selective action on the motor cortex. The action is unrelated to sedation since non-

TABLE 5 Comparison of Barbiturates

GENERIC NAME	TRADE NAME	R_1	R_2	R_3	X	DOSE
Long Acting (7 to 8 hours or more)						
Barbital	Veronal	$-C_2H_5$	$-C_2H_5$	H	O	0.3 to 0.5 Gm.
Mephobarbital	Mebaral	$-C_2H_5$	⬡	CH_3	O	0.1 to 0.2 Gm.
Phenobarbital	Luminal	$-C_2H_5$	⬡	H	O	0.1 to 0.2 Gm.
Intermediate Acting (6 to 8 hours)						
Amobarbital	Amytal	$-C_2H_5$	$-CH_2-CH_2-CH \begin{smallmatrix} CH_3 \\ CH_3 \end{smallmatrix}$	H	O	0.05 to 0.2 Gm.
Aprobarbital	Alurate	$-CH_2-CH=CH_2$	$-CH \begin{smallmatrix} CH_3 \\ CH_3 \end{smallmatrix}$	H	O	0.065 to 0.13 Gm.
Butabarbital	Butisol	$-C_2H_5$	$-\underset{\underset{CH_3}{\vert}}{CH}-CH_2-CH_3$	H	O	0.1 to 0.2 Gm.
Short Acting (4 to 6 hours)						
Pentobarbital	Nembutal	$-C_2H_5$	$-\underset{\underset{CH_3}{\vert}}{CH}(-CH_2)_2-CH_3$	H	O	0.05 to 0.1 Gm.
Secobarbital	Seconal	$-CH_2-CH=CH_2$	$-\underset{\underset{CH_3}{\vert}}{CH}-(CH_2)_2-CH_3$	H ‘	O	0.1 to 0.2 Gm.
Ultra-Short Acting						
Thiopental Sodium	Pentothal	$-C_2H_5$	$-\underset{\underset{CH_3}{\vert}}{CH}-(CH_2)_2-CH_3$	H	S	As needed

sedative doses are often effective and amphetamines can counteract the sedation without abolishing the anticonvulsant action. Phenobarbital is often combined with another anticonvulsant drug in the treatment of epilepsy.

Since many barbiturates are available for therapeutic use, the choice is based upon the requirements of the patient and the duration of action required. The use of barbiturates is regulated by the Drug Abuse Control Amendments.

A comparison of the commonly used barbiturates is presented in Table 5.

General Structure of Barbiturates
(See Table 5 for individual variations in this general structure.)

TOXICITY. Toxic effects may occur from prolonged use of the barbiturates as well as from a large overdose. Ten times the average therapeutic dose generally produces toxic effects, and death can occur from 15 times the therapeutic dose. When alcohol and barbiturates are used together, the effects of both are enhanced. Patients should be warned of this result.

A patient who is receiving phenobarbital and a coumarin anticoagulant may need a higher dose of the anticoagulant since phenobarbital increases the metabolic breakdown of coumarin anticoagulants. Adjustment of anticoagulant dosage is also necessary when phenobarbital is discontinued.

Barbiturates should not be employed in patients with porphyria as they often cause exacerbation of the disease.

Acute poisoning occurs often as a result of attempted suicide. About 20 per cent of hospital admissions for acute drug intoxication are cases of barbiturate poisoning. A deep coma ensues from large overdoses of barbiturates. This may be preceded by a period of delirium and hallucinations. Death is due to respiratory depression, and corrective therapy is directed toward minimizing this effect. Cardiovascular collapse does not occur until very late in the course of poisoning.

Bemegride is the drug of choice in acute barbiturate poisoning, although picrotoxin, nikethamide and even caffeine have been employed. Currently there is a trend to avoid giving central stimulants in barbiturate poisoning and to remove the drug instead via peritoneal dialysis. This latter method, although more inconvenient, is generally assumed to be safer because it circumvents the possibility of untoward effects from the stimulants.

Chronic poisoning or habituation to barbiturates creates a different picture. True addiction, although it has occurred, is relatively rare. More often the individual merely has a strong psychic dependence upon the drug and cannot tell the difference when the "little red sleeping pill" is filled with sugar rather than a barbiturate.

Symptoms of chronic barbiturate intoxication resemble those due to alcohol. These include sluggishness, difficulty in thinking, poor memory, faulty judgment, depression, crying, hostile and paranoid ideas and suicidal tendency.

Once barbiturate withdrawal has been accomplished under hospitalization, medical and psychiatric rehabilitative procedures should be instituted. At best the prognosis is uncertain because the strong psychic dependence upon the drug remains even after the physical withdrawal is accomplished.

NONBARBITURATE SEDATIVES AND HYPNOTICS

CHLORAL HYDRATE, U.S.P., B.P. (LORINAL, SOMNOS, NOCTEC). In doses used for hypnosis, chloral hydrate produces mild cerebral depression and a sleep greatly resembling physiologic sleep with little or no hangover.

It is readily absorbed from the gastrointestinal tract, and drowsiness occurs within 15 minutes followed by sleep within an hour.

Its use may cause a false positive test for glucose in the urine when Benedict's solution is used.

chloral hydrate

USES. Sometimes used for its sedative effect in the treatment of delirium tremens and in patients undergoing narcotic, barbiturate or alcohol withdrawal.

TOXICITY. Nausea and vomiting occur following oral administration. This results from a local irritation that may also increase peristalsis. Occasionally skin reactions and delirium have been noted: however, these effects are uncommon. Addiction to chloral hydrate has been known to occur, the symptoms being similar to chronic alcoholism but with more severe gastritis.

Chloral hydrate is contraindicated in patients with renal, hepatic or severe cardiac disorders, or peptic ulcer. It should be given with fruit juice or milk.

When chloral hydrate is combined with alcohol, the depressant effect is potentiated. This combination, known as a "Mickey Finn" or "knockout drops," is not used therapeutically.

DOSE. 500 mg. orally at bedtime as hypnotic.
250 mg. orally three times daily as sedative. 250 to 500 mg. rectally.

CHLORAL BETAINE (BETA-CHLOR). This betaine derivative of chloral hydrate has essentially the same properties as the parent compound.

DOSE. 250 to 500 mg. orally at bedtime.

ETHCHLORVYNOL, N.F. (PLACIDYL). Ethchlorvynol is a tertiary carbinol that produces effects ranging from light sedation through hypnosis. It is indicated as a mild hypnotic in the management of most forms of insomnia and as a daytime sedative in the management of mild anxiety or tension states, including pruritus or emotional factors associated with dermatologic disorders. It is of particular value when the use of barbiturates is inadvisable or contraindicated.

The drug should be protected from exposure to light.

TOXICITY. The sedative response may be exaggerated if the drug is taken with alcoholic beverages or other sedative-hypnotic drugs. Occasionally, a mild hangover, nausea, vomiting, syncope, dizziness, hypotension and muscular weakness are noted. If the drug is taken over a period of time, the dosage must be reduced gradually.

Overdosage may be treated with analeptic agents such as pentylenetetrazol. Peritoneal dialysis has been used successfully. The dosage of anticoagulants of coumarin type may need to be adjusted.

DOSE. 500 mg. orally at bedtime as a hypnotic.
100 to 200 mg. orally two or three times daily as a sedative.

ETHINAMATE, N.F. (VALMID). When doses sufficient for hypnosis are administered, a quiet, deep sleep is produced with little or no hangover. The drug is rapidly destroyed in the body tissues and has a duration of action of about four hours. Except for a small amount of the drug that may be excreted in the urine, the metabolic fate of ethinamate is unknown. Apparently detoxification does not occur in the liver because hepatic damage does not contraindicate its use. The drug is often used as a hypnotic in patients with liver or kidney damage when treatment with other sedatives would be dangerous.

TOXICITY. Addiction may occur upon prolonged use of this drug. Routine side effects are few. Extreme overdose produces death by respiratory depression. Dosage should be reduced gradually after prolonged administration.

DOSE. 0.5 to 1 Gm. orally at bedtime.

GLUTETHIMIDE, N.F., B.P. (DORIDEN). The action of glutethimide is similar to that of the short-acting barbiturates, and it may be used for the same conditions.

> **TOXICITY.** Skin rash and mild nausea have occurred. Bemegride has been found useful in the treatment of overdoses.
>
> Adjustment of a coumarin-type anticoagulant may be necessary.
>
> Repeated incidences of glutethimide abuse have occurred, thus it is now controlled federally as a dangerous drug. Withdrawal symptoms can occur following repeated use of the drug in high doses.
>
> **DOSE.** 500 mg. orally at bedtime as hypnotic.
> 250 mg. orally three times daily as sedative.

METHYPRYLON, N.F., B.P. (NOLUDAR). Methyprylon produces sleep within 30 minutes and has a duration of action of approximately six to seven hours. It is comparable to the intermediate barbiturates in use and effect.

> **TOXICITY.** Side effects are mild and include nausea, vomiting, constipation, drowsiness, excitation, vertigo, headache, pruritus, rash and diarrhea.
>
> **DOSE.** 200 to 400 mg. orally at bedtime as hypnotic.
> 50 to 100 mg. orally three or four times daily as sedative.

PROPIOMAZINE HYDROCHLORIDE (LARGON). Structurally and pharmacologically propiomazine is related to promethazine. In combination with promethazine and related compounds, propiomazine produces sedative, antiemetic and antihistaminic effects. The sedative effect of other central nervous system depressants is enhanced.

> **USES.** Used as a sedative and antiemetic for surgical and obstetric procedures.
>
> **TOXICITY.** Dizziness, hypotension and incoherency are not uncommon. Large doses may produce coma and shock.
>
> **DOSE.** 20 mg. I.M. or I.V. for sedation.

PARALDEHYDE U.S.P., B.P. Paraldehyde is a colorless liquid with a disagreeable odor and pungent taste. It is similar in effect to chloral hydrate and is likewise absorbed well from the gastrointestinal tract.

A hypnotic dose produces sleep in 10 to 15 minutes; larger doses produce analgesia. It may be used as a sedative and hypnotic in delirium tremens, bromide psychoses, alcohol or morphine withdrawal and obstetrics. Intramuscular injection is painful but is used when the patient is unable to take the drug orally. The drug should *not* be given subcutaneously because of the danger of sterile abscess and sloughing of tissue. It should be given deep I.M. into a large muscle, preferably using the Z-tract technique.

> **TOXICITY.** The drug should be used with caution in liver damage since this is the site of detoxification. Paraldehyde is a very safe hypnotic, however, and produces very little respiratory depression. Even a large overdose often does no more than prolong the sleep of the victim. When given intravenously, paraldehyde may produce circulatory collapse or pulmonary edema; thus this route should be reserved for extreme emergencies.
>
> Opened containers of paraldehyde are potentially very dangerous because it deteriorates upon standing and develops highly toxic peroxides. It should be stored only in tight, light-resistant containers. Partially filled containers should not be kept for any period of time since even the air in the container may be sufficient to cause the formation of peroxides.
>
> **DOSE.** 4 to 8 ml. given orally in juice or milk. 2 to 4 ml. I.M. as needed, 4 to 8 ml. rectally in retention enema.

FLURAZEPAM HYDROCHLORIDE (DALMANE). This synthetic hypnotic agent has been found to be useful in the treatment of all forms of insomnia, including primary difficulty in falling asleep, awaking during the night and early morning insomnia. The exact mechanism of action is not known; however, it is believed to act by increasing the arousal threshold in the thalamus, and reducing the response of this area of the brain to stimulation.

TOXICITY. As with most hypnotic agents, the action of this drug is potentiated by alcohol and other central depressants. Drowsiness, dizziness, staggering, ataxia, lethargy and disorientation have been reported. Mild gastrointestinal complaints occasionally occur such as nausea, vomiting, abdominal discomfort and diarrhea. It should not be used in pregnancy until further studies have been completed. Presently

TABLE 6   Sleep Aids and Other o-t-c-Sedatives†

PRODUCT	MANUFACTURER	METHAPYRILENE	SCOPOLAMINE	BROMIDES	OTHER
Alva-Tranquil 8-Hour Timed Release	Alva Labs	HCl 26 mg/tab	—	pot. bromide 518 mg	niacinamide 5 mg niacin 5 mg thiamine HCl 1 mg pot. salicylate 194.4 mg
Alva-Tranquil Regular	Alva Labs	HCl 10 mg/tab	—	pot. bromide 195 mg	pot. salicylate 85 mg thiamine HCl 2 mg niacin 4 mg niacinamide 4 mg
Bromo Seltzer	Warner-Lambert	—	—	pot. bromide 2½ gr/capful	acetaminophen 3 gr phenacetin 2 gr caffeine* sod. bicarbonate* citric acid*
Compoz	Jeffrey Martin	HCl 15 mg. plus pyrilamine maleate 10 mg/tab	aminoxide HBr. 0.15 mg	—	salicylamide 120 mg passion flower ext. 7.5 mg thiamine HCl 5 mg riboflavin 2 mg pyridoxide HCl 0.5 mg niacinamide 20 mg
Devarex	J.B. Williams	HCl 12 mg/cap	aminoxide HBr 0.15 mg	—	salicylamide 324 mg
Dormin	Dormin	HCl 25 mg/cap	—	—	—
Mr. Sleep	Jeffrey Martin	HCl 18.75 mg plus pyrilamine maleate 6.25 mg/tab	aminoxide HBr 0.2 mg	—	—
Neo-Nyte	Rabin-Winters	HCl 25 mg	aminoxide HBr 0.125 mg	—	—
Nervine	Miles	—	—	sod., pot. and ammonium bromides 9½ gr/cap or tab	niacinamide 7 mg thiamine 1 mg
Nytol	Block Drug	HCl 25 mg/tab	—	—	salicylamide*
San-Man	Plough	HCl 25 mg/tab	aminoxide HBr 0.25 mg	—	—
Sleep-Eze	Whitehall	HCl 25 mg/tab	HBr 0.125 mg	—	—
Somicaps	Am. Pharm. Co.	HCl 25 mg/tab	—	—	—
Sominex Capsules	J.B. Williams	HCl 50 mg/cap	aminoxide HBr 0.5/mg	—	salicylamide 200 mg
Sominex Tablets	J.B. Williams	HCl 25 mg/tab	aminoxide HBr 0.25 mg	—	salicylamide 200 mg
Sure-Sleep	American Labs	HCl 25 mg/tab	aminoxide HBr 0.25 mg	—	salicylamide 200 mg

its use in children has not been studied, thus it is not recommended for use in patients under 15 years of age.

DOSE. 15 to 30 mg. orally at bedtime.

OTHER SEDATIVES

Table 6 contains a list of sedatives and sleep aids that can be purchased without a physician's prescription.

TRANQUILIZERS

A relatively new pharmacologic group, the tranquilizers differ from the older sedatives in that they alleviate anxiety without seriously impairing mental ability. A sedated individual is drowsy, sometimes incoherent and has diminished reflex ability, whereas a tranquilized individual is most often able to go about his normal daily activities unimpeded by sedation or anxiety.

Needless to say, these agents have enabled a great step forward in medical progress. Mental patients, formerly uncommunicative and unresponsive, can now be calmed sufficiently so that they can discuss their problems and receive help. Many mental patients can now be treated on an outpatient basis for the same disorders that would have required hospitalization two decades ago.

THE PHENOTHIAZINES

The phenothiazines are all structurally similar and vary only by minor substitutes on the basic molecules. Since the discovery of the tranquilizing effects of chlorpromazine, many related phenothiazines have been developed and are available commercially.

The primary action of the phenothiazines is apparently a depression of the subcortical area of the brain. It is believed that they selectively inhibit the chemoreceptor "trigger" zone, the hypothalamus and the reticular formation, thus exerting their influence by interrupting the passage of impulses coming through this region to the cortex.

Depression of the chemoreceptor "trigger" zone enables the drugs to be used as antinauseants. This effect should be kept in mind when phenothiazines are used for neuropsychiatric disorders, since the antiemetic action may obscure the warning signs of toxicity from other drugs. In addition, some of these derivatives possess hypotensive, antispasmodic, sedative, antihistaminic, antitussive, antipruritic, hypothermic or weak adrenolytic properties.

They are used chiefly to treat symptoms associated with neuropsychiatric conditions, such as schizophrenia, manic-depressive states, paranoid psychoses and hysteria, and they are also useful in controlling the emotional disturbances and anxiety associated with other conditions, such as peptic ulcers, heart disease, menopausal anxiety, asthma, tension headaches, premenstrual tension and arthritis. Their use should never be substituted for nursing or medical intervention to discover the cause of a patient's anxiety and take steps to reduce it. Although many phenothiazines are useful in the treatment of nausea and vomiting, they should be used with extreme caution in the treatment of the morning sickness of pregnancy until more research has been carried out on the possible teratogenic effects of these and many other drugs.

Their ataractic (tranquilizing) and antiemetic effects make them useful in anesthesia and surgery because they allow smoother induction of anesthesia by decreasing anxiety and tension. In addition, tranquilizers potentiate the action of general anesthetics; thus a smaller dose of each may be given, which in turn reduces the risk of respiratory depression.

Refractory hiccoughs have also been successfully treated with the phenothiazines in some instances.

TOXICITY. Mild drowsiness is a relatively common side effect, especially when the drugs are given in large doses. Patients receiving these drugs should not drive automobiles or operate dangerous machinery. Liver damage is not uncommon, and agranulocytosis and other serious blood dyscrasias have been reported. Severe neurologic symptoms characterized by tonic convulsions have been noted especially in children.

Parkinsonian symptoms, such as tremors at rest, rigidity, shuffling gait and "pill-rolling" action of hands, occur after phenothiazines are taken for a period of time. This reversible "extrapyramidal syndrome" is more annoying than serious and disappears upon withdrawal of the drug. Patients should be reassured that these effects will indeed disappear. The symptoms may be minimized by concurrent administration of antiparkinsonian drugs.

Phenothiazines may potentiate the effects of alcohol, anesthetics, barbiturates or morphine and its derivatives.

Other side effects resemble those of atropine: dryness of the mouth, nasal congestion, constipation, miosis and mydriasis. Less frequent effects include dermatoses, dizziness, urinary difficulty, photosensitivity, tachycardia and postural hypotension. Postural hypotension is more frequent during the initial stage of therapy, when the drug is given intravenously or when large oral doses are given. In these instances the patient should be kept in a recumbent position for an hour after administration.

The nurse should avoid getting solutions on her hands, since contact dermatitis has been reported following contact with these agents.

Chlorpromazine hydrochloride, U.S.P., B.P. (Thorazine, Largactil, Megaphen).

Chlorpromazine is usually administered orally, but may be given by intramuscular injection. It should be injected deeply and slowly. Local irritation and pain at the injection site may be relieved by massage and by administering the drug in a 2% procaine solution. Postural hypotension is always an imminent danger when the parenteral route is chosen. The blood pressure should be checked before and after administration.

Patients should lie down for at least 30 minutes after the injection.

chlorpromazine hydrochloride

USES. In addition to its primary use in treating mental and emotional disturbances, chlorpromazine is also used in the treatment of hiccoughs. It may be administered for this condition during surgery in a saline solution as a slow intravenous infusion. It is also of value for the relief of vomiting, following surgical procedures or the administration of antineoplastic drugs.

Although chlorpromazine is supplied in suppository form, for practical and psychiatric reasons, it is not useful for repeated administration. The syrup and suppository forms are the most convenient for use in children, however. Solutions should be protected from light, and dark yellow solutions should not be used.

DOSE. 25 to 50 mg. orally or I.M. three times daily initially. The dose may be increased by 150 to 200 mg. daily until a satisfactory response is obtained. As much as 5000 mg. daily has been administered without serious side effects. The larger doses are used only in hospitalized patients, however.

Promazine hydrochloride, N.F., B.P. (Sparine).

The possibility of postural hypotension is considerably greater with promazine than with chlorpromazine, and it is not ordinarily used for long-term therapy. Rather it is employed in instances in which a temporary tranquilizing effect is desired. Patients should remain in bed for one half to one hour after parenteral administration, since serious hypotensive effects may result even after the first injection. Injections should be given slowly and deep into the muscle.

Arteriolar spasm and gangrene have occurred following intravenous injections of large doses.

A concentrated syrup is available for use when the administration of tablets is undesirable.

DOSE. 25 to 500 mg. orally or I.M. every 4 to 6 hours.

PROCHLORPERAZINE MALEATE, U.S.P., B.P. (COMPAZINE). Extrapyramidal symptoms, motor restlessness and dystonias are relatively common upon prolonged administration of prochlorperazine. Opisthotonos occurs in sensitive children and adults even upon short-term treatment or occasionally with the initial dose of this drug.

Prochlorperazine is used more often as a postoperative antiemetic than as a tranquilizer.

The syrup form should be protected from light; it should always be stored in a dark bottle and kept tightly closed at all times.

DOSE. 5 to 10 mg. orally or I.M. three or four times daily.

TRIFLUPROMAZINE HYDROCHLORIDE, B.P. (VESPRIN). Although most side effects are similar to those of chlorpromazine, there is a higher incidence of Parkinsonian symptoms with triflupromazine. Solutions should be protected from light, and discolored solutions should not be used.

DOSE. 10 to 25 mg. orally or I.M. twice daily.

TRIFLUOPERAZINE HYDROCHLORIDE, B.P. (STELAZINE). Trifluoperazine is available in tablets, in a concentrate solution and in an injectable form.

Extrapyramidal symptoms, motor restlessness and dystonias are common, especially at the higher dosage levels.

DOSE. 5 mg. orally or I.M. three times daily.

PERPHENAZINE, B.P. (TRILAFON). Perphenazine is available as tablets, including repeat-action tablets, as a syrup and as a liquid concentrate. Suppositories and an injectable preparation are also available; however,

they are rarely used since the oral route is generally satisfactory.

Perphenazine has good antiemetic action and few hypotensive and sedative effects.

DOSE. 2 to 16 mg. orally two to four times daily.

FLUPHENAZINE HYDROCHLORIDE (PERMITIL, PROLIXIN). Fluphenazine has fewer hypotensive and sedative effects than chlorpromazine, but parkinsonian symptoms are observed with prolonged use or high dosage levels.

It is available in tablets, as an elixir and in parenteral form. Solutions should be protected from light.

DOSE. 2.5 to 10 mg. orally daily.

MEPAZINE HYDROCHLORIDE (PACATAL). The action of mepazine is intermediate between the more potent tranquilizers, such as chlorpromazine, and milder agents, such as meprobamate. It has little or no effect on acute psychotic disturbances and is not as effective as chlorpromazine for long-term therapy.

Less sedation, drowsiness and depression are observed with mepazine than with chlorpromazine. The most common effects are atropine-like, although leukopenia and agranulocytosis have been observed on continued use.

Mepazine may be administered orally, intramuscularly or intravenously.

DOSE. For mild neuroses or tension, 25 mg. orally, I.M. or I.V. three or four times daily is usually sufficient. Psychotic patients may require as much as 400 mg. daily.

THIORIDAZINE HYDROCHLORIDE (MELLARIL). Since it has little if any antiemetic activity, thioridazine is not useful to control nausea. It may be used for most of the other conditions for which chlorpromazine is useful, however.

Since extrapyramidal symptoms are rare with thioridazine, it is often the drug of choice when patients are forced to discontinue use of the other phenothiazines because of these side effects. Dryness of the mouth is a common side effect. Postural hypotension has occurred on occasion following therapy.

DOSE. 20 to 800 mg. orally daily.

CARPHENAZINE MALEATE (PROKETAZINE). On a weight to weight basis, carphenazine is one of the less potent phenothiazine tranquilizers. It is used in the treatment of acute and chronic schizophrenia. It has a shorter duration of action than do many other agents.

All the toxic manifestations of chlorpromazine have been observed with carphenazine. Clinical use of carphenazine in pregnant patients is not recommended.

DOSE. 25 to 50 mg. orally three times daily.

NONPHENOTHIAZINE TRANQUILIZERS

AZACYCLONOL HYDROCHLORIDE, N.F. (FRENQUEL). Azacyclonol is an antihallucinatory drug indicated for the treatment of hallucinations and confusion such as those that occur in acute schizophrenia. It is also indicated for toxic psychoses and alcoholic hallucinations.

Unlike the phenothiazines, azacyclonol cannot be classified as a central nervous system depressant since it has no appreciable sedative or hypnotic effect in man.

TOXICITY. The toxicity is negligible. the only reported untoward effect is a mild rash, which disappears rapidly upon discontinuance of therapy.

DOSE. 20 to 100 mg. orally or I.M. three times daily.

MEPROBAMATE, N.F., B.P. (EQUANIL, MILTOWN). In addition to its usefulness as a mild tranquilizer, meprobamate has proved effective as a skeletal muscle relaxant for use in management of anxiety and tension occurring either alone or as accompanying symptoms. It is used as an anticonvulsant in petit mal epilepsy, although it is not effective in grand mal. There has been considerable controversy concerning the mechanism of action of this drug. Many current investigators consider it to be a simple central depressant rather than a true tranquilizer. It is still classified as a tranquilizer, however.

USES. Useful as a psychotherapeutic sedative in the treatment of psychoneurotic anxiety and tension states and in simple insomnia as well as prior to electroshock therapy.

TOXICITY. Dependence and habituation have been reported with this drug. It is especially noted in susceptible persons, such as alcoholics, former addicts and other severe psychoneurotics who have taken excessive doses for weeks or months. The drug should be withdrawn gradually rather than stopped abruptly because withdrawal symptoms are precipitated upon sudden withdrawal. Due to its abuse potential, this drug is now under federal control as a dangerous drug.

Tolerance to alcohol is lowered in patients taking meprobamate with slowing of reaction time and impairment of judgment and coordination when alcohol is taken.

Hypersensitivity reactions, such as skin eruptions, chills, fever, peripheral edema, nonthrombocytopenic purpura and bronchospasm, sometimes occur. Less commonly observed effects are gastric distress, severe diarrhea, proctitis, stomatitis, muscular paralysis, diplopia and paradoxical excitement. Transient leukopenia may occur. Other blood dyscrasias such as aplastic anemia and thrombocytopenia have been reported.

DOSE. 400 mg. orally three or four times daily.

CHLORDIAZEPOXIDE HYDROCHLORIDE, N.F. (LIBRIUM). Chlordiazepoxide is chemically unrelated to any other family of tranquilizers. In small oral doses the drug is effective in mild to moderate anxiety and tension, tension headache, preoperative and postoperative apprehension, premenstrual tension, menstrual distress, chronic alcoholism, behavioral disorders in children, and whenever anxiety and tension are concomitants of gastrointestinal, cardiovascular, gynecologic or dermatologic disorders. Larger doses of chlordiazepoxide are used to treat more severe anxiety and tension.

TOXICITY. The necessity of discontinuing therapy because of undesirable side effects has been rare. The chief side effect is drowsiness. Patients receiving the drug should not drive or operate machinery. Ataxia is common. Other effects include constipation, muscle tenderness and spasm, headache, dizziness, skin rash, confusion, lightheadedness, syncope, urinary frequency and menorrhagia. Caution must be exercised in administering chlordiazepoxide to individuals known to be addiction-prone, since prolonged administration of extremely large doses has caused addiction.

Any unused portion of the reconstituted parenteral solution should be discarded immediately.

The concomitant use of this drug with other psychotropic agents is not recommended; it is especially potentiated by the MAO inhibitors and phenothiazines as well as by alcohol.

DOSE. 10 to 25 mg. orally three or four times daily. 100 mg. I.M. every 6 hours. The patient should be kept recumbent after I.M. administration.

DIAZEPAM (VALIUM). Diazepam, which is related to chlorodiazepoxide, is useful in anxiety reactions stemming from stressful circumstances or whenever somatic complaints are concomitants of emotional factors. It is useful in psychoneurotic states manifested by anxiety, tension, fear and fatigue as well as in acute agitation due to alcohol withdrawal. In addition, diazepam may be of use to alleviate muscle spasm associated with cerebral palsy, athetosis and spinal cord injuries.

When injected intravenously or intramuscularly, diazepam has been shown to be extremely effective as an anticonvulsant. It is most useful when given by direct I.V. injection and the dose carefully titrated according to the condition of the patient. It may be used in status epilepticus or recurrent convulsive disorders.

It is not of value in dealing with psychotic patients manifesting anxiety, and should be avoided when there is reason to believe the patient is psychotic.

TOXICITY. It is necessary to limit the dosage to the smallest effective amount in elderly or debilitated patients to preclude the development of ataxia or oversedation. It is contraindicated in patients with glaucoma. Side effects include drowsiness, nausea, dizziness, excitement, sleep disturbances, hyperexcitability, hallucinations, blurred vision, diplopia, headache, incontinence, slurred speech, tremor and skin rash.

When used intravenously, apnea may occur. This lasts for a few moments only and should be controlled by bag breathing the patient during the episode. Equipment for this purpose should be available whenever the dose is administered intravenously.

It potentiates the action of phenothiazines, barbiturates, MAO inhibitors and alcohol.

Parenteral preparations should not be mixed in other solutions or mixed in the same syringe or bottle with other drugs.

DOSE. 2 to 5 mg. orally or I.M. two or three times daily. I.V. dose as required.

CHLORPROTHIXENE (TARACTAN). Chemically related to the phenothiazines, chlorprothixene has many of the same indications. It is, however, more active than chlorpromazine in inhibiting postural reflexes and motor coordination and less active in antihistaminic effects.

TOXICITY. The most frequent side effect is drowsiness. Tachycardia, postural hypotension, convulsions, constipation, dryness of the mouth, nervousness, insomnia and slight edema have also occurred. It is contraindicated in circulatory collapse and comatose states due to central depressants (alcohol, hypnotics, opiates, etc.).

DOSE. 10 mg. orally three or four times daily.

HYDROXYZINE PAMOATE, N.F. (ATARAX, VISTARIL). Hydroxyzine is used to treat anxiety and tension, psychomotor agitation and other emotional disturbances and as an adjunct in the treatment of alcoholism. It has been used effectively for behavioral problems and anxiety in children and in the management of allergic conditions, especially those associated with anxiety and tension, such as chronic urticaria, pruritus and asthma. In addition, it is effective as an anti-nauseant and as a mild anti-arrhythmic agent.

Hydroxyzine is potentiated by meperidine and barbiturates, and dosage must be adjusted when these are used concomitantly.

TOXICITY. No serious side effects have been noted. Transitory drowsiness, dryness of the mouth, headaches, itching and increased peristalsis have been reported. Hydroxyzine may potentiate meperidine, opiates, barbiturates and alcohol. Clinical observations have shown that the dosage requirement for anticoagulants is decreased when taken with hydroxyzine, but the reason for this phenomenon is unknown.

DOSE. 25 to 50 mg. orally or I.M. every four hours.

LITHIUM SALTS

Although not technically tranquilizers, lithium salts have proven quite effective in psychiatry, and they will be discussed in this section.

Lithium salts were used formerly in the treatment of gout and arthritis, but without much success. Recently, however, they have been found to be a useful adjunct in the treatment of the manic phase of manic-depressive disorders.

The exact mechanism of action is unknown, but it is believed that lithium re-places sodium in the cells, thus interfering with membrane transport. Patients in the manic phase appear to store exogenous lithium in the body's cells, and lithium appears in the urine only when the manic episode breaks. For acute attacks, it is necessary to use other therapy because three to ten days are required for onset of action of the lithium salts. They are of no benefit in the depressed stage of manic depression and are of only slight benefit in hyperactive states associated with other psychoses. They may have a beneficial effect even if the patient does not respond to phenothiazines.

There does not seem to be any deleterious effect to the use of lithium salts with other psychoactive drugs.

USE. The salts are used to treat the manic phase of manic depression.

TOXICITY. The accumulation of the salts in the blood must not exceed 1.7 mEq./L., and the level should be measured frequently during therapy. Muscular fasciculations, nausea, increased urinary output, dizziness, excessive drowsiness, tremors and other neurologic signs may occur. Lithium salts are contraindicated in patients with cardiac or renal disorders. An increased sodium intake, at least 4 Gm. extra per day, enhances excretion of lithium.

DOSE. As lithium carbonate—300 mg. orally three to six times daily.

ANALGESICS

NON-NARCOTIC ANALGESICS AND ANTIPYRETICS

Analgesics are agents that relieve pain by acting centrally to elevate the pain threshold without disturbing consciousness or altering other sensory modalities. Antipyretics are drugs that reduce elevated body temperatures. Because these actions are often found in the same drug, they are usually discussed together; nevertheless their pharmacologic activities are quite distinct.

All healthy persons are able to perceive

pain, but each person's interpretation of a painful sensation may be different. As previously noted, the point at which pain is perceived is termed the pain threshold. By raising this threshold (e.g., by the use of analgesic drugs) more painful stimuli are required before pain is perceived.

The mechanism by which analgesic drugs raise the pain threshold—alter the perception of pain—is not clearly understood. Most studies seem to indicate that these drugs act by interfering with pain impulses carried over sensory nerve tracts at subcortical levels of the brain and act peripherally to prevent inflammation.

Since many analgesics also serve as antipyretics, it has been suggested that this interference takes place in the vicinity of the thalamus, an area of the brain concerned with the relay of sensory impulses to the cerebral cortex. The wide variance in effectiveness of analgesics, however, suggests that perhaps they do not all act by the same mechanism.

Then, too, many drugs that relieve pain cannot be considered as analgesics per se. General anesthetics relieve pain by causing unconsciousness. Local anesthetics act by blocking nerve fibers. Antispasmodics are muscle relaxants and thus may relieve pain due to spasm. The adrenal corticoids relieve inflammation and pain associated with rheumatoid arthritis by an anti-inflammatory rather than an analgesic action.

Agents that are used chiefly for symptomatic relief of pain fall into two chief classes: narcotic analgesics and nonaddicting analgesics and antipyretics.

NURSING IMPLICATIONS IN RELIEF OF PAIN

The nurse has a very important role in relation to the administration of analgesics and the relief of pain in general. Most analgesics are ordered by the physician to be given p.r.n.—as needed or as indicated. Several factors must be taken into consideration by the nurse. First, the pain should be evaluated as to whether it is the same pain the patient has been experiencing or a sign of a new process or complication.

The *nature* and *location* of the pain should be recorded by the nurse. It is best to describe the pain in the patient's own words. The nurse should also record whether the analgesic relieves the pain. The analgesic should not be used as a substitute for other comfort measures, such as positioning and back care, and promoting the optimal comfort and well-being of the patient.

It should be remembered that greater relief is obtained from an analgesic when it is given at the first indication of pain rather than after waiting until the pain is severe. Patients should be taught to notify the nurse when they first experience pain.

The nurse must be aware of the different emotional and cultural reactions to pain that influence how a person perceives and expresses pain. The emotional reaction and importance given to the pain vary greatly in each individual.

A person who is stoic or feels that pain should be endured probably will not ask the nurse for an analgesic. A male patient may feel that he will be thought unmanly if he asks for pain relief. The nurse should offer analgesics to these patients if there are objective indications that the patient is experiencing pain, e.g., excessive perspiration, nausea, anxiety, tension and restlessness. Other patients, usually those who readily express their emotions, are unable to tolerate pain as well and may ask for analgesics more frequently.

It is essential that the nurse examine her own attitude toward pain, since her attitude influences her approach to the patient in pain. For example, the nurse who either consciously or unconsciously believes that a certain amount of pain should be endured, may tend to delay, or at least not be prompt, in administering a p.r.n. analgesic. The nurse may not be aware of her attitude and how it affects her patient care unless she examines her own feelings toward pain.

The nurse has several additional responsibilities when administering a narcotic analgesic. The validity of the physician's order must be checked. Orders for narcotics are valid only for a certain length of time, such as 24 or 48 hours, depending upon the hospital's regulations. The nurse must also check when the patient received the analgesic previously, since analgesics usually are not given any more frequently than every 3 to 4 hours. Any narcotic she administers must be entered in the special narcotic sheet or narcotic book as required by the Harrison Narcotic Act.

Because narcotics, and certain other analgesics are central nervous system depressants, precautions must be taken. The patient's respirations should be checked, especially before administering morphine. The drug should be withheld and the physician notified if the patient's respirations are less than 12 per minute.

Generally, patients receiving narcotics should be in bed because drowsiness or hypotension may be produced. At times bed rails may be indicated.

SALICYLATES

Although salicylic acid itself is so irritating that it may only be used externally, the salts and esters of the compound are so modified in their pharmacologic activity that they have proved very useful as analgesics and antipyretic agents. The salicylates exert their typical effects by virtue of their salicylic acid content, however. Differences in solubility and the degree of local irritation produced determine the therapeutic usefulness of the various compounds.

The antipyretic action of the salicylates is usually rapid and effective in febrile patients, but is rarely evident when the temperature is normal. When the salicylates are administered, heat production is not inhibited, but heat dissipation is increased because of increased peripheral blood flow and sweating. Marked sweating does not occur unless there is a fever, however. Body temperature is also somewhat lowered by radiation of heat.

By a selective depressant action, the salicylates alleviate certain types of pain. Since even large doses of salicylates produce no disturbances in cortical function, subcortical regions are assumed to be the location of analgesic activity. Headache, myalgia, arthralgia and other pains arising from integumental structures rather than visceral are

particularly well treated with salicylates, thus making them particularly effective in rheumatoid pain. The salicylates are inferior to codeine as analgesics, however.

Very often the salicylates, especially aspirin, are combined with other drugs for enhanced analgesic activity. Examples of these are:

Aspirin Compound (Empirin Compound, APC) = Aspirin, Phenacetin and Caffeine
Empirin Compound with Codeine
Anacin (Aspirin with Caffeine)
APC with Demerol
Trigesic (Aspirin, Acetaminophen and Caffeine)

In addition, salicylates are mild respiratory stimulants. As a result of induced hyperventilation, considerable changes in the acid-base balance of the blood may occur. Since more carbon dioxide is exhaled than normal, there is a preponderance of base in the blood with a resultant alkalosis. These effects are proportional to the dose administered and are reversible.

Oral doses of salicylates may result in epigastric distress because of local irritation. Recurrent use has caused gastritis and even gastric bleeding in susceptible individuals. Much research has been performed on this property of the salicylates. It has been shown that the size of the aspirin granules in the compressed tablets is related to the local irritation. Larger particles become trapped in the rugae of the stomach and cause irritation, whereas smaller particles are more rapidly solubilized and absorbed, producing less discomfort. Gastric irritation may be reduced by giving salicylates with food or after meals. Enteric-coated preparations may also be of value.

Buffering also aids solution of aspirin because it counteracts the acidity of the stomach, and hence decreases the opportunity for irritation and hastens absorption of the drug. Bufferin and Ascriptin are popular brands of buffered aspirin.

Some salicylate-induced nausea and vomiting has been demonstrated to be of central origin, however. In this case the buffering action would have no effect since its action is limited to the local effect in the stomach.

Individuals particularly sensitive to this central nauseant effect are simply intolerant to salicylates.

Other effects of the salicylates are lowering of elevated erythrocytic sedimentation rate, promotion of uric acid excretion, interference with immunologic processes and antirheumatic action.

The salicylates are rapidly absorbed from the upper gastrointestinal tract. Appreciable blood levels of sodium salicylate may be detected within 30 minutes of its oral administration. Aspirin is absorbed at a slightly slower rate. When absorbed, the salicylates are rapidly distributed throughout all body tissues. They are hydrolyzed in the tissues by enzymes, and products are excreted via the kidneys and may cause changes in the color of the urine. The presence of the drug in the urine may cause tests for glycosuria to be misinterpreted.

Contact with moisture can cause decomposition. The acetic acid produced causes the tablets to smell like vinegar. Aspirin and salicylates should not be stored in the bathroom where humidity and moisture are found.

TOXICITY. Considering the gross misuse and overuse of salicylates by Ameri-can consumers, the high incidence of toxic reactions to salicylates is not surprising. In adults the toxic effects usually result in little more than mild discomfort or inconvenience; however, in children, aspirin continues to be the leading cause of poisoning. Especially dangerous is the candy-type aspirin which, if left within the reach of children, is often consumed in large amounts with dangerous and even fatal effects.

Mild salicylate poisoning is called "salicylism" and is characterized by headache, dizziness, tinnitus, dimness of vision, confusion, lassitude, drowsiness, sweating, thirst, nausea, vomiting, diarrhea and dermatoses. Enteric-coated preparations are often employed to decrease the gastric irritation of the salicylates. Allergic reactions may be severe. Petechial hemorrhages are occasionally noted, but are minimized if adequate amounts of vitamin K are included in the diet.

In acute salicylate poisoning the symptoms progress to increased depression, stupor and coma. Cardiovascular

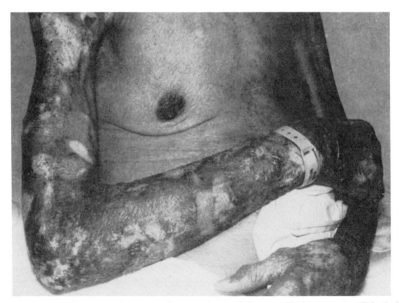

FIGURE 36. Allergic reaction to aspirin. (Grollman: *Pharmacology and Therapeutics,* Ed. 6. Lea & Febiger, Philadelphia, 1965.)

collapse, respiratory insufficiency and terminal asphyxial convulsions occur.

The nurse and the general public should be aware of the effects and possible side effects of these commonly used and self-prescribed drugs.

Salicylates' antipyretic effect may mask fever, an important symptom of illness. The ability of aspirin and salicylates to reduce prothrombin levels and therefore to increase bleeding tendencies should be considered by pregnant women about to deliver. This should also be considered when patients are placed on anticoagulant therapy, since they may be taking aspirin or other salicylates concurrently.

Consumer education is needed in order for the public to be able to assess the claims and advertising techniques used for these and other nonprescription drugs.

Patients who are allergic to aspirin or other salicylates should be aware of compounds in which these drugs are incorporated. Two commonly used combinations containing aspirin are A.P.C. and Darvon Compound.

Salicylate preparations and doses are as follows:

SALICYLIC ACID, U.S.P., B.P.   Used topically as a keratolytic agent.

METHYL SALICYLATE, U.S.P., B.P. (SWEET BIRCH OIL, OIL OF WINTERGREEN, GAULTHERIA OIL, BETULA OIL).   Used topically as a counterirritant.

ASPIRIN, U.S.P., ACETYLSALICYLIC ACID, B.P.   Used internally as an analgesic and antipyretic.

> **DOSE.**   0.3 to 0.6 Gm. orally or rectally every 4 to 6 hours.

SODIUM SALICYLATE, U.S.P., B.P.   Used as an analgesic and antipyretic.

> **DOSE.**   0.3 to 0.6 Gm. orally every 4 to 6 hours.

SALICYLAMIDE, N.F.   Salicylamide is structurally and pharmacologically very similar to aspirin. It is readily absorbed from the gastrointestinal tract and has analgesic effects equivalent to those of aspirin. It is less effective as an antipyretic, however.

Salicylamide may be administered to patients who are allergic to aspirin.

> **TOXICITY.**   The overall toxicity of salicylamide is relatively low. Gastrointestinal disturbances occur occasionally, and drowsiness and dizziness have been observed. In high overdosage, death occurs because of respiratory depression.

> **DOSE.**   300 to 600 mg. orally every 6 hours.

OTHER NON-NARCOTIC ANALGESICS

COLCHICINE, U.S.P., B.P.   Colchicine, an alkaloid from *Colchicum autumnale,* is still the drug of choice for gout, which is discussed in Chapter 19. The drug has no analgesic effect in other conditions and does not relieve other types of inflammation. It should be given promptly at the first indication of discomfort in gout, and often must be given in doses large enough to cause gastric irritation.

> **TOXICITY.**   Symptoms of overdose include severe abdominal pain, nausea, vomiting, diarrhea, shock, kidney damage and an ascending paralysis eventually causing death due to respiratory arrest.

> **DOSE.**   1 mg. orally every 2 hours until relief is obtained or the patient has nausea, vomiting, diarrhea or abdominal pain.

PROBENECID (BENEMID), U.S.P., B.P.   Probenecid was originally developed to inhibit the tubular secretion of penicillin, but it is not used for this purpose at present, since it is simpler and more economical merely to increase the dose of penicillin rather than to use two drugs to achieve a higher blood level of the antibiotic.

Probenecid was later found to be a potent uricosuric agent, however, and is currently employed for this purpose in the treatment of gout. The drug acts on the renal tubules to inhibit the reabsorption of uric acid. Concurrent administration of salicylates inhibits its action, however; thus they should never be administered at the same time.

> **TOXICITY.** Nausea, vomiting, skin rash and drug fever are observed as side effects to probenecid administration. Urate stones may form and cause renal colic. They can be prevented by keeping the urine alkaline and maintaining an adequate urinary output. It should also be kept in mind that acute attacks of gout may be precipitated by uricosuric agents, especially during the early phase of therapy. Concomitant administration of colchicine is useful in preventing these attacks, however. The drug causes a false positive reaction to Benedict's reagent, and may induce hypoglycemia in patients receiving sulfonurea drugs.

> **DOSE.** 250 mg. orally twice a day for one week, followed by 1 Gm. daily.

ACETANILID (ANTIFEBRIN). Acetanilid is roughly equivalent to the salicylates in mode of action and extent of analgesic and antipyretic activity. It lacks the antirheumatic activity of the salicylates, however, and is not generally employed to treat these conditions. Its use is generally restricted because of the toxic effects, but it is still used occasionally in combination with other drugs for potentiation of analgesic activity.

> **TOXICITY.** The most serious toxic effect of acetanilid is production of methemoglobin and consequent cyanosis. High concentrations of the drug may occasionally result in actual destruction of the corpuscles. In more serious cases, central nervous system stimulation, excitement and delirium may be noted, followed by depression and stupor, then coma and death.

> **DOSE.** 100 to 200 mg. orally three times daily.

PHENACETIN, U.S.P., B.P. (ACETOPHENETIDIN). Phenacetin is closely related to acetanilid in structure and in therapeutic as well as toxic effects.

Phenacetin, with aspirin and caffeine, is one of the ingredients of the commonly used APC compound. Rather recently it has been removed from commercial over-the-counter preparations (i.e., Anacin) because undesirable side effects (chiefly blood dyscrasias) have occurred with this drug.

> **DOSE.** 0.3 Gm. orally every 4 to 6 hours.

PHENYLBUTAZONE, N.F. (BUTAZOLIDIN). Phenylbutazone cannot be considered a simple analgesic and should never be administered casually. Patients should be carefully evaluated before treatment and should remain under close medical supervision.

The analgesic activity of phenlybutazone is inferior to that of the salicylates. It is used as an anti-inflammatory agent in the therapy of rheumatoid conditions.

> **TOXICITY.** This drug can severely depress granulocytopoiesis and deaths from agranulocytosis and aplastic anemia have occurred. It may also depress erythropoiesis. Nausea, diarrhea, vertigo, insomnia, euphoria, nervousness, hematuria, stomatitis, blurred vision and hepatitis have been observed. The drug also causes sodium retention and edema. The patient should be weighed daily and his sodium intake should be restricted. Patients should be advised to report the first signs of agranulocytosis: fever, sore throat, lesions in the mouth or black and tarry stools.

> It is contraindicated in patients with hypertension, cardiac, renal and hepatic dysfunction and in patients with a history of peptic ulcer. The dosage of coumarin anticoagulants and oral hypoglycemic agents may need to be adjusted.

> **DOSE.** 100 mg. orally three or four times daily.

ALKA-BUTAZOLIDIN. This compound contains phenylbutazone, aluminum hydroxide gel, magnesium trisilicate and homatropine methylbromide to reduce gastrointestinal disturbances. The dosage and pharmacologic actions are identical to those of phenylbutazone.

OXYPHENBUTAZONE (TANDEARIL). Although slightly modified from the original phenylbutazone molecule, this compound shows essentially the same effects and toxic symptoms as the parent compound.

DOSE. 100 mg. orally three or four times daily.

ACETAMINOPHEN, N.F. (TYLENOL). Acetaminophen provides effective analgesia in a wide variety of arthritic and rheumatic conditions involving musculoskeletal pain as well as other painful disorders, such as headache, dysmenorrhea, myalgias and neuralgias. It is also effective as an antipyretic and is employed in children for this purpose as well as in individuals allergic to salicylates.

TOXICITY. Acetaminophen has very few untoward effects. It does not produce the gastric irritation seen with salicylates and has no significant effects on the blood. Occasionally a mild dermatitis appears.

DOSE. 325 to 650 mg. orally every 4 hours.

PROPOXYPHENE HYDROCHLORIDE, U.S.P. (DARVON). A synthetic and relatively new addition to the analgesic field, propoxyphene is a unique agent in that, although it closely mimics the analgesic activity of codeine, it is nonaddicting. It is of particular value for pain associated with recurrent or chronic diseases and is comparable to the salicylates in antipyretic and antirheumatic activity.

TOXICITY. No contraindications to the use of propoxyphene have been reported. Huge doses may be accompanied by sedation, dizziness and somnolence. Occasionally a skin rash or gastrointestinal disturbance occurs, but it is uncommon.

If an overdose of propoxyphene is ingested, analeptic drugs (picrotoxin, amphetamine, caffeine sodium benzoate, etc.) should NOT be used since fatal convulsions may be produced. If

respiratory depression is present, supportive artificial respiration or small doses of nalorphine or levallorphan tartrate may be administered. Symptomatic treatment should also be provided.

DOSE. 32 to 65 mg. orally three or four times daily.

DARVON COMPOUND. This combination contains propoxyphene, 32 mg. (65 mg. in Darvon Compound-65); aspirin, 227 mg.; phenacetin, 162 mg.; and caffeine, 32.4 mg. The added ingredients potentiate the effects of propoxyphene, but the preparation must not be used it patients are hypersensitive to salicylates.

Caution must be observed not to confuse Darvon and Darvon Compound when pouring medications or transcribing doctors' orders.

DOSE. One or two capsules orally three or four times daily.

PENTAZOCINE HYDROCHLORIDE (TALWIN). This synthetic, non-narcotic analgesic is effective orally or parenterally with a potency of one half to one sixth that of morphine, and somewhat greater than that of meperidine on a weight basis.

As in the narcotic analgesics, pentazocine has some hypnotic effect and if given in repeated doses can decrease gastrointestinal motility. It is used as an analgesic to treat mild to severe pain, as a preoperative medication in adjunction to anesthesia, and in patients with chronic painful illnesses in order to avoid dependence on narcotics. Tolerance, as well as psychological and physical dependence on this drug will occur, however, as will withdrawal symptoms if the drug is discontinued suddenly after prolonged use. The dependence on this agent, however, is not as severe as the dependence on narcotics.

TOXICITY. Sedation, nausea, vomiting, constipation, vertigo, sweating, tachycardia, urinary retention, blurred vision, weakness, lethargy, paresthesias, tremors, confusion and hallucinations have been reported. Its use in obstetrics is not advised since respiratory depression of the newborn has been observed following administration. If respiratory depression occurs in an adult due to indiscriminate use of the drug, methylphenidate (Ritalin) is advised as an antidote.

DOSE. Oral—50 to 100 mg. every 3 to 4 hours. Subcutaneous, I.M. or I.V.—30 mg. every 3 to 5 hours.

NARCOTIC ANALGESICS

Narcotics are addicting drugs that may be either derived from natural sources, such as opium or cocaine, or prepared synthetically, such as meperidine and dolophine. In medical practice they are used for their powerful analgesic and hypnotic properties.

With the exception of cocaine, which is a central nervous system stimulant when taken internally, the narcotics as a group are classified as depressants. The euphoria or exaggerated sense of well-being is induced by depression of the higher brain centers and is the "kick" addicts are searching for when they begin the narcotic's habit. This euphoria is short-lived, however, and the addict soon finds that he must take increasingly larger and larger doses to experience this sensation. In later stages of addiction, the narcotic drug merely maintains the body's cells in a quasi-normal state, and euphoria is not experienced to any marked degree.

The legal aspects of narcotic administration are discussed in Chapter 1, and the sociological aspect and problems relating to narcotic addiction are discussed in Chapter 25. In this section the discussion is concerned merely with the pharmacologic effects of narcotics as they are employed in medical practice.

In order to understand the various aspects of narcotic use and misuse, it is necessary to distinguish between some closely related terms.

Addiction: the state in which the body's cells have become accustomed to functioning in the presence of a drug and carry on normal activities only in the presence of this drug. Withholding the addicting agent precipitates physical withdrawal symptoms.

Habituation: the state in which a psychological dependence upon an agent, such as a drug, has occurred. The habit of smoking is an example. Withholding the agent causes some mental anguish, perhaps, but no true physical withdrawal symptoms.

Dependence: the psychophysical state of an individual taking drugs routinely. "Drug dependence" is ordinary used with reference to the dependence of addiction, but may be loosely applied to habituation as well.

Tolerance: the ability of the body to endure steadily increasing doses of a drug; this increasing resistance to the usual effects of a drug is responsible for the successively larger doses required by narcotic addicts.

OPIUM ALKALOIDS

The dried juice of the opium poppy, *Papaver somniferum,* has been used for many centuries for its narcotic and analgesic properties.

The pharmacologically active constituents of opium are alkaloids. Although many of these alkaloids are present in crude opium, only three, morphine, codeine and papaverine, are currently used to any extent in medicine.

Morphine is by far the most important of the opium alkaloids and gives the crude drug its predominant characteristics. Many semisynthetic products may be formed by altering the basic morphine molecule. Codeine, as can be seen by its chemical structure, is merely methylmorphine. Dionin, heroin, dihydromorphinone, metopon and apomorphine are formed by similarly small changes in the morphine molecule. These synthetic and semisynthetic analogs all have pharmacologic activities similar to morphine but vary in potency and degree of activity.

Crude opium is commercially available as:

Opium Tincture, B.P. Dose. 0.6 ml. orally three times daily.

Paregoric, U.S.P., Camphorated Opium Tincture, B.P. Dose. 5 ml. orally three or four times daily.

Opium Powder. Dose. 60 mg. orally three or four times daily.

Opium and Belladonna Suppositories (B and O Suppositories). Dose. Opium 1 gr. Belladonna ⅛ gr. rectally three times daily.

These preparations are used chiefly as antidiarrhetics because the morphine content of the drug in the crude forms is not enough to warrant use as central nervous system sedatives and analgesics.

MORPHINE SULFATE, U.S.P., B.P., MORPHINE HYDROCHLORIDE, B.P. When full therapeutic doses of morphine are administered, euphoria, diminished activity and sluggishness are noted, followed by sleep. Severe pain is relieved, respiration is depressed, the pupils are constricted and peristalsis is decreased. Death, when it occurs following an overdose, is due to respiratory depression. Because of the depressant effect on respiration, the nurse should determine the patient's respiratory rate before administering morphine or other narcotics.

The relief of pain is the most outstanding effect of morphine and the one that is most often desired. It is highly selective in producing analgesia, and pain is relieved without excessive diminution of other sensations. It is especially effective in visceral pain, making it a drug of choice in postoperative medication.

Three components are observed in relief of pain by morphine:

1. The pain threshold is elevated, i.e., more painful stimuli are needed before the conscious self receives the "pain" signal. This factor operates more effectively when the drug is given before the painful stimulus is experienced. For this reason, following surgical procedures or whenever the patient is likely to experience pain, the drug should be given before the patient is tossing and turning in extreme distress.

2. Morphine alters the reactions to pain. Anxiety and fear no longer accompany pain when it is experienced. This factor is most important in pain relief, because it has been experimentally shown that much of the pain perceived is merely our own reaction to it.

3. Sleep is induced, which also raises the pain threshold.

Morphine is absorbed well from the gastrointestinal tract but is most often given hypodermically for rapid pain relief. It is eliminated mainly via the kidneys following conjugation and inactivation by the liver. Small amounts are also excreted via the lungs, feces, bile and sweat glands.

Since morphine readily crosses the placental barrier, it should not be used as an analgesic during or just prior to childbirth because respiratory depression may occur in the newborn. There have been reports of withdrawal symptoms in infants born to addicted mothers.

morphine

USES. The analgesic of choice for severe pain following major surgical procedures or for the pain of such conditions as renal or biliary colic or terminal cancer.

TOXICITY. Following a dose of morphine, muscular incoordination occurs, and the patient should not be allowed to get out of bed alone. Lightheadedness and vertigo are common complaints. The many and varied sites of action of morphine contribute to the unwanted side effects when it is used for analgesia. Respiratory depression is the most serious side effect. The decreased peristalsis causes constipation; nausea and vomiting occur on occasion and may be intensified by sudden movement.

The typical depressant activity of morphine is not always observed because some individuals exhibit idiosyncrasies to the drug, and evidence of central nervous system excitement is seen. Although this excitement is usually confined to nausea and vomiting, sometimes delirium and even convulsions may occur.

DOSE. 15 mg. I.M. every 4 to 6 hours.

CODEINE PHOSPHATE, U.S.P., B.P. Codeine has about one sixth the analgesic activity of morphine. The dosage response to codeine is unusual because increased analgesia occurs as expected with increase in doses up to 60 mg., but no further increase in analgesic activity is observed in most cases when doses over 60 mg. are administered.

USES. Codeine is employed for mild pain, cough and mild sedative effects.

TOXICITY. Toxic effects are less evident with codeine than with morphine. Respiratory depression is less prominent; instances of nausea, vomiting, constipation and constriction of the pupils are likewise less numerous.

Both tolerance and addiction occur to codeine, but it is rarely used by addicts because it does not produce the desired degree of euphoria.

DOSE. 30 mg. orally or I.M. every 4 to 6 hours.

DIHYDROMORPHINONE HYDROCHLORIDE (DILAUDID). The addition of two hydrogens to the basic morphine molecule increases the potency to four times that of morphine. The duration of action is shorter than the parent compound, however.

TOXICITY. Side effects and euphoria are less marked than with morphine.

DOSE. 1 to 4 mg. I.M. every 4 to 6 hours.

METHYLDIHYDROMORPHINONE HYDROCHLORIDE (METOPON). Methyldihydromorphinone is closely related to dihydromorphinone and in activity lies between it and morphine. The duration of action is similar to that of morphine.

TOXICITY. Euphoria is less evident than with morphine, and other toxic effects are not as marked.

DOSE. 6 mg. I.M. every 4 to 6 hours.

ETHYLMORPHINE HYDROCHLORIDE, N.F. (DIONIN). This drug's pharmacologic activity resembles that of codeine.

DOSE. 30 mg. I.M. every 4 to 6 hours.

DIHYDROCODEINONE BITARTRATE, N.F. (DICODID, HYCODAN). Although this drug's analgesic activity lies between codeine and morphine, the principal use of dihydrocodeinone is not as an analgesic; it is employed as a cough depressant and is available in tablet and syrup forms.

DOSE. 5 to 10 mg. orally every 4 to 6 hours.

HEROIN. No longer an official drug in the United States because of its extremely high rate of addiction, heroin is of interest only with regard to its extramedicinal use as the narcotic most commonly employed by addicts.

It is four to eight times as potent as morphine in analgesic activity, and intense euphoria accompanies its use. A certain atypical central nervous system excitation occurs with the administration of heroin, and it seems to persist to the satisfaction of the addict, even after tolerance has eliminated most of the euphoretic effects.

MEPERIDINE HYDROCHLORIDE, N.F., PETHIDINE HYDROCHLORIDE, B.P. (DEMEROL). The chief pharmacologic action of meperidine is upon the cerebrum to produce analgesia and sedation. It may be used for these effects in preoperative medication. Minor effects are exerted on smooth muscles, producing relaxation in some and contraction in others.

Euphoria is not marked with meperidine administration; thus it is not in as great demand by addicts as are morphine and heroin. Meperidine addicts are known, however. Analgesia may be obtained without the degree of sedation produced by morphine. Although meperidine does cause postural hypotension in patients unaccustomed to administration of narcotics, tolerance is gained to this effect, and meperidine may be used for ambulatory patients with chronic painful diseases.

When meperidine is used in therapeutic doses, the respiratory depression is not nearly as marked as with morphine. This agent is of greater benefit and safety for use in obstetrics. Extremely large doses depress respiration, however, which is the cause of death in poisoning.

> USES. For severe pain, primarily abdominal.

> DOSE. 50 to 100 mg. I.M. every 4 hours.

ALPHAPRODINE HYDROCHLORIDE, N.F. (NISEN-TIL). The analgesic activity of alphaprodine is between that of meperidine and morphine, although its duration of action is shorter. Untoward effects resemble those of morphine.

> DOSE. 40 to 60 mg. s.c. every 2 to 4 hours.

METHADONE, U.S.P., B.P. (DOLOPHINE). The pharmacologic action of methadone is similar to that of morphine except that it does not cause significant respiratory depression or addiction liability. Because its antitussive activity is quite pronounced, it is sometimes incorporated into cough preparations.

Methadone is used in withdrawal of addicts from morphine, or to maintain addicts during illness when withdrawal might be life-threatening. During the period in which the abstinence syndrome to morphine would occur, methadone is administered. When this latter drug is then withdrawn, the abstinence syndrome is not nearly as severe as would have been the case with morphine.

> DOSE. 5 to 15 mg. orally or I.M. every 4 to 6 hours.

LEVORPHANOL TARTRATE, N.F., B.P. (LEVO-DROMORAN). In all respects the pharmacologic effects of this synthetic narcotic parallel those of morphine. It may be administered both orally and parenterally for its analgesic effect.

> DOSE. 2 to 3 mg. I.M. or orally every 4 to 6 hours.

PAPAVERINE HYDROCHLORIDE, N.F., B.P. Although a derivative of opium. Papaverine is not generally employed for its effect on the central nervous system. It is discussed in Chapter 12.

NARCOTIC ANTAGONISTS

NALORPHINE HYDROCHLORIDE, U.S.P., B.P.; NALORPHINE (NALLINE). This semisynthetic analog of morphine is a specific antagonist to morphine rather than a compound with similar phamacologic effects. When given subsequent to morphine administration, nalorphine counteracts many of the actions of morphine and is especially useful in overcoming the respiratory depression of morphine overdosage. It is the specific antidote for morphine poisoning and should be readily available as an emergency drug.

Although nalorphine is somewhat effective in counteracting the effects of codeine and other morphine analogs, it does not counteract the respiratory depression of the barbiturates and other non-narcotic central nervous system depressants.

Nalorphine may be used as a rapid test for narcotic addiction because injection of nalorphine into an addict under the influence of a narcotic immediately precipitates withdrawal symptoms by counteracting the effect of the narcotic in the body. This speeds police investigation of suspected addicts, because considerable delay is caused while waiting for withdrawal symptoms to occur naturally. The appearance of withdrawal symptoms is unequivocal evidence of physical dependence on an addicting drug.

> DOSE. 3 mg. I.V. Dose is repeated as necessary.

LEVALLORPHAN TARTRATE, U.S.P. (LOR-FAN). Levallorphan is a narcotic antagonist which will prevent or overcome narcotic-induced respiratory depression, but has little if any effect on the analgesic effects of the narcotic.

When given intravenously, an initial reaction is obtained within one minute and lasts for 2 to 5 hours, increasing both the rate as well as the depth of respiration. It is believed that this mode of action is due to the ability of levallorphan to displace narcotics from effector sites on the cells of the respiratory center, thus returning to normal the central response to elevated carbon dioxide levels.

It is not effective against respiratory depression due to non-narcotic agents. Withdrawal symptoms may be precipitated if this agent is administered to addicts.

DOSE. 1 mg. I.V., followed at 3 minute intervals with additional doses of 0.5 mg. Total dose not to exceed 5 mg.

PLACEBOS

A placebo (Latin, "I shall please") is a pharmacologically inactive substance given for its psychological effect. Substances commonly used as placebos are vitamins, capsules containing sugar, and hypodermic injections of sterile water or physiologic saline.

The use of placebos is a practice that is widely misunderstood by nurses and other medical personnel. Placebos may be used in psychiatry and are occasionally used to relieve pain in certain patients.

When placebos are employed for the relief of pain, it is essential that the nursing and medical personnel understand that pain relief after the administration of a placebo does *not* mean that the pain was "all in the patient's head." The patient did experience pain and obtained relief from the placebo. The emotional and psychological aspects of pain are far from our understanding even today.

It must be remembered that there are two major components of pain. One is the perception of pain impulses. Certain analgesics act by raising the pain threshold and decreasing sensitivity to pain. The second component in pain is the emotional or psychological reaction to the pain that is felt. It is believed that the placebo affects this second component by altering the reaction to pain.

The effectiveness of a placebo depends greatly on the actions, attitudes and personality of the doctor and the nurse. The nurse who actually administers the placebo must believe in its effectiveness. It is also essential that the patient believe that he is being given a drug for the relief of pain. Often the prejudices and misunderstanding of personnel are a deterrent to the full effectiveness of a placebo.

ANTICONVULSANTS

Convulsive seizures (epilepsy) are due to an acute disturbance (focal or generalized) in cerebral function. This disturbance, although produced by an unknown cause, may be shown by tracings of brain wave patterns.

Studies have shown that small areas of diseased or traumatized tissue may be adversely affected by stimuli and may discharge electrical impulses in an abnormal manner. The spread of this discharge to other parts of the cerebrum results in loss of consciousness and convulsive phenomena. In susceptible individuals, seizures may be precipitated by such stimuli as sound, light or cutaneous stimulation. The reason these stimuli influence the tissues to discharge impulses in this manner is unknown. Precautions against seizures in such patients should be initiated by the nurse; for example, padded bed rails and equipment such as a mouth gag, suction equipment and an airway should be at the bedside.

Four types of epilepsy may be distinguished:

1. *Grand Mal.* Typical grand mal seizures are sometimes preceded by an aura and are characterized by a cry, loss of consciousness, falling and tonic-clonic contractions of the muscles of the extremities, trunk and head. Urinary and fecal incontinence may occur. The attack, which usually lasts two to five minutes, may be followed by deep sleep, headache or muscular soreness.

Focal or Jacksonian seizures are initiated by specific focal phenomena. The dysfunction may then spread to other parts of the brain, and loss of consciousness and convulsive movements may ensue.

2. *Petit Mal.* These seizures consist merely of a loss of consciousness for 1 to 30 seconds

with or without loss of muscular tone. The attack may occur several times daily, and often may go unnoticed by those around the individual.

3. *Psychomotor Epilepsy.* Psychomotor attacks are characterized by a loss of contact with the environment rather than a loss of consciousness. The individual may perform repetitious, purposeless movements, make unintelligible sounds, have disturbances in gait, etc. The victim is usually confused for a minute or two after the attack is ended.

4. *Epileptic Equivalents.* This term describes a group of disturbances that may occur in an individual who is subject to seizures. These include paroxysmal attacks of abdominal pain (abdominal epilepsy) and periods of mental cloudiness that may last for several hours.

In addition, convulsions may be caused by a number of other conditions such as generalized disturbances of cortical function associated with hypoglycemia, tetanus, poisoning, excessive hydration, protein shock, anaphylaxis and tremors. They may also occur as part of the withdrawal symptoms of narcotic or barbiturate addicts.

The effectiveness of antiepileptic drugs varies from case to case of epilepsy. Each patient must be individually evaluated in order that the drug, often combination of drugs, that is most effective in his particular case may be determined.

The patient should understand the necessity of continued drug therapy and medical supervision. He should also be advised of the danger of abruptly discontinuing the drug treatment and the potential effects of alcohol and physical and mental stress in precipitating seizures. Wearing a Medic Alert tag may be advisable. The patient and his family should receive encouragement and support, as well as instruction concerning his condition and therapy.

The mechanism of action of the various types of antiepileptic drugs is basically the same. They act both to prevent the abnormal foci from discharging and to depress excitability of various neuron circuits so that there is not a sufficient spread of impulses to precipitate an attack.

Four principal groups of drugs are used in epilepsy:

1. *Barbiturates.* All barbiturates do not have the same degree of effectiveness when used as anticonvulsants. Phenobarbital and mephobarbital are the ones generally most effective for this purpose and are especially effective in grand mal epilepsy. The major disadvantages to the barbiturates as antiepileptics are the sedation they produce, the possibility of habituation and the necessity of limiting the supply on hand with the suicide-prone. Sudden withdrawal from barbiturates has precipitated epileptic attacks; thus they should be withdrawn slowly.

DOSE. Phenobarbital, U.S.P. (Luminal) —30 mg. orally four times daily; 120 mg. I.M. three or four times daily.
Mephobarbital, N.F. (Mebaral)—30 mg. orally four times daily.
Primidone, U.S.P. (Mysoline)—0.25 to 2 Gm. daily.

2. *Hydantoins*

DIPHENYLHYDANTOIN SODIUM, N.F. (DILANTIN). Although primarily used in grand mal and psychomotor types of epilepsy, this agent has been observed to have many other useful pharmaceutical applications.

It has been found useful in the treatment of mood and behavior disorders by acting as a mild antidepressant, improving the sense of well-being and diminishing irritability. Prophylactically, it has been useful in controlling delirium tremens in acute alcohol withdrawal, and it has given relief from the symptoms of trigeminal neuralgia.

Given intravenously or orally, it has been shown to be effective in controlling cardiac arrhythmias, especially ventricular tachycardia and ventricular ectopic beats. It has not been of value in the treatment of atrial fibrillation or atrial flutter.

The mechanism of action of this drug has received considerable attention recently. It has been shown to stabilize nerve cells against hyperexcitability. This stabilizing effect has been observed in the peripheral nerve, the spinal cord, the neuromuscular junction and in the brain.

TOXICITY. The alkalinity of this agent causes gastrointestinal irritation, nausea and vomiting, but these effects are minimized if the drug is given with meals. Gingival hyperplasia (Fig. 37) is noted in a large percentage of patients. Careful mouth care and massage of the gums are important; the patient should notify his dentist that he is on hydantoin therapy. Acne-like skin eruptions occur, hypertrichosis and ataxia are seen and on occasion bone marrow depression produces rather severe megaloblastic anemia and aplastic anemia. It may be necessary to adjust the dosage of coumarin-type anticoagulants.

DOSE. Oral—100 mg. three times daily. I.V.—100 to 250 mg. at a rate not to exceed 50 mg. per minute. If a precipitate should form in I.V. administration, the injection should be stopped immediately.

Other Hydantoins:

DOSE. Ethotoin, B.P. (Peganone)—2 to 3 Gm. daily orally in divided doses. Mephenytoin (Mesantoin, Phenantoin)—200 to 600 mg. daily orally in divided doses.

3. *Oxazolidines.* The drugs in this group are used for treatment of petit mal seizures. Side effects are minor and can usually be controlled by regulating the dosage.

TOXICITY. A unique toxicity occurring in this group is that of visual disturbance. Patients may see halos around objects and have difficulties in color perception. Also evident are ataxia, drowsiness, nephrotoxicity and rarely bone marrow depression leading to aplastic anemia.

DOSE. Paramethadione, U.S.P., B.P. (Paradione)—900 mg. orally daily in divided doses.
Trimethadione, U.S.P. (Tridione)—1 to 2 Gm. orally daily in divided doses.

4. *Succinamides.* These, like oxazolidines, are used primarily for petit mal. These drugs probably produce side effects in more patients than do any of the other groups, however.

TOXICITY. 30 per cent of patients undergoing treatment with succinamides experience central nervous system effects such as headache, dizziness, excessive sedation, irritant action with nausea, vomiting, anorexia, skin eruptions and bone marrow depression leading to aplastic anemia.

DOSE. Ethosuximide (Zarontin)—0.5 Gm. orally in divided doses.
Methsuximide, N.F. (Celontin)—0.3 to 1.2 Gm. orally daily in divided doses.
Phensuximide, N.F. (Milontin)—0.5 to 1 Gm. two or three times orally daily.

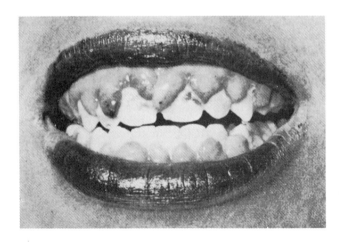

FIGURE 37. Gingival hyperplasia in a patient who had been receiving diphenylhydantoin over a period of one year. (Grollman: *Pharmacology and Therapeutics.* Ed. 6. Lea & Febiger, Philadelphia, 1965.)

MISCELLANEOUS DRUGS

AMINO-GLUTETHIMIDE (ELIPTEN). Structurally related to the sedative glutethimide, this amino derivative differs in that it does not appear to affect sensory areas significantly or to produce as much sedation as the parent compound. When combined with other anticonvulsant drugs, especially diphenylhydantoin and phenobarbital, it improves the degree of control and allows reduction in dosage, thus reducing the number and frequency of side effects. The drug may cause a false positive reaction for glycosuria in response to Benedict's reagent.

TOXICITY. Transient leukopenia and mild respiratory depression have been reported. In large dosages the drug may produce drowsiness, ataxia and generalized weakness, mental confusion, gastrointestinal disturbances, nausea, headache, anorexia and flushing. Skin rashes are quite common, usually appearing in five to eight days.

If the drug is withdrawn suddenly, there is usually a marked increase in frequency of seizures or even precipitation of status epilepticus. The dosage should be tapered off gradually.

DOSE.   250 mg. orally three times daily.

PHENACEMIDE (PHENURONE). Phenacemide is used in the control of psychomotor, grand mal and petit mal epilepsy as well as in the management of mixed seizures.

This is one of the most toxic anticonvulsants used therapeutically, and is employed only when the individual does not respond to the other drugs.

TOXICITY. Side effects include personality changes that may lead to attempted suicide and toxic psychoses. Liver damage and bone marrow depression occur and the latter leads to aplastic anemia and leukopenia. This drug should not be used in patients with a history of liver dysfunction and should be used with caution in patients with a history of psychiatric disorders. Anorexia, nausea, vomiting, abdominal distress, malaise, fever and rash also occur rather frequently. Blood counts and liver function tests should be done regularly during therapy. The urine test for sugar may be strongly positive.

Because of its effect on the cardiovascular system, the patient's vital signs should be checked frequently.

DOSE.   500 mg. orally three times daily.

SKELETAL MUSCLE RELAXANTS

Neuromuscular Blocking Agents

Neuromuscular blocking agents relax striated muscles. The milder agents may be used to relieve muscular spasm, whereas the more potent agents are employed to increase muscular relaxation during surgical procedures and orthopedic manipulation and to prevent trauma during electroshock therapy.

There are two general classifications of these drugs: those that act as hyperpolarizing agents at the myoneural junction, and depolarizing drugs, which lower the potential at the myoneural junction to a point at which further stimulation no longer produces contraction.

HYPERPOLARIZING AGENTS

Under ordinary circumstances, somatic nerve stimulation effects release of acetylcholine at the myoneural junction and causes depolarization of the muscle sole plate. The action potential spreads; the muscle contracts briefly and then relaxes. About the time the muscle relaxes, the acetylcholinesterase has destroyed the released acetylcholine and the end-plate repolarizes itself and is again receptive to stimulation.

Hyperpolarizing agents compete with the acetylcholine to maintain the receptor site in a state of polarization. This stability prevents acetylcholine from depolarizing the effector site. In addition to preventing further muscular contraction, normal muscle tonus is also interrupted.

The activity of these agents is potentiated by many general anesthetics; a smaller dose of each must be used when they are employed concurrently.

Antidotes for hyperpolarizing drugs are cholinergic agents, such as edrophonium chloride (Tensilon) and neostigmine (Prostigmin). Edrophonium chloride probably acts by displacing these drugs from the motor end-plate as well as inhibiting cholinesterase, whereas neostigmine acts only as a cholinesterase inhibitor, thus allowing the acetylcholine at the site to build up to a concentration at which it can effect depolarization of the membrane.

CURARE. The term curare is an Indian word meaning "poison" and has been applied to the large variety of arrow poisons that were used by the South American Indians.

d-tubocurarine

The characteristic action of curare, which owes its activity to tubocurarine, is muscular relaxation. It does not function when taken orally, but when injected intravenously acts within a minute or two. The first symptom of relaxation is haziness of vision, followed by bilateral drooping of the lids, with heaviness of the face and relaxation of the jaws. The inability to raise the head is followed by weakness or complete paralysis of spinal muscles, legs and arms. Shallowness of respiration is the last symptom to appear, and if allowed to progress, leads to death.

Because of the rapid destruction and excretion of the drug in the body, the action from a single dose usually does not exceed 15 or 20 minutes.

In addition to the relaxation of the skeletal muscles, a histamine-like peripheral action is also evidenced, probably because of the release of histamine in the body. This effect includes hypotension, bronchospasm, exocrine gland stimulation and hives. These conditions may be controlled with antihistamines.

Large doses of curare affect autonomic fibers as well as the skeletal muscles, with evidence of action at ganglia and postganglionic parasympathetic endings.

When used therapeutically, curare produces transient but useful relaxation in certain neurologic conditions, reducing hypertonia, tremor, incoordination, athetosis and dysarthria. It has been employed to produce improved relaxation in children with spastic cerebral palsy and in the diagnosis of myasthenia gravis. In the latter condition, a minute dose of curare greatly aggravates the muscular weakness and is considered diagnostic evidence of myasthenia gravis.

DOSE. Curare (Intocostrin)—50 units I.V.
Dimethyl tubocurarine chloride (Mecostrin)—2 mg. I.V.
Dimethyl tubocurarine iodide, N.F. (Metubine)—2 mg. I.V.
Tubocurarine chloride, U.S.P., B.P.—6 to 9 mg. I.V.

GALLAMINE TRIETHIODIDE, N.F. (Flaxedil). Although the pharmacologic effects of gallamine are very similar to those of curare, this drug is typified by a rapid onset and shorter duration of action, but it has no histaminic or autonomic effects.

TOXICITY. Since the molecule contains iodine, patients sensitive to iodine may develop a hypersensitivity reaction upon administration. Tachycardia occasionally occurs.

DOSE. 80 mg. I.V.

BENZOQUINONIUM CHLORIDE (MYTOLON). The action of benzoquinonium is similar to that of gallamine; however, it does have acetylcholinesterase activity and a polarizing effect. Salivation, bradycardia and bronchial constriction are observed when the drug is used.

DOSE. 12 mg. I.V.

DEPOLARIZING AGENTS

This group of skeletal muscle relaxants, in contrast to the hyperpolarizing agents, will of themselves initiate depolarization and the first muscular contraction. Following this, the receptor site is stabilized in the depolarized state from which it cannot recover until the action of the drug has worn off.

In very small doses the depolarizing agents have been used to treat myasthenia gravis. The drugs, given in amounts insufficient to initiate action, instead induce a mild state of depolarization, which sensitizes the receptor site to the endogenous acetylcholine and thus facilitates depolarization. If even slight overdoses are administered, however, the condition is much worsened because of excessive depolarization.

There are no good antidotes for the depolarizing agents. Cholinergic agents, such as edrophonium chloride, obviously only increase the depolarization if used as antidotes. Artificial respiration should be administered until the action of the drug is sufficiently diminished. Emergency equipment should be readily available.

DECAMETHONIUM BROMIDE (SYNCURINE, C-10). Decamethonium is about as potent as tubocurarine in its muscle relaxant ability. There are no histaminic side effects with this drug, however. General anesthetics do not potentiate its activity. Its duration of effect is intermediate between that of tubocurarine and succinylcholine. It does not act as a ganglionic blocking agent and has no cumulative effect after repeated doses.

Because of its short duration of action, decamethonium is often used in procedures such as endoscopy, endotracheal intubation and closure of the peritoneum following surgery.

Decamethonium has no use as a diagnostic agent in myasthenia gravis. In general, it has been replaced in therapy by succinylcholine chloride.

DOSE. 2 mg. I.V.

SUCCINYLCHOLINE CHLORIDE, U.S.P.; SUXAMETHONIUM CHLORIDE, B.P. (ANECTINE, QUELICIN, SUCOSTRIN). The shorter duration of action of succinylcholine permits a closer supervision of its effects when being employed during surgery. Other than the duration of action, the actions and effects are quite similar to decamethonium.

It is usually administered by continuous intravenous drip when prolonged relaxation is desired during a surgical procedure, but a single dose may be administered intravenously prior to electroshock therapy to reduce the chance of injury during convulsions.

The drug should be kept in the refrigerator and protected from light.

> **TOXICITY.** This drug has a low rate of toxic effects, but may cause respiratory depression in overdosage. Respirations should be monitored frequently during administration. There is no effective antagonist.

> **DOSE.** 20 mg. by I.V. drip at a rate insuring that no more than 2.5 mg. per minute is given to the patient.

Centrally Acting Muscle Relaxants

A number of drugs are administered orally to produce skeletal muscle relaxation by inhibiting reflexes in the central nervous system. They are not nearly as potent or effective as the neuromuscular blocking agents. Many people believe that any beneficial effect is as much due to the psychic effect of taking a medication as it is to the pharmacologic action of the drug. Drowsiness and sedation may be experienced initially; the patient should be cautioned against driving or using dangerous machinery.

CARISOPRODOL (SOMA, RELA). A central depressant, carisoprodol has a blocking effect on the interneurons. It appears to modify central perception of pain without abolishing peripheral pain reflexes. It is used in the symptomatic treatment of musculoskeletal disorders, such as bursitis, low back disorders, contusion, fibrositis, spondylitis, sprains and muscle strains.

Double blind studies with carisoprodol have shown conflicting results.

> **TOXICITY.** The chief side effect is drowsiness. Weakness, lassitude and a mild

skin reaction are occasionally observed. The effects may be potentiated by alcohol.

DOSE. 350 mg. orally four times daily.

CHLORMEZANONE (TRANCOPAL). Also useful as a tranquilizer, chlormezanone is of some value as a muscle relaxant. Its actions and toxicity resemble those of carisoprodol.

DOSE. 100 to 200 mg. orally three or four times daily.

CHLOROZOXAZONE (PARAFLEX). The action of this drug resembles that of carisoprodol. It is used orally as a moderately effective skeletal muscle relaxant.

TOXICITY. Side effects include nausea, vomiting, diarrhea, abdominal pain and constipation. Cutaneous hypersensitivity may occasionally occur.

DOSE. 500 mg. orally three or four times daily.

METAXALONE (SKELAXIN). Although clinical effectiveness as a muscle relaxant has not been established as yet, metaxalone is still used frequently for this purpose.

TOXICITY. This drug may produce hepatotoxic effects, leukopenia, hemoglobin depression, hemolytic anemia, gastrointestinal disturbances, central depression and accentuation of epileptic seizures. It is contraindicated in patients with epilepsy or impaired renal function.

DOSE. 400 mg. orally three or four times daily.

METHOCARBAMOL (ROBAXIN). Methocarbamol is used for the relief of muscular spasm and pain secondary to sprains or trauma.

TOXICITY. Patients experience flushing, blurred vision, a metallic taste in the mouth, lightheadedness and tension. It is contraindicated in patients with suspected renal pathology because it is excreted via the kidneys. The nurse should check the injection site for signs of irritation.

DOSE. 1 to 1.5 Gm. orally four times daily. 0.5 to 1 Gm. I.M. or I.V.

Similar agents used for muscle relaxation are:

Mephenoxalone (Trepidone) 400 mg. orally four times daily.
Phenaglycodol (Ultran) 400 mg. orally three times daily.
Styramate (Sinaxar) 200 mg. orally four times daily.

Muscle Relaxants Used in the Treatment of Parkinsonism

Parkinson's disease is a disease of the basal ganglia of the brain, which affects movement and control of the skeletal muscles and is characterized by slowness of movement, weakness, muscular rigidity and tremor. The patient usually has a wide-eyed, unblinking, staring expression. The muscles of the face are smoothed out and almost immobile. He walks with a slow, short, shuffling step and may break into a run spontaneously when pushed forward or backward. There is a pronounced slowness of all voluntary movements, particularly those carried out by the small muscles. Cramplike pains in the extremities and spine as a result of the rigidity and secondary joint changes are not uncommon. There usually are no mental changes unless the condition is secondary to diffuse disease of the brain. Sensation is intact and the reflexes are normal unless interfered with by muscular rigidity.

Symptoms similar to those of parkinsonism may result from prolonged therapy with the phenothiazine tranquilizers. Drugs used in Parkinson's disease are also used to alleviate these symptoms that mimic those of parkinsonism.

ETHOPROPAZINE HYDROCHLORIDE, B.P. (PARSIDOL). A phenothiazine derivative, ethopropazine is used in the treatment of Parkinson's disease and has an atropine-like blocking effect on the parasympathetic nerve endings. It is considered by some authorities to be the most effective agent available for the relief of major tremor and has a beneficial effect on rigidity. In general, however, the improvement in patients with Parkinson's disease is not entirely satisfactory. Generally, 20 to 30 per cent improvement is seen in 60 to 80 per cent of patients treated.

>**TOXICITY.** The overall incidence of side effects is high, and many patients do not tolerate a therapeutic dose. Drowsiness, dizziness and lassitude occur very frequently. Other side effects include blurred vision, dryness of the mouth, paresthesia, epigastric distress, headache, hypotension, confusion, ataxia and accentuation of parkinsonism. It should be administered with caution to patients with glaucoma, prostatic hypertrophy or pyloric obstruction.

>**DOSE.** 10 mg. orally four times daily.

MEPHENESIN N.F. (TOLSEROL); MEPHENESIN CARBAMATE (TOLSERAM). Mephenesin has been used to treat muscular aches and pains and certain types of tremors, such as those accompanying parkinsonism and acute alcoholism. It is used in psychotic states because of its sedative effects. The carbamate salt is slightly less potent, more slowly absorbed and longer acting than mephenesin itself.

The short duration of action of this drug is responsible for its limited usefulness. It is employed frequently as a drug in research to study motor disturbances.

>**TOXICITY.** Lassitude, leukopenia, nystagmus, diplopia and mild muscular incoordination have occurred during therapy. It may cause a local anesthetic effect on the tongue. The action of barbiturates and opiates may be intensified by mephenesin.

>**DOSE.** 1 to 3 Gm. orally three to five times daily.

ORPHENADRINE HYDROCHLORIDE (DISIPAL, NORFLEX). Orphenadrine reduces skeletal muscle spasm primarily through an atropine-like central action on cerebral motor centers or by its action in the medulla. It also has some postganglionic anticholinergic effects and some antihistaminic and local anesthetic action.

It is used in the symptomatic treatment of Parkinson's disease. As with the other drugs of this type, tolerance to orphenadrine may develop upon prolonged use.

>**TOXICITY.** Atropine-like side effects, gastrointestinal disturbances, skin reactions and central nervous system stimulation with confusion and hallucinations have occurred. It should be administered with caution to patients with tachycardia, glaucoma, urinary retention or prostatic hypertrophy.

>**DOSE.** 100 mg. orally twice daily.

PROCYCLIDINE HYDROCHLORIDE (KEMADRIN). In the symptomatic treatment of Parkinson's disease, procyclidine appears to relieve muscular rigidity better than it does tremor. It may be combined with other agents for more effective therapy of the disease.

The toxic effects resemble those of orphenadrine.

>**DOSE.** 2.5 mg. orally three times daily.

TRIHEXYPHENIDYL HYDROCHLORIDE (ARTANE). This synthetic agent exerts a direct inhibitory effect upon the parasympathetic nervous system, and causes a relaxation of skeletal muscles. It is useful in Parkinsonism, in the prevention or treatment of extrapyramidal effects of the phenothiazines, and is effective against the tremor and rigidity associated with both these conditions.

The toxic effects resemble the other drugs in this class.

>**DOSE.** 2 mg. orally three or four times daily.

BENZTROPINE METHANESULFONATE (COGENTIN). Benztropine is employed orally or parenterally for the relief of tremor and rigidity associated with Parkinson's Disease, and likewise is of value in treating the Parkinson-like effects following the use of phenothiazine tranquilizers.

The other symptoms of Parkinson's Disease, i.e., the mask-like facies, oculogyric crises and sialorrhea may be relieved with therapy, but to a lesser extent.

TOXICITY. Sedation, dryness of the mouth, blurred vision, nausea, dermatoses, constipation, depression and visual hallucinations have been reported. It should be used with extreme caution in patients with glaucoma since mydriasis is produced, thus aggravating this condition.

DOSE. 1 to 6 mg. orally or I.M. daily.

NURSING IMPLICATIONS IN PARKINSONISM

The improvement in mobility produced by the actions of these muscle-relaxing drugs may cause a sudden increase in the demand for cardiac output. This is especially true in patients receiving L-Dopa, where improvement is apt to be somewhat rapid and dramatic. Therefore, patients should be cautioned to resume activity gradually, and only under adequate supervision.

The atropine-like side effects of several drugs used in Parkinson's Disease can contribute to the development of constipation and difficulty in urination. The nurse should check frequently on the patient's bowel and bladder output in order to prevent these complications.

Patients with progressive neurological disease and their families need psychological and emotional support. The nurse should keep in mind that the mask-like appearance of the face results in the patient's inability to express pain, discomfort or many of the human emotions that are usually conveyed by changes in facial expression.

GUIDE FOR THE NURSING ASSESSMENT OF A PATIENT RECEIVING AN ANALGESIC

I. Why is the patient receiving an analgesic? Where is the location of the pain? What are the characteristics of the pain? How does the patient describe it? Has the pain changed in character or location? Has the cause of the pain been determined?

II. What is the patient's emotional and psychological reaction to the pain? Does he express pain readily or does he avoid requesting pain relief? What does this pain mean to this patient? What are the beliefs and/or misconceptions about the use of pain-relieving drugs, especially narcotics?

III. Is the analgesic effective in relieving the patient's pain? Is there lessening of muscle tension, perspiration, restlessness? Does the patient indicate he is experiencing pain relief? Are nursing measures to help in pain-relief being carried out (e.g., change of position, diversion, back care, reducing anxiety)?

IV. Is the analgesic administered for optimal effect? How often does the patient require the analgesic? Is the analgesic administered whenever possible before the pain becomes severe? Is administration coordinated whenever possible with painful or uncomfortable measures, such as coughing and deep breathing, dressing changes, etc.?

V. Has the patient experienced any side effects of the analgesic? Are there indications of central nervous system depression? Is there excessive sedation? Are bedside rails in place? Are respirations adequate in rate and depth? Has the patient experienced dizziness or other signs of hypotension? If the analgesic is an opium derivative, are urinary and bowel function adequate? What is the patient's addiction liability, i.e., does he have a history of drug abuse; have requests for analgesia increased rather than decreased as expected? Could the narcotic be alternated with a non-narcotic analgesic to reduce possibility of addiction? Is the patient receiving other drugs which may affect the action and effect of this analgesic?

VI. What are the learning needs of the patient? Does he understand the need to request an analgesic before the pain is severe? Does he understand the appropriate use of the analgesic, especially if it is a narcotic? Have misconceptions and fears been determined and clarified?

GUIDE FOR THE NURSING ASSESSMENT OF A PATIENT RECEIVING A HYPNOTIC

I. Why does this patient need a hypnotic? Does he require a hypnotic routinely at home or only during hospitalization? What is the patient's usual bedtime ritual? What is his usual pattern and schedule of sleep at home? In the hospital, is the patient sleeping or inactive during the day, so that sleep at night is disturbed?

II. Is the hypnotic effective in providing restful sleep? Does the patient awake during the night? Is a longer-acting hypnotic needed? Are nursing measures, such as back rub and quiet environment, employed to promote sleep? Are measures used when possible to allow for the patient's usual nighttime ritual?

III. Has the patient experienced any side effects from the hypnotic? Has he experienced morning hangover effect? Does it interfere with his functioning? Are other drugs, such as alcohol, avoided to prevent potentiation of effect? Is there indication of undue central nervous system depression? Are drug interactions likely with other drugs the patient is receiving? Has the patient experienced side effects common to this particular hypnotic? Does the patient show a tendency toward dependence on this hypnotic or hypnotics in general?

IV. What are the learning needs of the patient and his family? Does he understand the dangers of drug abuse? Is he aware of the dangers of alcoholic intake in conjunction with a hypnotic? Does the patient understand the dangers of overdosage? Does he understand the need to keep these drugs out of the reach of children? Does he understand the advisability of not leaving the hypnotic at the bedside because of the danger of accidental overdosage when in a semi-awake state?

GUIDE FOR THE NURSING ASSESSMENT OF A PATIENT RECEIVING A SEDATIVE OR TRANQUILIZER

I. Why is this patient receiving this drug? Has the underlying cause of anxiety or stress been determined? Have nursing measures been taken to assess and determine this? Has the patient been encouraged to express his feelings and anxieties? What is the patient's attitude toward taking this drug? Has the patient exhibited any suicidal tendencies?

II. Is this drug being administered in a therapeutic manner? Is the scheduling of dosage producing optimal effect? If the drug is given on a p.r.n. basis, have nursing measures been used to determine why the drug is needed, or to decrease the need for the drug? What nursing measures can be used to enhance the drug effect in the patient? Does the patient have his own supply of the drug or a similar drug which he may be taking without the physician's knowledge?

III. Is this drug producing the intended effect in the patient? What was the patient's previous behavior? Have the patient's affective responses changed? Is there a lessening of depression? If so, is the patient being observed for suicidal attempts? Has the patient's activity increased or decreased? Is the patient more receptive to interaction? Has his degree of social interaction changed? Does the patient have an increased interest in his environment? Has there been an improvement in the patient's appearance and hygiene? Have the patient's sleeping and eating patterns improved?

IV. Is the patient experiencing any side effects from this drug? Is the patient drowsy or excessively sedated? Are safety measures, such as side rails and supervision of ambulation, needed? Has the patient been cautioned against using dangerous machinery or driving a car? Is the sedation interfering with the patient's work or normal functioning? Is the patient receiving other drugs which may affect the action of this drug (e.g., alcohol)? Does the patient have any of the side effects commonly associated with this drug? Is this patient likely to develop psychologic dependence on this or similar drugs?

V. What are the patient's learning needs? Does the patient need to learn the sources of his anxiety or basis for his behavior? Does the patient need to learn new ways of coping with stress and change? Does the patient understand the purpose of this drug? Does the patient know what signs and symptoms should be reported and which ones are expected? Has the patient been advised to avoid foods or drugs, such as alcohol, which may alter this drug's effect? Does the patient understand the need for continued medical supervision and the dangers of self-medication?

QUESTIONS FOR DISCUSSION AND REVIEW

1. What do you think about the advisability of routinely taking central nervous system stimulants, such as No-Doz (active ingredient caffeine) or Dexedrine, to stay awake and study? How would you explain the effects of these drugs to a friend who is using them?

2. How do the psychic energizers differ from the central nervous system stimulants?

3. How do tranquilizers differ from sedatives? Sedatives from hypnotics?

4. What symptoms would you expect in a patient who is awakening from general anesthesia using ether?

5. Explain the difference between chlorpromazine, phenobarbital and morphine regarding:

    A. addiction   C. tolerance

    B. habituation   D. dependence

6. What do you understand by the term "pain threshold"?

7. Analyze T.V. commercials and other advertisements dealing with nonprescription hypnotics, sedatives, and analgesics. Consider truthfulness and accuracy of claims, misleading or confusing statements and the extent to which they encourage drug use.

8. What objective signs would indicate that a patient is experiencing pain?

BIBLIOGRAPHY

Adams, E.: Barbiturates. *Sci. Amer., 198*:60, 1958.
Adriani, J.: Local anesthetics. *Amer. J. Nurs., 59*:86, 1959.
Adriani, J.: Reactions to local anesthetics. *J.A.M.A., 196*:405, 1966.
Adriani, J. and Zepernick, R.: Anesthesia for infants and children. *Amer. J. Nurs., 64*:107, 1964.
AMA Drug Evaluations. Chicago, American Medical Association, 1971.
Ataractic and Hallucinogenic Drugs in Psychiatry. WHO Technical Report Series No. 152. Geneva, Switzerland, World Health Organization, 1958.
Balme, H. W.: The relief of pain. *Nurs. Mirror, 128*:22, (February 7) 1969.
Barnard, J.: Understanding and treating the patient in pain. *R.N.,* May, 1967, p. 73.
Beecher, H. K.: Anesthesia. *Sci. Amer., 196*:70, 1957.
Best, C. H. and Taylor, N. B.: *The Physiological Basis of Medical Practice.* 6th Ed. Baltimore, The Williams and Wilkins Co., 1965.
Billars, K. S.: You have pain? I think this will help. *Amer. J. Nurs., 70*:2143, (October) 1970.
Boyd, E. M.: The safety and toxicity of aspirin. *Amer. J. Nurs., 71*:964, (May) 1971.

Breckenridge, F. J. and Bruno, P.: Nursing care of the anesthetized patient. *Amer. J. Nurs., 62*:76, (July) 1962.

Brokken, B., et al.: L-Dopa: a nursing adventure. *Nurs. Clin. N. Amer., 4*:733, (December) 1969.

Brumlik, J. and Moretti, L.: The effect of diphenylhydantoin on nerve conduction velocity. *Neurology, 16*:1217, 1966.

Carnes, M. A.: Postanesthetic complications. *Nurs. Forum, 4*:46, 1965.

Carozza, V. J.: Understanding the patient with epilepsy. *Nurs. Clin. N. Amer., 5*:13, (March) 1970.

Chambers, W. G. and Price, G. G.: Influence of the nurse upon the effects of analgesics administered. *Nurs. Res., 16*:228 (Summer) 1967.

Chinitz, A., Seelinger, D. F. and Greenhouse, A. H.: Anticonvulsant therapy in trigeminal neuraligia. *Amer. J. Med. Sci., 252*:62, 1966.

Claghorn, J. L. and Schoolar, J. C.: Propoxyphene hydrochloride, a drug of abuse. *J.A.M.A., 196*:1089, 1966.

Connel, P. H.: Clinical manifestations and treatment of amphetamine type dependence. *J.A.M.A., 196*:718, 1966.

Council on Drugs: A chloral hydrate complex. *J.A.M.A., 190*:1123, 1964.

Crawford, E. W.: Changing patterns in anesthesia and nursing problems. *AORN J., 4*:88, (March-April) 1966.

Dekornfeld, T. J.: Aspirin. *Amer. J. Nurs., 64*:60, (December) 1964.

Dingle, H. R.: Antihypertensive drugs and anesthesia. *Anesthesia, 21*:151, 1966.

DiPalma, J. R. (ed.): *Drill's Pharmacology in Medicine.* 4th Ed. New York, McGraw-Hill Book Co., 1971.

DiPalma, J. R.: L-Dopa, new hope for C.N.S. disease. *R.N., 34*:63, (March) 1971.

Dobkin, A. B. and Po-Giok Su, J.: Newer anesthetics and their use. *Clin. Pharmacol. Ther., 7*:648, 1966.

Done, A. K.: Salicylate poisoning. *Amer. J. Med., 36*:167, 1964.

Dowatt, D. D.: Drugs and anesthesia. *Nurs. Mirror, 128*:31, (April 18) 1969.

Dundee, J. W.: Clinical pharmacology of general anesthetics. *Clin. Pharmacol. Ther., 8*:91, 1967.

Edwards, R. E.: Abuse of central nervous system stimulants. *Amer. J. Hosp. Pharm.,* March, 1965, p. 145.

Essig, C. F.: Clinical aspects of barbiturate and sedative drug abuse. *Amer. J. Hosp. Pharm.,* March, 1965, p. 140.

Falconer, M. W., et al.: *The Drug, the Nurse, the Patient.* 4th Ed. Philadelphia, W. B. Saunders Co., 1970.

Fangman, A. and O'Malley, W. E.: L-Dopa and the patient with Parkinson's Disease. *Amer. J. Nurs., 69*:1455, (July) 1969.

Friend, D. G.: Sedative hypnotics. *Clin. Pharmacol. Ther., 1*:5, 1960.

Gardner, R.: Amphetamine dependence and misuse. *Nurs. Mirror, 130*:22, (March 6) 1970.

Gates, M.: Analgesic drugs. *Sci. Amer., 215*:131, (November) 1966.

Goldberg, L. I.: Monamine oxidase inhibitors. *J.A.M.A., 190*:456, 1964.

Goodman, L. S. and Gilman, A.: *Pharmacological Basis of Therapeutics.* 4th Ed. New York, Macmillan Co., 1970.

Goss, C. M. (ed.): *Gray's Anatomy of the Human Body,* 28th Ed. Philadelphia, Lea and Febiger, 1966.

Goth, A.: *Medical Pharmacology.* 3rd Ed. St. Louis, C. V. Mosby Co., 1968.

Govoni, L. E. and Hayes, J. E.: *Drugs and Nursing Implications.* 2nd Ed. New York, Appleton-Century-Crofts, 1971.

Greiss, F. C., Jr.: Obstetric anesthesia. *Amer. J. Nurs., 71*:67, (January) 1971.

Guzman, F. and Lim, R. K. S.: The mechanism of action of the non-narcotic analgesics. *Med. Clin. N. Amer., 52*:3, 1968.

Hershberg, P. I.: Does morphine deserve a primary role in coronary care therapy? *Amer. Heart J., 77*:289, 1969.

Hilmi, K. I. and Reagan, T. J.: Relative effectiveness of antiarrhythmic drugs in the treatment of digitalis-induced ventricular tachycardia. *Amer. Heart J., 76*:365, 1968.

Horwitz, D., et al.: Monamine oxidase inhibitors, tyramine, and cheese. *J.A.M.A., 188*:1108, 1964.

Isbell, H., et al.: Chronic barbiturate intoxication. *Arch. Neurol. Psychiat., 64*:1, 1950.

Jacobson, J.: The management of patients taking drugs prior to anesthesia. *Amer. Ass. Nurs. Anesth. J., 36*:433, (December) 1968.

Jaffe, J. H.: Narcotics in the treatment of pain. *Med. Clin. N. Amer., 52*:33, 1968.

Kaufman, M. A. and Brown, D. E.: Pain wears many faces. *Amer. J. Nurs., 61*:48, 1961.

Keele, C. A. and Neil, E.: *Samson Wright's Applied Physiology.* 11th Ed. London, Oxford University Press, 1965.

Kramer, J. C., et al.: Amphetamine abuse. *J.A.M.A., 201*:305, 1967.

Kuzava, B. A.: Innovar and its components: fentanyl and droperidol. *Amer. Ass. Nurs. Anesth. J., 38*:134, (April) 1970.

Lasagna, L.: The pharmacological basis for the effective use of hypnotics. *Pharmacol. Physicians, 1(2)*:1, 1967.

Livingston, S.: Antiepileptic drugs. *Amer. J. Nurs., 63*:103, (October) 1963.

Lynn, F. H. and Friedhoff, A. J.: The patient on a tranquilizing regimen. *Amer. J. Nurs., 60*:234, 1960.

Main, R. J. and Richardson, A. W.: *Physiology.* 2nd Ed. St. Louis, C. V. Mosby Co., 1953.

Maloney, E. M. and Johnannesen, L.: How the tranquilizers affect nursing practice. *Amer. J. Nurs., 57*:1144, 1957.

Marston, A. E.: Drugs in current use in psychiatric medicine. *Nurs. Mirror, 127*:24, (November) 1968.

Martin, W. R.: Some clinical aspects of addiction to narcotic analgesics. *Amer. J. Hosp. Pharm.,* March 1965, p. 133.

McBride, M. A. B.: The additive to the analgesic. *Amer. J. Nurs., 69*:974, (May) 1969.

McCaffery, M. and Moss, F.: Nursing intervention for bodily pain. *Amer. J. Nurs., 67*:1224, (June) 1967.

Millichap, J. G.: Anticonvulsant drugs. *Postgrad. Med., 37*:22, 1965.

Minckley, B. B.: Physiologic hazards of position changes in the anesthetized patient. *Amer. J. Nurs., 69*:2606, (December) 1969.

Minor, R. W. (ed.): The regulation of hunger and appetite. *Ann. N.Y. Acad. Sci., 63*:144, 1955.

Modell, W.: The search for a morphine substitute. *Amer. J. Nurs., 57*:1565, 1957.

Murphree, H. B.: The use of potent analgesics. *Amer. J. Nurs., 63*:104, (September) 1963.

Oswald, I.: Drugs and sleep. *Pharmacol. Rev., 20*:273, 1968.

Pain: Part I: Basic concepts and assessment. (Programmed instruction). *Amer. J. Nurs., 66*:1085, (May) 1966.

Pain: Part II: Rationale for intervention. (Programmed instruction). *Amer. J. Nurs., 66*:1345, (June) 1966.

Pansky, B. and House, E. L.: *Review of Gross Anatomy.* New York, Macmillan Co., 1964.

Ranson, S. W. and Clark, S. L.: *The Anatomy of the Nervous System.* 10th Ed. Philadelphia, W. B. Saunders Co., 1959.

Rodman, M. J.: Advances in treating Parkinsonism. *R.N., 32*:59, (September) 1969.

Rodman, M. J.: The central nervous system stimulants. *R.N., 30*:85, (September) 1967.

Rodman, M. J.: Drugs for neuromuscular pain and spasm. *R.N., 29*:62, (May) 1966.

Rodman, M. J.: Drugs for pain problems. *R.N., 34*:59, (April) 1971.

Rodman, M. J.: Pain-relieving drugs in labor and delivery. *R.N., 27*:95, 1964.

Rosati, R. and Wallace, A. G.: Electrophysiologic effects of diphenyl-hydantoin on the heart of awake dogs. *Amer. J. Cardiol., 19*:147, 1967.

Sadove, M. S. and Albrecht, R. F.: Sedatives and tranquilizers in the treatment of pain. *Med. Clin. N. Amer., 52*:47, 1968.

Shore, P. A. and Brodie, B. B.: A concept for a role of serotonin and norepinephrine as chemical mediators in the brain. *In* Shuster, L. (ed.): *Readings in Pharmacology.* Boston, Little, Brown and Co., 1962.

Shore, P. A., Pletscher, A., Tomick, E. G., et al.: Role of brain serotonin in reserpine action. *Ann. N.Y. Acad. Sci., 66*:609, 1957.

Stuart, D. M.: To depress the craving for food. *Amer. J. Nurs., 62*:88, 1962.

Stubbs, D. H.: Anesthesiology—what nurses should know about it. *AORN J., 4*:75, 1966.

Symposium: Post-anesthetic complications. *Anesthesiology, 22*:657, 1961.

Tantum, K. R., et al.: The scope and challenge of modern anesthesia. *Nurs. Clin. N. Amer., 3*:591, (December) 1968.

Tewari, S. N., et al.: A comparison of non-barbiturate sedatives in elderly patients. *Nurs. Time, 66*:178, (February) 1970.

Vandam, L. D.: Anesthesia. *Ann. Rev. Pharmacol., 6*:379, 1966.

Wintrobe, M. M., et al.: *Harrison's Principles of Internal Medicine.* 6th Ed. New York, McGraw-Hill Book Co., 1970.

Wise, R. P.: Muscle disorders and the relaxants. *Brit. J. Anesth., 35*:558, 1963.

Youmans, W. B.: *Fundamentals of Human Physiology.* 2nd Ed. Chicago, Year Book Medical Publishers, Inc., 1962.

Chapter 12 Drugs That Affect the Autonomic Nervous System

Important Concepts Discussed

1. The autonomic nervous system is composed of efferent nerves, which control involuntary bodily functions.

2. When a nerve impulse reaches an effector site, the organ or tissue is stimulated or depressed by the chemical release at the nerve ending.

3. Drugs may mimic or inhibit the effects of the autonomic nervous system.

4. Skeletal muscle relaxants may enhance or inhibit the activator chemical at the neuromuscular junction. Antidotes must be chosen carefully to counteract the specific effect of the drug at the effector site.

5. The nonspecific actions of most of these drugs produce side effects for which the nurse must observe, so that she may design nursing interventions to alleviate them.

The autonomic nervous system, one of the systems of the body that serves to maintain homeostasis, is composed of a series of efferent nerves leading from the central nervous system to control the heart, glands and smooth muscles of the body. It is divided into two parts; the sympathetic and parasympathetic nervous systems, which are distinguishable by their site of origin within the central nervous system and by their activities. By a delicately balanced system of checks and balances, these two opposing systems work to control and coordinate the various functions of virtually all structures of the body except skeletal muscle.

Unlike the somatic nerves, which supply the skeletal muscles, the autonomic nerves are not myelinated and their synapses do not occur solely within the central nervous system, but are found in ganglia located just outside the spinal cord or very near their effector organs.

Almost every autonomic pathway consists of two neurons. The axon of the cell body within the central nervous system is called the preganglionic fiber; the axon that passes away from the ganglion is termed the postganglionic fiber.

The Sympathetic Nervous System

The sympathetic nervous system, which arises from the thoracolumbar region of the spinal cord, is characterized by relatively short preganglionic fibers, because the ganglia of this system are located very near the spinal cord. In the parasympathetic system, on the other hand, the fibers arise from the cranial and sacral portions of the central nervous system, and the ganglia are located very near or even within the organ innervated.

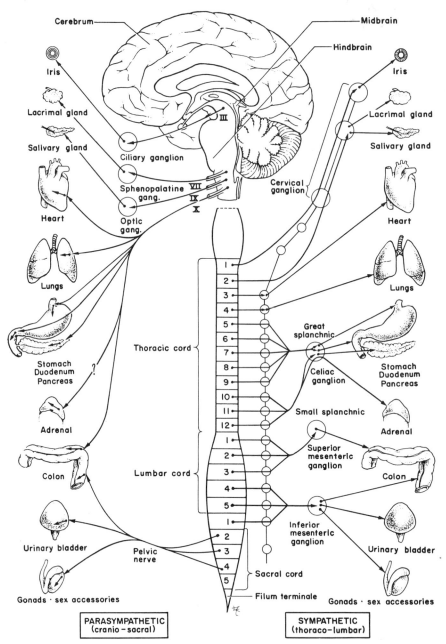

FIGURE 38. Autonomic nervous system. (Villee: *Biology.* Ed. 6. W. B. Saunders Co., Philadelphia, 1972.)

The parasympathetic system is considered vital to life. Removal of the sympathetic system, however, would not of itself cause death, but the body could no longer cope with unusual circumstances such as cold and anoxia; thus conditions that would ordinarily be tolerated as a matter of course may prove serious and even fatal to the sympathectomized animal.

The two systems differ also in their manner of control. The parasympathetic system has discrete control over various organs, whereas the sympathetic system acts by mass firing in emergency situations. The "fight-or-flight" reaction, which occurs upon sympathetic stimulation, includes the following:

1. There is a pilomotor reaction, i.e., the body hair "stands on end." This, of course, is not as noticeable in humans as in some animals such as the cat.

2. The pupils of the eye are dilated.

3. Bronchi dilate to enable entry of more air.

4. The heart rate increases.

5. The gastrointestinal tract relaxes so that digestion can be postponed until the emergency is over. This relaxation includes the gall bladder and urinary bladder. Blood is shunted away from the gastrointestinal tract and is consequently available to the skeletal muscles.

6. The gastrointestinal sphincters contract to prevent continued digestion.

7. Blood vessels constrict over most of the body to produce an over-all elevation in blood pressure. Exceptions to this general rule, however, are the coronary and skeletal muscle blood vessels. These are dilated under the influence of epinephrine, thus providing additional nutrients and oxygen to muscles that must perform additional work during exertion.

8. Sweat glands increase secretion.

9. Glycogen is broken down to form glucose; thus the blood sugar level is elevated.

The sympathetic system organizes the body for environmental conditions of emergency whenever the body may be subjected to unusual stress. When the body is performing strenuous work or exercise, in danger, in extreme temperatures, or under painful stimuli and following hemorrhage or asphyxia, the sympathetic system is in an augmented state of excitement. It is also hyperactive under conditions of strong emotions, such as love, fear and rage.

Psychosomatic symptoms are often manifestations of prolonged stress or anxiety. If an individual is unduly anxious for a period of time, the heart rate may increase under the influence of the sympathetic nervous system, the blood pressure may be elevated, perspiration increases, digestion may be delayed, etc. Contrary to the opinion of many individuals, physiological changes produced by psychosomatic causes are as real as those produced by organ and tissue pathology.

Along with the widespread action of the peripheral sympathetic system under conditions of stress, the adrenal medulla is also stimulated to release epinephrine into the blood where it is transmitted throughout the body. Many of the gross symptomatic changes are a result of this circulating epinephrine.

In addition to the widespread emergency responses produced by the sympathetic nervous system, under normal circumstances it aids in the regulation of heat loss from the body. This control is accomplished by decreasing the number of sympathetic impulses to the surface blood vessels, thus permitting them to dilate and increase the radiation of heat from the body, and by increasing perspiration and cooling the skin by evaporation. Blushing is another result of inhibition of the sympathetic vasoconstrictor tone.

The Parasympathetic Nervous System

Considerably unlike the widespread action of the sympathetic system, the parasympathetic system is more localized in its actions. Typically it affects single organs or, in some cases, small groups of organs without affecting others. The parasympathetic system more directly protects and maintains the internal environment. It constricts the pupil

TABLE 7 Responses of Effector Organs to Nerve Impulses

ORGAN	SYMPATHETIC	PARASYMPATHETIC
Eye		
Pupil	Dilate	Constrict
Ciliary muscles	Relax for far vision	Accommodates for near vision
Smooth muscle of orbit	Constrict	————
Blood vessels		
Coronary	Dilate	Dilate
Genitalia	Constrict	————
Muscle (at rest)	Constrict	————
Cerebral	Constrict	Dilate
Pulmonary	Constrict	Dilate
Visceral	Constrict	Dilate
Heart		
S-A node (rate)	Increase	Decrease
Pilomotor muscles	Contract	————
Bronchi	Relax	Constrict
Gastrointestinal tract		
Smooth muscle	Relax	Constrict
Secretions	Inhibit	Increase
Sphincters	Constrict	Relax
Gall bladder	Relax	Contract
Urinary bladder		
Detrusor	Relax	Contract
Trigone and sphincter	Contract	Relax
Uterus		
Pregnant	Stimulate	Stimulate
Nonpregnant	Stimulate	Variable
Spleen	Constrict	————
Liver		
Glycogenolysis	Increase	————
Bile secretion	Decrease	Increase
Pancreas		
Isles of Langerhans	————	Secretion
Exocrine cells	————	Secretion
Salivary glands	Mucous secretion	Watery secretion
Adrenal medulla	Secretion	————
Vas deferens, seminal glands	Decrease secretion	Increase secretion

of the eye in bright light; it elicits secretions of the salivary glands by an unconditioned reflex when food enters the mouth or by a reflex conditioned by the sight or smell of food.

In the digestive processes, the parasympathetic vagus nerve may have a somewhat wider action. By reflex action the stomach may be stimulated to secrete gastric juice along with enhanced secretion of pancreatic juice and bile. The motility of the walls of the stomach and intestine is augmented; the sphincters of the stomach are inhibited and relaxed in turn to aid in the flow of the gastric contents.

The parasympathetic action on the heart is to slow its rate. The vagus nerve, which acts as a continuous brake on the heart's action, is an effector nerve of the parasympathetic nervous system.

Parasympathetic fibers contract the urinary bladder and the internal bladder sphincter. The smooth muscles of the bronchi are constricted and the secretion of mucus is increased.

Table 7 provides a summary of the various actions of the divisions of the autonomic nervous system on effector organs in the body.

Transmitter Chemicals of the Autonomic Nervous System

Considerable research has revealed that transmission of the neural impulses at all ganglia and at the site of the effector organ is accomplished by chemical substances.

Acetylcholine is released by the cholinergic fibers, which include preganglionic sympathetic and parasympathetic fibers, postganglionic parasympathetic fibers and a few postganglionic sympathetic fibers, e.g., those to the sweat glands and pilomotor muscles. The somatic (voluntary) nerve fibers, those to the skeletal muscles, are also cholinergic fibers.

$$H_3C\overset{O}{\overset{\|}{C}}-O-CH_2CH_2-\overset{+}{N}\overset{CH_3}{\underset{CH_3}{-CH_3}}$$
acetylcholine

Norepinephrine is secreted by the adrenergic fibers, which include most of the postganglionic sympathetic fibers.

Both acetylcholine and norepinephrine are manufactured by the body via enzymatic processes. Almost immediately upon the release of these chemicals due to nervous system stimulation, other enzymes destroy them. Since the effector chemical is destroyed by the time the muscle fiber has recovered from the stimulation they produced, only one contraction is caused by the release of the effector chemical under normal conditions.

Acetylcholine is destroyed by the enzyme acetylcholinesterase (also called cholinesterase). Norepinephrine is broken down in a two-step process by two enzymes: catechol-o-methyl transferase and monoamine oxidase (MAO).

There are many ways of interfering with the activity of the autonomic nervous system. The postganglionic fiber transmission in the sympathetic or parasympathetic system may be enhanced or inhibited, or the nerve transmission could be blocked at the ganglia. In each case activity would be altered to a greater or lesser extent depending upon the drug used, dosage employed, conditions under which it is performed and the mode of administration.

CHOLINERGIC DRUGS

Cholinergic drugs, drugs having the same effect as stimulation of the cholinergic fibers, are of three types:

Cholinomimetic drugs. These drugs replace or have the same effect as acetylcholine. (Acetylcholine itself is not used therapeutically because it is destroyed too rapidly in the body.)

Reversible antiesterases. These drugs inhibit acetylcholinesterase, but their action may be reversed.

Irreversible antiesterases.

CHOLINOMIMETIC DRUGS

Cholinomimetic drugs are primarily derivatives of acetylcholine. In general they are employed to stimulate depressed cholinergic nerves, to antagonize the action of an overactive or stimulated sympathetic nervous system or to improve transmission of impulses at the myoneural junction of skeletal muscles.

General therapeutic uses for cholinomimetic drugs are as follows:

1. To dilate peripheral blood vessels. These drugs are used for symptomatic relief of vascular spasm in conditions such as Raynaud's disease or intermittent claudication.

2. To slow the heart beat through a vagal effect. These drugs may be used in the treatment of sinus tachycardia; however, they are not effective if the tachycardia is due to organic disease.

3. To treat glaucoma through constriction of the ciliary muscle, thus relieving conges-

tion of the canal of Schlemm, which drains excess fluid from the eye.

4. To restore accommodation of the eye after use of mydriatic agents.

5. To treat postoperative atony of the bladder and urinary retention.

6. To treat myasthenia gravis and curare poisoning.

7. To relieve certain muscle spasms.

All cholinomimetic drugs are not equally effective in all these areas, however. Some tend to be more specific for one or two effects and are used to treat these conditions. Specificity is a desired characteristic of pharmacologic agents, because unwanted side effects often occur if the drug is a general rather than a specific effector.

> **TOXICITY.** The toxicity of the cholinomimetic drugs is dependent upon the number of sites they affect, i.e., whether they are muscarinic, nicotinic or both in their effects on cholinergic nerve endings.

Muscarinic and nicotinic drugs, so-called because their effects resemble the pharmacologic effects of muscarine and nicotine, both affect cholinergic nerve endings. The muscarinic drugs act only on the postganglionic parasympathetic nerve endings, whereas the nicotinic drugs act at the ganglia of both systems and at somatic nerve endings as well, producing first a stimulation then a depression of the site. Muscarinic effects include bradycardia, dyspnea, epigastric disorders, nausea, vomiting, increased salivation and sweating and disturbances in visual accommodation. Nicotinic effects include muscular twitching and action on the central nervous system producing restlessness, insomnia and confusion.

Atropine blocks the muscarinic effects, but not the nicotinic effect. Tetraethylammonium chloride (TEA) blocks the nicotinic effect at the ganglia; curare blocks it at the skeletal muscles.

METHACHOLINE CHLORIDE, N.F. (MECHOLYL). Methacholine is closely related to acetylcholine, and its actions are similar but more persistent than those of acetylcholine. It produces powerful stimulation of the cholinergic system, including slowing the heart, lowering the blood pressure, constricting the bronchioles, dilating the blood vessels and increasing peristalsis.

It is useful for the treatment of selected cases of paroxysmal atrial tachycardia and for the treatment of chronic superficial ulcers, Raynaud's disease, scleroderma and other vasospastic conditions of the extremities.

> **TOXICITY.** Side effects include nausea, vomiting, involuntary defecation, peripheral vasodilation and profuse sweating. In susceptible persons it has been known to precipitate asthmatic attacks. Heart block, atrial fibrillation and cardiac arrest may occur occasionally. Atropine counteracts these effects.

Care should be taken when injecting methacholine to be sure that it is in subcutaneous tissues, since it should not be given intramuscularly or intravenously. The drug should be prepared immediately prior to injection since it is quite unstable.

Because of methacholine's vasodilating effect, the patient should be in a recumbent position for the injection and for about 30 minutes afterwards. Vital signs should be checked before and after injection. Atropine and other emergency drugs and equipment should be readily available in case of toxic effects.

> **DOSE.** 200 to 600 mg. orally two or three times daily. 2.5 to 40 mg. subcutaneously twice daily.

BETHANECHOL CHLORIDE, U.S.P. (URECHOLINE). Although similar in action to acetylcholine, bethanechol is less toxic and less active. It is used in the treatment of postoperative abdominal distention, urinary retention and gastric retention following vagotomy. It may also be used in the treatment of megacolon, neurogenic bladder atony, gastric atony and retention following gastric surgery. It differs from methacholine in that it does not exhibit any ganglion stimulating effects.

> **TOXICITY.** Usually the side effects consist of abdominal cramps, flushing or

sweating. It should not be given intramuscularly or intravenously because of the excessive parasympathetic stimulation that would be induced. Other effects, such as malaise, salivation, headache, diarrhea, asthmatic attacks and fall in blood pressure, may occur. In general it exhibits fewer and less severe side effects than methacholine. Atropine is an effective antidote.

DOSE.   10 to 30 mg. orally three or four times daily. 2.5 to 5 mg. subcutaneously two or three times daily.

CARBACHOL, U.S.P., B.P. (DORYL, CARCHOLIN).   Because of its insusceptibility to hydrolysis by acetylcholinesterase, carbachol is the most powerful drug of this group, but it is also potentially quite toxic. The chief use of carbachol is in glaucoma in which the eye does not respond to simpler and milder drugs.

TOXICITY.   Carbachol seems to have less cardiac action than does methacholine, but it is more potent generally with greater degrees of muscarinic and nicotinic effects. Gastrointestinal symptoms, such as cramps, diarrhea and nausea, are usually rather prominent, as well as hypotension and the precipitation of asthmatic attacks.

DOSE.   1 or 2 drops of 0.75 to 3% solution in eye four times daily.

PILOCARPINE NITRATE, U.S.P., B.P.; PILOCARPINE HYDROCHLORIDE, U.S.P.   Pilocarpine is the leaf alkaloid obtained from *Pilocarpus jaborandi* and *P. microphyllus*. It exhibits most of the muscarinic effects of acetylcholine; particularly responsive are the sweat and salivary glands. It is primarily employed for its miotic effect to relieve glaucoma; its other actions are rarely therapeutically important and usually constitute undesirable side effects. For this reason, pilocarpine is not as useful as the other drugs in this class.

The drug should be protected from exposure to light.

TOXICITY.   Muscarinic effects occur as mild toxic reactions. Most notable are

salivation, lacrimation, sweating, nausea, vomiting, diarrhea, tenesmus, blurred vision, slowed pulse and dyspnea. When poisoning occurs, death is usually a result of respiratory failure or pulmonary edema. Atropine is an effective antidote.

DOSE.   5 to 10 mg. orally or subcutaneously. Ophthalmic preparation: 1 or 2 drops of a 0.5 to 3 per cent solution every 2 or 3 hours.

REVERSIBLE ANTIESTERASES

Before any appreciable cholinergic action may be obtained, 50 per cent of the tissue cholinesterase must be inactivated. Since 90 per cent inactivation causes death, there is a narrow margin of safety for these drugs, which is even more serious with the irreversible antiesterases.

Tissue antiesterases are apparently destroyed uniformly throughout the body; there is no predilection for destroying those in one area in preference to another. Since specificity for an effector organ cannot be guaranteed, the resultant actions of these drugs are not always the same; effectors tend to differ in their degree of sensitivity to the enzyme.

Small doses probably act only at the postganglionic parasympathetic endings; larger quantities produce an effect at the ganglia and skeletal muscle myoneural junctions. Still larger doses act at the least sensitive effectors in the central nervous system.

PHYSOSTIGMINE SALICYLATE, U.S.P., B.P. (ESERINE).   An alkaloid obtained from the seed of *Physostigma venenosum Balfour,* which is also called the Calabar bean, physostigmine is an effective acetylcholinesterase inhibitor in body fluids and tissues. It prevents enzymatic hydrolysis of acetylcholine and allows it to exert its characteristic action more intensely. This action includes not only the muscarinic actions of acetylcholine on smooth muscles, secretory glands and the heart, but also actions on the nicotinic effectors in the skeletal muscles and autonomic ganglia. For this reason the effects of physostigmine are not always entirely predictable.

The main pharmacologic actions of physostigmine concern the pupil of the eye and the intestine; the others are usually regarded mainly as side effects. It causes pupillary constriction, constriction of the muscle of accommodation and blurring of vision for 12 to 36 hours after the drug is administered. The constriction of the pupil provides for the relief of glaucoma by decreasing congestion at the entrance of the canal of Schlemm; the constriction of the muscle of accommodation is useful in restoring accommodation following the local instillation of mydriatic drugs for an eye examination. Many physicians prefer not to use physostigmine in this manner, however, and simply allow the more gradual return to accommodation and pupil reflexes by natural means as the action of the mydriatic drug wears off.

The tone and motility of the gastrointestinal tract are increased, peristalsis is exaggerated and bowel evacuation may result when physostigmine is administered.

Only clear, colorless solutions of the drug should be used.

> **TOXICITY.** An overdose of physostigmine produces violent peristalsis, nausea, vomiting, colic, defecation, skeletal muscle twitching, nystagmus, pin-point pupils, blurred vision, bronchiolar constriction, urgency and difficulty of voiding, excessive perspiration and low blood pressure. Death may occur if pulmonary edema or central respiratory paralysis occurs. Atropine is an effective antidote.

> **DOSE.** Miotic: 1 drop of a 0.02 per cent solution two to six times daily. Intestinal uses: 1 to 2 mg. orally; 0.5 to 1 mg. subcutaneously.

NEOSTIGMINE BROMIDE, U.S.P., B.P.; NEOSTIGMINE METHYLSULFATE, U.S.P., B.P. (PROSTIGMIN). Neostigmine is a synthetic analog of physostigmine. Their actions are similar but neostigmine has less effect on the circulatory system, the eye and glandular activity, but it has a rather selective action on the bowel, the urinary bladder and skeletal muscle.

It is used occasionally postoperatively to dispel flatus from the gastrointestinal tract and to restore peristalsis. Although more effective agents are available, neostigmine is sometimes used to treat atony of the urinary bladder, enabling complete emptying.

When the patient's condition warrants treatment of this type, neostigmine is used to allay the symptoms of myasthenia gravis. This disease of unknown origin is characterized by a physiological derangement of the conduction of the normal impulse at the myoneural junction of skeletal muscle. It is believed to be due to either a lack of acetylcholine or an increase of cholinesterase at the junction. The outstanding symptoms of this condition are abnormal fatigability and muscular weakness that is increased by their use. After rest, their strength returns; thus the patient feels strongest in the morning and becomes tired and weak toward evening. The muscles of the neck, throat, lips, tongue, face and eyes are primarily involved. The course of the disease is variable and there may be prolonged remissions. Some cases are rapidly fatal as a result of pulmonary infections and respiratory failure; in others the life span is little affected.

Patients with myasthenia gravis may be allowed to adjust their drug dosage and frequency to a certain degree, depending on their individual needs and activity. Usually a larger dosage is needed toward the later part of the day. A particular problem in drug dosage and scheduling may arise if the patient's condition is such that, because of excessive weakness in the morning, he is unable to give himself the first dose of the day.

The scheduling of drug dosage should be planned so that the patient has sufficient muscle strength for eating, chewing and swallowing at meal time. When given orally, it may be necessary to crush the tablet if the patient is experiencing dysphagia.

The patient may develop a myasthenic crisis suddenly, without any evident cause. Severe muscular weakness and respiratory failure develop; these symptoms may be difficult to differentiate from those of cholinergic crisis caused by overdosage of an anticholinesterase.

Neostigmine is often used as a diagnostic

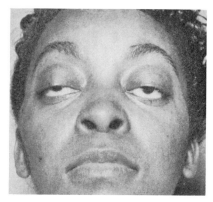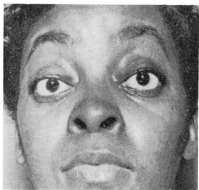

FIGURE 39.   The effect of neostigmine in myasthenia gravis. (Grollman: *Pharmacology and Therapeutics*. Ed. 6. Lea & Febiger, Philadelphia, 1965.)

agent for myasthenia gravis. After the muscular weakness is determined, the patient is given an intramuscular injection of 1.5 mg. neostigmine and 0.6 mg. atropine. A positive response is characterized by a rapid disappearance of the weakness in one half to one hour after the injection, with the return of the symptoms in four to eight hours.

It was also used as a test for pregnancy in the past. If the patient is not pregnant, menstruation usually occurs within 72 hours after intramuscular injection of the drug for three days.

TOXICITY.   The toxic effects of neostigmine are similar to those of physostigmine. Atropine is an effective antidote.

DOSE.   Therapeutic for myasthenia gravis: 0.5 mg. I.M. three or four times daily or 15 mg. orally two or three times daily. Gastrointestinal disorders: 0.25 to 0.5 mg. I.M. three times daily.

PYRIDOSTIGMINE BROMIDE, U.S.P., B.P. (MESTINON).   This drug has a smoother and slightly more prolonged action than neostigmine. It is used in the symptomatic treatment of myasthenia gravis and in cases of neostigmine intolerance. The side effects resemble those of physostigmine, but they are not as severe.

DOSE.   600 mg. orally daily, in four or five divided doses.

AMBENONIUM CHLORIDE (MYTELASE).   On a weight to weight basis, ambenonium is about three times as potent as neostigmine. It is rapidly absorbed from the gastrointestinal tract and is used chiefly in the treatment of myasthenia gravis and postoperative abdominal distention and urinary retention.

TOXICITY.   Adverse effects, other than those seen with physostigmine, include nervousness, dizziness, headache and confusion.

It is contraindicated in patients receiving mecamylamine because a muscle reaction consisting of inability to swallow and extreme muscle weakness ensues.

DOSE.   5 to 25 mg. orally three or four times daily.

BENZPYRINIUM BROMIDE, N.F. (STIGMONENE).   This synthetic agent is very similar to neostigmine in actions and side effects. Also like neostigmine, it is used to decrease postoperative abdominal distention and urinary retention.

DOSE.   2 mg. I.M. every 3 hours.

EDROPHONIUM CHLORIDE, U.S.P., B.P. (TENSILON).   Although edrophonium chloride may be used as a diagnostic agent for myasthenia gravis, its chief pharmacologic use is as an antidote for curare poisoning. Preparations of edrophonium should be on hand whenever curare or tubocurarine is administered during surgical procedures.

Curare and tubocurarine affect skeletal muscles by preventing the depolarization of the motor end-plate (which is necessary for the muscle to contract in response to a nervous impulse). Edrophonium, because of its action as an anticholinesterase, prolongs the effect of acetycholine at the motor end-plate and allows enough of the transmitter chemical to build up for stimulation and muscle contraction to occur.

Edrophonium should never be given as an antidote for succinylcholine or decamethonium, however, because these drugs exert their effect in just the opposite manner—by causing depolarization of the motor end-plate (and one contraction), but thereafter preventing repolarization which is necessary before another contraction can occur. Edrophonium, by allowing acetylcholine to build up (which also causes muscle contraction by depolarizing the end-plate), only enhances the effect of the skeletal muscle relaxant in this case and may cause death.

The patient's pulse should be checked frequently during treatment with this drug, and equipment should be available in the event of respiratory distress.

> **TOXICITY.** Edrophonium should be used with caution. When the drug is administered in large doses, its action overcomes the effect of curare to an extent that it may act like succinylcholine and again cause skeletal muscle relaxation. Side effects include bronchiolar spasm, bradycardia, cardiac dysrhythmias and increased salivation.
>
> **DOSE.** 10 mg. I.V. as needed.

IRREVERSIBLE ANTIESTERASES

The irreversible antiesterases are distinguished from the reversible agents in that they have a longer duration of action and are also quite different structurally from acetylcholine.

These drugs, alkyl phosphates, were first used in World War I as nerve gases. Now, although they are chiefly used in insecticides, they are still applied in the eye to produce miosis and to aid in the treatment of glaucoma. Because of the number of side effects incurred with systemic use of these agents, they are restricted to topical application.

ISOFLUROPHATE, N.F. (DIISOPROPYL FLUORO-PHOSPHATE, DFP, FLOROPRYL). This drug is a potent anticholinesterase and exhibits many of the muscarinic and nicotinic actions of acetylcholine. The miotic effect is more potent and prolonged than with pilocarpine, neostigmine or physostigmine.

It is used chiefly for glaucoma that is not amenable to therapy with the milder miotic agents.

> **TOXICITY.** Even upon local administration, toxic effects are noticeable. Headache, photophobia, aching of the eyes, blurred vision and twitching of the eyelids often occur. Atropine is used as an antidote.
>
> **DOSE.** 1 to 3 drops of a 0.01 to 0.1% solution in the eye one to three times daily.

DEMECARIUM BROMIDE (HUMORSOL). Demecarium is used chiefly in the treatment of glaucoma and strabismus. One must watch for the possible development of iris cysts during therapy.

> **DOSE.** 1 or 2 drops of a 0.125 to 0.25% solution in the eye one to three times daily.

ECHOTHIOPHATE IODIDE, U.S.P. (PHOSPHOLINE IODIDE). Like demecarium, this drug is also employed in the treatment of glaucoma. Iris cysts may develop during therapy, however.

> **DOSE.** 1 or 2 drops of a 0.06 to 0.25% solution in the eye one to three times daily.

Other irreversible antiesterases, such as mintacol (Bayer 600), tetraethyl pyrophosphate (TEPP) and octamethyl pyrophosphoramide (OMPA), are used only as insecticides because they are too toxic for human use.

CHOLINERGIC BLOCKING AGENTS

Many agents inhibit cholinergic nerve endings. The net effect is sympathetic action because the two systems oppose each other at all times.

These agents inhibit the action of acetylcholine at the receptor sites, producing a reversible blockade. The degree of blocking with a certain dose depends upon the action of the particular agent on a specific receptor site and also upon whether the site is being overstimulated at the time.

Cholinergic blocking agents may be quaternary, tertiary or secondary amines. The quaternary amines are used primarily as ganglionic blocking agents. They penetrate membranes only slightly and are very poorly absorbed when given orally. The quaternary amines are not fat soluble and, therefore, do not produce a noticeable effect on the central nervous system. They are not greatly altered in the body and, for the most part, are excreted in the urine almost completely in the active state.

Secondary and tertiary amines undergo quite a different metabolism in the body. These are absorbed quite well when taken orally, are fat soluble and thus have an effect on the central nervous system, are almost completely metabolized in the body and are eliminated in an inactive state.

General therapeutic uses of the cholinergic blocking agents are as follows:

1. To relax sphincter muscles in the eye and produce mydriasis. Paralysis of the ciliary muscle also occurs, causing cycloplegia and blurring of vision. The use of anticholinergics is ordinarily contraindicated in glaucoma because an increase in intraocular pressure is very often a side effect even with drugs that are rather specific for a certain part of the body. When anticholinergic drugs are given, the ocular effects may be minimized somewhat by applying miotic agents locally.

2. To inhibit postganglionic vagal neurons to the stomach and decrease gastric motility and secretion in patients with peptic ulcers. Ideally, for this purpose a drug should be long-acting, fairly well absorbed when given orally and relatively free from side effects. Tolerance should not readily develop. (Tolerance does develop to some of these drugs, however, but may be circumvented by changing to another drug within this group.)

3. To treat gastrointestinal spasms caused by an overactive parasympathetic system.

4. Incorporated into cathartic preparations to minimize excessive griping action.

5. To treat biliary, renal and urinary colic.

6. To treat enuresis by relaxing the urinary bladder so that the micturition reflex occurs less readily.

7. To relax smooth muscles of the bronchi and reduce secretions. This area is not blocked well by the anticholinergic drugs, however. The sympathetic agents are usually employed for this purpose.

8. To inhibit the vagus nerve and consequently affect cardiac muscle. These drugs may restore rhythm to the heart when there is a temporary heart block.

9. To reduce secretory activity prior to anesthesia.

10. For central nervous system action. Some anticholinergics, e.g., atropine, have a stimulating effect on the central nervous system.

11. To produce twilight sleep, which is used especially in obstetrics.

12. To treat motion sickness when antisecretory, antispasmodic or central nervous system effects may be beneficial.

13. To relieve involuntary muscular twitching in Parkinsonism. These agents are also used for Parkinson-like syndromes, such as those produced as a side effect of tranquilizer therapy.

Toxic effects of the anticholinergic drugs include dry mouth, blurred vision, tachycardia, difficulty in initiation of urination, constipation and central nervous system effects.

Because of the non-specific nature of drug action, many side effects, which are often discomforting and annoying to some patients, accompany the use of these drugs. Many times patients are not aware that some of the side effects are expected; a simple explanation may alleviate much of their concern. Patients may need a great deal of encouragement to continue with the drug therapy if the side effects are particularly distressing to them.

Nursing measures should be instituted to help reduce discomfort and prevent the development of some of these side effects. Dryness of the mouth may be alleviated to some degree by having the patient use gum or hard candy to increase salivation. The urine output should be recorded and excessive urinary retention prevented. Bowel regularity should also be checked, and nursing measures taken to prevent the development of constipation.

The patient should be observed for increasing restlessness and delirium which may necessitate a reduction in dosage. The pulse rate should be checked periodically in order to detect tachycardia.

BELLADONNA ALKALOIDS

Belladonna consists of a mixture of alkaloids from *Atropa belladonna* (deadly nightshade) and other plants. These alkaloids, atropine, hyoscyamine and scopolamine, all produce anticholinergic effects when applied locally as in the eye or when administered systemically in oral or parenteral preparations.

Atropine is used more often than the other two alkaloids; thus it will be discussed in detail. The actions and effects of hyoscyamine and scopolamine closely parallel those of atropine.

ATROPINE SULFATE, U.S.P., B.P. Atropine is quite typical of the anticholinergic agents and is an antidote for the muscarinic effects of cholinergic drugs. It is used in the eye to produce mydriasis and to paralyze the ciliary muscle and produce loss of accommodation. It is quite useful in eye examinations. It must be used with extreme caution in patients with glaucoma, because intraocular pressure may be markedly increased.

When administered systemically, atropine

atropine sulfate

stimulates the central nervous system, causing the patient to become restless, talkative or even delirious. Stimulation of the respiratory center occurs, making breathing faster and easier. Atropine's action, however, is not adequate to counteract respiratory depression, such as that which occurs with an overdose of depressant drugs, and may even deepen the depression in such cases.

The anticholinergic effect of atropine lessens the inhibitory influence of the vagus on the heart and, consequently, increases the heart rate.

It produces a marked relaxation of the smooth muscle of the gastrointestinal tract, and for this reason it is often employed in oral preparations for intestinal hypermotility. It does not affect the secretion of bile, but it has an antispasmodic effect on the gallbladder and the bile duct.

Because of inhibition of parasympathetic nerve endings in the respiratory tract, atropine decreases secretions of the nose, pharynx and bronchial tubes. It relaxes the bronchial muscles, increasing the ease of respiration. In general, however, when immediate and dramatic relaxation of the bronchioles is required, as in severe asthmatic attacks, atropine is not sufficient. The sympathetic drugs, such as epinephrine, are usually employed for this purpose.

The nerves to the sweat glands, although sympathetic, are an exception to the rule in that acetylcholine is secreted at the postganglionic nerve ending. Atropine has an inhibitory influence on these sympathetic nerves as well as the cholinergic parasympathetic nerve endings. As a result, the skin becomes hot and dry.

Atropine causes a decrease in salivary secretion, and the mouth becomes dry. The patient becomes quite thirsty and sometimes has difficulty swallowing. A dry mouth is perhaps the most common complaint of patients receiving anticholinergic therapy. It does not warrant discontinuing the drug in most cases, however, and patients usually tolerate it very well when they become accustomed to this side effect.

Atropine is used quite often as a preanesthetic medication. In addition to the inhibition of mouth and respiratory secretions, the mild stimulation of the heart is considered beneficial.

Atropine is occasionally used to relieve biliary and renal colic as well as to relieve pylorospasm, spastic colon and hypertonicity of the urinary bladder and ureters. The belladonna alkaloids have been used to relieve dysmenorrhea, but the effect is often unsatisfactory.

TOXICITY. The side effects of atropine are the same as those for the general class of anticholinergic drugs. Atropine may also cause "atropine fever," producing elevated temperature. It may also cause a rash or flushing of the skin, which is more common when the drug is given to children. Toxic doses produce stupor and coma.

Scopolamine is often given with a narcotic or barbiturate to produce "twilight sleep" in obstetrics. Scopolamine causes amnesia and produces delirium if given in the presence of pain. Bedside rails and close supervision by the nurse are usually indicated when scopolamine is used in obstetrics.

DOSE. Atropine: 0.5 mg. orally, subcutaneously, I.M. or I.V.; in the eye in a 0.5 to 3% solution.
Hyoscyamine: 0.25 to 1 mg. orally or subcutaneously
Scopolamine: 0.6 mg. orally or subcutaneously; in the eye in a 0.2% solution.

BELLADONNA TINCTURE, U.S.P., B.P. The tincture of belladonna is an alcohol-water solution of the belladonna alkaloids. It should be stored away from heat and light. It is given orally for its antispasmodic effect on the gastrointestinal tract. It is often combined with a digestant vehicle, such as elixir of lactated pepsin.

DOSE. 0.6 ml. orally three times daily $\frac{1}{2}$ hour before meals and at bedtime.

HYOSCYAMUS, N.F. Obtained from the plant *Hyoscyamus niger* (henbane), this alkaloid is very similar to atropine and scopolamine in effect, but it is not used to any extent at present.

DOSE. 200 mg. orally.

SYNTHETIC ATROPINE-LIKE DRUGS

HOMATROPINE HYDROBROMIDE, U.S.P., B.P.; HOMATROPINE METHYLBROMIDE (NOVATRIN, MESOPIN). The pharmacologic effects of homatropine closely resemble those of atropine; however, homatropine is not a central nervous system stimulant. It is less toxic than atropine and likewise less potent. It is used for many of the same purposes as atropine.

DOSE. Homatropine hydrobromide: in the eye in a 1 to 2% solution.
Homatropine methylbromide: 5 mg. orally three or four times daily.

METHSCOPOLAMINE BROMIDE, N.F. (PAMINE, LESCOPINE). Methscopolamine bromide is employed chiefly for its antispasmodic and antisecretory effects on the gastrointestinal tract. It reduces peristalsis, slows the emptying of the stomach and suppresses gastric acidity.

It is used to treat hypermotility of the gastrointestinal tract, hyperacidity and peptic ulcers.

TOXICITY. Aside from the general toxic symptoms produced with oral anticholinergic drugs, methscopolamine may have a curare-like effect on smooth muscle because of its ganglionic blocking action.

DOSE. 2.5 to 5 mg. orally four times daily, before meals and at bedtime. 0.25 to 1 mg. subcutaneously or I.M. every 6 to 8 hours.

METHANTHELINE BROMIDE, N.F. (BANTHINE). Methantheline is very similar in effect to atropine. Although it is still sometimes used in the treatment of gastric hypermotility and hypersecretion, it is not very effective and has been replaced by more effective agents.

DOSE. 50 to 100 mg. orally, I.M. or I.V. four times daily.

PROPANTHELINE BROMIDE, U.S.P., B.P. (PRO-BANTHINE). This analogue of methantheline is considerably more effective than the parent compound as an anticholinergic agent. Consequently, it has replaced methantheline to a very great extent.

It is usually administered orally for treatment of intestinal hypermotility or peptic ulcer, but may be administered intramuscularly as well. Parenteral preparations should be stored away from heat and light.

DOSE. Oral—15 mg. four times daily, usually with meals and at bedtime. I.V. or I.M.—30 mg. every 6 hours.

Other anticholinergic drugs with similar effects are incorporated in Table 8.

ADRENERGIC DRUGS

The adrenergic drugs are used for a variety of actions, both central and peripheral. Their actions are not as specific as those of the cholinergic agents, however, and tend to overlap considerably with unwanted side effects. Therapeutic uses of the adrenergic drugs are as follow:

1. In circulatory emergencies. Following administration of an adrenergic drug, the cardiac output is increased, force and rate of the heartbeat are increased and there is an increase in systolic blood pressure. (A secondary effect due to pressor receptors in the carotid artery and aortic arch could actually cause slowing of the heart, however. This may be prevented with atropine.)

2. To treat bronchial asthma, particularly status asthmaticus. There is an increase

---

TABLE 8   Anticholinergic Drugs

GENERIC NAME	TRADE NAME	DOSE
Anticholinergics employed chiefly for their mydriatic effect in the eye:		
Eucatropine	Euphthalmine	2 to 10% solution
Cyclopentolate	Cyclogyl	0.5 to 5% solution
Bistropamide	Mydriacyl	0.5 to 1% solution
Anticholinergics employed chiefly for spasmolytic and antisecretory effects on the gastrointestinal tract:		
Adiphenine	Trasentine	75 mg. orally three times daily before meals.
Amprotropine	Syntropan	50 to 100 mg. orally three or four times daily.
Dicyclomine	Bentyl	20 mg. orally four times daily.
Diphemanil	Prantal	100 mg. orally every 4 to 6 hours.
Glycopyrrolate	Robinul	1 mg. orally three times daily.
Hexocyclium	Tral	25 mg. orally four times daily.
Isopropamide	Darbid	5 mg. orally every 12 hours.
Mepenzolate	Cantil	25 mg. orally four times daily.
Methscopolamine nitrate	Skopolate, Skopyl	5 mg. orally before meals and at bedtime.
Oxyphencyclimine	Daricon	10 mg. orally in morning and at bedtime.
Oxyphenonium	Antrenyl	5 mg. orally four times daily.
Pentienate	Monodral	10 mg. orally four times daily.
Pipenzolate	Piptal	5 mg. orally three times daily and 5 to 10 mg. at bedtime.
Piperiodolate	Dactil	50 mg. orally before meals and at bedtime.
Tricyclamol	Elorine, Tricoloid	100 mg. orally four times daily.
Tridihexethyl	Pathilon	50 mg. orally four times daily.
Valethamate	Murel	10 mg. orally three or four times daily.
Anticholinergics employed in the treatment of parkinsonism are:		
Benztropine	Cogentin	0.5 mg. orally daily.
Biperiden	Akineton	2 mg. orally three times daily.
Caramiphen	Panparnit	12.5 mg. orally three times daily.
Chlorphenoxamine	Phenoxene	50 mg. orally three times daily.
Cycrimine	Pagitane	5 mg. orally three times daily.
Ethopropazine	Parsidol	10 mg. orally four times daily.
Orphenadrine	Disipal	50 mg. orally three times daily.
Procyclidine	Kemadrin	7.5 mg. orally three times daily.
Trihexyphenidyl	Artane, Pipanol	1 mg. orally daily.

in the size of the airway, and vasoconstriction occurs in blood vessels of the bronchial mucosa. The major disadvantage to the use of these agents is their short duration of effect and the excessive drying of secretions, which causes irritation of the passages.

3. To produce local vasoconstriction. These agents are combined with local anesthetics to prolong anesthesia and reduce local bleeding.
4. To shrink nasal mucosa in rhinitis. Disadvantages to the use of adrenergic drugs here are the short duration of effect and the subsequent rebound effect, which often produces more congestion than formerly.
5. To treat allergic responses, such as serum sickness and hay fever.
6. In the eye to reduce conjunctival congestion, to control bleeding during surgery and to reduce intraocular pressure because vasoconstriction prevents or slows formation of fluid. (The mydriatic effect overcomes the beneficial effects of vasoconstriction upon intraocular pressure, however.)
7. Combined with atropine and applied to the eye to break up adhesions between the iris and lens. This combination would affect both the radial and sphincter muscles of the iris; thus a stronger force would be applied during dilation of the pupil.

EPINEPHRINE (ADRENALIN, SUPRARENIN).

Since epinephrine is the natural hormone of the sympathetic nervous system, the general group of sympathetic effects is produced when epinephrine is administered therapeutically.

Epinephrine is ineffective if applied to intact skin, but produces marked vasoconstriction if applied topically to the mucous

epinephrine

membranes or injected into tissues. It is used to lessen vasodilation and hyperemia of the conjunctiva, to reduce congestion of the nasal mucous membranes and following surgery of the eye, ear, nose and throat. If epinephrine is injected with a local anesthetic the resulting vasoconstriction prolongs the action of the anesthetic. Many commercial preparations contain epinephrine for this purpose. Although it is valuable in arresting capillary bleeding, it is not effective in massive or arterial hemorrhage.

The heart rate is accelerated following an injection of epinephrine because it stimulates the myocardium and the conducting tissue, resulting in stronger contractions and more complete emptying of the heart chambers. This effect, with the marked vasoconstriction in many blood vessels of the body, produce an elevation of the blood pressure. Large doses of epinephrine also cause constriction of the blood vessels of the skeletal muscles, thus producing an extreme rise in blood pressure. Under physiologic conditions or moderate doses of the drug, the skeletal muscle blood vessels are dilated, whereas many of the other vessels of the body (notably the splanchnic blood vessels) are constricted.

Following the administration of epinephrine, a brief period of hypotension ensues before the blood pressure returns to normal. This reversal of effect on the blood vessels explains the increased amount of nasal congestion experienced when the brief effect of epinephrine in nasal preparations wears off.

Because of its relaxant effect on the smooth muscles in the respiratory tract, epinephrine is often used to relieve acute asthmatic attacks. The patient or a member of his family may be taught to administer epinephrine by injection in the event of a severe asthma attack at home. It is the most effective agent known to treat status asthmaticus.

The smooth muscles of the gastrointestinal tract are relaxed by epinephrine, whereas the sphincters are contracted. Thus, the net effect is a slowing of the rate at which intestinal contents are moved through the tract. Because of the short duration of action of epinephrine, however, therapeutic doses administered to improve the heart rate, blood pressure, etc. do not noticeably alter peristalsis for any clinically significant period.

TOXICITY. Epinephrine is a very potent drug and even a small overdose can produce disastrous results. An overdose can produce ventricular fibrillation and death, especially in the presence of a malfunctioning heart. Because of the various strengths and types of preparation, the nurse should be very careful that she has the correct preparation for the route to be used.

Patients receiving epinephrine very often have a feeling of oppression, especially a fear of death. Tachycardia and palpitations, along with dizziness and a throbbing type of headache, add to anxiety. Symptoms of poisoning are more evident in patients predisposed to anxiety or in those with hypertension or hyperthyroidism. The milder toxic symptoms may be relieved by discontinuance of the drug, whereas the more severe reactions must be treated symptomatically.

Epinephrine is contraindicated in hypertensive and hyperthyroid patients. It should not be used concurrently with some general anesthetics, such as chloroform and cyclopropane, because these agents also have cardiac effects; simultaneous administration of epinephrine greatly enhances the possibility of ventricular fibrillation.

Solutions which are brown in color or have a precipitate should not be used. Urine tests for glycosuria may become positive.

COMMERCIAL PREPARATIONS

Epinephrine solution, U.S.P.; Adrenalin solution, B.P. *Dose.* Applied topically in a 1:1000 solution.

Epinephrine injection, U.S.P., B.P.; Adrenalin injection, B.P. *Dose.* 0.2 to 1 mg. of a 1:1000 solution subcutaneously or I.M. as needed.

Epinephrine bitartrate, U.S.P. *Dose.* For ophthalmic use in a 2% solution.

Epinephrine inhalation, U.S.P. *Dose.* The 1:100 solution is used to treat asthmatic conditions when administered by oral inhalation.

Sterile epinephrine suspension, U.S.P. (Epinephrine in oil injection). *Dose.* 0.2 to 0.5 cc. of a 1:500 solution I.M.

LEVARTERENOL BITARTRATE INJECTION, U.S.P.; NORADRENALINE ACID TARTRATE, B.P. (NOREPINEPHRINE, LEVOPHED, ARTERENOL). The effects of levarterenol (norepinephrine) are somewhat different from epinephrine. In instances in which epinephrine causes vasodilation, norepinephrine gives widespread constriction, thus elevating the systolic and diastolic pressures.

This difference in therapeutic action may be explained by the two types of receptors in the smooth muscle of the blood vessels. These receptors, termed alpha (α) and beta (β), differ considerably in their response to epinephrine and levarterenol.

The beta receptors are more sensitive than the alpha receptors to epinephrine. Thus, with very small doses of epinephrine, only the beta receptors respond, causing vasodilation instead of the expected vasoconstriction. If the dose is increased the alpha receptors are stimulated and the resultant vasoconstriction overcomes the weaker effect of the beta receptors. This explains the reflex lowering of blood pressure as most of the epinephrine is metabolized by the body, since as the circulating levels of epinephrine decrease, once again only the more sensitive beta receptors are being stimulated.

Levarterenol, on the other hand, stimulates only the alpha receptors, thus no vasodilation is observed in small doses of this drug, and no hypotension occurs before the blood pressure returns to normal.

This variation in effect between epinephrine and levarterenol permits levarterenol's use in a number of instances in which epinephrine is undesirable, if not actually harmful; e.g., epinephrine may never be used to counteract the hypotension incurred by an overdose of a tranquilizing or hypotensive drug because the beta effect will be additive to the hypotension already incurred and a fatal hypotensive effect may result.

Levarterenol does not change the cardiac rate and output; overall effects are rather that of essential hypertension. It does not increase oxygen utilization, elevate blood sugar or stimulate the anterior pituitary to release ACTH as does epinephrine. There is no therapeutically significant effect on the bronchiolar musculature; thus levarterenol is not used in status asthmaticus.

The chief therapeutic use is in the treatment of circulatory collapse. If the decrease in blood pressure is due to diminished blood volume, however, whole blood should be used rather than levarterenol.

> TOXICITY. Because of the potent vasoconstrictor effect of this drug, care should be taken to prevent the undiluted drug's contacting the skin. Extravasation of an I.V. fluid containing levarterenol may cause sloughing of tissue. The blood pressure and intravenous flow rate must be monitored continuously in order to maintain the desired vasoconstriction without producing toxicity. A drop in blood pressure may occur if the drug is stopped too abruptly.

> Overdosage produces marked hypertension, photophobia, headache, chest pain, and vomiting.

> DOSE. 4 to 8 mg. in 1000 ml. of 5% dextrose solution I.V.

MEPHENTERMINE SULFATE, N.F., B.P. (WYAMINE). The vasopressor effect of mephentermine is similar to that of epinephrine, except that it has a more prolonged duration of action. It may be taken orally for a mild hypertensive effect.

> DOSE. Oral—10 to 30 mg. three times daily. Parenteral—15 to 30 mg. I.M. or I.V.

METARAMINOL BITARTRATE, N.F. (ARAMINE). Metaraminol is often preferred to levarterenol as a vasopressor agent because it is not nearly as damaging to tissue if accidentally extravasated.

It may be administered intramuscularly if the intravenous route is not feasible in particular cases.

> DOSE. 0.5 to 5 mg. I.V.

Nursing implications. When a patient is receiving levarterenol or metaraminol by intravenous infusion, the nurse has several very important responsibilities. Precautions must be taken to prevent and detect early infiltration of the solution both because of the interruption of the drug administration to the patient and the sloughing of tissue that may result. The site should be checked frequently for swelling or blanching.

When the patient's blood pressure has been elevated and stabilized at the desired level, the doctor usually specifies the rate of flow of the infusion and the desired blood pressure range. The nurse must then adjust the rate of flow of the infusion according to blood pressure determinations. This requires the measurement of the blood pressure every five minutes. The rate of flow of the infusion can be affected by many factors, such as change in position of the patient's arm if the infusion is by arm. A frequent check of the blood pressure is, therefore, essential to prevent the patient from having either severe hypotension or severe hypertension.

It is essential that the infusion bottle be very clearly labeled with the amount and name of the drug.

METHOXAMINE HYDROCHLORIDE, U.S.P. (VASOXYL). The chief use of this synthetic adrenergic agent is as a vasopressor drug. It exhibits fewer side effects than epinephrine.

> DOSE. 5 to 10 mg. I.M.

EPHEDRINE SULFATE U.S.P.; EPHEDRINE HYDROCHLORIDE, N.F., B.P. (EPHEDRON, IONEPHRIN). This drug, obtained from *Ephedra vulgaris*, has been used for thousands of years by primitive peoples. It is believed to cause adrenergic action by prolonging the life of the adrenergic mediator; thus its action is somewhat analogous to the action of acetylcholinesterase on the parasympathetic system.

Unlike epinephrine, ephedrine is absorbed quite well from the gastrointestinal tract, and it is given orally as well as parenterally. Although it is not as potent as epinephrine, it has a more prolonged action on the heart and blood vessels.

Ephedrine is relatively effective in stimulating the central nervous system. Its action is exerted mainly on the cerebral cortex and medulla where it stimulates the respiratory center.

When applied locally to the eye it has mydriatic action. Its action on the smooth muscle of the bronchioles resembles that of epinephrine, but it is less potent. For this effect it is incorporated into many oral anti-asthmatic drugs. When taken over a period of time in preparations of this type, ephedrine causes slowing of peristalsis and delayed emptying of the stomach, because of its inhibitory effect on the gastrointestinal smooth muscles.

Ephedrine is used in cough preparations, nasal decongestants, and mydriatic preparations and for the treatment of narcolepsy. The patient's pulse should be checked frequently during therapy with this drug. If possible, ephedrine should not be given near bedtime because the central nervous system stimulation it produces can lead to insomnia.

TOXICITY. The central nervous system and cardiac stimulation produced necessitates caution when ephedrine is used in patients with cardiac conditions. Insomnia, headache, dizziness, tremors, sweating and palpitation are also produced. Urinary retention is occasionally a problem.

Although tolerance has been known to develop in instances in which ephedrine is used for a period of time, it is not extensive, and habituation to this drug has not been observed.

DOSE. Oral—25 mg. three or four times daily. In the eye—3 to 4 % solution or ointment.

ISOPROTERENOL HYDROCHLORIDE, U.S.P.; ISOPROTERENOL SULFATE, N.F. (ISUPREL, NORISODRINE, ALUDRINE). Isoproterenol is more effective than epinephrine as a bronchodilator although it has less effect on the smooth muscle of the blood vessel. For this reason it is used to treat bronchospasm during anesthesia, to treat asthma and in preparations to shrink the nasal mucosa.

It stimulates the heart; thus it is occasionally used to increase the heart rate in patients with heart block. It has some benefit in the treatment of allergic conditions.

The drug should always be protected from light, and only clear, colorless solutions should be used.

TOXICITY. The heart stimulant effect may give rise to severe tachycardia in overdosage or in susceptible persons. Precordial pain, palpitation, flushing, headache, tremor and nausea may occur with therapy. It is contraindicated in patients with insufficient coronary blood flow.

DOSE. 10 to 15 mg. sublingually three or four times daily. 0.2 to 1 mg. I.V. as required. By inhalation, 5 to 15 inhalations of a 1:200 solution or 3 to 7 inhalations of a 1:100 solution.

METHOXYPHENAMINE HYDROCHLORIDE, U.S.P. (ORTHOXINE). Methoxyphenamine is not as stimulating to the central nervous system as is ephedrine. It is routinely used in the treatment of asthma. Since it is absorbed well from the gastrointestinal tract it is usually administered orally.

DOSE. 50 to 200 mg. orally three times daily.

PHENYLEPHRINE HYDROCHLORIDE, U.S.P., B.P. (NEO-SYNEPHRINE). Although phenylephrine is less potent than epinephrine, it is generally longer lasting and has more specificity of action. It has no effect on the central nervous system.

It is used chiefly as a nasal decongestant in the treatment of sinusitis, vasomotor rhinitis and hay fever.

Parenterally it acts as a vasopressor and may be used in the treatment of hypotension. Local discomfort may occur at the site of injection. Its action is not sufficiently prolonged to be of use when a hypertensive effect must be sustained over a considerable period of time; levarterenol or a similar agent is preferable.

It is occasionally used as a mydriatic agent when pupil dilation without cycloplegia is desired.

Any unclear solution should not be used.

> **DOSE.** Parenteral—0.1 to 1 ml. of a 1% solution.
> In the eye—2.5% solution.
> Application to nasal mucosa—0.25 to 1% solution.

NAPHAZOLINE HYDROCHLORIDE, N.F. (PRIVINE). Although this drug is more potent than ephedrine as a nasal decongestant, more "rebound" congestion is produced. Nevertheless, its chief therapeutic use is in nasal preparations.

> **DOSE.** 0.1 to 0.5% solution intranasally.

TETRAHYDROZOLINE HYDROCHLORIDE, N.F. (TYZINE). Tetrahydrozoline resembles naphazoline in therapeutic effect. A sedative effect that may lead to a light comatose condition is noted especially in children; thus it should not be used in excessive doses or for prolonged periods of time in pediatric patients.

> **DOSE.** 0.05 to 0.1% solution intranasally.

CYCLOPENTAMINE HYDROCHLORIDE, N.F. (CLOPANE). The activity of this drug resembles that of tetrahydrozoline; it is used chiefly in nasal preparations to relieve nasal congestion.

> **DOSE.** 0.05 to 0.1% solution intranasally.

ETHYLNOREPINEPHRINE HYDROCHLORIDE (BRONKEPHRINE). This agent has a great deal of specificity for the smooth muscle of the respiratory tract; it is used chiefly as a bronchial vasodilator.

> **DOSE.** 0.5 ml. I.M. or S.C. as needed.

NYLIDRIN HYDROCHLORIDE (ARLIDIN). The primary effect of nylidrin is that of peripheral vasodilation; it affects the beta rather than the alpha receptors. It is useful in the treatment of Raynaud's and Buerger's diseases and intermittent claudication.

> **DOSE.** 6 mg. orally three or four times daily.

ISOXSUPRINE HYDROCHLORIDE (VASODILAN). Like nylidrin, isoxsuprine is a smooth muscle relaxant. It is useful in the treatment of peripheral vascular disorders and is occasionally employed to relieve dysmenorrhea.

> **DOSE.** 10 to 20 mg. orally three times daily.

METHAMPHETAMINE HYDROCHLORIDE, U.S.P., METHYLAMPHETAMINE HYDROCHLORIDE, B.P. (DESOXYN, DESOXYEPHEDRINE). In this synthetic derivative of ephedrine, the central stimulant effect is greatly increased. Both elevation of the blood pressure and nasal decongestion are observed when the drug is employed.

It is used in anti-obesity preparations as an anorexigenic.

> **DOSE.** 5 to 10 mg. orally or two or three times daily. The last dose should be given at least six hours before bedtime to avoid producing insomnia.

BENZPHETAMINE HYDROCHLORIDE (DIDREX). The chief use of benzphetamine is as an anorexigenic. Sympathomimetic effects are observed upon continued use; thus it should not be given to hypertensive patients.

> **DOSE.** 25 to 50 mg. orally three times daily.

Other sympathomimetic (adrenergic) drugs that may be used as anorexigenics are:

Diethylpropion Hydrochloride (Tenuate, Tepanil)—25 mg. orally three or four times daily before meals and in midevening.

Phendimetrazine Tartrate (Plegine)—35 mg. orally three times daily before meals.

Phenmetrazine Hydrochloride, N.F. (Preludin)—25 mg. orally two or three times daily before meals or 75 mg. once daily.

Phentermine (Ionamin)—15 mg. in the morning.

ADRENERGIC BLOCKING AGENTS

Although sympathetic stimulation is blocked with these drugs, they are generally not as specific or as useful as the parasympathetic blocking agents.

The main blocking action is on the smooth muscle, causing relaxation. The blood pressure is lowered, and there is increased tone and activity of the gastrointestinal tract. There is little effect on the heart, however. Most of the cardiac effects are on the atrioventricular rather than on the sinoatrial node.

The hyperglycemic reaction is blocked, as are the glands of internal and external secretion and the release of ACTH.

One of the most important uses of the adrenergic blocking agents is in the diagnosis of pheochromocytoma (tumor of the adrenal medulla). If hypertension is due to a tumor of this type, marked lowering of blood pressure is observed following the injection of an adrenergic blocking agent.

Adrenergic blocking agents are also moderately successful in the treatment of essential hypertension, peripheral vascular diseases, glaucoma and cardiac arrhythmias.

The ergot alkaloids although technically adrenergic blocking agents, are used for this effect primarily to promote uterine contraction. (These drugs are discussed in the chapter dealing with the endocrine system, however, because their effect closely parallels that of oxytocin, a natural hormone.)

Adrenergic blocking agents used to diagnose pheochromocytoma are:

Phentolamine Hydrochloride (Regitine)—5 mg. I.V.

Piperoxan (Benodaine)—15 to 20 mg. I.V.

Adrenergic blocking agents used to treat peripheral vascular disease are:

Phenoxybenzamine Hydrochloride (Dibenzyline)—10 to 20 mg. orally three times daily.

Tolazoline Hydrochloride (Priscoline)—50 mg. orally three times daily.

Azapetine Phosphate (Ilidar)—50 mg. orally three times daily.

Guanethidine Sulfate, U.S.P., B.P. (Ismelin)—10 to 25 mg. orally three or four times daily.

> **TOXICITY.** Nasal congestion, tachycardia, symptoms of gastrointestinal stimulation such as diarrhea or irritation, postural hypotension and central nervous system stimulation have been observed.

GANGLIONIC BLOCKING AGENTS

The ganglionic blocking agents inhibit both adrenergic and cholinergic effects by a nicotinic type of depression of the autonomic ganglia. They are used in cases of extreme hypertension, i.e., malignant hypertension. In cases in which the other hypotensive agents are not effective, these drugs are the agents of choice. They should not be used to treat simple hypertension, however, because untoward effects are common.

Additional uses are in the prediction of the effects of sympathectomy (occasionally performed for severe hypertension) and in the diminution of bleeding in delicate surgery by lowering the blood pressure.

Frequently stimulation, followed by depression, is observed when ganglionic blocking agents are employed; thus the hypertension gets worse before it gets better.

> **TOXICITY.** Dry mouth, constipation, difficulty in defecation and urination, cycloplegia and postural hypotension are often observed.

NICOTINE. Nicotine is used in animal experiments but is not a therapeutic agent for humans. It first stimulates then depresses the autonomic ganglia, skeletal muscle and the central nervous system, especially the medullary centers for emesis, respiration and vasoconstriction. In overdosage death is due to respiratory depression.

Nicotine is employed primarily as an insecticide. The toxic effects may be observed if enough of the insecticide is inhaled or ingested.

TOXICITY. Although nicotine is absorbed from tobacco, toxic effects are usually minimal because it is excreted rapidly enough to prevent accumulation of poisonous amounts. Symptoms of mild toxicity include nausea, vomiting and stimulation of the central nervous system producing restlessness, insomnia, irritability and dizziness. In more severe poisoning, there is excessive initial stimulation of the central nervous system, which proceeds to depression with concurrent depression of the respiratory and vasomotor centers.

TETRAETHYLAMMONIUM CHLORIDE (TEA, ETAMON). TEA is used in the treatment of peripheral vascular diseases, such as thromboangiitis obliterans (Buerger's disease), arteriosclerosis obliterans, and other conditions, such as herpes zoster, thrombophlebitis, Raynaud's disease, trench foot and immersion foot. TEA should be used with caution because it promptly lowers blood pressure in both normal and hypertensive patients, and peripheral vascular collapse may ensue.

TOXICITY. Dyspnea, weakness, slowing of speech, difficulty in muscular movement, dryness of the mouth and loss of ocular accommodation occur. It should be used with extreme caution in patients with severe hypertension, especially in the presence of poor renal function or high diastolic blood pressure. It is not suitable for the routine treatment of hypertension because its action is very transitory. It is contraindicated in patients with recent coronary thrombosis and should be used with extreme caution in elderly patients and those with arteriosclerosis.

DOSE. 200 to 500 mg. orally or I.V. two or three times daily. (Dosage should be individualized depending on response.)

HEXAMETHONIUM SALTS (BISTRIUM BROMIDE, BISTRIUM CHLORIDE, ESOMID CHLORIDE, METHIUM CHLORIDE). Several salts containing the hexamethonium ion are used medicinally, including the bromide, chloride, iodide and bitartrate salts.

As a ganglionic blocking agent, hexamethonium interrupts the effect of the central nervous system on the vascular system, producing vasodilation and inhibition of gastric secretion and gastrointestinal motility. The potency of hexamethonium is several times that of TEA, and it has a more prolonged duration of action.

DOSE. Chloride salt—50 mg. I.M. every 6 hours; 125 mg. orally four times daily. Bromide salt—66.6 mg. I.V. every 6 hours.

PENTOLINIUM TARTRATE, B.P. (ANSOLYSEN). Pentolinium is about one and a half times longer acting than hexamethonium. The effect on blood pressure is similar to that of hexamethonium except that the onset of action is somewhat slower and the recovery is somewhat prolonged.

It may be administered orally as well as parenterally.

DOSE. 20 mg. orally three times daily. (Maximum daily dose is 1 Gm.). 2.5 to 3.5 mg. I.M or s.c. every 6 hours (may be increased gradually to 30 to 60 mg. daily).

TRIMETHAPHAN CAMSYLATE TRIMETHAPHAN CAMPHORSULPHONATE, B.P. (ARFONAD). Trimethaphan is about 30 times as potent as and has a duration about twice that of TEA salts. It has little or no curare-like action and has little effect on intestinal tonus or gastric motility. Its use is limited for the most part to the anesthetist who must control blood pressure at a hypotensive level, as in certain types of cranial surgery. Because the duration of action is relatively short, it is best administered by continuous intravenous drip.

DOSE. 10 to 50 mg. I.V. initially, then as needed.

CHLORISONDAMINE CHLORIDE (ECOLID). Chlorisondamine may be administered orally to treat moderate to severe diastolic hypertension. It should not be administered for the treatment of mild, labile hypertension. When it is used in conjunction with reserpine, thiazide diuretics or other hypotensive agents, the dosage of each drug must be reduced because synergistic action occurs.

DOSE. 50 to 100 mg. orally twice daily. 1 to 10 mg. subcutaneously or I.M.

QUESTIONS FOR DISCUSSION AND REVIEW

1. Why do some individuals blush when embarrassed? Explain the physiological mechanism behind this phenomenon.
2. Explain in detail how the heart is caused to beat faster when an individual perceives that he is in danger.
3. Explain the differences between the control exerted upon the body by the central nervous system and the autonomic nervous system.
4. What symptoms would a patient have if his parasympathetic nervous system is stimulated for any reason? What nursing measures would be indicated?
5. What symptoms would a patient have if his sympathetic nervous system is stimulated for any reason? What nursing measures would be indicated?
6. Why is atropine commonly used as a pre-anesthetic agent?
7. Why are the cholinergics used in the treatment of glaucoma?
8. What are the nurse's responsibilities when a patient is receiving Levophed or Aramine?
9. For each of the groups of drugs discussed in this chapter, outline the common side effects and the nursing measures that may be taken to alleviate or prevent them.

BIBLIOGRAPHY

Best, C. H. and Taylor, N. B.: *The Physiological Basis of Medical Practice.* 6th Ed. Baltimore, The Williams and Wilkins Co., 1965.
Boura, A. L. A. and Green, A. F.: Adrenergic neuron blocking agents. *Ann. Rev. Pharmacol.,* 5:183, 1965.
DiPalma, J. R. (ed.): *Drill's Pharmacology in Medicine.* 4th Ed. New York, McGraw-Hill Book Co., 1971.

Finger, K. F.: A review of drugs used in the treatment of hypertension. *Wisconsin Pharm.*, January, 1965, p. 20.

Friend, D.: Gastrointestinal anticholinergic drugs. *Clin. Pharmacol. Ther., 4*:559, 1963.

Goodman, L. S. and Gilman, A.: *Pharmacological Basis of Therapeutics.* 4th Ed. New York, Macmillan Co., 1970.

Goth, A.: *Medical Pharmacology.* 3rd Ed. St. Louis, C. V. Mosby Co., 1964.

Govoni, L. E. and Hayes, J. E.: *Drugs and Nursing Implications.* 2nd Ed. New York, Appleton-Century-Crofts, 1971.

Gray, H.: *Anatomy of the Human Body.* 27th Ed. Philadelphia, Lea and Febiger, 1959.

Haggerty, R. J.: Levarterenol for shock. *Amer. J. Nurs., 58*:1243, 1958.

Hunter, A. R. and Miller, R. A. (ed.): Symposium on adrenergic drugs and their antagonists. *Brit. J. Anesth., 38*:666, 1966.

Ingelfinger, F. J.: Anticholinergic therapy of gastrointestinal disorders. *New Eng. J. Med., 268*:1454, 1963.

Kaufman, M. A.: Autonomic responses as related to nursing comfort measures. *Nurs. Research, 13*:45, (Winter) 1964.

Keele, C. A. and Neil, E.: *Samson Wright's Applied Physiology.* 11th Ed. London, Oxford University Press, 1965.

Lucchesi, B.: Antiarrhythmic effects of beta adrenergic blocking agents. *Ann. N.Y. Acad. Sci., 139*:940–951, 1967.

Main, R. J. and Richardson, A. W.: *Physiology.* 2nd Ed. St. Louis, C. V. Mosby Co., 1953.

Pansky, B. and House, E. L.: *Review of Gross Anatomy.* New York, Macmillan Co., 1964.

Rosenberg, R.: The use and abuse of vasopressors. *Surg. Clin. N. Amer., 44*:155, 1964.

Schwab, R. S.: The pharmacologic basis of treatment of myasthenia gravis. *Clin. Pharmacol. Ther., 1*:319, 1960.

Smith, V. M.: Newer anticholinergic drugs. *Med. Clin. N. Amer., 48*:399, 1964.

Von Euler, V. S.: Epinephrine and norepinephrine: action and uses in man. *Clin. Pharmacol. Ther., 1*:65, 1960.

Wintrobe, M. M., et al. (eds.): *Harrison's Principles of Internal Medicine.* 6th Ed. New York, McGraw-Hill Book Co., 1970.

Wurtman, R. J.: Catecholamines. *New Eng. J. Med., 273*:637, 1965.

Youmans, W. B.: *Fundamentals of Human Physiology.* 2nd Ed. Chicago, Year Book Medical Publishers, Inc., 1962.

Chapter 13 Drugs That Affect the Heart and Circulatory System

Important Concepts Discussed

1. *Drugs affect the heart by altering its rate and strength of contraction.*

2. *Drugs affect the blood vessels by changing the vasoconstrictor tone of the smooth muscle.*

3. *The oxygenation of all tissues is dependent on a sufficient cardiac output and the adequacy of the arterial blood vessels.*

4. *Nursing assessment and interventions are essential in order to maintain the patient's optimal cardiovascular function.*

Disorders of the heart are of great medical importance, and they assumed pharmacologic importance as drugs were discovered to correct or at least diminish many of them. In order to appreciate how the cardiac drugs affect the heart, however, it is necessary to have a working knowledge of cardiac physiology.

CARDIAC PHYSIOLOGY

The circulation of blood throughout the body depends on systematic contractions of the cardiac muscle. The tissues involved in the special system responsible for the heart beat are the sinoatrial (S–A) node, the atrioventricular (A–V) node, the atrioventricular bundle (bundle of His) and the branches of the bundle of His (the Purkinje fibers).

The S–A node, about three fourths inch in length, is embedded in the muscle of the right atrium. It is a neuromuscular structure consisting of specialized cardiac muscle fibers embedded in connective tissue with a few nerve cells and fibers. The S–A node is the pacemaker of the mammalian heart and emits electrical impulses which, when carried to the muscle cells of the heart, cause them to contract.

The A–V node lies in the right atrium at the lower part of the interatrial septum. Its microscopic structure closely resembles that of the S–A node, and the strength of its impulse is second only to that of the S–A node. If the S–A node is destroyed or severely inhibited, the A–V node may assume the role of pacemaker for the heart. The two nodes are apparently connected only by atrial muscle.

The A–V bundle, first described by His, is a well defined bundle of muscular bridges that is responsible for the conduction of impulses throughout the heart. This bundle

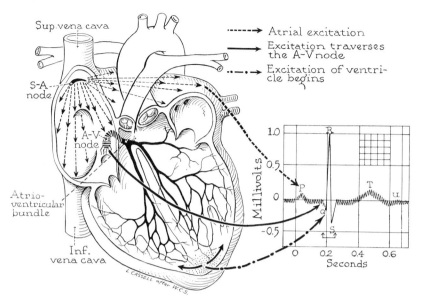

FIGURE 40. Correlation of the electrocardiogram with the spread of the excitation wave. (From King, B. G. and Showers, M. J.: *Human Anatomy and Physiology.* Ed. 6. W. B. Saunders Co., Philadelphia, 1969.)

originates at the A–V node and extends to the upper part of the interventricular septum where it divides into a right and a left branch, each going to the corresponding ventricle. The muscle cells composing the ventricular branches of the system have special features differing from those of the bundle stem. These peculiar cells, swollen in appearance, were described by Purkinje and have long been known by his name. The Purkinje system penetrates deeply into the ventricular muscle and is responsible for conduction of the contraction impulse to this tissue.

Disorders of the pacemaker and conducting system are many and varied. Cardiac arrhythmia and fibrillation are conditions in which the normally regular beat of the heart is replaced by irregularly spaced, rapid or purposeless contractions. Arrhythmia, the less dangerous of the two, is characterized by an irregular rhythm, whereas fibrillation is a state in which various areas of the cardiac muscle contract independently rather than as a unit. Instead of contracting with enough force to eject the blood into the rest of the circulatory system, the quivering contraction is purposeless. Fibrillation is rapidly fatal.

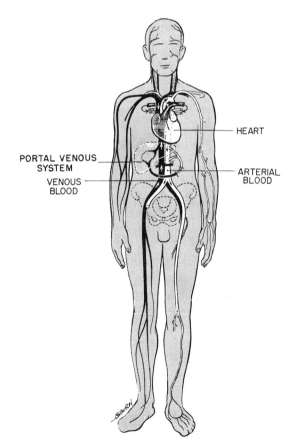

FIGURE 41. Circulatory system. (Guyton: *Function of the Human Body.* Ed. 3. W. B. Saunders Co., Philadelphia, 1969.)

In the normally functioning heart, with ventricular systole, or contraction, blood is forced from the left ventricle into the aorta and is distributed to the capillary beds in all parts of the body. The capillary blood is collected in veins and is returned to the right atrium of the heart via the vena cava. With contraction of the atria, blood is again forced into the ventricles. From the right ventricle, blood is carried to the lungs for oxygenation and returns to the left atrium via the pulmonary vein, ready for distribution to peripheral body parts once again.

Although many drugs can alter cardiovascular function, only those that have their main pharmacologic effect on the cardiovascular system will be discussed in this section. The others will be described elsewhere in connection with their other important pharmacodynamic properties.

CARDIAC GLYCOSIDES

Digitalis. The cardiac action of digitalis, or foxglove, was first reported to the medical world in 1785 by William Withering, physician and botanist of Birmingham, England. The professional curiosity of the English physicians of that time had been greatly aroused by the amazing cures of dropsy that were effected by an elderly woman in Shropshire who treated her patients with a jealously guarded family recipe. The formula was finally obtained by William Withering, and digitalis was discovered to be the active ingredient. His discovery must have awakened a latent poetic talent, for he soon described his "wonder drug" as follows:

THERAPEUTIC INDICATIONS FOR DIGITALIS

The Foxglove's leaves, with caution given,
Another proof of favouring Heav'n
Will happily display;
The rapid pulse it can abate;
The hectic flush can moderate
And, blest by Him whose will is fate,
May give a lengthen'd day.

Although digitalis was first acclaimed chiefly for its relief of dropsy, or edema, later studies revealed that its primary action was on the heart, and the diuresis that occurred with treatment, merely followed as a logical effect of improved circulation.

ACTIVE INGREDIENTS. Official digitalis is the dried leaf of the flowering foxglove plant, *Digitalis purpurea,* although *Digitalis lanata* is also used in some preparations.

The active constituents of these plants are glycosides. Each glycoside is an aglycone or "genin" combined with one to four molecules of sugar. Although the aglycone, or nonsugar portion, is the pharmacologically active part, this fraction of the molecule is not administered alone, because the attached sugars are necessary for the water solubility and cell penetrability needed for an optimal therapeutic effect.

The dried, powdered leaves of *D. purpurea* contain at least three cardiac glycosides: digitoxin, gitoxin and gitalin. Of these, digitoxin is by far the most important. *D. lanata* contains three precursor glycosides: lanatosides A, B, and C, which may be further hydrolyzed to give digitoxin, gitoxin and digoxin respectively. *D. lanata* is used chiefly for the lanatoside C and the digoxin components.

MODE OF ACTION. Digitalis acts primarily on the heart to (1) increase the force of systolic contraction, (2) slow conduction and lengthen the refractory period through the atrioventricular node and bundle of His and (3) increase vagal activity, which slows the heart. Secondary effects are a decrease in heart size, changes in cardiac output, and electrocardiographic changes.

The enlargement (dilation and hypertrophy) of the diseased heart is a compensatory reaction. Cardiac dilation, whether under physiologic conditions or associated with heart disease, is the means whereby the heart mobilizes its reserves of energy. The most common causes of cardiac hypertrophy are valvular disease and hypertension; less common causes are hyperthyroidism, adherent pericardium, anemia and congenital cardiac defects.

When a heart is persistently unable to maintain an adequate circulation during rest or mild exertion, the condition is called chronic or congestive heart failure. The chief manifestations of this condition are raised venous pressure, dyspnea, cyanosis, congestion and consequent enlargement of the spleen and liver, oliguria, albuminuria and edema. The edema (dropsy) was long thought to be a primary disease rather than the secondary effect of congestive heart failure.

The cardiac output in congestive heart failure is often less than normal and the diseased myocardium responds to a lesser degree than does normal heart muscle to an increase in venous pressure. As the myocardium fails, blood accumulates in the chambers of the heart and it dilates.

Digitalis was used to treat edema before its mechanism of action was understood. The present view is that digitalis does not affect urine flow except insofar as it improves the hemodynamics of heart failure. With increased force of systolic contraction and elevated cardiac output, venous return is increased as well. Thus blood is forced through the circulatory system more rapidly, and excretion of urine via the kidneys is facilitated.

Increased force of systolic contraction is the basic effect of digitalis at therapeutic dose levels during congestive heart failure. The increased force results in more complete emptying of the ventricles at systole and correspondingly greater output per beat. The slowing of the heart is due in part to slower conduction through the cardiac muscle, but to a greater extent to the enhanced vagal impulses to the heart.

ABSORPTION AND EXCRETION. The absorption of a single oral dose of digitalis begins within two hours after administration, and its maximal effect is reached within six to eight hours. When given intravenously, cardiac glycosides begin to exert their action within 10 minutes.

In the blood, cardiac glycosides are bound by serum albumin and then concentrated in various tissues of the body. Heart muscle does not selectively accumulate digitalis glycosides; their presence in the heart muscle merely has more effect than it has in other tissues. The exact fate of digitalis glycosides in man is unknown; however, their detoxification by the liver seems most likely. Only very small amounts are destroyed and excreted daily. This slow rate of excretion is the basis for the cumulative effects and the eventual poisoning that may occur from repeated doses. Following the initial large "digitalizing dose" of the drug in which optimal amounts of digitalis are stored in the heart, only small maintenance doses need be taken daily to replace the small amounts excreted. (See subsequent dosage schedule for digitalis preparations.)

TOXICITY. Many toxic effects of digitalis are merely extensions of its therapeutic actions. For this reason, a "nontoxic" digitalis does not exist. The optimal effective dose is very slightly less than that which has toxic effects; thus continual watchfulness for symptoms of toxicity is necessary.

Some of the earliest toxic effects of digitalis are disturbances in vision and gastrointestinal upsets. Vision is often blurred, white borders may appear on dark objects and objects may appear frosted. Color vision is often disturbed; chromatopsia is most common for yellow and green.

The gastrointestinal disturbances include anorexia, nausea, vomiting, diarrhea and abdominal discomfort. When the drug is discontinued, these effects disappear within a few days. Alteration in cardiac rate and rhythm occurs in some cases of overdosage. The

TABLE 9   A Comparison of Digitalis Preparations

	DIGITALIS LEAF	DIGITOXIN	DIGOXIN	LANATOSIDE C	GITALIN
Average adult digitalizing					
Dose: Oral	1.5 Gm.	1–2 mg.	2–3 mg.	5–10 mg.	5 mg.
I.M.	——	1–2 mg.	1–2 mg.	1–2 mg.	——
I.V.	0.3–0.4 Gm.	1–2 mg.	1–1.5 mg.	1–2 mg.	5–6 mg.
Average maintenance dose	0.1 Gm.	0.1–0.2 mg.	0.5 mg.	0.5–1.5 mg.	0.5 mg.
Onset of action from					
oral dose	3–4 hrs.	2–4 hrs.	1 hr.	variable	2–4 hrs.
Maximal effect from					
oral dose	12–24 hrs.	12–24 hrs.	6 hrs.	6 hrs.	8–10 hrs.
Onset of action from					
I.V. dose	1–2 hrs.	½–2 hrs.	5–10 min.	5–10 min.	1 hr.
Maximal effect from					
I.V. dose	12–24 hrs.	8–9 hrs.	1–2 hrs.	1–2 hrs.	8–9 hrs.
Duration of action	14–21 days	14–21 days	3 days	2–3 days	7–20 days

most prominent effect is an excessive slowing of the heart. For this reason it is necessary to take the pulse (preferably the apical pulse) for one full minute before administering each subsequent dose. If the apical pulse is below sixty, or there is any great change in rate or rhythm, the dose of the drug should be withheld and the physician notified.

Headache, fatigue, malaise and drowsiness are quite common symptoms of overdosage and occur early in the course of digitalis intoxication. Generalized muscle weakness and easy fatigability may be particularly prominent. Mental symptoms include disorientation, confusion, aphasia and even delirium and hallucinations. The neuropsychiatric effects are especially likely to develop in elderly arteriosclerotic patients. The exact physiological effects of digitalis in this area are unknown, however.

A potassium deficiency or a high calcium blood level increases the danger of toxicity. Oral calcium preparations and vitamin and mineral supplements containing calcium salts should not be taken concurrently with digitalis administration. Thiazide diuretics should not be given with digitalis because the potassium loss they cause enhances the toxic effects of digitalis.

STANDARDIZATION.   Because of the wide variance in potencies of the many preparations of digitalis, there was an obvious need for standardization. For many years the response of the cat was used to standardize digitalis. The cat unit, or the amount of digitalis that effects a predetermined response in the cat, has been replaced by the official U.S.P. digitalis unit, using the pigeon as a standard test animal. The U.S.P unit represents the potency of 0.1 Gm. of digitalis powder, approximately the average daily maintenance dose.

Variations in potency of U.S.P. digitalis still occur; this necessitates caution in changing from one commercial brand to another, and a patient whose maintenance dose is well-regulated on one U.S.P. product cannot be shifted indiscriminately to another in the belief that the same dose can be prescribed. Furthermore, one digitalis preparation injected intravenously usually has a greater effect than if it were given orally; two products of comparable intravenous potency may differ greatly from each other when administered by mouth because of the wide variations in the degree of absorption from the gastrointestinal tract.

The nurse should be very careful that she is administering the correct digitalis preparation and dosage, because names of the preparations are quite similar. Their dosage, onset of action and length of action vary greatly, however.

PREPARATIONS OF *Digitalis purpurea* (PURPLE FOXGLOVE)

Powdered Digitalis, U.S.P.; Prepared Digitalis, B.P.

Digitalis Tincture, N.F.

Digitalis Tablets

Digitora Tablets: A mixture of the cardiac glycosides in the digitalis leaf.

Digitoxin, U.S.P., B.P. (Crystodigin, Digitaline Nativelle, Purodigin)

Gitalin (Gitaligin): A mixture of cardiac glycosides

$C_{18}H_{31}O_9$

digitoxin

PREPARATIONS OF *Digitalis lanata* (WHITE FOXGLOVE)

Lanatoside C, N.F. (Cedilanid)

Deslanoside, N.F. (Cedilanid-D): Chemically derived from lanatoside C, this preparation is somewhat more water soluble and is the form preferred for parenteral administration.

Digoxin, U.S.P., B.P. (Lanoxin)

Acetyldigitoxin (Acylanid)

COMBINATIONS OF DIGITALIS PRINCIPLES

Digilanid. This is a mixture of lanatosides A, B and C. Its action closely resembles official whole digitalis leaf.

> **DOSE.** Digitalizing—3 to 6 mg. orally.
> Maintenance—0.33 to 0.66 mg. orally daily.

Digalen. Digalen is a purified mixture of the cardiac glycosides in digitalis leaf. Its effect is comparable to whole leaf.

> **DOSE.** Digitalizing—10 to 15 units orally.

> Maintenance—0.8 to 1.6 units orally daily.

Digifolin. This preparation contains the natural mixture of cardiac glycoside of digitalis leaf from which the therapeutically inert material has been separated. The action is very similar to the whole leaf.

> **DOSE.** Digitalizing—10 to 15 units orally.
> Maintenance—0.8 to 1.6 units orally daily.

OUABAIN INJECTION, U.S.P., B.P. (G-STROPHANTHIN).

Ouabain is a crystalline glycoside obtained from the seeds of *Strophanthus gratus* or from the wood of *Acokanthera schimperi.* This glycoside has all the pharmacologic actions of digitalis, but unlike digitalis, ouabain is not absorbed from the gastrointestinal tract and thus must be given intravenously. This may account in part for its infrequent use. The onset of action occurs in a few minutes with the peak about $1\frac{1}{2}$ hours after administration. Ouabain is used when a rapid effect is desired, such as in emergency treatment of acute heart failure, supraventricular arrhythmia or atrial flutter.

> **TOXICITY.** Symptoms of toxicity resemble those of digitalis.

> **DOSE.** Digitalizing—1 mg. I.V.
> Maintenance—Usually maintenance is carried out with a digitalis glycoside rather than with ouabain.

SQUILL. The dried, fleshy bulb of this "sea onion," *Urginea maritima,* exhibits cardiac action comparable to that of digitalis and ouabain. Scillaren is a mixture of the two natural glycosides (component A and component B) occurring in fresh squill. The drug is available only for oral administration.

> **TOXICITY.** The toxic potential is comparable to that of digitalis.

> **DOSE.** Digitalizing—9.6 to 14.4 mg. orally.
> Maintenance—0.8 to 3.2 mg. orally daily.

NURSING IMPLICATIONS

An important role of the nurse in caring for a patient receiving digitalis preparations is to observe for indications of toxicity. Since digitalis may cause excessive slowing of the heart, the nurse should count the patient's pulse before she administers a dose. The pulse should be counted for one full minute in order to detect any irregularities. If it is below 60 beats per minute, or if there is a great change in the pulse, the dose should not be given until the physician is notified. The apical pulse is preferable for a more accurate indication of cardiac rate, since weaker contractions of the heart may not be perceptible at the radial artery. Taking the apical-radial pulse to determine the pulse deficit may be indicated in order to evaluate cardiac arrhythmias and cardiac efficiency. The pulse rate and other characteristics should be recorded along with a notation that the digitalis dose was administered or omitted.

Since there may be little difference between the digitalizing dose and the toxic dose, the nurse should be alert for indications of toxicity. When the patient is receiving maintenance doses of digitalis preparations which have a long duration of action (e.g., Digitoxin), toxicity may develop gradually from the overlapping effects of repeated doses.

Other conditions may affect the development of toxicity in a particular patient. If the patient has hypokalemia or hypercalcemia, the effect of digitalis on the myocardium is increased. The nurse should be aware of the symptoms and laboratory tests which reflect these electrolyte disturbances in order to prevent the development of digitalis toxicity. Since many patients who are receiving digitalis are also on diuretic therapy, the possibility of fluid and electrolyte disturbances from the diuretic drug must be considered in relation to their effect on cardiac action and digitalis therapy. A further discussion of fluid and electrolyte balance is found in Chapter 19.

Oral preparations of digitalis should be given preferably with or after meals in order to prevent the possibility of gastric irritation. When preparations are given intramuscularly, the nurse should insure that they are given deep into the muscle because of the problem of tissue irritation. When given intravenously, digitalis glycosides should be given slowly and the patient should be observed carefully.

Other measures to promote optimum cardiac function and to prevent the occurrence of congestive heart failure are important in the total care of the patient. Diuretics and dietary sodium restrictions may be prescribed in order to decrease or prevent the development of excess fluid which places added stress on the heart. The effect of physical stress on cardiac function may be reduced by restricting the patient's activity; the degree of restriction depends on the patient's condition and may range from strict bedrest to curtailment of only extreme types of physical activity. The emotional and psychological causes of stress must also be identified and relieved whenever possible. Reassuring the patient and explaining his care and treatment will do much to alleviate some of this stress.

Observations for the effectiveness of the digitalis therapy should be made. There should be a general slowing of the pulse rate, and the improved circulation resulting from the more forceful heart contraction should be reflected in the relief of the symptoms of congestive heart failure. The patient should feel less fatigue and should gain increasing strength. Visible edema, such as in the legs and ankles, should decrease gradually. The patient should experience relief from dyspnea and orthopnea, and skin color should improve. A decrease in weight would reflect the increased renal excretion of excess fluid. This secondary diuretic effect of digitalis can also be measured by maintaining and assessing the record of the patient's intake and output.

The patient needs to understand the purpose of his drug therapy and total plan of care. The nurse should insure that the patient who is taking digitalis at home knows the importance and necessity of taking the drug as prescribed. Patients have been known to omit doses and then take two or three doses at once to "make up" for the doses missed. If the patient or a family member is capable, he may be taught to take his pulse each day. The patient should be advised of the symptoms that should be reported to his physician and of the necessity of continued medical supervision. Symptoms which the patient should report include those of digitalis toxicity as well as signs and symptoms that may indicate congestive heart failure. Because of the many interrelationships involved in congestive heart failure, the patient must also understand his underlying condition and other aspects of the therapeutic plan, such as sodium restrictions, the degree of activity advised and other drug therapy.

ANTIARRHYTHMIC AND ANTIFIBRILLATORY AGENTS

The antiarrhythmic and antifibrillatory agents are drugs that act to restore normal sinus rhythm to the heart. Arrhythmias may be caused by any condition which affects the irritability or sensitivity of the heart to nervous impulses. Electrolyte imbalances may cause or precipitate arrhythmias. Arrhythmias frequently are caused by ischemia or infarct of the myocardial tissue, resulting in disturbances of the electrical conduction pathways in the heart. Stimulation of the autonomic nervous system may also influence cardiac rate and the development of various types of arrhythmias.

Arrhythmias usually result in a very rapid or very slow heart rate. Other arrhythmias may produce a radial pulse rate within normal range; they are detected by apical pulses, auscultation, or electrocardiogram interpretation. The efficiency of the heart may be affected by some arrhythmias. A few arrhythmias are dangerous and may be rapidly fatal, or cause congestive heart failure and cardiogenic shock.

In caring for the patient with a cardiac arrhythmia, the nurse should observe the patient's general status as well as indications of the arrhythmia. The patient's arrhythmia may be visualized and checked by the use of a cardiac monitor if one is available. The

apical-radial pulse may be used to determine the pulse deficit which will reflect the efficiency of the heart's contractions. The patient's apical pulse should be counted before administering each dose of an antiarrhythmic agent.

The patient's general cardiac status should be observed closely for indications that the arrhythmia is affecting the cardiac output. The nurse should observe particularly for signs of pulmonary edema, congestive heart failure and cardiogenic shock.

In coronary care units and other specialized units, nurses who have had advanced and specialized training usually take a greater responsibility in the administration of certain cardiac drugs by the intravenous route. These nurses give the drugs on the basis of their identification of certain arrhythmias reflected in electrocardiographic changes on the cardiac monitor.

QUINIDINE SULFATE, U.S.P., B.P.   Quinidine, an optical isomer of quinine, is one of the natural alkaloids obtained from Cinchona bark. It has many of the pharmacologic properties of quinine, but its actions on cardiac muscle are more specific and more effective than those of quinine.

USES.   Quinidine prolongs the refractory period of the heart muscle, decreases its irritability and rate of conductivity and depresses the activity of the vagus nerve. In digitalized hearts, quinidine may cause various and often unpredictable abnormalities of rhythm, including cardiac arrest.

Quinidine is absorbed rapidly from the upper gastrointestinal tract, and maximal cardiac effects are usually obtained within three hours with residual effects persisting six to eight hours or more. It is excreted via the kidneys.

TOXICITY.   Like all cinchona alkaloids, quinidine in large doses can cause the condition known as "cinchonism," which in its mildest form consists of ringing in the ears, headache, nausea and slightly disturbed vision. After larger doses, symptoms also involve the gastrointestinal tract and the central nervous system, with headache, fever, confusion, nausea, vomiting and pain. Hypersensitivity reactions occur occasionally. Fatalities sometimes occur from cardiac standstill or ventricular fibrillation. Quinidine is contraindicated in patients who have had severe cinchonism, in patients with severe infection, such as bacterial endocarditis, and in those with chronic valvular disease or heart block.

Apical pulse should be checked before administering the drug. Oral doses are given before meals in order to promote maximum absorption. When given intravenously, quinidine should be injected very slowly.

DOSE. Oral—200 to 400 mg. three to five times daily for one to three days. I.V.—300 to 500 mg.

PROCAINAMIDE HYDROCHLORIDE, U.S.P., B.P. (PRONESTYL). The amide of procaine is an effective antiarrhythmic agent, particularly in patients with abnormal ventricular rhythms. It has a longer duration of action than procaine because it is not hydrolyzed as readily and it is less toxic and has fewer central nervous system effects.

procainamide hydrochloride

Procainamide has essentially the same cardiac effects as quinidine. Excitability of both the atria and the ventricles is depressed and conduction in the atria, bundle of His and ventricles is slowed because of the prolonged refractory period.

Intravenous administration of procainamide causes hypotension that is more pronounced when the initial blood pressure is high and when the drug is injected rapidly. This effect is usually not produced by oral administration. The blood pressure should be checked before and during intravenous therapy.

The local anesthetic effects of procainamide are comparable to those of procaine, except that, like many amides, the drug is poorly effective for the blocking of nerve trunks.

Procainamide is rapidly absorbed from the gastrointestinal tract. Approximately 60 per cent is excreted unchanged by the kidneys, much of the rest is slowly hydrolyzed by plasma esterases.

Solutions of the drug may become slightly yellow, without any pharmacologic alteration, but any solution that is brown should be discarded.

TOXICITY. Ventricular tachycardia or even fibrillation similar to that produced by quinidine may occur. In patients with conduction disturbances, procainamide causes additional depression of conduction. When it is given orally, gastrointestinal upsets occur, such as nausea, vomiting, diarrhea and anorexia. Mental depression and hallucinations have been reported. Frequent blood examinations during therapy are essential because fatal agranulocytosis has been reported following prolonged use of procainamide.

The only absolute contraindication to its use is hypersensitivity to the drug; the other dangers must be balanced against the patient's condition and the beneficial effect expected to be attained by administration of the drug.

DOSE. Oral—250 mg. 3 or 4 times daily. I.V.—100 mg. slowly in I.V. drip.

XYLOCAINE HYDROCHLORIDE (LIDOCAINE). Orginally developed as a local anesthetic, xylocaine has been shown to be extremely effective as an antifibrillatory agent when administered intravenously. It is believed to exert its effect by increasing the threshold for stimulation in the ventricles during diastole, or the relaxation phase of the heart. It is often employed in cardiac intensive care units most particularly for the period immediately following myocardial infarctions, when the damaged myocardium may go into fibrillation. Ventricular fibrillation if not corrected within a very short period will lead to death. Constant monitoring with an electrocardiograph is necessary when this drug is administered so that the dose can be carefully titrated.

TOXICITY. Xylocaine is metabolized by the liver and excreted by the kidney, thus predisposing liver or kidney disorders may allow toxic accumulations of the drug; the dosage should be lowered accordingly if this agent is to be used under these conditions. Drowsiness, dizziness, tinnitus, blurred vision, vomiting, twitching, tremors, convulsions, hypotension, cardiovascular collapse and bradycardia may occur with overdosage.

DOSE. 50 to 100 mg. I.V. at a rate of 25 to 50 mg./minute. No more than 300 mg. may be administered in a one hour period. I.V. infusions may be given at a rate of 1 to 4 mg./minute.

PROPANOLOL HYDROCHLORIDE (INDERAL). Propanolol is an antiarrhythmic agent which exerts its effect due to its action as a beta-blocker. The beta type of adrenergic or sympathetic receptor is present in the myocardium and is responsive to circulating norepinephrine. Sympathetic stimulation in the form of circulating norepinephrine produces acceleration in rate and strength of cardiac contraction; however, it is believed that in certain instances this same hormonal stimulation may be responsible for producing arrhythmias in susceptible individuals. This drug acts by competing with norepinephrine for the beta receptor sites, thus preventing excessive stimulation with the sympathetic hormones. There is a reduction in heart rate and force of contraction, which counteracts cardiac hyperactivity. Propanolol does not interfere with the action of digitalis, and may be used with digitalis in some instances. It may be used in atrial flutter and fibrillation, in paroxysmal atrial tachycardia and in the control of extrasystoles, both atrial and ventricular.

Prior to surgery for pheochromocytomas, this agent will protect the heart from the effects of excessive circulating levels of epinephrine and norepinephrine. It is usually used in combination with an alpha-blocker such as phentolamine (Regitine) or phenoxybenzamine (Dibenzyline) when given preoperatively for this purpose. If an alpha-blocker were not used concomitantly, the alpha receptors would go unopposed and excessive and dangerous hypertension could result.

TOXICITY. This drug is contraindicated in bronchial asthma and allergic rhinitis (since responsiveness to epinephrine and norepinephrine is often necessary in the acute control of these diseases.) It is also contraindicated in patients on MAO inhibitors, in congestive heart failure and cardiogenic shock. Side effects noted are nausea, vomiting, diarrhea, lassitude, skin rash, paresthesias of the hands, hallucinations and alopecia.

DOSE. Oral—10 to 30 mg. three times daily. I.V.—1 to 3 mg. administered with EKG monitoring. Rate should not exceed 1 mg./minute.

VASODILATORS AND ANTIHYPERTENSIVE AGENTS

Various types of drugs are used to produce vasodilation in certain conditions in order to increase the blood supply to tissues or to lower the person's blood pressure.

Hypertension is a condition in which a person's blood pressure is elevated persistently above normal. A systolic pressure greater than 150 mm. Hg. or a diastolic pressure above 90 mm. Hg. are considered indicative of hypertension. Measures must be taken to reduce the hypertension because of the increased stress placed on the cardiovascular system and the resulting physiologic changes.

Essential hypertension is the term used to describe hypertension for which there is no evident pathologic basis such as renal disease or pheochromocytoma. Sodium appears to have some role in essential hypertension, since sodium restriction and the use of diuretics usually results in a decrease in blood pressure. Other drugs used in hypertension are directed to the relaxation and dilation of arterioles.

When patients are receiving antihypertensive drugs, the blood pressure and pulse should be checked frequently in order to assess drug effect and also to observe for too great or too rapid a drop in the blood pressure. Postural hypotension may occur and may require close supervision of the patient.

The nurse should be observant for factors which may be contributing to the patient's hypertension. Emotional and psychological stress may cause an increased sympathetic response resulting in vasoconstriction and elevation of the blood pressure. Sedatives or tranquilizers may be needed. A quiet environment and plan of care which allows periods of rest for the patient is of particular importance during periods of extreme hypertension. Stimulants, such as tobacco and caffeine, should be avoided.

The drugs to be discussed in this section dilate the blood vessels and consequently lower blood pressure, but they do not accomplish the effect through the autonomic nervous system. The agents that act via the autonomic nervous system have been previously discussed.

THE NITRITES

The basic action of the nitrites in the body is to relax smooth muscles, especially those of the smaller blood vessels. Therefore, a fall in blood pressure is their most characteristic effect. The speed and extent of the decline depends on the dose and preparation of nitrite used, the route of administration, the original level of the blood pressure and the individual's susceptibility to the drug.

The nitrites exert no direct effect on the myocardium. Cardiac output is either not altered or decreased only slightly. The coronary vasodilation produced by the nitrites improves the deficient blood supply to the heart. When they are used in angina pectoris, the functional pain due to myocardial ischemia is relieved, and the heart is able to work more efficiently.

Amyl nitrite may be absorbed from the lungs and is often supplied as "perles," which are easily crushed in a handkerchief for inhalation of the vapors when an angina attack is imminent. Relief is usually obtained within one minute. It is inactivated almost immediately by the gastric hydrochloric acid when taken orally, and it is poorly effective when administered hypodermically. Nitroglycerin is usually administered sublingually in the form of soluble tablets, because absorption through the mucous membrane is more effective than if the drug is swallowed. Erythrityl tetranitrate and mannitol hexanitrate are slowly absorbed from the gastrointestinal tract. This accounts for their delayed onset of action and prolonged effect.

Nitroglycerin is one of the few medications that a patient is usually allowed to have at his bedside if ordered by his physician. The number of tablets should be counted and should be checked each day to determine how many the patient has used and to replenish the supply if necessary. The patient should have a fresh supply and should keep them in a tightly sealed container since exposure to air may decrease their effectiveness. Patients should be instructed to be in a sitting or lying position when they take these tablets because of the danger of fainting or dizziness from hypotension. They should also be instructed to report the occurrence of pain. The nurse should assess the characteristics of the pain, the circumstances precipitating the anginal attack and whether it was relieved by the nitroglycerin. If relief is not obtained, the physician should be notified immediately since this may indicate coronary occlusion.

TOXICITY

When present in excess, the nitrite ion oxidizes hemoglobin to methemoglobin, causing cyanosis and functional anemia by lowering the blood's oxygen-carrying power. Headache, increased intraocular pressure, syncope and cardiovascular collapse have been noted. Following large doses of nitrites, cardiovascular collapse is due to the pooling of blood on the venous side of the circulatory system and is not due to arteriole dilation. Indeed, there may be reflex constriction of the arterioles in an attempt to maintain blood pressure. This constriction may even produce a "paradoxical anginal attack" from an overdose of drug given to treat the condition.

The smallest effective dose of the nitrites should always be given, because the body rapidly builds a tolerance to these drugs. Within several weeks the tolerance is quite pronounced, but it is quickly lost when the drug is discontinued. During this time, the nitrite is replaced with another drug until the patient again becomes susceptible to the nitrite's effects.

PREPARATIONS AND DOSES

Amyl Nitrite, N.F.—0.2 ml. by inhalation.

Glyceryl Trinitrate, U.S.P., B.P. (Nitroglycerin, Trinitrin)—0.1 to 1 mg. sublingually.

$$CH_2-O-NO_2$$
$$CH-O-NO_2$$
$$CH_2-O-NO_2$$

glyceryl trinitrate

Sodium Nitrite, U.S.P.—30 to 60 mg. orally every 3 or 4 hours.

Erythrityl Tetranitrate (Cardilate)—15 to 60 mg. orally every 4 to 6 hours.

Mannitol Hexanitrate (Nitranitol)—16 to 64 mg. orally every 4 to 6 hours.

Pentaerythritol Tetranitrate (Peritrate, Pentritol)—10 to 20 mg. orally three or four times daily.

Isosorbide Dinitrate (Isordil)—5 to 10 mg. every 4 hours.

VERATRUM ALKALOIDS

Veratrum is an ancient drug that was used in the Middle Ages in sorcery and mystical rites; it has also been used as a crow poison, an insecticide, an emetic, a local counterirritant, a cardiotonic and an adjunct in the treatment of fever and eclampsia.

The veratrum alkaloids are a family of substances from plants belonging to the suborder Melanthaceae. The species usually employed as sources of the alkaloids are *Veratrum album*, *V. viride*, and *V. sabadilla*. The composition of mixtures of the veratrum alkaloids varies greatly from preparation to preparation and is determined by the species, the habitat and the part of the plant employed.

The principal effect of the alkaloids on the cardiovascular system is called the Bezold effect—a reflex decrease in blood pressure and heart rate. The hypotension results from peripheral vasodilation and not from a decrease in cardiac output. Perhaps this results in large part from reflex inhibition of the central vasomotor center. The afferent impulses of this reflex inhibition appear to arise in the carotid sinuses, the left ventricle and the lungs, but delineation of the efferent pathway is unclear. The drugs are not adrenergic or ganglionic blocking agents.

Doses of veratrum alkaloids larger than those required to affect the cardiovascular system produce a direct central depression of respiration and a direct bronchoconstrictor effect.

The alkaloids act on nerve fibers and skeletal muscle to produce a prolonged secondary tetanus following the normal initial twitch induced by single direct or indirect stimulation. The contraction is associated with a repetitive discharge of impulses in the muscle fibers. Veratrine appears to promote potassium leakage from cells and to interfere with the movement of sodium across the neuronal membrane in its repolarization.

TOXICITY

The range between the therapeutic and toxic doses of veratrum alkaloids is quite narrow. Parenteral administration necessitates careful regulation of dosage and close observation for blood pressure changes and for respiratory depression. Atropine should be available as an antidote. Other toxic effects may include nausea, vomiting, excessive salivation and perspiration, hiccups, numbness and tingling in the extremities, flushing, confusion, blurred vision and gastrointestinal upsets.

Although the incidence of side effects is greater when the drug is given orally, they are generally less severe and transitory. The appearance of toxic effects during parenteral administration very often necessitates discontinuation of the drug.

ALKAVERVIR (VERILOID). Alkavervir is a mixture of alkaloids from *V. viride*.

> **DOSE.** 3 to 5 mg. orally three times daily.

CRYPTENAMINE ACETATES (UNITENSEN). A selective isolation of alkaloids from *V. viride* is carried out to produce cryptenamine. It is available in oral and injectable forms. Parenteral therapy is restricted to hospitalized or closely supervised patients and is employed in eclampsia (convulsive toxemia), hypertensive crisis (encephalopathy), pre-eclampsia (nonconvulsive toxemia) and pre-eclampsia with underlying essential hypertension.

> **DOSE.** Oral—2 mg. twice daily. Parenteral—1 mg. diluted with 20 ml. of 5% dextrose solution and infused at the rate of 1 ml./minute.

PROTOVERATRINE A (PROTALBA). Protoveratrine A is one of the alkaloids from *V. album.*

> **DOSE.** 200 to 400 mcg. orally four times daily.

PROTOVERATRINE A AND B MALEATES (VERALBA, PROVELL MALEATE). This mixture of two alkaloids from *V. album* may be administered orally, intravenously or intramuscularly. When given intravenously, the patient should be kept flat for at least an hour, and his blood pressure and pulse should be monitored frequently.

> **DOSE.** Oral—500 mcg. four times daily. I.M.—120 to 400 mcg. every 4 to 8 hours. I.V.— 100 mcg. diluted with 10 ml. saline and administered at a rate of 0.5 ml./min. for 8 min. Smaller doses may be administered every 2 minutes thereafter for a total dose of 80 to 160 mcg.

RAUWOLFIA SERPENTINA

The powdered root of this shrub has been used for centuries for many disorders, especially for certain types of mental disorders. Although it is an effective tranquilizer, at present more clinical attention is given to its cardiovascular effects, i.e., a reduction of arterial blood pressure and a slowing of the heart rate. Conventional doses do not cause direct peripheral vasodilation or adrenergic or ganglionic blocking.

The drug has a tranquilizing effect on the central nervous system, resulting in a reduction in spontaneous activity with relaxation. Unlike the barbiturates, which act by a general central nervous system depression, rauwolfia appears to merely reduce attention and responsiveness to external stimuli, thus tranquilizing rather than sedating the individual.

Rauwolfia is adequately absorbed from the gastrointestinal tract, but there is a slow onset of action, suggesting that the drug may act indirectly. Similarly, when the medication is withdrawn, the hypotension and bradycardia may persist for several weeks. It is theorized that the drug acts by blocking afferent impulses that normally stimulate sympathetic vasopressor reflexes near the level of the hypothalamus and by decreasing the reactivity of the peripheral sympathetic nervous system. It also decreases the level of circulating epinephrine and norepinephrine. Excretion appears to be via the kidney.

TOXICITY

Side effects are mild when they appear and usually do not necessitate the withdrawal of the drug. They include lethargy, nasal congestion, weakness and diarrhea. Large doses may increase gastric secretion, and produce mental depression and cause difficulty in peptic ulcer patients. When possible they should be administered after meals. The drug passes the placental barrier and may affect the fetus. This drug should be used with caution in bronchial asthma patients since this condition may be aggravated by the drop in catecholamine level.

Rauwolfia serpentina, N.F. (Raudixin). Whole root.

> **DOSE.** 50 to 100 mg. orally three times daily.

Alseroxylon (Rauwiloid). This is a partially purified mixture of the sedative-antihypertensive alkaloids.

> **DOSE.** 2 to 4 mg. orally daily.

Reserpine, U.S.P., B.P. (Rau-Sed, Serpasil, Reserpoid, Sandril). Reserpine is probably the preparation that is used in most instances for its cardiovascular and tranquilizing effects.

> **DOSE.** Hypotensive—0.1 to 1.0 mg. orally or I.M. daily. Tranquilizing—2 to 5 mg. orally daily.

reserpine

Syrosingopine (Singoserp). This drug is a synthetic analogue of reserpine and is less potent than the parent compound.

> **DOSE.** 1 to 2 mg. orally daily.

Other vasodilators and antihypertensive agents

Hydralazine hydrochloride, N.F., B.P. (Apresoline). This agent is a hypotensive drug, but it is less effective than reserpine. It reduces pathologically elevated blood pressure and yet increases cardiac output and blood flow through the kidneys.

The mechanism of action of hydralazine has been subject to much debate. It has been shown to exert an antihypertensive effect as a result of renal vasodilation, but many believe there is a direct general relaxation of vascular smooth muscle as well. This is widely accepted as being the predominant mode of action.

It is of value in essential and malignant hypertension as well as in hypertension of pregnancy and that which persists after sympathectomy. It is contraindicated in angina pectoris because of its cardiac stimulation. Hydralazine is often combined with reserpine in the therapeutic management of hypertension.

> **TOXICITY.** The incidence of untoward effects from hydralazine is high. Headache, palpitation, nausea and vomiting are the most common side effects. Postural hypotension, nasal congestion, flushing, paresthesias, dizziness and muscle cramps occur occasionally. Dermatoses and blood dyscrasias occur rarely. Chronic administration of large doses causes an acute rheumatoid state in approximately 10 per cent of cases; this disappears when the drug is withdrawn, however. Skin reactions resembling those of lupus erythematosus have been reported occasionally.

> **DOSE.** Oral—25 mg. four times daily after meals and at bedtime; and may be gradually increased to 100 mg. four times daily.

> I.M. or I.V.—20 to 40 mg. every 6 hours with careful monitoring of blood pressure.

Methyldopa (Aldomet). This antihypertensive compound is a decarboxylase inhibitor and interferes with the formation of both norepinephrine and serotonin, thus indirectly lowering the blood pressure via the autonomic nervous system. It is recommended for patients with sustained moderate to severe hypertension.

> **TOXICITY.** A transient sedation sometimes occurs during early therapy. Aggravation of angina pectoris has been reported as have occasional instances of nasal congestion, gastrointestinal disturbances, fever and reversible jaundice. The use of methyldopa is contraindicated in active hepatic disease. It is not recommended for patients with mild or labile hypertension that is responsive to mild sedation or thiazide therapy.

> **DOSE.** 0.5 to 2 Gm. orally daily.

MEBUTAMATE (CAPLA). Chemically related to meprobamate, this drug has similar pharmacological effects. Mebutamate appears to lower blood pressure by a selective action on vasomotor control centers in the brain stem and on vasomotor tracts in the spinal cord. It is useful in treating mild hypertension.

TOXICITY. Drowsiness, dizziness, headache, weakness and mild gastrointestinal disturbances may occur.

DOSE. 300 mg. orally three or four times daily.

PAPAVERINE HYDROCHLORIDE, N.F., B.P. Unlike the rest of the opium alkaloids, papaverine is non-narcotic and non-addicting. Its main actions are exerted on cardiac and smooth muscle. It acts directly on the heart muscle to depress conduction and prolong the refractory period. Smooth muscles, espe-

papaverine hydrochloride

cially of the larger arteries, are relaxed. Little is known of its fate in the body or its exact mechanism of action.

USES. Papaverine has been employed for severe cardiac pain due to coronary occlusion and for peripheral vasodilation. It is not as dependable as the nitrites for the treatment of angina pectoris, but it has been employed for this condition.

TOXICITY. Although the toxicity of papaverine is low, the drug should be injected slowly since cardiac arrhythmias and fatal apnea may result from rapid injection. Other side effects are flushing, sweating and mild constipation. The drug should be injected cautiously when the heart muscle is depressed. Solutions that are cloudy should not be used.

DOSE. 0.1 Gm. orally three or four times daily.

30 to 60 mg. I.M. or I.V. one to three times daily.

DIOXYLINE PHOSPHATE (PAVERIL). The structure of dioxyline differs only slightly from that of papaverine, but its pharmacologic activity is greatly enhanced. The actions and uses are the same as those for papaverine.

DOSE. 200 to 300 mg. orally three or four times daily.

CYCLANDELATE (CYCLOSPASMOL). Cyclandelate exerts a direct, papaverine-like effect on smooth muscles, especially those of the arterial walls. It is used in the management of occlusive vascular disease and vasospastic conditions.

TOXICITY. Flushing, tingling of extremities, headache, gastrointestinal disturbances and tachycardia have been reported but appear to be of little consequence.

DOSE. 200 mg. orally four times daily.

DIPYRIDAMOLE (PERSANTIN). The mode of action of dipyridamole is unknown, but it appears to act on the coronary vessels and the myocardial cells to increase coronary blood flow without significantly changing blood pressure or heart rate. It is used for the treatment of coronary insufficiency, angina pectoris and in postmyocardial infarction therapy. It is not recommended in the acute phase of myocardial infarction because it has not been fully evaluated in this condition.

TOXICITY. Headache, dizziness, weakness, gastrointestinal disturbances and dermatoses have been reported. It should be used cautiously in patients with hypertension.

DOSE. 25 to 50 mg. orally two or three times daily.

ISOXSUPRINE HYDROCHLORIDE (VASODILAN). Isoxsuprine has been administered orally, intramuscularly, intravenously, subcutaneously and intraarterially to patients with peripheral vascular disease. It appears to be useful as a myovascular relaxant for the relief of symptoms due to arterial insufficiency in patients with peripheral vascular disorders. In addition, it is useful in the treatment of cerebral vascular insufficiency and uterine hypermotility and spasm. In women with acute, debilitating dysmenorrhea, it relieves cramps without producing noticeable side effects.

TOXICITY. Toxic effects have occurred chiefly with extremely large doses. They include tachycardia, hypotension, nausea, vomiting and fainting.

DOSE. 10 to 20 mg. orally three or four times daily.

ANTILIPEMIC AGENT

CLOFIBRATE (ATROMID-S). Clofibrate appears to lower blood cholesterol by interfering with the rate of biosynthesis. Elevated blood phospholipid and triglyceride levels are also reduced, but normal levels do not seem to be affected. Females appear much more susceptible to the action of this drug than males and show greater reduction in the blood levels of lipids with similar doses.

It is well absorbed orally and is used in the treatment of hypercholesterolemia and/or hypertriglyceridemia. Treatment of familial lipid disorders has generally proved to be of little value. When the drug is withdrawn, there is a rapid return of blood lipids to or above pretreatment levels within two to three weeks. It is not generally believed to be of long term benefit in the treatment or prevention of atherosclerosis.

TOXICITY. Nausea, vomiting, diarrhea, headache, weakness, lethargy, dermatoses, pruritis, alopecia, muscle cramping, leukopenia and agranulocytosis have been reported. It should be administered with caution to patients with diabetes mellitus as hypoglycemic episodes have occurred. Doses of anticoagulants should be reduced to one-third to one-half the original dose when administered with this drug, as clofibrate also causes prolonged prothrombin time.

DOSE. 500 mg. orally four times daily.

NURSING IMPLICATIONS IN PERIPHERAL VASCULAR DISEASE

When a patient with peripheral vascular disease is receiving a vasodilator to increase the peripheral blood flow, the nurse should observe closely for evidence of increased circulation. The pedal and popliteal pulse should be checked bilaterally for their presence, strength and equality of strength. The skin color should reflect increased tissue oxygenation as evidenced by a decrease in cyanosis or blanching of the skin, increased warmth and sensation and decreased numbness and tingling.

Patients should be taught measures to promote optimal circulation, such as avoiding caffeine and tobacco, long periods of sitting and girdles or round garters. Measures should also be taken to prevent skin breakdown and injury which could easily lead to infection and gangrene if the blood supply is not sufficient. Patients should be taught to inspect their feet daily for signs of injury and to apply lotions to their skin if dry. Tepid water only should be used in soaking their feet because of the decrease in sensation which could lead to accidental burning without their realizing it.

SCLEROSING AGENTS

Modern therapists often advise surgical procedures for varicose veins. Sclerosing agents are still used to some extent, however, in the obliteration of the varicosities. They act to sclerose or destroy the functional capabilities of the veins into which they are injected. Collateral circulation must subsequently transport the blood that formerly was carried via the varicosed vein.

SODIUM MORRHUATE, U.S.P. Sodium morrhuate, a combination of the sodium salts of the fatty acids of cod liver oil, is quite effective in sclerosing veins. Contraindications to its use include incompetency of the collateral deep veins of the lower extremities, active or recent phlebitis, tuberculosis, hyperthyroidism, cardiac decompensation and pregnancy.

DOSE. 1 ml. of a 5% solution injected

I.V. The maximal amount at any site should not exceed 2 ml.

SODIUM PSYLLIATE, N.F. (SYLNASOL). In addition to its use for varicosities of the lower extremities, sodium psylliate also scleroses internal hemorrhoids that are not prolapsed or thrombosed. It is a combination of the sodium salts of the fatty acids from psyllium (*Plantago ovata*).

DOSE. 0.1 to 6 ml. of a 5% solution injected I.V. once or twice weekly.

SODIUM TETRADECYL SULFATE (SODIUM SOTRADECOL). Like sodium psylliate, sodium tetradecyl sulfate is used to sclerose varicose veins and internal hemorrhoids.

DOSE. Used in 1, 3 or 5% solution. No more than 6 ml. of 5% solution and proportional amounts of lower concentrations should be used.

GUIDE FOR THE NURSING ASSESSMENT OF A PATIENT RECEIVING A DIGITALIS GLYCOSIDE

I. Why is the patient receiving this drug? What is the pathophysiology underlying the need for digitalis? What signs and symptoms did or does the patient have? How long has the patient been receiving digitalis?

II. Is the digitalis drug being administered correctly? Is the correct dosage and preparation being given? Is the apical or apical-radial pulse determined before each dose is administered? Is the dose being withheld if the pulse is below 60 or has changed greatly in rate or characteristics? If administered orally, is the digitalis drug given with or after meals to decrease gastric irritation? If given intramuscularly, is it given deep into the muscle? If given intravenously, is it given slowly and the patient observed closely?

III. Is the digitalis preparation producing the desired effect? Is there a decrease in the pulse? Is it stronger and more regular? Is there a decrease in the pulse deficit, if present previously? Do the interpretations of electrocardiograms indicate improvement in cardiac function? Is there evidence of increased efficiency of cardiac function? Is there a decrease in respiratory rate, dyspnea, orthopnea, rales and other signs of pulmonary edema? Is there an improvement in general skin color? Is there a decrease in visible edema, such as in the legs and other dependent areas? Has there been a decrease in the patient's weight? Does the patient's intake and output record indicate increased urinary output? Does the patient show an increased sense of well-being and increasing strength? What other measures are being used to promote the intended effect on cardiovascular function (e.g., diuretics, low sodium diet, restrictions on activity)?

IV. Does this patient have any side effects of digitalis therapy? Has the pulse decreased below 60 beats per minute? Has there been a great decrease or increase in the pulse rate, or change in rhythm and strength? Does the patient complain of visual disturbances or gastrointestinal disturbances such as nausea, vomiting or diarrhea? Is the patient receiving a digitalis preparation with a long duration of action which may produce a cumulative effect with repeated doses? What other drugs is the patient receiving, especially diuretics, which may influence the effect of digitalis? What are the patient's serum potassium and calcium levels? What other conditions does the patient have which may cause fluid and electrolyte imbalance and thereby affect cardiac action or sensitivity to digitalis?

V. What are the patient's (and family's) learning needs? Does he understand the purpose of the medication? Does he understand the necessity of taking the drug as prescribed? Does he understand how often he should take it? Would it be feasible to teach this patient or a member of his family to take his pulse daily or at certain intervals? Does the patient know the signs and symptoms he should report to his physician? Does the patient understand other aspects of the therapeutic plan such as diet, other drugs and activity? Does he understand the need for continued medical supervision?

QUESTIONS FOR DISCUSSION AND REVIEW

1. What warning symptoms are indicative of an overdose of digitalis? Under what circumstances is this most likely to occur?

2. Explain the differences in the modes of action of digitalis and quinidine in bringing about a decrease in heart rate.

3. Explain the mechanism by which nerve impulses cause the heart to beat.

4. What are the indications that digitalis is producing the desired effect in a patient in severe congestive heart failure? How does digitalis relieve the symptoms of congestive heart failure?

5. What is a pulse deficit and what is its meaning if it is present?

6. Review the procedure for obtaining an apical-radial pulse.

7. Outline a teaching plan for a patient who will be taking digitalis at home.

8. Outline a teaching plan for a patient who will be taking nitroglycerin sublingually for angina pectoris.

9. Outline a teaching plan for a patient who is taking a vasodilator for arterial insufficiency in his legs.

10. What are the nursing responsibilities in caring for a patient with essential hypertension?

BIBLIOGRAPHY

AMA Drug Evaluations. Chicago, American Medical Association, 1971.

Bernstein, H.: Drug treatment of cardiac arrhythmias. *Amer. J. Nurs., 64*:118, (July) 1964.

Best, C. H. and Taylor, N. B.: *The Physiological Basis of Medical Practice.* 6th Ed. Baltimore, The Williams and Wilkins Co., 1965.

Braunwald, E. and Klocke, F. J.: Digitalis. *Ann. Rev. Med., 16*:371, 1965.

Brest, A. N. and Moyer, J. H. (eds.): *Cardiovascular Drug Therapy.* New York, Grune and Stratton, 1965.

Brunner, L. S., et al.: *Textbook of Medical-Surgical Nursing,* 2nd. Ed. Philadelphia, J. B. Lippincott Co., 1970.

Conn, H. L., Jr.: Quinidine as an antiarrhythmic agent. *Med. Clin. N. Amer., 48*:286, 1964.

Conn, R.: Newer drugs in the treatment of cardiac arrhythmias. *Med. Clin. N. Amer., 51*:1223, 1967.

Doherty, J. E.: The clinical pharmacology of digitalis glycosides: a review. *Amer. J. Med. Sci., 255*:382, 1968.

Dollery, C. T.: Alpha-methyldopa (Aldomet) in the treatment of hypertension. *Med. Clin. N. Amer., 48*:335, (March) 1964.

Drugs used in the care of the cardiac patient. *Nurs. Clin. N. Amer., 4*: 645, (December) 1969.

Estes, J. W. and White, P. D.: William Withering and the purple foxglove. *Sci. Amer., 212*:110, (June) 1965.

Finnerty, F. A., Jr.: Newer antihypertensive drugs. *Med. Clin. N. Amer., 48*:329, 1964.

Fisch, S.: Antianginal drugs. I. The therapeutic role of coronary vasodilators. *Amer. Heart J., 71*:281, 1966.

Fisch, S.: Antianginal drugs. II. Human pharmacology of nitroglycerin. *Amer. Heart J., 71*:417, 1966.

Fisch, S.: Antianginal drugs. III. Clinical use of nitroglycerin. *Amer. Heart J., 71*:564, 1966.

Fisch, S.: Antianginal drugs. IV. The long-acting nitrates. *Amer. Heart J., 71*:712, 1966.

Fisch, S.: Antianginal drugs. V. Monamine oxidase (MAO) inhibitors. *Amer. Heart J., 71*:837, 1966.

Fisch, S.: Antianginal drugs. VI. Beta-adrenergic blocking drugs. *Amer. Heart J., 72*:131, 1966.

Frieden, J.: Lidocaine as an antiarrhythmic agent. *Amer. Heart J. 70*:713, 1965.

Goodman, L. S. and Gilman, A.: *Pharmacological Basis of Therapeutics.* 4th Ed. New York, Macmillan Co., 1970.

Goss, C. M. (ed.): *Gray's Anatomy of the Human Body.* 28th Ed. Philadelphia, Lea and Febiger, 1966.

Goth, A.: *Medical Pharmacology.* 3rd Ed. St. Louis, C. V. Mosby Co., 1968.

Govoni, L. E. and Hayes, J. E.: *Drugs and Nursing Implications.* 2nd Ed. New York, Appleton-Century-Crofts, 1971.

Kayden, H.: Clinical use of procaine amide. *Amer. Heart J., 70*:567, 1965.

Kayden, H.: The current status of procaine amide in management of cardiac arrhythmias. *Progr. Cardiovasc. Dis., 3*:331, 1961.

Kayden, H.: Pharmacology of procaine amide. *Amer. Heart J., 70*:423, 1965.

Keele, C. A. and Neil, E.: *Samson Wright's Applied Physiology.* 11th Ed. London, Oxford University Press, 1965.

Koch-Weser, J.: Mechanism of digitalis action on the heart. *New Eng. J. Med., 277*:417, 1967.

Laude, J. and Burckhardt, D.: Digitalis intoxication. *Hosp. Med., 3*:23, (February) 1967.

Luchi, R. J., Helwig, J. and Conn, H. L., Jr.: Quinidine toxicity and its treatment. *Amer. Heart J., 65*:340, 1963.

Lyon, A.: Antiarrhythmic drugs. II. Clinical uses of quinidine. *Amer. Heart J., 69*:834, 1965.

Lyon, A.: Quinidine toxicity. *Amer. Heart J., 70*:139, 1965.

Lyon, A. and DeGraff, A.: Antiarrhythmic drugs. I. Mechanisms of quinidine action. *Amer. Heart J., 69*:713, 1965.

Main, R. J., and Richardson, A. W.: *Physiology.* 2nd Ed. St. Louis, C. V. Mosby Co., 1953.

Mercer, E. N. and Osborne, J. A.: The current status of diphenylhydantoin in heart disease. *Ann. Intern. Med., 67*:1084, 1967.

Moser, M.: Use and abuse of antihypertensive agents. *G.P., 35*:87, 1967.

Pansky, B. and House, E. L.: *Review of Gross Anatomy.* New York, Macmillan Co., 1964.

Rodman, M. J.: Drugs for congestive heart failure and arrhythmias. *R.N., 30*:51, (November) 1967.

Rodman, M. J.: Drugs for managing high blood pressure. *R.N., 32*:73, (May) 1969.

Rodman, M. J.: Drug management in peripheral vascular disease. *R.N., 29*:61, (August) 1966.

Rodman, M. J.: Drugs used in coronary and cerebral vascular diseases. *R.N., 29*:63, (September) 1966.

Ruthen, G. C.: Diphenylhydantoin in cardiac arrhythmias. *Amer. Heart J., 70*:275, 1965.

Spittell, J. A., Jr. (ed.): Symposium on treatment of venous disorders. *Mod. Treatm., 2*:1061, (November) 1965.

Weatherall, M.: Ions and the action of digitalis. *Brit. Heart J., 28*:497, 1966.

Wintrobe, M. M., et al.: *Harrison's Principles of Internal Medicine.* 6th Ed. New York, McGraw-Hill Book Co., 1970.

Youmans, W. B.: *Fundamentals of Human Physiology.* 2nd Ed. Chicago, Year Book Medical Publishers, Inc., 1962.

Chapter 14 Blood Coagulants and Anticoagulants

Important Concepts Discussed

1. *The mechanism of blood clotting is complex and involves a series of reactions.*

2. *Blood clotting may be inhibited or decreased either by inhibiting the formation of the clotting substances in the liver or by interfering with the peripheral action of these substances.*

3. *Blood clotting may be accelerated or increased either by increased formation of the liver precursors or by administration of the clotting factors therapeutically.*

4. *Nursing observations to detect bleeding are essential when anticoagulants are administered.*

If blood stands in a test tube for five or six minutes, it loses its fluidity and becomes a jelly. If this jelly, or clot, is magnified many times it is seen to contain a mesh of delicate fibrils, among which are entangled the red and white blood cells and many platelets. The fibrils are composed of fibrin, a substance formed by the conversion of fibrinogen of the plasma from a soluble to an insoluble form by the action of thrombin.

A very intricate mechanism is involved in the coagulation of blood. For clarity, the various blood clotting factors will be listed, some of which have more than one synonym.

    I Fibrinogen
   II Prothrombin
 III Thromboplastins—from lung, brain, platelets and other tissues
 IV Calcium
  V Ac-globulin
      Labile factor
      Proaccelerin, inactive and active

 VI Precursor of factor VII (This factor is generally not listed in the blood clotting mechanism; both the precursor and factor VII are generally termed together as factor VII.
 VII Proconvertin, inactive and active
      Serum prothrombin conversion (SPC)
      Stable factor
VIII Antihemophilic globulin (AHG)
      Thromboplastinogen
      Antihemophilic factor A
 IX Plasma thromboplastin component (PTC)
      Christmas factor B
      Antihemophilic factor B
  X Stuart factor
      Prower factor
 XI Plasma thromboplastin antecedent (PTA)
 XII Hageman factor
XIII Fibrin stabilizing factor (FSF)

Blood clotting sequence for intrinsic blood clotting:

Hageman F. (XII) $\xrightarrow{}$ Activated Hageman F.

PTA (XI) $\xrightarrow{\text{Act. Hageman F.}}$ Activated PTA

Christmas F. (IX) $\xrightarrow[\text{Calcium}]{\text{Act. PTA}}$ Act. Christmas F.

Antihemophilic F. (VIII) $\xrightarrow[\text{Act. Christmas F.}]{\text{Phospholipid, Calcium}}$

Act. Antihemophilic F.

Stuart F. (X) $\xrightarrow[\text{Calcium}]{\text{Act. Antihemophilic F.}}$ Act. Stuart F.

Proaccelerin (V) $\xrightarrow[\text{Act. Stuart F.}]{\text{Phospholipid, Calcium}}$

Act. proaccelerin

Prothrombin (II) $\xrightarrow[\text{Calcium}]{\text{Act. proaccelerin}}$ Thrombin

Fibrinogen $\xrightarrow{\text{Thrombin}}$ Fibrin

The clotting mechanism which occurs after tissue injury differs only slightly from the above scheme. The extrinsic sequence for blood clotting begins with the release of tissue thromboplastin (III) as shown:

Pro-SPC (VII) $\xrightarrow{\text{tissue thromboplastin}}$ Act. Pro-SPC

Stuart F. (X) $\xrightarrow{\text{Act. Pro-SPC}}$ Act. Stuart F.

The rest of the sequence follows as above from the activation of factor (X) to the formation of fibrin.

Prothrombin is synthesized in the liver in the presence of vitamin K. A vitamin K deficiency would inhibit the blood clotting mechanism at this point. The conversion of prothrombin to thrombin is accelerated by the presence of plasma accelerator globulin (Ac-globulin), which is also known as Factor V or the labile factor of blood because it disappears from stored plasma. The blood protein fibrinogen, under the influence of thrombin, forms the long fibrin strands of the blood clot.

SCREENING TESTS FOR COAGULATION DISORDERS

Various screening tests are used to determine where the source of difficulty lies when a patient has a clotting disorder. Some defects may be treated by specific therapy; thus, diagnosis is essential.

BLEEDING TIME. The bleeding time is the interval required for effective hemostasis to occur following a standardized wound of the capillary bed. The Ivy method is generally employed, in which a blood pressure cuff maintains a pressure of 40 mm. mercury on the upper arm, and an incision 2 mm. in length and depth is made just below the antecubital fossa. The blood is blotted on filter paper every 30 seconds, and the end point is marked when the blood ceases to stain the filter paper.

Prolonged bleeding time may be found in disorders of the small blood vessels, particularly that of impaired contractility, without demonstrable defects in the blood clotting mechanism itself. In thrombocytopenia, or platelet deficiency, a prolonged bleeding time may likewise be observed, due to the absence of normal plugging of small wounds by platelet aggregates.

WHOLE-BLOOD CLOTTING TIME. The clotting time is defined as the time required for a firm clot to be formed in freshly shed blood placed in glass tubes. The normal clotting time when the tubes are placed in a water bath at 37° is within the range of 4 to 10 minutes. The clotting time is a nonspecific test and is subject to a wide range in errors due to faulty techniques.

PROTHROMBIN TIME. The prothrombin time is one of the more important and useful of all clotting tests. It was originally meant to reflect prothrombin concentration, measured by its activation to thrombin following the addition of thromboplastin and calcium, and the subsequent formation of visible fibrin. Subsequent studies have shown, however, that many variables may be involved which affect the outcome of the prothrombin time. It remains a useful, though crude screening test and is employed almost exclusively to measure the amount of anticoagulation obtained by therapeutic anticoagulants.

For more detailed analyses of blood clotting disorders, more specific and complicated screening tests may be performed, such as the prothrombin-consumption test, partial thromboplastin time and fibrinogen concentration tests. These are discussed in hematology manuals.

BLOOD COAGULANTS

The role of vitamin K in blood coagulation has been discussed in the chapter on vitamins; thus it will not be covered specifically in this section.

FIBRINOGEN, U.S.P. (PARENOGEN). The fibrinogen fraction may be recovered from human plasma by precipitation with organic solvents under controlled conditions of pH, ionic concentration and temperature. It is prepared commercially in a vacuum-dried frozen state, readily soluble in sodium chloride for intravenous infusion.

Since thrombin must act upon fibrinogen to form a clot, a serious deficiency in the amount of circulating fibrinogen would interfere with blood coagulation. Excessive fibrinolysin, causing hypofibrinogenemia, occurs in rare instances, as in premature separation of the placenta with intrauterine fetal death, in metastatic, prostatic or pancreatic carcinoma and following extensive surgical procedures, especially thoracic or prostatic. This condition has been attributed to the entrance of fibrinolysin into the circulation, inactivating most of the plasma fibrinogen, and leaving the blood thereafter incoagulable. Other theories have attributed the deficiency to the presence of fibrinolytic agents in the blood that prevent the formation of an adequate clot.

Greatly reduced fibrinogen levels have been noted in pernicious anemia, myelogenous leukemia, erythremia, widespread destruction of the bone marrow from metastases or other causes, scurvy, pellagra, extensive burns, infectious diseases, malignancies and impaired absorption from the gastrointestinal tract. The cause of the fibrinogen deficiencies in these states is unknown. Only rarely is hypo- or afibrinogenemia congenital.

In general, a plasma fibrinogen level of less than 50 mg. per 100 ml. is critical and is an indication for immediate fibrinogen therapy.

The dry powder should be refrigerated, and the liquid should be given immediately after preparation.

TOXICITY. The presence of viruses within fibrinogen has remained a definite hazard despite ultraviolet irradiation of the compound. Because the presence of homologous serum jaundice virus or hepatitis viruses cannot be determined, the virus should be assumed to be present, constituting a definite hazard to be weighed against the consequences of withholding the use of fibrinogen.

DOSE. 2 to 6 Gm. intravenously.

CARBAZOCHROME SALICYLATE (ADRENOSEM, ADRESTAT). Carbazochrome salicylate is quite an effective hemostat in conditions characterized by increased capillary permeability, which allows oozing of blood.

It has no effect on blood clotting time or prothrombin or vitamin K levels. It does not affect massive hemorrhage or arterial bleeding. It has no sympathomimetic action and does not raise blood pressure or cardiac rate or output. Its action results solely from its ability to prevent or correct abnormal capillary permeability.

USES. It is particularly effective in the treatment of conditions such as idiopathic purpura, prevention of retinal hemorrhage, prevention of postoperative bleeding following nasopharyngeal, prostatic and bladder surgery and in epistaxis and pulmonary bleeding.

TOXICITY. Toxicity is minimal. Sensitivity reactions may result from repeated use. Intramuscular administration sometimes causes transitory pain at the site of injection.

DOSE. 1 to 5 mg. orally or I.M. four times daily.

AMINOCAPROIC ACID (AMICAR). Aminocaproic acid acts very specifically to inhibit the activity of profibrinolysin (plasminogen activator substance) and fibrinolysin (plasmin). This drug should be administered only in the presence of high fibrinolysin levels (hyperplasminemia). In most cases, the use of fresh whole blood, fibrinogen infusions and other emergency measures is also required.

Aminocaproic acid has been used in systemic hyperplasminemia associated with surgical complications following heart surgery and portacaval shunt, in carcinoma of the lung, prostate, cervix or stomach, in abruptio placentae and in hematologic disorders such as aplastic anemia.

If it is accepted that fibrinolysis is a normal process, potentially active at all times to dissolve fibrin clots and thereby ensure the fluidity of blood, it must also be accepted that inhibition of fibrinolysin by aminocaproic acid may result in clotting or thrombosis. However, there is no conclusive evidence in the few reported cases of intravascular clotting that followed this treatment. Rather, it appears that such intravascular clotting was most likely a result of the fibrinolytic disease being treated.

When adminstered intravenously aminocaproic acid should be given slowly in 5% dextrose solution, sodium chloride injection or balanced electrolyte injection.

> **TOXICITY.** Side effects may include nausea, cramps, diarrhea, dizziness, malaise, tinnitus, headache and rash. They are mild, however, and disappear upon withdrawal of the drug.
>
> Reduced dosage is recommended for patients with cardiac, liver or renal impairment. It is contraindicated in patients with active intravascular clotting, possible fibrinolysis and bleeding.
>
> **DOSE.** 4 to 5 Gm. orally or I.V. initially, then 1 to 1.25 Gm. every hour until a plasma level of 130 mcg./ml. is obtained.

PROTAMINE SULFATE U.S.P., B.P. Although protamine sulfate is a weak anticoagulant, it is used medically to inactivate heparin. Because of protamine's positively charged molecules it neutralizes the negatively charged heparin, inhibiting it by a colloidal effect.

> **USES.** The chief use of protamine is to treat heparin overdosage; however, it is also used in hemorrhagic diseases, such as hemorrhage accompanying leukemia, menorrhagia, postpartum

bleeding and following irradiation. In some of these disorders the presence of a circulating anticoagulant similar to heparin has been demonstrated.

The drug should be refrigerated.

> **TOXICITY.** Embolic vascular phenomena have been produced experimentally in animals using large doses of protamine. Sensitivity reactions have occurred during its administration.
>
> **DOSE.** Heparin overdosage—1% solution, administered slowly I.V. over a period of 1 to 3 minutes. Hemorrhagic disorders—4 to 5 mg./kg. body weight I.V. daily.

LOCAL HEMOSTATICS

THROMBIN, B.P. Thrombin is a sterile protein substance that is prepared from bovine prothrombin by interaction with thromboplastin in the presence of calcium. It is the only substance needed to cause the formation of a fibrin clot in the presence of plasma fibrinogen.

> **USES.** Thrombin is used topically either alone or with fibrin foam as a hemostatic agent to arrest capillary bleeding and as a tissue "glue" to obliterate a dead space after surgical excision of tissue and to facilitate the adherence of skin grafts. Thrombin will not arrest hemorrhage from a spurting artery; it must be ligated surgically.
>
> Thrombin must not be injected, because intravenous administration causes intravascular clotting and embolism. It can be administered orally either in milk or in antacid preparations as an adjunct in the control of upper gastrointestinal bleeding.
>
> It should be stored in powder form between 2 and 8° C. After reconstitution into solution form, it is stable for only 8 hours at room temperature or 48 hours if refrigerated.
>
> **TOXICITY.** Homologous serum hepatitis has been traced to a preparation of

human thrombin used as a hemostatic in neurosurgical procedures. It is an antigenic substance and may induce sensitivity reactions when administered orally.

DOSE. 1000 to 10,000 units topically or orally.

CELLULOSE, OXIDIZED, U.S.P., B.P. (OXYCEL). Oxidized cellulose exerts its hemostatic effect by the formation of an artificial clot of cellulosic acid. This clot acts like the fibrin fibrils to trap the solid constituents of blood and arrest bleeding. The addition of thrombin does not enhance its activity. If applied dry, the oxidized cellulose is absorbed in two to seven days; absorption of large amounts of the blood-soaked material may take six weeks or longer.

USES. Oxidized cellulose is used to control moderate bleeding and also as a temporary packing or implant following surgical procedures. It should not be used for permanent packing in fractures because it inhibits bone regeneration. Since cellulosic acid inhibits epithelialization, it should not be used as a surface dressing for a prolonged period of time.

ABSORBABLE GELATIN SPONGE, U.S.P., B.P. (GELFOAM). The ability of this gelatin sponge to take up as much as 50 times its weight of blood or water renders it quite valuable in the control of capillary oozing. It is most effective when moistened with thrombin.

When implanted in a wound, it is absorbed in four to six weeks.

OXIDIZED REGENERATED CELLULOSE, U.S.P. (SURGICEL). This cellulose product is available in knitted fabric strips and carded fiber pads especially developed to make it useful in controlling bleeding after surgery. It may be used for implants in cardiac surgery, for cranial hemorrhage and for many otolaryngologic procedures.

It is most effective when applied dry, and it is neither necessary nor desirable to impregnate it with other hemostatic agents.

ANTICOAGULANTS

Anticoagulant drugs inhibit blood clotting by affecting factors in the clotting mechanism. They are used to prevent the coagulation of blood for transfusion and to prevent and arrest the extension of thromboembolic disorders.

Because of the interference with the blood clotting mechanism when the patient is taking anticoagulants, there is always the danger of hemorrhage. Laboratory tests, such as prothrombin time and bleeding time, should be monitored closely. The patient's vital signs should be checked carefully and frequently, since they may reflect the presence of internal hemorrhage. The stools and urine should be observed for blood. The skin should be checked for petechiae or hematoma formation.

Patients may receive anticoagulants on an outpatient basis. In this case, the patient and his family must be taught to be alert for signs of bleeding and to notify the physician immediately. A patient should carry a card with him at all times stating that he is on anticoagulant therapy, in case of an accident. He should be cautioned against the possible consequences of cuts, scratches and/or bruises.

SODIUM HEPARIN INJECTION, U.S.P., HEPARIN INJECTION, B.P. (PANHEPARIN, LIQUAEMIN, LIPO-HEPIN). Heparin is used therapeutically for the prevention and treatment of coronary thrombosis, thrombophlebitis and other thromboembolic disorders, frostbite, vascular surgery and blood transfusions. According to one theory regarding its mode of action, heparin appears to inactivate thromboplastin, thereby preventing the conversion of prothrombin to thrombin. It also increases the agglutinability of the platelets.

Heparin is involved in the disappearance of lipids from the blood; it is used as a lipemia-clearing agent in atherosclerosis, angina pectoris, hyperlipemic states and xanthoma tuberosum.

Since heparin is ineffective when taken orally, it must be injected. For this reason, after anticoagulant therapy is initiated with the rapidly acting heparin, one of the orally effective anticoagulants is used to continue therapy, since the oral route is greatly preferred by most patients. All oral forms of anticoagulants have a delay of several hours before onset of action occurs, however; they cannot effectively replace heparin when immediate anticoagulant action is needed. It is important to give heparin promptly at the time specified to maintain a consistent, optimum degree of anticoagulation.

Although heparin can be given intramuscularly, it is usually given subcutaneously at a 90 degree angle in the fat pad above the iliac crest, either anteriorly or posteriorly. The subcutaneous route frequently causes hematoma formation. The injection should be carefully given to avoid any unnecessary trauma because of the patient's tendency to bleed. A narrow gauge needle should be used to minimize the trauma. The site of injection should not be massaged after injection; gentle, but firm, pressure should be applied instead to prevent hematoma formation.

The sites of injection should be carefully rotated. Injection should not be made into a bruised area or within two inches of a scar or the umbilicus.

TOXICITY. The chief toxicity of heparin is concerned with overdosage and dangerously prolonged clotting times. In surgical cases, particular attention must be paid to hemostatic procedures, and following the operation, the nurse must be alert for signs of concealed bleeding or hematoma formation. Hypersensitivity may be manifested by urticaria, conjunctival itching, lacrimation, and fever. Because clotting time, not bleeding time, is affected, patients receiving heparin may shave with a razor.

Heparin is contraindicated in pregnancy and during childbirth, following surgery of the brain or spinal cord and in the presence of active bleeding.

Protamine sulfate is an effective antidote.

DOSE. 10,000 to 12,000 units s.c. every 8 hours. Under some circumstances it may be administered I.V.

BISHYDROXYCOUMARIN, U.S.P. (DICUMAROL). Bishydroxycoumarin lengthens the prothrombin time by retarding prothrombin production in the liver. (Prothrombin time is the coagulation time of plasma under specified test conditions. It is a measure of the concentration of prothrombin in the blood.) It is used in the prophylaxis and treatment of intravascular clotting and as an adjunct to heparin therapy.

bishydroxycoumarin

Following oral administration of this drug, there is a latent period of 24 to 72 hours before the effects are manifested. Its effects tend to be cumulative, and the prothrombin time of patients on bishydroxycoumarin therapy should be checked at frequent intervals, daily if possible. In the normal individual, the prothrombin time is about 15 seconds, depending on the method used and the type of thromboplastin employed. Under the influence of anticoagulant drugs, the prothrombin time is increased to 22 to 35 seconds, which is generally considered to be an effective and safe range. If the prothrombin time is increased beyond this range, the dosage should be decreased.

When drug therapy is initiated, the patient's prothrombin time is checked daily and the next dose determined on the basis of the test results. Orders for these anticoagulants are therefore written on a daily basis until the patient's prothrombin level is stabilized. Periodic laboratory tests are always done throughout the entire time the patient is receiving the drugs.

TOXICITY. The main toxic effect of bishydroxycoumarin is hemorrhage due to dangerously decreased prothrombin levels in the blood. It is contraindicated in patients with hemorrhagic tendencies, blood dyscrasias, ulcerative lesions of the gastrointestinal tract, diverticulitis, colitis, threatened abortion, recent brain and spinal cord surgery, vitamin K deficiency and liver disease. It should be used with caution during pregnancy and lactation because of the danger of producing hypoprothrombinemia in the infant.

The action of coumarin anticoagulants is affected by a large number of drugs. The dose of the anticoagulant may need to be adjusted when the patient receives another drug or stops taking a drug.

Fresh whole blood and vitamin K are antidotes.

DOSE. Regulated by the prothrombin time. May give 200 to 300 mg. orally initially, followed by 50 mg. daily as a maintenance dose.

SODIUM WARFARIN, U.S.P. (COUMADIN, PANWARFIN, ATHROMBIN-K). Warfarin is a synthetic anticoagulant. Like the other coumarin derivatives, it interferes with blood clotting, depressing the prothrombin activity of the blood by interfering with the utilization of vitamin K.

The onset of action of warfarin is more rapid than that of bishydroxycoumarin, and the duration of effect is about equally long.

After parenteral or oral administration, the onset of action occurs in about 12 hours, with therapeutic levels being attained within 24 hours. The peak effect occurs in about 36 hours, and the duration of action varies from two to five days. No therapeutic advantage is gained by parenteral administration of the drug if the patient is able to take oral medication.

Warfarin has the same indications, contraindications and toxic effects as bishydroxycoumarin. Its main advantages over the latter are the faster onset of action and the smaller doses required.

Recent studies have shown that there is a depression of anticoagulant activity in warfarin-treated patients who are also receiving griseofulvin therapy. The anticoagulant activity should be carefully monitored

when these two drugs are administered concurrently.

DOSE. Initial—40 to 60 mg. I.V. or orally. Maintenance—5 to 10 mg. daily.

Other anticoagulants with similar uses and action are:

Acenocoumarol (Acenocoumarin, Sintrom)
Dose. Initial—16 to 28 mg. orally. Maintenance—2 to 10 mg. daily.
Anisindione (Miradon)*
Dose. Initial—300 mg. orally. Maintenance—75 to 150 mg. daily.
Ethyl Biscoumacetate (Tromexan)
Dose. Initial—1.5 Gm. orally. Maintenance—600 to 900 mg. daily.
Phenindione (Danilone, Hedulin)*
Dose. Initial—200 to 300 mg. orally. Maintenance—50 to 100 mg. daily.
Phenprocoumon (Liquamar)
Dose. Initial—21 to 30 mg. orally. Maintenance—6 to 9 mg. daily.

FIBRINOLYSIN, HUMAN (ACTASE, THROMBOLYSIN). Fibrinolysin (plasmin) is the naturally occurring enzyme of blood plasma that breaks down the long fibrin molecules into small polypeptides that may readily be excreted. It is obtained commercially from fractionated plasma.

Although it aids in the dissolution of clots, it does not prevent further clot formation.

The effect of fibrinolysin in thrombophlebitis, phlebothrombosis and pulmonary embolism is questionable when therapy is not instituted until after the clot has formed. Obviously, the earlier therapy is instituted the more favorable are the results; treatment is often disappointing if it is undertaken five days or more after the clot is formed.

TOXICITY. Fever is the most common side effect of fibrinolysin therapy and usually occurs three to eight hours after infusion is begun. This reaction may be minimized by the administration of sedatives, antipyretics or antihistamines

---

*These drugs may cause the urine to become orange or red in color, which may give the false impression that the patient has hematuria.

before or during infusion. Less frequent toxicity symptoms are hypotension, tachycardia, chills, nausea, vomiting and dizziness.

DOSE. 50,000 units in I.V. infusion over a two hour period. If necessary, three doses may be given over a five day period.

GUIDE FOR THE NURSING ASSESSMENT OF A PATIENT RECEIVING AN ANTICOAGULANT

I.   Why is the patient receiving the drug? Where is the locus of clot formation?

II.   How is the anticoagulant being administered? Is it being administered correctly? Is the dosage accurate? Are laboratory results obtained before the next dose is ordered? Is the correct technique being used if it is heparin that is being given subcutaneously? Are sites rotated and selected properly?

III.   What are effects of the anticoagulant? Has the patient had any indication of thrombus or emboli? Do laboratory tests indicate that the desired degree of anticoagulation is being maintained? Are other drugs the patient is receiving increasing or decreasing the effect of the anticoagulant, if it is a coumarin derivative? Does the patient have any indications of bleeding? Are the vital signs stable? Are there any visible bruises or petechiae? Is there hematuria (pink, red or smoky urine)? Is there bleeding in the gums? Are the stools black and tarry, or guaiac positive for blood? What antidote should be available to counteract the effects of this drug?

IV.   What are the patient's (and family's) learning needs? Does he understand why he is receiving an anticoagulant? Does he understand the need for continual medical supervision and accurate administration? Is he aware of the signs and symptoms of bleeding that should be reported? Is he aware of the advisability of carrying an identification card or Medic Alert tag? Does he understand the necessity of avoiding trauma and cuts?

QUESTIONS FOR DISCUSSION AND REVIEW

1.   Diagram the blood clotting mechanism.

2.   Show on your diagram of the blood clotting mechanism how the following prevent or aid coagulation:

a.	heparin	d.	vitamin K
b.	bishydroxycoumarin	e.	thrombin
c.	warfarin	f.	absorbable gelatin sponge

3. Which coagulant would be best for:
    a. arterial bleeding
    b. bleeding following tonsillectomy
    c. hyperfibrinolysis
    d. surgical implant
4. How would severe liver damage affect blood clotting?
5. What part does vitamin K play in blood coagulation?
6. What signs and symptoms should the nurse be alert to in a patient receiving anticoagulants?
7. What are the laboratory tests and normal values used in your hospital to serve as guidelines for:
    a. heparin therapy
    b. coumarin anticoagulant therapy
8. Outline a teaching plan for a patient who is to take coumadin at home.

BIBLIOGRAPHY

AMA Drug Evaluations. Chicago, American Medical Association, 1971.

Antihemophilic factor (human). *Amer. J. Nurs., 68*:131, 1968.

Cohn, H. D.: Hemostasis and blood coagulation. *Amer. J. Nurs., 65*:116, 1965.

Coles, M.: Haemophilia today. *Nurs. Times, 65*:1415, (November 6) 1969.

Council on Drugs: An antifibrinolytic agent, aminocaproic acid (Amicar). *J.A.M.A., 191*:489, 1965.

Dallman, P. R. and Pool, J. G.: Treatment of hemophilia with factor VIII concentrates. *New Eng. J. Med., 278*:199, 1968.

Deykin, D.: The use of heparin. *New Eng. J. Med., 280*:937, 1969.

Drapeau, J.: The nurse and the hemophiliac patient. *Canad. Nurs., 63*:38, (July) 1967.

Fletcher, R.: Anticoagulant treatment. *Nurs. Times, 64*:1646, (December 6) 1968.

Gaston, L. W.: The blood clotting factors. *New Eng. J. Med., 270*:236, 290, 1964.

Goodman, L. S. and Gilman, A.: *Pharmacological Basis of Therapeutics.* 4th Ed. New York, Macmillan Co., 1970.

Goss, J. E. and Dickhaus, D. W.: Increased bishydroxycoumarin requirements in patients receiving phenobarbital. *New Eng. J. Med., 273*:1094, 1965.

Goth, A.: *Medical Pharmacology.* 3rd Ed. St. Louis, C. V. Mosby Co., 1968.

Govoni, L. E. and Hayes, J. E.: *Drugs and Nursing Implications.* 2nd Ed. New York, Appleton-Century-Crofts, 1971.

Handley, A. J.: Anticoagulant therapy. *Nurs. Mirror, 129*:20, (July 25) 1969.

Hunninghake, D. B. and Azarnoff, D. C.: Drug interactions with warfarin. *Arch. Int. Med., 121*:349, 1968.

Israel, H. L., et al.: Fibrinolysin treatment of thromboembolism. *J.A.M.A., 188*:628, 1964.

Jorpes, J. E.: Heparin: its chemistry, pharmacology and clinical use. *Amer. J. Med., 33*:692, 1962.

Keele, C. A. and Neil, E.: *Samson Wright's Applied Physiology*. 11th Ed. London, Oxford University Press, 1965.

Lewis, J. H. and Bayer, W. L.: Therapy in coagulation defects. *Med. Clin. N. Amer., 51*:1241, 1967.

MacDonald, M. G. and Robinson, D. S.: Clinical observations of possible barbiturate interference with anticoagulation. *J.A.M.A., 204*:97, 1968.

Main, R. J. and Richardson, A. W.: *Physiology*. 2nd Ed. St. Louis, C. V. Mosby Co., 1953.

Meyer, O.: Treatment with anticoagulants. *Cardiovasc. Nursing,* (May-June, 1968).

Olwin, J. H. and Koppel, J. L.: Anticoagulant therapy. *Amer. J. Nurs., 64*:107, (May) 1964.

Pansky, B. and House, E. L.: *Review of Gross Anatomy*. New York, Macmillan Co., 1964.

Robinson, D. J. and MacDonald, M. G.: The effect of phenobarbital administration on the control of coagulation achieved during warfarin therapy in man. *J. Pharmacol. Exp. Ther., 153*:250, 1966.

Rodman, M. J.: Drugs that affect blood coagulation. *R.N., 32*:59, (July) 1969.

Seale, A. L.: The nurse's responsibility in anticoagulant therapy. *Nurs. Clin. N. Amer., 1*:325, (June) 1966.

Wasserman, A. J., et al.: Anticoagulants in acute myocardial infarction. *Amer. Heart J., 71*:43, 1966.

Wintrobe, M. M., et al. (eds.): *Harrison's Principles of Internal Medicine*. 6th Ed. New York, McGraw-Hill, 1970.

Youmans, W. B.: *Fundamentals of Human Physiology*. 2nd Ed. Chicago, Year Book Medical Publishers, Inc., 1962.

Chapter 15 Hormone and Hormone-like Substances

Important Concepts Discussed

1. *The endocrine system is composed of a highly interrelated group of glands that control many metabolic functions.*

2. *Insufficient endocrine secretion can be supplemented by hormones from natural and synthetic sources.*

3. *Overactive endocrine glands may be controlled in some cases by specific inhibitory drugs.*

4. *Most hormonal activity is ultimately under the control of the pituitary gland and is greatly influenced by the central nervous system.*

5. *Careful observations by the nurse are important in assessing the hormonal effect.*

6. *Education of the patient is an important role of the nurse when hormones must be administered for extended periods of time in hormone replacement therapy.*

The endocrine system is composed of a complex, interrelated group of glands—specialized epithelial structures that produce hormones. These hormones, which regulate metabolic activities of the organism, are passed directly into the blood either as a result of nervous stimulation or in response to the action of another hormone upon the endocrine gland.

The following generalities may be applied to hormones:

1. None of the hormones is believed to initiate cellular reactions. The organ or tissue influenced by the hormone reacts by increasing or decreasing the rate of its inherent activity.

2. Most hormones are not secreted at a constant rate. Some hormones are cyclic (gonadotropins), some are secreted in response to the diet (insulin) and others are secreted in greater amounts as a result of stress (adrenal cortical hormones).

3. Hormones exert their effects in catalytic concentrations. Very small amounts of these materials produce major physiologic changes in body functions. This hormonal property has advantages and disadvantages, since if the body inactivates the hormone too slowly, symptoms of overdosage may develop.

4. Hormones may produce their effects in three ways:

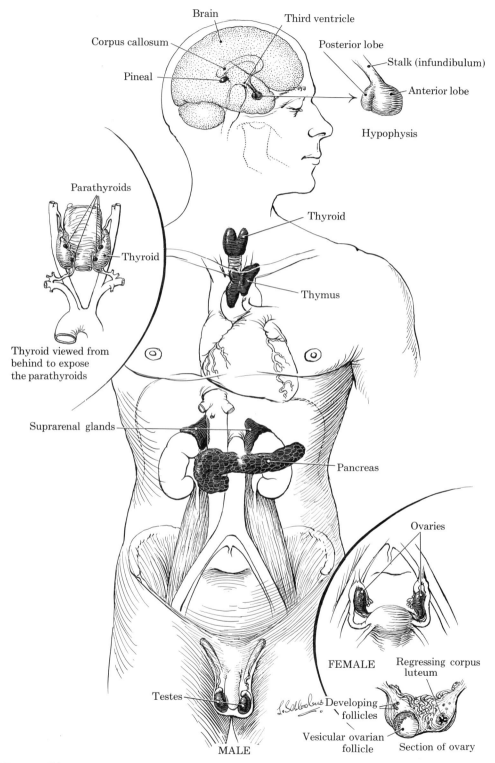

FIGURE 42. Diagram of the endocrine system. (*Dorland's Illustrated Medical Dictionary*. Ed. 24. W. B. Saunders Co., Philadelphia, 1965.)

A. They may act directly upon a target organ; e.g., epinephrine acts on blood vessels *in vivo* and *in vitro*.

B. Some hormones may act not on a target organ, but on another endocrine gland; e.g., luteinizing hormone (LH) from the anterior pituitary influences the interstitial cells of the testes to secrete testosterone, a hormone that then acts upon target organs to produce the secondary sex characteristics.

C. A few hormones are conditionally acting, depending upon the sensitivity of the target organ. In some cases the target organ must be influenced first by another hormone; e.g., progesterone has a marked effect upon the uterus following pretreatment with estrogen.

Endocrine hormones, then, are responsible for a great many regulatory processes in the body. Overall control is due in large part to the pituitary gland, which secretes the tropic hormones to other endocrine glands. Feedback to the pituitary occurs when secretion occurs from the target endocrine glands and the output of the tropic hormones is decreased. Upon stimulation by the pituitary, the other endocrine glands are able to regulate such functions as growth, metabolic rate, sexual development and electrolyte and glucose balance in the blood.

Exogenous hormones are used therapeutically to replace or increase the natural supply of hormone. In the event of destruction of the pituitary or any other endocrine gland, life and relative homeostasis can be maintained by hormone administration. In a few instances, e.g., insulin, these hormones are still obtained by natural sources; however, in most cases chemical synthesis is possible, more economical and more readily controlled than animal sources.

HORMONES OF THE PITUITARY GLAND

The pituitary gland, or hypophysis, is a small structure about the size of a pea, which lies in a cavity in the sphenoid bone between the cerebrum and the nasopharynx. It is divided into two parts: the neurohypophysis, and the adenohypophysis. The neurohypophysis, sometimes called the pars nervosa or the main part of the posterior pituitary, is formed by a downgrowth of nervous tissue from the brain. The adenohypophysis origi-

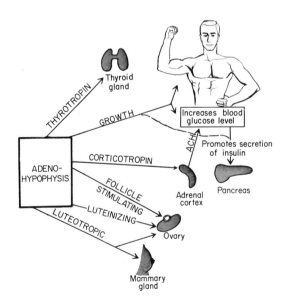

FIGURE 43. Metabolic functions of the adenohypophyseal hormones. (From Guyton: *Textbook of Medical Physiology.* Ed. 4. W. B. Saunders Co., Philadelphia, 1971.)

nates in Rathke's pouch, a small portion of oral epithelium that grows upward during fetal life to meet and adhere to the neurohypophysis.

There are three divisions of the adenohypophysis:

1. The *pars distalis,* which is the largest portion, or the anterior pituitary. All known hormones secreted from the adenohypophysis originate in this portion.

2. The *pars tuberalis,* which is a cloak of cells around the infundibular stalk or "stem" of the hypophysis.

3. The *pars intermedia,* which is a narrow band of cells structurally different from the cells of the pars distalis and lies between the pars distalis and neurohypophysis. Some research workers have proposed the theory that a melanocyte-stimulating hormone (MSH) is secreted by the pars intermedia and affects skin pigmentation. It seems to be much more active in fish and reptiles than in humans, however, and there is still controversy concerning its source.

The anterior lobe of the pituitary consists of the pars distalis and the pars tuberalis. The posterior lobe consists of the pars intermedia and the processus infundibuli, a portion of the neurohypophysis.

HORMONES FROM THE PARS DISTALIS (ANTERIOR PITUITARY)

Recent evidence indicates that secretion from the pars distalis is under the ultimate control of the hypothalamus. Neurosecretory material from the hypothalamus enters the hypophyseal portal system, which is the principal blood supply to the pars distalis, and stimulates various hormone-producing cells to secrete hormones.

Because of this relationship with the central nervous system, pituitary secretion is influenced by conditions such as stress, trauma or violent emotional reactions, and in turn can alter many body functions to meet these emergencies.

The secretions of the anterior pituitary are also greatly influenced by the concentration of other hormones circulating in the blood. A high concentration of the thyroid hor-

mone, for instance, would inhibit the secretion of the thyrotropic hormone from the anterior pituitary. Corticosteroids when administered therapeutically have a similar effect upon the secretion of the adrenocorticotropic hormone (ACTH).

Much of the hormone activity of the body is ultimately controlled by the anterior pituitary, and for this reason it is often called the master gland of the body. It secretes tropic hormones that are named for the endocrine glands they influence, e.g., the thyrotropic, gonadotropic and adrenocorticotropic hormones regulate the secretions of the thyroid, gonads and adrenal cortex respectively.

It is not known precisely how many hormones are secreted by the anterior pituitary, but at least six extracts with specific action have been isolated. These hormones are the growth hormone (somatotropin, GH), thyroid-stimulating hormone (thyrotropin, TSH), adrenocorticotropic hormone (ACTH), follicle-stimulating hormone (FSH), luteinizing hormone (LH) and prolactin (lactogenic hormone, LTH).

It has been postulated that the anterior pituitary secretes other hormones in addition to these six, because extracts of the gland have been prepared that have had other effects on the body. These substances have not been purified, however, and the effects are considered by some to be side effects of the known hormones.

GROWTH HORMONE (SOMATOTROPIN, GH). The growth hormone controls general body growth and bone growth and increases the amount of cellular protein. Experimental evidence has shown, however, that the growth hormone alone is not sufficient to attain completely normal growth; thyroid hormone must also be present. This hormone also affects fat metabolism. It decreases tissue fat by removing it from the periphery and redistributing it, especially to the liver and kidneys.

Because of the effects of growth hormone on carbohydrate metabolism, it was formerly called the "diabetogenic hormone." When administered to experimental animals, growth hormone causes:

1. Release of hepatic glucose.

2. Increased secretion of insulin from the pancreas (due to the elevated blood sugar level).

3. Increased glucose uptake by the tissues (due to the increase in circulating insulin).

Excessive secretion of growth hormone during the normal growth period results in giantism. This condition occurs most often in men and produces oversized but well-proportioned individuals, some growing to a height of eight feet or more. Most pituitary giants do not live beyond 30 years of age.

The presence of excessive growth hormone after epiphyseal closure of the long bones can cause growth of only the soft tissues and cartilage of the body. In the late stages of this condition, known as acromegaly, the affected individual has a grotesque appearance with large spadelike hands and feet, thickening of the skin, and enlargement of the tongue, lips, nose, ears, jaw and skull. Acromegaly ordinarily affects those between the ages of 20 and 40 years, the first noticeable symptom often being an increased hat size. The condition is slow to develop, however, and progresses over a period of many years.

A deficiency of growth hormone results in stunted growth, or pituitary dwarfism. These individuals have normal body proportions but are often sexually underdeveloped.

The growth hormone has recently been obtained as a crystalline protein, and experiments with the hormone are being conducted on a very small scale. The commercial availability of this hormone is very limited, since the growth hormone from cattle and other domestic animals is not effective in humans. The hormone obtained from monkeys and other primates is somewhat effective in humans, but the supply is very limited. It will probably not be available for large scale clinical use until it can be synthesized chemically.

THYROTROPIN (TSH, THYTROPAR). Thyrotropin increases the activity of the thyroid

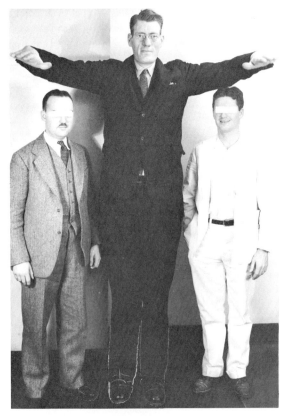

FIGURE 44. Giantism caused by hypersecretion of growth hormone. (Courtesy of Dr. E. Perry McCullagh in Villee: *Biology*. Ed. 6. W. B. Saunders Co., Philadelphia, 1972.)

gland and causes it to release the thyroid hormone. Removal of the pituitary brings about atrophy of the thyroid gland. The gland decreases in size, and the thyroid follicle cells subsequently become flattened.

The commercial product (Thytropar) is the powdered purified hormone of the bovine pituitary. Its stimulating action on the thyroid is useful for both diagnostic and therapeutic purposes.

> **USES.** When TSH is used as a diagnostic agent, the effect is evaluated by comparing the radioactive iodine uptake by the thyroid gland and the protein bound iodine level in the blood before TSH administration with readings taken 24 hours after administration. This TSH diagnostic evaluation can distinguish between inadequate anterior pituitary influence on the thyroid and primary dysfunction of the gland itself. Thyrotropin is used therapeutically to treat myxedema and simple goiter.

> **DOSE.** 10 units diluted in 2 ml. of sodium chloride and injected I.M. or S.C.

ADRENOCORTICOTROPIC HORMONE, U.S.P. (ACTH, CORTICOTROPIN, CORTROPHIN).
Adrenocorticotropic hormone (ACTH) stimulates the adrenal cortex to release corticosteroids. Injection of ACTH reduces the amounts of cholesterol and ascorbic acid in the adrenal cortex, presumably because they are used in the synthesis of the steroids. Without ACTH stimulation, atrophy of the adrenal cortex occurs.

Atrophy of the adrenal cortex becomes a problem in the therapeutic administration of the corticosteroids because the high level of circulating drugs causes a reciprocal inhibition of the adrenal cortex. In the event that an emergency situation arises when the therapeutic dose of the corticosteroid is being reduced or withdrawn, the atrophied adrenal cortex is not able to secrete sufficient hormones for the body to adapt to the emergency. Supplemental corticosteroids must always be given. Serious consequences and even death may result under conditions of even relatively mild stress.

In a normally functioning adrenal cortex,

the peripheral effects produced upon administration of ACTH are the same as those produced by administration of cortisone or hydrocortisone. Because its action depends on the functional integrity of the adrenals, ACTH is of no value in Addison's disease except as a diagnostic agent.

Oral administration of ACTH is not useful because it is destroyed by the gastric juices. Topical application is of no benefit, since the substance acts only on and through the adrenal glands.

> **USES.** ACTH is used in the treatment of gout, rheumatoid arthritis, rheumatic fever, lupus erythematosus, asthma and eye and skin diseases. The clinical effects are similar to those of the glucocorticoids; the glucocorticoids are usually given because closer dosage regulation and more predictable effects may be obtained with these agents.

> **DOSE.** I.M.—10 to 20 units every 6 to 8 hours. I.V.—5 to 20 units dissolved in 500 ml. of 5% glucose or isotonic saline solution and given over an 8 hour period.

FOLLICLE STIMULATING HORMONE (FSH); LUTEINIZING HORMONE (LH).
Two gonadotropic hormones are liberated by the anterior pituitary: the follicle stimulating hormone (FSH) and the luteinizing hormone (LH), which is also known as the interstitial cell–stimulating hormone (ICSH.)

Both hormones are liberated in the male and in the female, and there is a difference only in the sex organs that they influence. In the female the FSH is responsible for the development of graafian follicles in the ovaries; LH controls the development of the corpus luteum after the follicle has ruptured as well as the release of estrogens and progesterone.

In the male, FSH increases the size of the seminiferous tubules, whereas LH stimulates the interstitial cells of the testes to produce the male sex hormone, testosterone.

PROLACTIN (LACTOGENIC HORMONE, LUTEOTROPIC HORMONE, LTH).
Prolactin appears to exert a maturing influence on the secreting cells of the mammary gland following

their proliferation under the influence of progesterone and estrogen. It has little if any effect on immature mammary glands.

Experimental evidence indicates that neither FSH nor LH could completely account for the secretion of the corpus luteum. The active principle from the anterior pituitary that stimulates the large amount of progesterone secretion during the early months of pregnancy was given the name "luteotropin." As prolactin was more rigorously purified, it was discovered that prolactin and this luteotropic factor were the same secretion, and the synonym luteotropic hormone or LTH was applied to prolactin.

No commercial preparations of this hormone are available at present.

HORMONES FROM THE POSTERIOR PITUITARY

The posterior pituitary, like the anterior pituitary, is quite dependent upon the hypothalamus for its secretory properties. In the case of the posterior pituitary, however, this relationship is more direct. Microscopic studies have failed to show any evidence of secretory cells in the neurohypophysis, although it is abundantly supplied with nerve fibers. Further studies have shown that the secretions from the posterior pituitary originate in the hypothalamus in the supraoptic and periventricular nuclei and are passed to the posterior pituitary via the supraopticohypophyseal nerve tract. The posterior pituitary, then, merely acts as a storage place for the hormones and releases them upon proper stimulation.

When an aqueous extract of the posterior pituitary is administered parenterally, it produces three responses: (1) uterine muscular stimulation (oxytocic effect), (2) peripheral vascular constriction (pressor effect) and (3) increased renal water absorption (antidiuretic effect).

Two hormones, oxytocin and vasopressin, have been isolated from the posterior pituitary and are responsible for these effects. The pharmacologic activity of these hormones overlaps, even in pure preparations, because oxytocin has some vasopressor activity and vasopressin has oxytocic activity.

Vasopressin, also known as the antidiuretic hormone, has antidiuretic effects that are much more marked than its pressor effects, however. The vasopressor effects are ordinarily seen only in unphysiologic or therapeutic doses of this hormone.

VASOPRESSIN INJECTION, U.S.P., B.P. (ANTIDIURETIC HORMONE, ADH, PITRESSIN). Vasopressin, like oxytocin, has oxytocic and pressor effects. Its most therapeutically important activity, however, is its ability to increase the reabsorption of water from the cells of the distal convoluted tubules and the thin portion of Henle's loop in the kidneys. Because of this activity it has received its synonym, the antidiuretic hormone.

When this hormone is absent, diabetes insipidus occurs. In this disease there is a decreased ability to reabsorb water filtered in the glomerulus of the kidney, and the urine volume increases from the normal 1 to 2 liters to 10 to 25 liters per day. The patient suffers from excessive thirst and drinks copiously.

Vasopressin is prepared commercially in an aqueous injectable form that can be administered subcutaneously or intramuscularly and in the form of vasopressin tannate, an oily solution that has a more prolonged effect in the body. The tannate form must be completely dissolved before the dose is withdrawn. Prolonged rotation of the ampule may be necessary to ensure that all particles are in suspension; otherwise, a serious error in dosage may occur.

Posterior pituitary powder is dried pituitary gland that, when snuffed, is absorbed from the nasal mucous membrane and checks the polyuria of diabetes insipidus. It is often more acceptable to the patient than repeated injections that are necessary to control the condition.

TOXICITY. Vasopressin can cause spasm of the coronary arteries. It must be administered with caution to patients with inadequate coronary circulation (i.e., angina pectoris). Water retention and occasionally water intoxication may occur. Accurate records of the patient's fluid intake and output should be kept, and he should be weighed daily. Large doses may cause intestinal and uterine cramps.

DOSE. Aqueous vasopressin (20 units/ml.)—1 ml. s.c. or I.M. Vasopressin tannate (5 units/ml.)—0.3 to 1 ml. I.M. Posterior pituitary powder—10 to 20 units as snuff inhalation.

OXYTOCIN INJECTION, U.S.P., B.P. (PITOCIN, SYNTOCINON). Posterior pituitary injection, particularly oxytocin, produces rhythmic contractions of the uterine musculature. The effects of oxytocin depend upon whether the patient is pregnant, and sensitivity to the extract increases as gestation progresses.

USES. Oxytocin is used to induce labor and to shorten it in selected cases. In addition, it constricts the uterus and decreases hemorrhage after delivery of the placenta.

The use of oxytocin is contraindicated in the first stage of labor, because severe laceration and trauma to the still rigid cervix can cause death of both mother and child.

Oxytocin promotes the ejection of milk from lactating breasts by stimulating the contractile tissues in the mammary gland. It has no effect on actual milk production.

TOXICITY. Overdosage may produce uterine tetany followed by increasing clonic contractions. The drug is contraindicated in patients with cardiovascular disease and those who have previously had a cesarean section and if there is a malpresentation of the fetus, or if rupture of the uterus threatens. The blood pressure and pulse should be taken frequently during administration and a check made on the fetal heart tones every 15 minutes. The frequency, strength and duration of uterine contractions should be noted because fetal blood and oxygen are decreased by prolonged uterine contractions.

DOSE. 0.1 to 1 ml. I.M. For induction of labor give 1 ml. containing 10 units in 1000 ml. of 5% dextrose in water slowly by I.V. drip. The patient must be watched very carefully.

Oxytocic Drugs

Several drugs from plant and synthetic sources are classified as oxytocic drugs because of their pharmacologic resemblance to oxytocin. These drugs generally are used for their effect on the smooth muscle of the uterus, but like oxytocin have the undesirable side effect of also causing constriction of the smooth muscles of the peripheral blood vessels.

The ergot alkaloids and their synthetic analogs are the most widely used oxytocic drugs.

ERGOT, N.F. Ergot is obtained from the fungus *Claviceps purpurea,* a parasitic growth found naturally on rye and other grains. Before its pharmacologic and toxic properties were widely known, it was the cause of widespread poisoning in instances in which it was a contaminant in flour prepared from these grains. Whole villages were at times subjected to the toxic and even fatal effects of widespread vasoconstriction if a local baker happened to have ergot fungus in the rye he used to bake bread.

Both levorotatory and dextrorotatory forms of these alkaloids are present in natural sources of ergot, but only the levorotatory form is active pharmacologically. Since the alkaloids are prepared synthetically at present, commercial preparations have only the levo forms.

Three groups of alkaloids have been isolated from ergot: the ergotamine group (of which ergotamine is the principal alkaloid used), the ergobasine group (of which ergonovine is the principal alkaloid) and the ergotoxine group. This latter group contains three alkaloids, but since they offer no different or advantageous pharmacologic effects over ergotamine, these are not used in therapy at present.

ERGOTAMINE TARTRATE, U.S.P., B.P. (GYNERGEN). Although ergotamine exerts a constricting effect on the smooth muscle of the uterus and its blood vessels, the principal use of this alkaloid in therapy is in the treatment of migraine headaches.

Migraine headaches are believed to be produced by a combination of emotional factors and a hereditary predisposition to vascular instability. The aura or warning signs before the onset of a headache are produced by a transient vasoconstriction of one or more cerebral vessels, followed by a pulsating dilation of one or more extracranial vessels and a painful compression of surrounding structures. If ergotamine is taken orally or parenterally at the beginning of an attack, the dilation and consequent pain are often minimized. It is less effective if it is taken when the attack is already well under way, since edema and swelling of the vessel walls is believed to occur in addition to the vasodilation. Simple smooth muscle constriction, therefore, is not the total answer to the problem.

Routine prophylactic use of ergotamine is not recommended because of the high incidence of ergotism, or chronic poisoning, from its prolonged use.

Ergotamine has largely been replaced by ergonovine in the treatment of postpartum hemorrhage.

TOXICITY. Acute toxic effects from ergot or its alkaloids are rare, although they may occur in cases of attempted abortion when large doses are taken. The symptoms are abdominal cramps, vomiting, diarrhea, rapid pulse, headache, mental confusion and unconsciousness. Uterine hemorrhage and abortion may result from such overdosage.

Chronic poisoning, or ergotism, is not uncommon, since it is usually due to overdosage or certain disease states that increase the sensitivity to these alkaloids. Epidemics of chronic poisoning caused by ingestion of contaminated grain are rare today owing to improved agricultural procedures.

Ergotism causes gangrene by a prolonged constriction of the blood vessels and the filling of the blood vessels with a substance that blocks circulation.

Vascular stasis in the toes, fingers, hands and feet causes drying and death of the tissues, whereupon the phalanges break off with neither pain nor bleeding. Prolonged constriction of the retinal vessels causes blindness. Convulsions may occur. Treatment of poisoning is accomplished by withdrawal of the drug and symptomatic therapy.

DOSE. 2 mg. I.M., orally or sublingually. Oral doses may be repeated at 30 minute intervals, to a total of 6 mg. in 24 hours and not more than 12 mg. in a week.

DIHYDROERGOTAMINE (D.H.E. 45). Obtained by hydrogenating ergotamine, this synthetic compound is also useful in the treatment of migraine. It is somewhat less toxic than ergotamine and has a lower incidence of side effects.

DOSE. 1 mg. I.M. or I.V.

METHYSERGIDE MALEATE (SANSERT). Methysergide is a partially synthetic compound that is structurally related to lysergic acid butanolamide (methylergonovine) and is administered for its inhibitory or blocking effects on serotonin. Although it has some residual oxytocic properties, its primary pharmaceutical use is in the prevention of vascular or migraine headaches. When taken regularly, it is believed to inhibit serotonin effector sites, which may be responsible for the vascular instability in times of stress or emotional tension. It reduces the frequency and severity of these headaches and appears to be the most useful drug available for this purpose. It has little or no effect in the treatment of actual attacks of migraine or histamine headaches, however.

TOXICITY. The most common side effects upon continued therapy with methysergide are nausea, vomiting, epigastric pain, dizziness, muscular cramps in the lower extremities following exertion (due to vasoconstriction) and drowsiness. Patients should be advised to report numbness, coldness or pain in their hands or feet. In recent years an unexplained but not infrequent side effect has been reported—that of retroperitoneal fibrosis upon long term therapy with this drug. The fibrosis has a tendency to block the ureters bilaterally and produce subsequent hydroureter and hydronephrosis. Periodic pyelograms should be performed for this reason on all patients taking this drug routinely. It is contraindicated in pregnancy, arteriosclerosis and in constrictive peripheral vascular disorders.

DOSE. 2 mg. orally three times daily, preferably with meals.

Ergonovine maleate, U.S.P. (Ergotrate). Although ergonovine, like ergotamine, has generalized vasoconstrictive effects, it has a greater selectivity for uterine musculature for which it is used exclusively.

It is used, administered orally, for the prevention and treatment of postabortal and postpartum hemorrhage in nonemergency situations. The injectable form is intended primarily for intramuscular use immediately postpartum to hasten uterine contraction and lessen bleeding. Intravenous administration is restricted to patients in whom hemorrhage is excessive and emergency situations that warrant administration by this route.

An initial tetanic contraction of the uterus is obtained, followed by successive minor relaxations and contractions. The rhythmic contractions usually continue for three or more hours after injection.

TOXICITY. Nausea, vomiting, allergic reactions and extreme elevations of blood pressure have been observed following administration of ergonovine. The systemic hypertensive effect is noted especially following intravenous administration and is exaggerated if another vasoconstrictor has been administered previously.

Confusion occasionally arises between ergotamine and ergonovine, particularly since the trade name of the latter drug is Ergotrate. Nurses should be especially mindful of this name similarity, since it has been the cause of rather serious errors in the ordering and administration of these drugs.

The expiration date of ergonovine should be checked carefully because the injectable form deteriorates with age.

DOSE. 0.2 mg. orally, I.M. or I.V.

Methylergonovine maleate, U.S.P. (Methergine). This synthetic compound is very similar to ergonovine in its therapeutic and toxic effects, although it has a more prolonged constrictive effect on the muscles of the uterus. It is reputed to have fewer systemic vasoconstrictive effects than ergonovine, but when the drug is given to susceptible persons, these effects are demonstrated nevertheless. The patient's blood pressure and pulse should be checked frequently, especially after intravenous administration.

Administration of methylergonovine instead of ergonovine is based largely upon the personal preference of the physician.

Rather rapid deterioration of the injectable form occurs when exposed to heat and light; thus it should be protected from these elements and should not be used if discoloration occurs.

DOSE. 0.2 mg. orally, I.M. or I.V.

HORMONES OF THE PANCREAS

In addition to being an exocrine or duct gland responsible for the liberation of digestive enzymes, the pancreas is also an endocrine gland because of the clusters of hormone-secreting cells, the islets of Langerhans, that are scattered irregularly throughout the substance of the gland.

These islets of endocrine tissue are composed of three types of cells—the alpha, beta and delta cells. The alpha cells secrete glucagon and the beta cells secrete insulin, but the function of the delta cells is unknown.

Glucagon, U.S.P. Glucagon is a polypeptide that is a product of the alpha cells of the islets of Langerhans. It acts directly on the liver to increase blood glucose by inducing a breakdown of stored liver glycogen, and in addition by stimulating liver gluconeogenesis from protein. In this way it can increase hepatic glucose output even in the absence of stored liver glycogen, a function that becomes important in starvation.

Glucagon is frequently employed to terminate diabetic insulin reactions and to terminate insulin shock therapy. It has a clinical advantage in that it can be administered intramuscularly. The venous sclerosing effect of intravenously administered glucose for these conditions is avoided, as well as potential kidney damage from extremely high blood glucose levels following intravenous administration of 50 per cent glucose solutions.

It has recently been found to be of value in the treatment of essential hyperlipemia of nondiabetic patients. When 1 mg. of glucagon is administered one hour following meals, there is a rapid decrease in serum cholesterol and esterified fatty acids in the serum. Since hyperlipemic patients usually develop atherosclerosis, although no cause-and-effect relationship has been established, this use of glucagon may prove to have many clinical benefits.

In most patients with hypoglycemia a clinical response to intramuscular glucagon is observed with a rise in blood sugar within 20 minutes. Occasionally, although there is almost invariably a rise in blood sugar, it does not rise above hypoglycemic levels. In these cases, intravenous glucose must be administered.

Blood glucose is not usually raised to a level far above normal; thus if an insulin reaction is due to a long-acting insulin, additional oral glucose should be given to prevent recurrent attacks of hypoglycemia. This may be given in the form of orange juice or soft drinks.

TOXICITY. Nausea, vomiting, allergic phenomena, hypotension and occasional secondary hypoglycemia.

DOSE. 1 mg. s.c., I.M. or I.V.

INSULIN

Insulin, the hormone secreted by the beta cells of the islets of Langerhans, is composed of two chains of amino acids joined by disulfide linkages. After many years of research, investigators derived the chemical formula for insulin in 1955, but it was not synthesized until 1964. Further research will most probably provide a synthetic insulin that may be used for the treatment of diabetes mellitus. This would be very advantageous, since slight modifications could be made in the molecule to restore its effectiveness in individuals who have become immune to insulin through antibody production.

Removal of the pancreas or destruction of the islets of Langerhans by alloxan (producing alloxan diabetes) produces the following effects:

1. There is decreased glucose tolerance. Normally the blood sugar is about 100 mg. per cent. When a moderate dose of glucose is administered orally or intravenously, the blood glucose level in a normal individual may reach 130 mg. per cent, and then return to normal within one hour. In a diabetic, however, the same dose of glucose may cause a rise in blood glucose to 400 mg. per cent, and this level may persist for three or four hours, causing many unfavorable secondary effects.

2. Glucose is not deposited in the liver and muscle in normal amounts, thus there is hyperglycemia, which exceeds the renal threshold for reabsorption of glucose, and glycosuria occurs with resultant kidney damage. Since the osmotic properties of sugar cause excess excretion of water in the urine, the urine volume increases and the patient is dehydrated and thirsty.

3. Glucose is not oxidized for energy.

4. Gluconeogenesis occurs as one attempt to meet the body's energy needs. Because of the breakdown of ingested and body proteins the level of nonprotein nitrogen in the urine is increased. Very often the diabetic has a negative nitrogen balance.

5. There is an increased mobilization of fat from the storage depots since fat utilization for energy is increased. The ketone bodies that are intermediate products of fat oxidation (acetoacetic acid, beta-hydroxybutyric acid and acetone) increase in the blood and are formed more rapidly than the body can metabolize them.

Since these ketone bodies are acidic, much of the basic reserve of the body, sodium bicarbonate, is used to buffer them. This imbalance in the buffer system causes a lowering of blood pH, or acidosis. If severe enough, acidosis produces the comatose state known as diabetic coma.

Partial excretion of these ketone bodies occurs via the lungs; a sweet, fruity odor can often be detected on the breath of an uncorrected diabetic.

The hyperglycemia that occurs with diabetes mellitus may be controlled adequately in most instances by the administration of exogenous insulin.

Insulin, either endogenous or exogenous, acts primarily by enabling glucose to leave the blood stream and cross cell membranes, there to be utilized for energy or stored as glycogen. The disease process of diabetes mellitus, however, appears to be more widespread than first believed and in spite of rigid control of blood glucose levels the other physical and physiological malfunctions that occur with this disease continue to progress. Atherosclerosis occurs to a greater extent in the diabetic than in the normal population, which is the reason many diabetics have coronary occlusions at an early age. The inelastic blood vessels accentuate the development of hypertension. Sclerosis of the retinal arteries, hemorrhages and microinfarcts of the retina and cataracts occur, with the development of many serious visual problems. Circulation is poor in the extremities, leading to the formation of slow healing skin ulcerations with even minor trauma to the leg and foot. The ulcerations often progress to gangrene, and amputation is then necessary. Diabetic patients should always be instructed to wear well-fitting shoes and stockings and to take immediate care of minor lesions. The toenails should be carefully trimmed and patients should be instructed to consult their physicians immediately for care of ingrown toenails, corns and callouses that occur. Progressive kidney changes occur, and renal damage may be sufficient to cause death in some instances.

In patients with diabetes that is difficult to control with insulin, many physicians prefer to allow moderate hyperglycemia rather than to risk hypoglycemic episodes or insulin shock, which may occur with wide variations in blood glucose levels following the administration of insulin. The concurrent symptoms of diabetes are not appreciably increased by insulin doses that allow glucose to spill into the urine at some time during the day. It is believed by many investigators that the sclerosis of kidney blood vessels seen in diabetes is an independent phenomenon and is not directly related to blood glucose levels.

Even after an acceptable dose of insulin has been established, the patient should be aware that unusual activity or changes in the carbohydrate content of his diet will alter his insulin requirements. Although febrile illnesses may in some instances reduce the insulin requirements, infections may increase the requirements. Any patient who must undergo surgery, even though he may have been previously regulated on oral hypoglycemic agents, should be changed to insulin injections because the insulin requirement is often increased by administration of a general anesthesia and in times of stress.

INSULIN SHOCK

Insulin shock is produced by extremely low blood glucose levels and may be brought about by changes in body insulin requirements as previously discussed or by an accidental overdosage of insulin. The first symptoms are trembling, confusion and sweating, accompanied by shallow, rapid breathing. Drowsiness proceeds to coma unless glucose is administered. Diabetic patients should be thoroughly acquainted with the symptoms of impending insulin shock and should be instructed to carry sugar cubes or have ready access to sugar, orange juice or other high carbohydrate beverages should such symptoms occur.

Since a diabetic patient becomes unconscious when an insufficient amount of insulin is present (diabetic coma) and when too much insulin is administered (insulin shock), the symptoms distinguishing these two conditions are extremely important. Table 10 is a comparison of symptoms helpful in determining which condition exists. In some

TABLE 10 Insulin Reactions

	DIABETIC COMA *acidosis*	REGULAR INSULIN REACTION *shock*	PROTAMINE ZINC OR NPH INSULIN REACTION
ONSET:	Slow (days) in adults. Fairly rapid in children.	Sudden, rapid (minutes). Reaction occurs in daytime.	Insidious, slow (hours). Reaction occurs in evening.
SYMPTOMS:	Weakness, mental dullness.	Trembling, mental confusion, weakness, drowsiness, nervousness.	Weakness, drowsiness, nervousness, trembling, irritability.
	FREQUENTLY: Nausea, vomiting, no appetite, thirst.	FREQUENTLY: NO nausea; hunger, NO abdominal pain.	OCCASIONALLY: Nausea, vomiting.
	Hot dry skin, abdominal pain, dim vision.	Cold, clammy skin, double vision.	FREQUENTLY: Headache, hunger, NO abdominal pain.
	Deep, labored breathing, air hunger, loss of consciousness.	Normal or shallow breathing, loss of consciousness.	Cold, clammy skin, double vision.
	Fruity odor on breath.		Normal or shallow breathing, loss of consciousness.
TREATMENT:	Check urine—high sugar content. Call doctor—he will prescribe REGULAR INSULIN.	Check urine—may contain sugar. Keep patient awake and give sugar or orange juice. Call doctor.	Check urine—most likely sugar-free. Give sugar or orange juice for fast effect, and milk, crackers or bread for prolonged effect. Call doctor.

cases, however, these symptoms cannot be readily defined. In the treatment of an unconscious diabetic in whom a rapid diagnosis is not possible, it is preferable that the error should be made on the side of safety, that is, by administration of intravenous glucose. With an already elevated blood glucose level, the patient will not be appreciably harmed by additional glucose. A rapid response should occur if the patient is in insulin shock. Additional insulin given to a patient already in insulin shock may be sufficient to cause death. Except in an extreme emergency in which no physician is available, the nurse should not attempt to administer drugs to an unconscious diabetic.

COMMERCIAL PREPARATIONS OF INSULIN

There are five types of insulin preparations, all obtained from the pancreas of domestic animals. The basic action of all is alike; they differ mainly in the time of onset of action and the duration of effect in lower-

ing blood sugar. These preparations are standardized to contain 40, 80 or 100 units per ml. The dosage is regulated by the patient's requirements. Insulins should be refrigerated, but should not be frozen. Expiration dates on insulin labels should be checked.

INSULIN INJECTION, U.S.P., B.P. (REGULAR INSULIN). This is a clear, aqueous solution of insulin. When injected, it takes effect rapidly (within one hour) but has a very short duration of action. Thus, in order to maintain the diabetic, injections would have to be given every three or four hours. Regular Insulin is used in insulin shock therapy and is the form administered to patients in diabetic coma since rapid action is desired in both instances.

Often, when the physician writes the insulin orders for a diabetic patient, he provides for additional units of regular insulin to be given if the urine test before a meal indicates glycosuria or ketonuria. He orders a specific number of units of regular insulin to be given for each degree of glycosuria. An additional amount is usually ordered if the urine is positive for acetone. The additional units of regular insulin are considered necessary to "cover" the additional carbohydrate the patient will consume with the next meal.

Urine samples to be tested for glycosuria and ketones should be obtained about one half hour before the meal and at bedtime. The patient should empty his bladder completely about 30 minutes before the specimen is to be collected. This insures that the urine testing will reflect the patient's present level of glycosuria rather than the sugar excreted previously.

Other drugs which the patient is receiving may cause inaccurate results in tests for glycosuria. A different type of urine test may be needed.

EXAMPLE:

If urine is 1 + ... no insulin
            2 + ... 5 units regular insulin
            3 + ... 10 units regular insulin
            4 + ... 15 units regular insulin

If acetone is present, add 5 units regular insulin.

ISOPHANE INSULIN SUSPENSION, U.S.P. (NPH INSULIN). NPH insulin, an abbreviation for neutral protamine Hagedorn insulin, was named after its discoverer. It is a cloudy suspension of fine crystals prepared by the reaction of protamine with insulin. The insoluble precipitate resulting from the reaction provides effective insulin blood levels for 28 hours, but there is a two hour delay in onset after the dose is given, which is the reason NPH insulin is not used when immediate action is desired. The more uniform blood sugar level provided by the longer-acting insulins is preferable for regulating diabetic patients, however. This type of insulin is often given in combination with regular insulin for management of the diabetic patient with only one injection daily. NPH insulin is never given intravenously.

Before preparing the injection of NPH insulin, one should rotate the vial gently between the palms to be sure that the particles are suspended evenly. Neglecting to do this, or causing bubbles by shaking, may result in inaccurate dosage. If a precipitate is still present after mixing, the insulin should not be used.

NPH insulin should be given one half to one and a half hours before breakfast. Its peak of action occurs 10 to 20 hours after administration. It may be necessary to provide for a snack in the afternoon to prevent hypoglycemia. There is also the possibility of hypoglycemia occurring during the night because of the prolonged action of NPH insulin.

PROTAMINE ZINC INSULIN SUSPENSION, U.S.P., PROTAMINE ZINC INSULIN INJECTION, B.P. Another long-acting insulin, protamine zinc insulin is quite similar in effect to NPH insulin. It requires six to eight hours for onset of action after the dose is administered; the peak of action is reached in 16 to 24 hours but effects persist for 24 to 36 hours. Usually the individual can be maintained on one injection daily, because the previous dose covers the time span necessary for onset of action. It is given subcutaneously and should never be given intravenously. PZI insulin should be rotated gently before withdrawal from the vial to be sure that it is evenly suspended.

GLOBIN ZINC INSULIN INJECTION, N.F., B.P. Prepared from the hemoglobin of beef blood, globin zinc insulin is intended primarily for patients who are sensitive to protamine. The onset of action is in one or two hours; the duration of action is 24 hours. Its effects are comparable to those of protamine zinc insulin. Globulin zinc insulin should never be given intravenously. Any solution that is cloudy should not be used.

LENTE, SEMI-LENTE AND ULTRA-LENTE INSULIN. The action of zinc on insulin under specific conditions gives us three forms of the delayed-action insulin. The product formed from the reaction is relatively insoluble at the pH of blood. It should never be given intravenously. Semi-lente has the smallest particle size and, therefore, the shortest duration of action (12 to 16 hours) with an onset of action in one to two hours. Ultra-lente has the largest particle size and has a duration of action of 36 hours with an onset time of four hours. Lente insulin is prepared by mixing the other two forms and has a duration of action of 24 to 28 hours with an onset time of two to three hours.

As mentioned previously, it is often advisable to mix a short-acting insulin such as regular insulin with a longer acting form such as NPH or protamine zinc to cover immediate insulin needs and to provide day-long requirements in one injection. There is no great danger from incompatibilities due to this mixing process, because the time and temperature necessary for changing regular insulin to the longer acting forms are not present in the syringe at room temperature.

The lente insulins contain no sensitizing substances. They can therefore be used by patients who are allergic to other types of insulin.

DOSE. 5 to 50 units or more.

THE NURSE'S ROLE IN RELATION TO INSULIN THERAPY AND DIABETES

Insulin (and oral hypoglycemic agents) is only one aspect in the treatment of the patient with diabetes. The diet of the diabetic is equally important and must be closely aligned with the drug therapy. A very delicate balance must be maintained between the carbohydrate intake and the amount of insulin administered in order to prevent hyperglycemia or hypoglycemia.

The timing of meals must coincide with the time during which the insulin or oral agents are in effect. Insulin should usually not be given without consulting the doctor if the patient is permitted no oral intake, unless he has an intravenous infusion with glucose or will have eaten by the time the insulin exerts its effect.

Likewise, if a patient has received his insulin, his carbohydrate intake must be assured according to the planned diet. If the patient does not eat all of his meal, a supplement or substitution must be made to avoid hypoglycemia or insulin shock. Special problems arise, such as when the diabetic patient vomits his meal and is unable to retain food. The doctor should be notified immediately so that an intravenous infusion can be started to provide the patient with carbohydrate and electrolytes.

Great care is necessary in preparing and administering insulin. The type of insulin ordered should be checked carefully with the label on the vial. The strength of the insulin preparation should be noted and the dose measured according to the appropriately calibrated insulin syringe. For example, U 40 insulin should be measured with a syringe calibrated for U 40; U 80 should be measured with a syringe calibrated for U 80. The dose can also be measured with a tuberculin syringe calibrated in minims, in which case it is necessary to determine the number of minims of the particular strength of insulin that are needed to give the required dose. (See Chapter 4 for instructions on determining the dosage in minims.) Care should be taken that all air is removed from the syringe when measuring the dose, since this interferes with the accuracy of the dose, particularly when a small volume is administered.

Insulin is usually administered by subcutaneous injection using a 90 degree angle. Because of the necessity for daily or even more frequent injections, it is very important that the sites of injection be carefully rotated in order to prevent atrophy of the subcutaneous tissue. A record and plan for rotation of sites should be kept and carefully followed. The usual sites for injection are the lateral aspects of the arms, the abdomen and the anterior portions of the thigh. Patients should be taught injection technique. A member of the family should also be taught to administer insulin in the event that the patient is unable to do so.

Because of the diabetic's increased susceptibility to infection, strict aseptic technique is essential. The diabetic must be taught how to clean and sterilize equipment at home. Syringes and needles should be boiled for 20 minutes. Disposable syringes and needles may also be used.

Insulin must be kept cool. This may present a problem to diabetics when they are traveling. Some have solved this problem by placing the insulin vial in a thermos bottle with cold water. Insulin should not be

1. With thumb and index finger of one hand, stretch the skin away from clean area selected for injection and cleanse area with an alcohol swab. Using a circular motion, wipe injection area from the center out toward the edge of injection site.

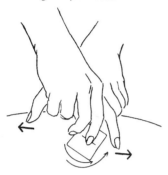

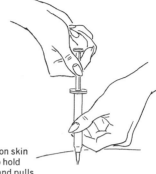

3. Release pressure on skin and use freed hand to hold syringe while other hand pulls back slightly on plunger.

If blood appears in bottom of syringe barrel, pull unit out of skin slightly — 1/16 to 1/8 inch — to remove needle tip from blood vessel. Pull back slightly on plunger again. If more blood appears, select new injection site. Replace the needle if you do this because the first one is contaminated.

2. Keeping skin stretched, grasp syringe firmly near its tip with other hand, taking care not to touch sterile needle.

Quickly thrust needle straight into injection site, as illustrated. Thrust needle in up to its hub.

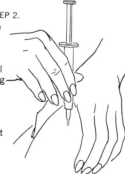

ALTERNATE METHOD TO STEP 2.

2a. If injection is to be made into an area with only a thin layer of fat, pinch a fold of skin between fingers, rather than stretching skin. This will keep needle from penetrating into a muscle.

Taking care not to touch sterile needle, grasp syringe firmly near its tip.

Quickly thrust needle straight into injection site, as illustrated. Thrust needle in up to its hub.

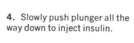

4. Slowly push plunger all the way down to inject insulin.

5. Hold alcohol swab close to needle hub. Withdraw syringe and attached needle rapidly, in a straight line.

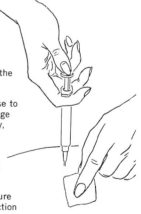

6. As needle comes out of skin, quickly place alcohol swab over injection site.

7. Briefly apply firm pressure on alcohol wipe over injection site.

8. Record injection site and do not use it again for at least 14 days.

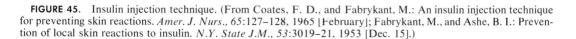

FIGURE 45. Insulin injection technique. (From Coates, F. D., and Fabrykant, M.: An insulin injection technique for preventing skin reactions. *Amer. J. Nurs.*, 65:127–128, 1965 [February]; Fabrykant, M., and Ashe, B. I.: Prevention of local skin reactions to insulin. *N.Y. State J.M.*, 53:3019–21, 1953 [Dec. 15].)

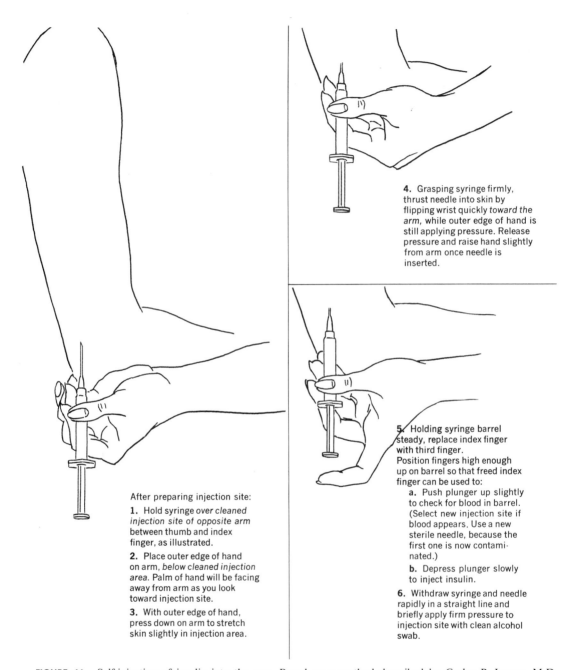

4. Grasping syringe firmly, thrust needle into skin by flipping wrist quickly *toward the arm*, while outer edge of hand is still applying pressure. Release pressure and raise hand slightly from arm once needle is inserted.

After preparing injection site:

1. Hold syringe *over cleaned injection site of opposite arm* between thumb and index finger, as illustrated.

2. Place outer edge of hand on arm, *below cleaned injection area*. Palm of hand will be facing away from arm as you look toward injection site.

3. With outer edge of hand, press down on arm to stretch skin slightly in injection area.

5. Holding syringe barrel steady, replace index finger with third finger. Position fingers high enough up on barrel so that freed index finger can be used to:

    a. Push plunger up slightly to check for blood in barrel. (Select new injection site if blood appears. Use a new sterile needle, because the first one is now contaminated.)

    b. Depress plunger slowly to inject insulin.

6. Withdraw syringe and needle rapidly in a straight line and briefly apply firm pressure to injection site with clean alcohol swab.

FIGURE 46. Self-injection of insulin into the arm. Based on a method described by Carlos P. Lamar, M.D. (*J.A.M.A.*, April 29, 1950, p. 132), this technique utilizes the hand as a self-injector for entering arm injection sites at approximately a 90° angle (From *The H Line*, Vol. I, No. 6–7, Summer-Fall, 1967. Becton-Dickinson and Co., Rutherford, N.J.)

frozen, however. Allowing the insulin to warm to room temperature before it is injected is advised as a means of reducing subcutaneous tissue atrophy.

Patients with diabetes should always carry sugar with them in case they have a hypoglycemic reaction. They should also carry an identification card stating that they are diabetic. Many times diabetics in diabetic coma have been thought to be intoxicated because of the acetone odor of the breath.

It is usually the responsibility of the nurse, after securing permission and information from the physician, to initiate a teaching plan for the diabetic and his family. This plan should include an explanation of the basic facts of his disease, insulin and techniques of administration, urine testing, diet, signs and symptoms of diabetic coma and insulin shock and indicated action. The general hygienic measures and means to help prevent the many complications of diabetes mellitus should also be included.

ORAL HYPOGLYCEMIC AGENTS

Since insulin is rapidly destroyed in the gastrointestinal tract, it must always be administered parenterally. The prospect of daily injections for the rest of their lives, is a bleak one for many diabetic patients. The disease presents many inconveniences in traveling and even in daily living because of the necessity for keeping needles and syringes sterile and ready for use and having the appropriate insulin preparation available and under refrigeration at all times.

A ready solution to many of these problems would be the availability of an appropriate insulin-like agent that could be administered orally. It has been known since the late 1870's that guanidine, when administered orally, produces muscle cramps and lowers blood sugar. The biguanides, which were developed from guanidine, were used for the treatment of diabetes mellitus until insulin became available. The biguanides were unsatisfactory and produced many serious side effects; the convenience of oral administration did not give them an overall advantage over the safer insulin.

In the 1950's the sulfonylureas, also hypoglycemic agents, were developed and have gained great popularity in the treatment of diabetes. They have not proved to be of benefit in diabetes that appears in childhood or even in severe diabetes that has its onset later in life. Since it is presumed that their mechanism of action is based on their ability to cause insulin release from the pancreas, they could be expected to perform well only in the presence of functional pancreatic islet tissue. Other drugs that the patient is receiving may produce hypoglycemia. Included in this group are salicylates, alcohol, sulfonamides, butazolidin, and MAO inhibitors.

Mild diabetes should be regulated by diet alone, if possible, and only if this therapy is inadequate should oral hypoglycemics be used. In some cases these agents may be used in addition to insulin to aid in the smooth, overall control of the disease.

TOLBUTAMIDE, U.S.P., B.P. (ORINASE). Although tolbutamide is a derivative of the sulfonamides, it has no antibacterial action. Its outstanding pharmacologic effect is the ability to lower blood sugar levels by promoting the release of insulin from the pancreatic beta cells. The drug has no value if no beta cells are present; it is obviously not a substitute for insulin in all types of diabetic patients.

$$SO_2NH-\overset{\overset{\displaystyle O}{\|}}{C}-NH-C_4H_9$$

tolbutamide

Tolbutamide is most successful in the treatment of mild forms of diabetes that develop in middle age. If there are complications in therapy, however, such as severe trauma or major surgery, supportive insulin therapy is necessary.

TOXICITY. Tolbutamide is contraindicated in patients having juvenile or growth-onset types of diabetes, unstable or brittle diabetes or a history of diabetic coma. It is also contraindicated in maturity-onset diabetes complicated by ketosis, acidosis, diabetic coma, fever, severe trauma, gangrene, Raynaud's disease or serious impairment of renal, hepatic or thyroid function.

Hypoglycemia is the most serious side effect of tolbutamide. Other side effects include gastrointestinal disturbances, allergic skin manifestations and alcohol intolerance. The latter effect is due to the inhibition of the enzyme alcohol dehydrogenase, which breaks down alcohol within the body. Without this enzyme a cumulative effect of alcohol is readily obtained. Patients should be made aware of these effects when taking this drug. Leukopenia has been noted in some patients.

Because of reported incidences of cardiovascular complications when tolbutamide is administered, it is now recommended for use only when diet control and insulin are ineffective in controlling diabetes.

DOSE. 3 Gm. orally the first day, 2 Gm. the second day and 1 Gm. the third day, preferably given in divided doses after meals. Maintenance dose is usually between 0.5 and 1.5 Gm. daily.

CHLORPROPAMIDE, U.S.P. (DIABINESE). Chlorpropamide is also an oral hypoglycemic agent that has an effect on the pancreatic beta cells similar to that of tolbutamide.

Unlike tolbutamide, which is inactivated in the body, chlorpropamide is slowly excreted unchanged in the urine. It has a longer duration of action than tolbutamide and is about twice as potent. Like tolbutamide, it is most effective in maturity-onset diabetes.

TOXICITY. Although the side effects are generally of a short duration, they may be more severe than noted with tolbutamide. Severe hypoglycemia has occurred, as has thrombocytopenia, dermatoses, jaundice, gastrointestinal and neurologic disturbances, alcohol intolerance and blood dyscrasias.

DOSE. 500 mg. orally daily initially in one dose before or with breakfast. Maintenance dose is 250 to 500 mg. daily.

ACETOHEXAMIDE (DYMELOR). Acetohexamide is rather closely related to tolbutamide and chlorpropamide in pharmacologic action, although it is not quite as potent as chlorpropamide. The toxic side effects are similar.

DOSE. 0.25 to 1.5 Gm. orally daily.

PHENFORMIN (DBI). Unlike the other three oral hypoglycemic agents, phenformin does not stimulate the beta cells to release insulin. Its exact mode of action is not completely understood, but it apparently acts peripherally to aid in the utilization of glucose.

Phenformin is often combined with insulin to aid in the control of brittle diabetes.

TOXICITY. Nausea, vomiting and diarrhea and a metallic taste occur occasionally but usually disappear with reduction of the dosage. It should be administered with caution to individuals with hepatic disorders.

DOSE. Initial—25 mg. orally twice daily; maintenance—50 to 150 mg. daily.

Very recent developments in the study of diabetes mellitus have brought about some interesting speculations. It has been observed that in maturity-onset diabetes (the diabetes that occurs after 30 years of age), the blood level of insulin, rather than being decreased, is actually higher than normal, and the blood sugar level is also elevated. The elevated insulin level would explain the continual hunger these patients experience, leading to a failure to stay on corrective diets.

Most likely further research will reveal that, although these individuals have sufficient insulin in the blood, they are merely unable to utilize it. Perhaps a whole new field of diabetic therapy will follow in the wake of this new scientific discovery; at any rate, it poses many unanswered questions.

THYROID HORMONES AND ANTITHYROID DRUGS

The thyroid gland is a bilobed structure located on each side of the larynx. It consists of many hollow spheres, called follicles, which store thyroglobulin.

The thyroid gland has a tremendous avidity for iodide. After the iodide is trapped, it is oxidized to iodine and used to iodinate tyrosine, an amino acid also found in high concentrations in the thyroid follicles. Two molecules of tyrosine are first coupled, and the iodine atoms are added successively to the molecule.

Following iodination, the products, chiefly triiodothyronine (T_3), which contains three iodine atoms, and thyroxine (T_4), which has four iodine atoms, are stored in the thyroid follicles in the form of thyroglobulin until they are released into the blood. The thyroid gland can store several weeks' supply of these thyroid hormones, as is evidenced by the fact that it takes about this long for symptoms to develop following administration of antithyroid drugs.

The actions of the thyroid gland are multiple but involve chiefly the following:

1. Calorigenesis. Stimulation of heat production and oxygen consumption resulting in an elevated basal metabolic rate (BMR) is perhaps the most fundamental effect of the thyroid hormone. The BMR is used as an index of thyroid activity. After thyroid removal, there is a gradual decrease in metabolism and heat production. A low point is reached about two months after surgery and results in a BMR 35 to 40 per cent below normal.

2. Growth and differentiation. The effect of the thyroid hormone on growth and differentiation is said to be different from its effect on energy metabolism. The retardation of growth is not as severe following thyroidectomy as it is following a deficit of growth hormone, but thyroid hormone and growth hormone are both needed for normal growth and development.

3. Protein metabolism. As long as the individual is in physiologic balance, the thyroid hormones are protein anabolic agents.

There is increased nitrogen retention, protein anabolism and growth. If an excess of these hormones is administered, however, just the opposite effect occurs, and the hormones enhance protein catabolism. Hyperthyroid individuals have an increased nitrogen excretion and a negative nitrogen balance. Regardless of how much these individuals eat, there is a gradual weight loss.

4. Cardiovascular system. An increase of thyroid hormone increases oxygen consumption and carbon dioxide production. The body, in an effort to rid itself of this excess heat, increases the cardiac output and heart rate. The blood pressure may be elevated slightly or it may remain normal.

A thyroid deficiency, or hypothyroidism, may be due to primary or secondary causes. A primary deficiency may be due to either direct failure of the thyroid gland or a lack of sensitivity to thyrotropin. A secondary deficiency would be due to failure of the anterior pituitary to secrete thyrotropin. The net result of the metabolic disorders due to the lack of thyroid hormone would be the same in either case, however. When thyroid hormone is deficient or absent in young children, usually because of a lack of iodine or a failure of the gland to develop, cretinism results (Fig. 47, A). The child, a cretin, exhibits retarded mental and physical growth, has an enlarged tongue, coarse features, malformed bones, a distended abdomen and puffy skin. If therapy with the thyroid hormone is begun in sufficient time (before 6 months of age), the child is able to develop normally. If treatment is not begun until later, however, permanent mental and physical disorders will persist.

If a thyroid deficiency becomes evident in adulthood, the condition is known as myxedema (Gull's disease) (Fig. 47, B). It is characterized by increasing lethargy, thick, puffy skin, mental deterioration, obesity, loss of hair and lowered metabolic rate. Since normal development had occurred prior to the onset of the disease, few permanent effects persist after thyroid therapy is instituted. Results are best, of course, if treatment is begun early in the course of the disease.

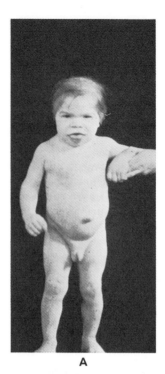

A

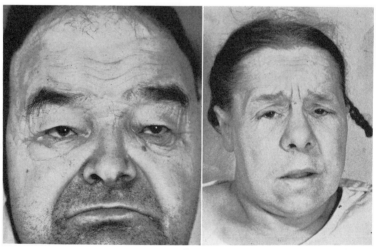

B

FIGURE 47 A & B.   Photos of cretinism (Bronstein, et al., Am. J. Med. Sci.) and myxedema (Williams, R. H., and Bakke, J. L., in Williams: *Textbook of Endocrinology*. Ed. 4. W. B. Saunders Co., Philadelphia, 1968.)

Simple goiter is produced by a lack of iodine and is seen relatively frequently in areas in which the iodine content of soil and water is low. Since iodine is incorporated into the thyroxin molecule, no hormone can be manufactured without it. Because of the scarcity of the element, the gland enlarges in an attempt to retain as much of the iodine of the blood as possible. Subsequent iodine therapy does not cause the enlarged thyroid to diminish in size, but halts further growth. Surgical procedures are necessary to remove the enlarged portion of the gland.

Hypertrophy of the thyroid gland produces an opposite picture—that of exophthalmic goiter (Graves' disease). In this condition, the thyroid need not be noticeably enlarged, but it produces excess hormone with a resulting increased BMR, increased production of heat, loss of weight, increased heart rate and blood pressure, nervousness and exophthalmos. The protrusion of the eyes, which is characteristic of this condition, is caused by hypertrophy of the connective tissue behind the eyeball. The progress of this hypertrophy is halted by therapy, but the protrusion already present remains. Hyperthyroidism may be treated by surgery or x-ray therapy or by destruction of a portion of the gland with antithyroid drugs.

When patients are receiving drugs which affect thyroid function, there is always the possibility of inducing too great an effect, resulting in the patient having the opposite type of thyroid condition. The nurse should observe for indications of hyperthyroidism in patients receiving thyroid replacement therapy, as well as observing for the reduction of the symptoms of hypothyroidism. Conversely, the patient receiving antithyroid drugs should be observed for indications of too great a reduction in thyroid function.

THYROID PREPARATIONS

THYROID, U.S.P., B.P.   The entire defatted and dried thyroid glands of domestic animals may be incorporated directly into tablets for oral administration. The glands are standardized on the basis of their iodine content.

The adult with myxedema can readily be maintained on the correct amount of thyroid hormone and can remain normal with a natural life expectancy. The U.S.P. preparation of thyroid gland in tablet form is usually the most inexpensive form of therapy. It is the form most commonly used for individuals who must remain on supplemental thyroid hormone throughout their lives. Because longstanding hypothyroidism may have undesirable side effects, including a predisposition to atherosclerosis, a full replacement dose should be administered whenever possible. Patients need to understand that they will require replacement therapy throughout their lives.

In childhood, the treatment regimen is the same as in adults except that every attempt should be made to administer the largest dose that can be tolerated without ill effects to ensure normal growth and development. Very often a full adult dose is required to accomplish this end. The measure of success in treating cretinism is directly related to the age at which therapy is instituted. If no thyroid gland develops in the fetus, the deficiency probably dates from the fetal age of three months because little thyroid hormone is transferred across the placenta from the maternal blood.

thyroxin

Thyroid hormones are sometimes used in the treatment of obesity. At best, this therapy should be a temporary measure to increase the basal metabolic rate and the burning of calories. Since most cases of obesity are due simply to overeating rather than to any underlying endocrine disorder, this method of treatment is not without disadvantages, and signs of thyrotoxicosis rapidly appear if therapy is continued for a prolonged period of time. For this reason, the Food and Drug Administration has prohibited the use of even small amounts of thyroid hormone in proprietary drugs for obesity.

In addition to symptomatic hypothyroidism, thyroid preparations may be used for treatment of menstrual disturbances related to thyroid dysfunction and in combination with other therapeutic measures in the treatment of habitual abortion, sterility and certain dermatologic conditions. Its efficacy in the treatment of these latter conditions varies greatly.

When administered orally, thyroid hormone is readily absorbed from the gastrointestinal tract, but a latent period of at least 24 hours occurs before therapeutic effects are observed. The maximal effects may not be seen for 10 days to two weeks; when dosage increments are given they must not be prescribed until the maximal effects of the previous dosage level are observed. Because of the cumulative effects of the hormone, effects may persist for as long as four to eight weeks after the drug is withdrawn.

Since thyroid hormone gradually deteriorates in the presence of heat, light and moisture, the tablets should not be kept for an extended period of time before use. They may become hardened and insoluble and, therefore, will not be absorbed completely. Ordinarily no more than a three months' supply should be dispensed to a patient at one time.

TOXICITY. Toxic symptoms are due to the cumulative effects of the drug in the body and resemble the effects of hyperthyroidism: hypertension, tachycardia, chest pain, dyspnea, nervousness, tremor, insomnia, increased basal metabolic rate and weight loss. The pulse should be checked before and during the administration of thyroid preparations, and the dose should be withheld from an adult with a pulse of 100 beats or more per minute.

DOSE. 30 to 200 mg. orally daily.

THYROGLOBULIN (PROLOID). Thyroglobulin tablets consist of a mixture of triiodothyronine and tetraiodothyronine, which are extracted from the thyroid glands of domestic animals. Although it does not have the impurities and inert substances present in the preparations of whole thyroid gland, it does not have the specificity or predictability of action that the synthetic preparations have. A double standardization is performed on thyroglobulin extracts—one for therapeutic potency in animals and the other for iodine content.

Thyroglobulin may be used whenever thyroid hormone is indicated. Its use rather than the other available preparations is determined by the physician's preference.

TOXICITY. Toxic reactions are similar to those experienced with the powdered thyroid preparation.

DOSE. 60 to 180 mg. orally daily.

SODIUM LEVOTHYROXINE, U.S.P. (TETRAIODO-THYRONINE, T$_4$, SYNTHROID, LEVOID). Thyroxine is the principal secretion of the thyroid gland and, in the blood, is bound to plasma proteins. Only the levorotatory form is prepared commercially since the dextrorotatory form has little or no activity.

There is a lag of one to two days before the effects of orally administered thyroxine are detectable. It is not believed to be the ultimately active form of the hormone at the cellular level. Thyroxine probably acts upon oxidizing enzymes in the body because it increases the metabolism and oxygen consumption of nearly all cells and tissues.

Since this active principle is prepared synthetically, biological assay is not required for determination of potency. One hundred mcg. (0.1 mg.) of sodium levothyroxine is clinically equivalent to 30 to 60 mg. of the powdered thyroid gland.

TOXICITY. Side effects of sodium levothyroxine resemble those of hyperthyroidism and may include palpitation, anginal pain, dyspnea, headache, hypertension, diarrhea, nervousness and mental agitation. Since it has a slow onset of action, symptoms of overdosage may not appear for one to three weeks. If signs of overdosage appear, the drug should be discontinued for two to six days and then resumed at a lower dosage. It should be used with caution in patients in whom hypertension would be hazardous, such as in angina pectoris and cardiovascular or peripheral vascular disorders. It is contraindicated in patients with nephrosis, adrenal insufficiency or recent myocardial infarctions.

DOSE. 50 to 100 mcg. orally daily for one to three weeks, then increased in increments of 50 to 100 mcg. every one to three weeks until the desired response is obtained. The maintenance dose is usually 150 to 400 mcg. daily.

✓SODIUM LIOTHYRONINE, U.S.P. (TRIIODOTHY-RONINE, T$_3$, CYTOMEL). In this synthetic preparation, the levo form is also employed because it is more than twice as active as the racemic mixture of liothyronine. Sodium liothyronine is readily absorbed from the gastrointestinal tract. It is more loosely bound to plasma proteins than is thyroxine; thus it is more readily available to the tissues and has a faster onset of action. Although the exact mechanism of action of liothyronine has not been determined, it appears to be the ultimately active thyroid hormone at the cellular level, being absorbed directly by the target cells immediately after conversion from levothyroxine.

Sodium liothyronine sometimes increases the sperm count and motility and has been used with variable success in the treatment of male infertility. Like other thyroid preparations, it has been employed for gynecologic disorders, such as amenorrhea, premenstrual tension and dysmenorrhea. Quite beneficial effects in the regulation of the menstrual periods have been attained, particularly in younger women but only if the gynecologic symptoms are due to a deficiency of thyroid hormone.

Twenty-five mcg. of liothyronine is equivalent to about 65 mg. of crude thyroid gland.

>TOXICITY. Because of liothyronine's rapid onset of action, beneficial effects as well as symptoms of overdosage, such as tachycardia and excitability may appear within 24 to 48 hours after oral administration. The more rapid effects may allow rapid attainment of a euthyroid state in hypothyroid individuals as well as a rapid cessation of side effects when the drug is withdrawn.

>DOSE. 5 to 25 mcg. orally daily. Dosage is then increased at one or two week intervals until a satisfactory level has been attained.

ANTITHYROID DRUGS

The antithyroid drugs are administered to decrease or inhibit the production of thyroid hormone. Since they do not counteract the effects of circulating thyroid hormone, they are of little value in the immediate treatment of toxicity symptoms of hyperthyroidism. Therapeutic benefits are not observed until the reserve stores of thyroid hormone are depleted.

✓ PROPYLTHIOURACIL, U.S.P., B.P. Propylthiouracil decreases thyroxine production presumably by inhibiting the oxidation of iodide, a step necessary before iodine can be used in the synthesis of thyroxine. A time lag of several days to weeks may occur before the antithyroid effects appear since there is no effect on the thyroxine already present in the gland. Since iodide uptake is not decreased by this drug, studies of the radioactive iodine uptake by the thyroid gland remain the same.

propylthiouracil

Propylthiouracil is used in the treatment of hyperthyroidism in cases in which surgery is not feasible because of the patient's age or physical condition, and it may be used prior to surgery to make the patient a better surgical risk. When propylthiouracil is administered preoperatively, iodine, in the form of strong iodine solution (Lugol's solution), is usually given concurrently for seven to ten days prior to surgery in order to prevent the extreme vascularity and tendency to hemorrhage during surgery that tend to be produced when propylthiouracil is administered alone for a period of time. When propylthiouracil is used as a substitute for surgery, thyroid hormone is often administered with it to maintain a euthyroid condition.

>TOXICITY. This drug should be stored in light-resistant containers. Hyperplasia of the thyroid gland occurs frequently if antithyroid drugs are administered for a prolonged period of time since the secretion of thyrotropic hormone from the anterior pituitary is increased because of the thyroid hormone deficiency.

>Agranulocytosis is the most serious toxic effect of propylthiouracil therapy, but leukopenia and thrombocytopenia may also occur. For this reason, periodic blood counts should be made dur-

ing therapy, and the patient should be instructed to report symptoms of agranulocytosis, such as sore throat or fever. Skin rashes, urticaria, swelling of the cervical lymph nodes, gastrointestinal disturbances, hepatic damage, arthralgia, visual disturbances, headache, drowsiness and vertigo occur occasionally.

Antithyroid drugs should not be used during pregnancy or lactation unless absolutely necessary for the health or survival of the mother. The drug has been shown to pass the placental barrier with deleterious effects on the unborn child.

DOSE. 300 mg. orally initially, then 50 to 100 mg. daily.

IOTHIOURACIL SODIUM (ITRUMIL SODIUM). This iodinated derivative of thiouracil is very similar in action and effect to propylthiouracil and methylthiouracil. Because it contains iodine, it does not produce the extreme vascularity and friability seen when the other thiouracil compounds are administered alone.

Iothiouracil may be used preoperatively in the treatment of hyperthyroidism and in cases in which surgery is contraindicated. The concurrent administration of iodine is not necessary with this derivative.

TOXICITY. As with propylthiouracil and methylthiouracil, the most serious side effects of this drug are blood dyscrasias. Periodic blood counts should be made during therapy. Gastrointestinal and dermatologic disorders are observed frequently. It is contraindicated in pregnant or lactating women.

DOSE. 300 mg. orally daily in three or four divided doses.

METHIMAZOLE, U.S.P. (TAPAZOLE). Although the actions and effects of methimazole are very similar to those of propylthiouracil, this drug is approximately 10 times as potent as propylthiouracil on a weight to weight basis. The therapeutic effects of methimazole usually appear within

a few days after therapy is begun, but it is usually more difficult to stabilize the patient when it is used alone. It is usually employed in cases in which the patient has become refractory to other antithyroid drugs.

TOXICITY. Side effects and contraindications are the same as those for propylthiouracil.

DOSE. 10 to 30 mg. orally daily.

METHYLTHIOURACIL, U.S.P., B.P. (METHIACIL, MURACIL, THIMECIL). Methylthiouracil is closely related to propylthiouracil in structure and action. On a weight to weight basis, however, methylthiouracil is somewhat more potent and toxic, which is the reason it is seldom used in preference to propylthiouracil or methimazole. It may be useful, however, in patients who are refractory to other antithyroid drugs.

TOXICITY. Methylthiouracil produces a higher incidence and greater severity of side effects than does propylthiouracil or methimazole. Agranulocytosis, leukopenia and thrombocytopenia occur with great frequency. For this reason, blood cell counts should be made periodically during therapy. Dermatologic disturbances and gastrointestinal irritation occur upon continued therapy. It is contraindicated during pregnancy and lactation.

DOSE. 200 mg. orally daily in four divided doses for two months, then maintenance dose based on basal metabolic rate.

IODINE, U.S.P. A small amount of iodine is essential for the formation of thyroid hormones and is used in the prophylaxis and treatment of hypothyroidism. In large doses, however, it has just the opposite effect—that of inhibiting thyroid secretion and producing involution of the gland, making it less friable and vascular prior to surgery. Iodine solutions may be administered alone prior to thyroidectomy, but more often they are combined with other antithyroid drugs. When administered with other antithyroid drugs, iodine has an additive antithyroid action that enables the patient to become euthyroid more quickly than if one antithyroid drug were used alone.

The basal metabolic rate decreases at about the same rate when iodine is administered as when the thyroid gland is removed surgically. Maximal effects are usually observed after 10 to 15 days of administration. Iodine temporarily promotes storage of thyroid hormones in the thyroid gland and lowers the amount released into circulation. This inhibition is short-lived, however, and hyperthyroid symptoms are likely to reappear in a few weeks, because of the release of excessive amounts of stored thyroid hormones.

Careful and accurate measurement of the prescribed dosage is important because of the small volumes to be administered.

> **TOXICITY.** The use of iodine solution is contraindicated in patients with tuberculous lesions since it is believed that it causes a breakdown of the healing process. It is also contraindicated in patients with laryngeal edema, swelling of the salivary glands or increased salivation upon previous exposure to iodine since symptoms often precede toxic manifestations or slow healing skin ulcers of iododerma.

> **DOSE.** Strong Iodine Solution, U.S.P. (Lugol's Solution)—0.3 ml. orally three times daily. Saturated Solution of Potassium Iodide (SSKI)—0.5 to 1 ml. orally daily.

✓ **RADIOACTIVE IODINE (I^{131}).** The use of radioactive iodine in the control of hyperthyroidism is discussed in the chapter devoted to radioactive drugs.

THE PARATHYROID HORMONES

The role of the parathyroids in the control of the blood calcium level is well known. Serious and even fatal consequences result when the parathyroids are removed during thyroidectomy. Within 24 hours after removal of the parathyroids the calcium level of the blood falls precipitously and the patient becomes restless with involuntary muscular twitchings and spasms leading to tetany. Following the sustained tonic phase of the tetanic convulsion, there is a short period of apparent recovery, followed by a series of convulsions and recoveries, with increased weakness. If the hypocalcemic convulsions are not treated with intravenous calcium injections, a coma and death ensue because of spastic contraction of laryngeal and respiratory smooth muscle and consequent respiratory failure.

Parathyroid hormone promotes increased absorption of calcium by the gastrointestinal tract, decreased urinary excretion of calcium and increased mobilization of calcium from bone, thus raising the calcium blood level by three mechanisms.

If parathormone is given in excess to embryonic limb rudiments in tissue culture there is a disappearance of osteoblasts (bone-forming cells), increased formation of osteoclasts (bone-removing cells), a marked dissolution of the bony matrix and replacement of bone with connective tissue. These effects are also observed in hyperparathyroidism in humans in the disease called osteitis fibrosa cystica, which is marked by an excessively high blood calcium level due to dissolution of bone.

The greatly increased amount of serum calcium in the body fluids as a result of these mechanisms eventually leads to deposits of calcium in abnormal places, such as the kidneys, intestinal wall, heart, lungs and skin where they can be painful as well as dangerous.

Recent evidence suggests the existence of two parathyroid hormones. The former theory, which held that parathormone is released when the calcium level is low and not released when it is high, was disproved by a series of animal experiments in which the parathyroids were removed. It was found that a second hormone, calcitonin, is apparently released when the serum calcium levels are elevated. It is now suggested that a dual response is concerned with the mechanism of maintaining optimal calcium blood levels. The source of calcitonin, however, is controversial. Some workers believe that it arises from the thyroid gland and have named it "thyrocalcitonin," whereas others maintain that it is a second hormone of the parathyroids. Further research will no doubt elucidate the matter.

Drugs used to treat parathyroid disorders

PARATHYROID INJECTION, U.S.P. (PAROIDIN). This parathyroid extract for injection is obtained from the parathyroids of domestic animals and relieves symptoms of hypocalcemic tetany and increases the blood calcium level by mobilizing calcium from the bones. The plasma calcium level begins to rise about four hours after injection of the extract and reaches its maximal level in 12 to 18 hours, returning to normal within 24 hours.

Associated with the increased serum calcium and decreased urinary excretion, there is increased urinary excretion of inorganic phosphate. Calcium and phosphate values in the urine are usually reciprocal; if one is increased, the other is invariably decreased. The reason for this phenomenon is unknown.

The use of parathyroid hormone in tetanic convulsions should be restricted to patients in whom the level of serum calcium has been reduced. It is not beneficial in the treatment of tetany in which the serum calcium level is normal. Since repeated administration of the exogenous hormone leads to tolerance and loss of therapeutic effect, dihydrotachysterol or calciferol (synthetic vitamin D preparations) should be substituted for the hormone as soon as possible, since both are effective in raising serum calcium levels. Parathyroid hormone is usually administered with calcium salts.

TOXICITY. Overdosage with parathyroid hormone leads to hypercalcemia and removal of calcium from bone, followed by vomiting, diarrhea, loss of muscle tone and coma. Blood calcium determinations should be made frequently during therapy because there is only a narrow range of safety.

DOSE. 50 to 150 units s.c. or I.M.

initially, then 20 to 40 units every 12 hours.

DIHYDROTACHYSTEROL, U.S.P. (A.T. 10, HYTAKEROL). Dihydrotachysterol, one of the substances having vitamin D activity, is used primarily to elevate blood calcium levels in hypocalcemia. It increases the serum calcium level primarily by promoting urinary excretion of phosphate and reciprocally promoting mobilization of calcium from bone. Unlike calciferol, which increases blood calcium levels chiefly by promoting increased intestinal absorption, this compound has only slight effects on intestinal absorption.

Dihydrotachysterol has a slower onset of action than does the parathyroid hormone and requires seven to ten days of therapy for full therapeutic effect. It is effective only by oral administration and may be used alone or with other agents to raise serum calcium levels in various hypocalcemic states. It is not used in emergency situations because the intravenous calcium salts are required to raise dangerously low calcium levels.

TOXICITY. Since the therapeutic dose is very close to the toxic dose, the drug should be administered with extreme accuracy. Blood and urine calcium levels should be checked regularly. Toxic symptoms of overdose are due to hypercalcemia; thirst, headache, vertigo, tinnitus, anorexia, nausea, vomiting, abdominal cramps, polyuria, albuminuria, ataxia and stupor. Should these symptoms occur, saline cathartics should be administered with a high fluid intake. In conditions threatening life, sodium citrate may be administered intravenously to chelate the calcium in the blood. This procedure is hazardous, however, and should be performed with the utmost care to prevent hypocalcemic reactions.

DOSE. 0.25 mg. orally daily for several days, then 0.25 to 1.0 mg. weekly. Therapy should be supplemented with daily oral doses of 10 to 15 Gm. of calcium in the form of lactate or gluconate salts.

CALCIUM SALTS. The use of calcium salts in the treatment of hypocalcemia is discussed in Chapter 6.

HORMONES OF THE ADRENAL GLANDS

The adrenal glands, located above the kidneys, are composed of an outer cortex and an inner medulla, which have distinct physiological functions.

The medulla secretes two closely related hormones, epinephrine and norepinephrine. Epinephrine increases the heart rate, blood pressure and blood glucose level and decreases liver glycogen. It causes dilation of the pupils of the eyes, pilomotor reactions and dilation of most blood vessels. Norepinephrine has much weaker effects on blood sugar and heart rate, but it is a more powerful vasoconstrictor. The specific actions and effects of these hormones are discussed at greater length in the chapter on the autonomic nervous system.

The adrenal cortex is more complex than the medulla and secretes a number of hormones with different types of activity. The cortex is composed of three zones: the outer, zona glomerulosa, a middle, zona fasciculata, and the inner, zona reticularis. Cells are formed by mitosis in the outer layer and are pushed in toward the zona reticularis where they degenerate and disappear.

Approximately 30 hormones, all steroid, have been extracted from the adrenal cortex. In general, they may be grouped into three categories:

1. glucocorticoids, which among other actions stimulate the conversion of proteins to carbohydrates.

2. mineralocorticoids, which regulate sodium and potassium metabolism.

3. Androgens, which have male sex hormone activity.

Hydrocortisone is the most potent glucocorticoid, and aldosterone is the most potent mineralocorticoid. Desoxycorticosterone, however, is also very potent as a mineralocorticoid. Adrenosterone and dehydroepiandrosterone are typical adrenal androgens.

Addison's disease. Hypofunction of the adrenal cortex results in the condition known as Addison's disease. It is characterized by increased urinary excretion of sodium, bicarbonate, chloride and water, with retention of potassium. The loss of sodium produces acidosis, and the loss of body fluid leads to lowered blood pressure with a decrease of rate of blood flow. There is a decrease in the blood sugar concentration and in the glycogen content of liver, muscle and other tissues. Anorexia is accompanied by nausea, vomiting, and gastrointestinal discomforts. Muscle fatigue is evident, the basal metabolism decreases and the individual is less able to withstand stress. Death occurs within a few days after complete removal of the adrenal glands.

Cushing's syndrome. Hypersecretion of the adrenal cortex causes Cushing's syndrome. Sodium, chloride, water and carbohydrate metabolism is upset. Females may develop male characteristics, including increased body hair and fat, an enlarged clitoris and amenorrhea. Muscles are weak and become wasted, bones fracture easily and excessive glucocorticoids produce a condition that resembles diabetes mellitus. Acne, hypertension, edema, striae and thinning of the skin, hyperpigmentation of the skin and nails, ecchymoses, impairment of glucose tolerance, negative nitrogen balance, alkalosis and mental disturbances are also produced.

Partial removal of the adrenals can alleviate this condition, or supplementary hormones may be given therapeutically following total removal of the gland, and the individual may lead a nearly normal life.

Adrenogenital syndrome. A third disease, the adrenogenital syndrome, results from an interruption in the metabolism of hydrocortisone, which leads to increased production of adrenal androgens. The androgens produce precocious sexual maturity in males and masculinization in females.

Glucocorticoids Used in Therapy

HYDROCORTISONE, U.S.P., B.P. (COMPOUND F, CORTEF, CORTRIL, HYDROCORTONE). Hydrocortisone is one of the glucocorticoids that affects protein and carbohydrate metabolism, promoting gluconeogenesis, hyperglycemia, glycosuria, a loss of protein from many organs and a negative nitrogen balance. It also affects fat metabolism by inhibiting lipogenesis in the liver and causing atypical deposition of fatty tissue in the abdomen, shoulder areas and face (moon-face).

hydrocortisone

Hydrocortisone affects the electrolyte balance by promoting retention of sodium and excretion of potassium and increasing the urinary excretion of creatine and uric acid. It inhibits the activity of the lymphatic system, produces lymphopenia and reduces the size of enlarged lymph nodes. There is a decrease in circulating eosinophils, and antibody production decreases.

Hydrocortisone and other glucocorticoids alter the normal inflammatory responses of the body, which may be advantageous in the control of arthritis, but are deleterious in the case of tuberculosis or peptic ulcers, allowing progression of these disorders. The development of granulomatous tissue is slowed and wound healing is prolonged.

Following absorption, hydrocortisone is distributed to most tissues and crosses the placenta but accumulates only in the liver, where it is conjugated prior to excretion via the kidneys.

This hormone is used therapeutically in the treatment of collagen diseases, including rheumatoid arthritis, disseminated lupus erythematosus, periarteritis nodosa, dermatomyositis and scleroderma. Hydrocortisone is only palliative in these conditions, however. Upon discontinuance of the drug the symptoms promptly recur, and cartilage and bone destruction may even progress while the individual is under steroid therapy. The condition is merely not as debilitating as it would be without the benefit of the drug.

Hydrocortisone produces prompt remission of acute symptoms of rheumatoid arthritis, and after one or two weeks the blood sedimentation rate usually falls to normal levels. Upon discontinuance of the drug, symptoms begin to reappear within 48 hours.

Hydrocortisone is often combined with aldosterone and sodium chloride in the treatment of adrenal insufficiency. Neoplasms of the lymphatic system, such as lymphosarcoma, leukemia and Hodgkin's disease, sometimes show temporary response to hydrocortisone.

This drug may be used topically, orally and parenterally to relieve all types of allergic reactions. Here again relief is only symptomatic, but ordinarily disorders of this nature are temporary; the patient may remain largely symptom-free while the allergy runs its natural course.

TOXICITY. The most serious side effect of hydrocortisone therapy is the inhibition of the anterior pituitary production of ACTH and the consequent atrophy of the adrenal cortex. Intermittent injections of ACTH during therapy alleviate this condition somewhat. Hydrocortisone therapy should never be discontinued abruptly, but tapered off gradually to allow time for recovery of the adrenal cortex. Adrenal insufficiency may still be encountered in periods of stress, such as injections, trauma or surgery, for as long as two years following discontinuing the drug. Supplemental corticoids should be administered under these circumstances.

When hydrocortisone and related glucocorticoids are administered over a period of time, symptoms of Cushing's

TABLE 11   Glucocorticoid Preparations and Comparable Doses

GENERIC NAME	BRAND NAMES	DOSE
Betamethasone	Celestone	0.6 mg.
Cortisone Acetate, N.F., B.P.	Compound E, Cortogen, Cortone	25 mg.
Dexamethasone, N.F., B.P.	Decadron, Deronil, Gammacorten	0.75 mg.
Flurandrenolone	Cordran	0.05% topically.
Fluocinolone	Synalar	0.025% topically.
Fluprednisolone	Alphadrol	1 mg.
Hydrocortisone, U.S.P., B.P.	Compound F, Hydrocortone, Cortef, Cortril	20 mg.
Methylprednisolone, N.F.	Medrol	4 mg.
Paramethasone	Haldrone	2 mg.
Prednisolone, U.S.P., B.P.	Delta-Cortef, Hydeltra, Meticortelone, Paracortol, Sterane	5 mg.
Prednisone, U.S.P., B.P.	Deltasone, Deltra, Meticorten, Paracort	5 mg.
Triamcinolone	Aristocort, Kenacort	4 mg.

syndrome appear if a high hormone level is maintained.

Except in emergency situations, hydrocortisone and all other glucocorticoids are contraindicated in patients with peptic ulcers, psychoses, acute glomerulonephritis, herpes simplex of the eye, vaccinia or varicella, and tuberculosis (active or arrested). They should be used with caution in diabetes mellitus, hypertension, congestive heart failure, chronic nephritis, thrombophlebitis, osteoporosis, convulsive disorders, infectious diseases, diverticulitis and renal insufficiency. They should rarely be used during pregnancy since adrenal insufficiency in the mother and newborn at the time of delivery is a possibility.

DOSE.   Very individualized. In arthritis 60 to 80 mg. orally daily. I.V.—100 to 250 mg. every 6 to 8 hours as required.

Other glucocorticoids have therapeutic actions similar to hydrocortisone. Many of the newer synthetic forms are active in much smaller doses, however, and the incidence of side effects is lower.

Table 11 is a comparison of some glucocorticoids. The doses given are equivalent doses of the various drugs shown merely to indicate therapeutic potency. The doses used in therapy vary greatly according to the severity of the condition being treated.

NURSING IMPLICATIONS

The nurse has many important responsibilities in caring for the patient receiving large doses of glucocorticoids because of the many side effects produced. Some glucocorticoid preparations may have overlapping mineralocorticoid effects and cause sodium and fluid retention and potassium excretion. The patient's blood pressure should be checked routinely. An accurate record of intake and output, daily weight and observation for edema are indicated. A low sodium diet and potassium supplements may be ordered.

The patient's appearance, as in Cushing's syndrome, may be affected. The moonface, "buffalo hump" and truncal fat may result from the mobilization of fat to these areas. There may be hirsutism and acne from an excessive androgenic effect as well. The patient must be reassured that these changes in appearance will begin to disappear when the drug is withdrawn.

The gluconeogenesis promoted by glucocorticoids raises the blood glucose level and creates a negative nitrogen balance. A high protein diet may be needed. The urine should be checked routinely for sugar and acetone since "steroid diabetes" may result from the elevated blood glucose level. Diabetic patients receiving steroids will probably require the administration of additional insulin.

Because glucocorticoids suppress the inflammatory response certain nursing measures are needed. The patient must be protected as much as possible from sources of infection since his lymphatic system is usually depressed and healing is delayed. The usual signs and symptoms of inflammation, such as redness, heat, swelling and pain, may be "masked" by glucocorticoids.

Because of the tendency of glucocorticoids to promote the formation of peptic ulcers, several preventive measures may be taken. A bland diet and ulcer regimen may be instituted. Oral preparations should be given with or immediately after meals to decrease gastric irritation.

Steroid therapy may cause emotional or psychological changes in some patients. Patients may experience an exaggeration of previous neurotic or psychotic tendencies. Emotional changes may also occur as the drug is withdrawn. The nurse should observe and record any changes in the patient's behavior when he is taking steroids or they are being gradually withdrawn.

When glucocorticoids have been given over a period of time, the drug should not be discontinued abruptly. The dosage should be gradually reduced so that the patient's adrenal glands are stimulated gradually into hormone production. The return of complete adrenal function may take a period of time during which unusual stress may precipitate an Addisonian-like crisis. Patients who are undergoing surgery and have had steroid therapy terminated within the past 12 to 18 months may need a supplemental dose of glucocorticoid to meet the stress response in surgery.

If a patient is receiving steroids as replacement therapy, as in Addison's disease or after adrenalectomy, it is vital to the patient's life that he receive his medication.

Patients should carry identification tags with this type of information at all times. If the patient's adrenal function is only slight or absent, it is very important that he and his family and also the nurse understand that stress (physical, emotional or psychological) increases his need for steroids. This need may be evidenced by nausea and vomiting, arthralgia and decreased blood pressure.

Mineralocorticoids Used in Therapy

DESOXYCORTICOSTERONE ACETATE, U.S.P., DEOXYCORTONE ACETATE, B.P. (CORTATE, DOCA, PERCORTEN). This mineralocorticoid, unlike the glucocorticoids, is inactive when given orally since it is destroyed in the gastrointestinal tract. It causes increased retention of sodium and water and increased potassium excretion presumably by altering the mechanism by which these substances are reabsorbed or excreted by the kidneys.

DOCA is used with glucocorticoids in the treatment of adrenal insufficiency. Following an increase in blood volume due to water retention there is an increase in cardiac output and blood pressure. It has the glucocorticoid effects of promoting a negative nitrogen balance and increasing absorption of fat and glucose from the gastrointestinal tract.

TOXICITY. Toxic effects are related to water retention and include edema, pulmonary congestion, cardiac failure and hypertension. In addition there are mild glucocorticoid side effects as previously described.

DOSE. 1 to 5 mg. daily I.M. or buccally (placed under the tongue or against the cheek and allowed to dissolve).

FLUDROCORTISONE ACETATE (FLORINEF). Oral administration of fludrocortisone produces therapeutic effects similar to those of DOCA by promoting sodium retention. It is useful in the treatment of Addison's disease.

DOSE. 1 or 2 mg. orally daily.

HORMONES FROM THE GONADS

The gonads, or sex glands, of the male and female are responsible for production of the germ cells necessary for reproduction and the sex hormones that bestow secondary sex characteristics upon the individual at puberty. As stated previously, the testes and ovaries are acted upon by the same gonadotropic hormones, FSH and LH from the anterior pituitary, but differ in their respective responses to this stimulation.

FEMALE REPRODUCTION SYSTEM

At puberty, FSH from the anterior pituitary stimulates the development and maturation of the graafian follicles in the ovaries. The follicles, developed from columns of germinal epithelial cells that grow downward toward the center of the ovary from the surface layer, contain a large cell or ovum in the center surrounded by a single layer of cells. Numerous primary graafian follicles are found in ovaries of fetuses and children. Under the influence of LH, the cells surrounding the primitive ovum produce the female hormone estradiol. Estradiol is responsible for the development of the secondary sex characteristics of the female and the changes in the accessory organs of reproduction during the first part of the menstrual cycle.

The removal of the ovaries of a young female animal prevents it from becoming sexually mature. The accessory organs fail to develop, menstruation does not occur, secondary sex characteristics do not appear and the sex instinct is never manifested. Injections of the female sex hormone into such an animal correct all the effects of oophorectomy.

As the graafian follicle matures or ripens, it becomes distended with accumulated fluid and moves outward to the surface of the ovary. It projects from the surface as a small cystlike swelling, which eventually bursts, under the influence of LH, and discharges the ovum. This process is known as ovulation and occurs about every 28 days.

The cavity of the ruptured follicle fills with a clot of blood that is soon replaced by a mass of cells filled with a yellow, fatlike material called lutein. The mass is now called the corpus luteum and, under the continual developmental stimulation of LH from the anterior pituitary, the corpus luteum produces another hormone, progesterone, which prepares the uterus for the reception of the fertilized ovum.

Progesterone is responsible for the uterine changes characteristic of the last half of the menstrual cycle (thickening of the uterine wall, increased supply of blood vessels, etc.), the development of the placenta, the maturation of the mammary glands during pregnancy, the multiplication of the uterine muscle fibers and the inhibition of uterine contraction until parturition.

If fertilization of the ovum does not occur, the corpus luteum disintegrates and the unfertilized ovum as well as the thickened uterine lining pass off in the menstrual flow. If fertilization occurs, the corpus luteum continues to increase in size until the latter months of pregnancy, and its hormone continues to influence the growth and functional integrity of the placenta and uterus.

As parturition approaches, the corpus luteum disintegrates, the uterus contracts because the inhibiting influence of progesterone is no longer present and birth occurs.

Progesterone may be administered parenterally in the event that the corpus luteum disintegrates before the pregnancy is completed. If administered in sufficient time, it may halt the progress of a threatened abortion.

During pregnancy, hormones resembling the gonadotropic hormones are produced by the placenta. These anterior pituitary-like hormones (APLH) or chorionic gonadotropins are present in the urine and are the basis for the urine pregnancy test. Occasionally APLH preparations are used therapeutically, but they have no advantage over agents that are easier to manufacture and less expensive.

FEMALE HORMONE THERAPY

ESTROGENS

Estrogens (natural and synthetic) may be administered therapeutically for replacement therapy in a variety of conditions:

Menopausal syndrome. The purpose of therapy in this case is to relieve the various physiological effects of a decline in natural hormone production. The doses required for relief vary from woman to woman and from time to time in an individual. They should be used in minimal doses during menopause merely to lessen the extremely undesirable effects of the transition period, but not to prolong the natural body adjustment, which must be made eventually.

Sexual infantilism. Estrogen therapy in sexual infantilism promotes the development of the uterus and the secondary sex characteristics. In most cases, therapy must be continued for a prolonged period of time.

Dysmenorrhea. Although estrogens are occasionally employed for dysmenorrhea, their therapeutic value here is questionable, except from a psychological point of view.

Inhibition of lactation. In high blood concentration, estrogens produce a reflex inhibition of the lactogenic hormone, thus suppressing lactation. They are employed in instances in which a mother prefers not to nurse her infant.

Inhibition of breast cancer. High blood concentration of estrogens are beneficial in the treatment of breast cancer since they reflexly inhibit the mammary glands, but they are not a substitute for surgery.

Inhibition of prostate carcinoma. Prostate carcinoma is often aggravated by testosterone; thus, therapy of this malignancy is treated by local excision, orchiectomy and low doses of estrogen. Doses are regulated so that minimal if any feminization occurs.

Estrogen therapy may cause nausea, vomiting, diarrhea, fluid retention and edema.

ESTRADIOL CYPIONATE, N.F. (DEPO-ESTRADIOL). Estradiol cypionate is an esterified derivative of estradiol, the natural female estrogen, which is available in an oily solution for intramuscular use only. Following injection, the estrogen is released slowly and therapeutic effects persist for about three to four weeks.

DOSE.   Initially 1 to 5 mg. is given I.M. as a single weekly dose for two to three weeks. A single dose every three to four weeks is usually sufficient for maintenance.

ESTRADIOL DIPROPIONATE, N.F. (OVOCYLIN). This derivative of estradiol is somewhat less subject to metabolic transformation in the body tissues than is estradiol and is absorbed and eliminated more slowly. It should not be used in instances in which potent and prolonged action is undesirable. It is probably most useful in postoperative management following oophorectomy and in the management of severe menopausal symptoms. It is also used to treat kraurosis vulvae, pruritus vulvae and senile vaginitis.

DOSE.   Initially 1 to 5 mg. I.M. as a single weekly dose for two to three weeks, then 1 to 2.5 mg. every 10 to 14 days.

ESTRADIOL VALERATE (DELESTROGEN). This valeric acid ester of estradiol is available in an oil solution for intramuscular injection, after which its estrogenic effects persist for approximately two to three weeks. It is readily adaptable as a source of estrogens during the first portion of the menstrual cycle.

DOSE.   20 mg. I.M. initially, followed in two weeks by 5 mg. in combination with a progestogen. After two more weeks the cycle may be repeated.

ESTROGENIC SUBSTANCES, CONJUGATED, (AMNESTROGEN, CONESTRON, PREMARIN). This naturally occurring, water-soluble conjugated form of mixed estrogens is obtained from pregnant mares' urine. The principal estrogens present are sodium estrone sulfate and sodium equilin sulfate.

The oral preparations in many cases produce fewer gastrointestinal side effects than do other synthetic estrogens such as diethylstilbestrol. It is acceptable for long term therapy following oophorectomy or for postmenopausal symptoms.

In addition to its use for estrogen replacement therapy, this estrogenic preparation is used intravenously for the control of hemorrhage.

Intravenous injection into experimental animals increases the level of circulating prothrombin and accelerator globulin and decreases antithrombin activity. The therapeutic effects of the preparation when used to treat abnormal surgical bleeding are believed to be due to its ability to increase acid mucopolysaccharides in the intercellular ground substance and thus aid hemostasis.

The intravenous preparation may be safely used in male patients without untoward feminizing effects, since it is rapidly eliminated from the body. Feminization occurs on long term therapy, however.

DOSE. Oral—1.25 to 2.5 mg. daily; intravenous—20 mg.

ESTRONE, N.F., OESTRONE, B.P. (THEELIN). Estrone is a synthetic estrogen that is prepared as an aqueous or oily suspension for intramusclar use. In addition, it is available as a vaginal suppository for the treatment of senile vaginitis. It has largely been replaced by other estrogenic products for treatment at present.

DOSE. Intramuscular—200 mcg. to 1 mg. one or more times weekly. Suppository—200 mcg.

ETHINYL ESTRADIOL, U.S.P., ETHINYLOESTRADIOL, B.P. (ESTINYL, ETICYLOL, DIOGYN-E, LYNORAL, ORESTRALYN). This synthetic estrogen is prepared from estrone and is one of the most potent estrogens. It is the drug of choice in instances in which massive estrogenic therapy is indicated since it may be prescribed in smaller doses than many other estrogenic compounds.

TOXICITY. Headache, nausea and vomiting occur more frequently than with conjugated estrogens when administered orally.

DOSE. 50 mcg. orally one to three times weekly for hypo-ovarianism. 20 to 50 mcg. is given one to three times daily for the control of menopausal symptoms.

CHLOROTRIANISENE, N.F. (TACE). Chlorotrianisene has the unusual property of being stored in the body fat after gastrointestinal absorption. It is slowly liberated from these storage depots and is gradually metabolized in the liver to an estrogenic compound that is more potent than the parent compound.

Chlorotrianisene is given quite frequently for the inhibition of lactation and for supplemental or replacement estrogen therapy. It is not recommended for use in the treatment of mammary cancer occurring five years or more past menopause because uterine bleeding occasionally occurs and may obscure the warning signs of uterine carcinoma in this age group.

DOSE. 12 to 25 mg. orally daily.

DIETHYLSTILBESTROL, U.S.P., STILBOESTROL, B.P. (STILBESTROL). This synthetic estrogen derivative possesses greater activity than natural estrogens and may be administered orally, parenterally or in the form of ointments and suppositories. The drug is very sensitive to light, and parenteral solutions may discolor upon standing.

TOXICITY. Although side effects are few when diethylstilbestrol is administered parenterally, they are fairly common when the oral route is used because absorption of the drug into the blood is more rapid than when it is administered parenterally. The most common side effects are nausea, vomiting and headache. The enteric coated form is most often used in an attempt to decrease the undesirable gastrointestinal side effects, but they still occur with an appreciable frequency.

DOSE. 500 mcg. to 1 mg. orally daily. Suppositories—100 to 500 mcg. vaginally once daily.

DIENESTROL, N.F., DIENOESTROL, B.P. (RESTROL, SYNESTROL). Dienestrol has the same action and effects as diethylstilbestrol, but it appears to be tolerated better following oral administration. It is less effective than diethylstilbestrol in inducing withdrawal bleeding in the treatment of amenorrhea, but it is useful in the control of the symptoms of menopause and in suppression of lactation.

It is used quite often as a hormonal suppressant in the treatment of inoperable mammary and prostatic carcinoma.

DOSE.   0.5 to 1.5 mg. orally daily.

METHALLENESTRIL (VALLESTRIL).   Methallenestril produces the same estrogenic effects as other synthetic estrogen compounds, although it is only one tenth as potent as diethylstilbestrol when administered orally.

It has the same side effects and contraindications as diethylstilbestrol.

DOSE.   3 to 6 mg. orally daily.

HEXESTROL.   This synthetic estrogen has actions and effects very similar to diethylstilbestrol. It is employed chiefly to inhibit lactation.

DOSE.   200 mcg. orally three times daily.

PROGESTOGENS

In addition to progesterone, the natural hormone secreted by the corpus luteum, many synthetic progestogens are employed therapeutically. Progesterone is inactive when administered orally; the synthetic compounds are employed when oral administration is desired.

Progestogens are useful in the treatment of functional uterine bleeding involving a hyperplastic nonsecreting endometrium, primary and secondary amenorrhea and in a few cases of infertility in which malfunction of the corpus luteum is suspected. They have also been employed in the treatment of habitual abortion, but the beneficial effects are questionable.

Most progestogens suppress ovulation, but the preparations employed most often for this purpose are discussed in the section on oral contraceptives.

PROGESTERONE, N.F., B.P. (LIPO-LUTIN, LUTO-CYLIN, PROGESTEROL, PROGESTIN, PROLUTON). Although progesterone is the natural hormone secreted by the corpus luteum, most commercial preparations are prepared synthetically. When administered intramuscularly, this compound induces secretory

progesterone

changes in the endometrium, stimulates the growth of the mammary glands and relaxes uterine smooth muscle.

The drug should be protected from light.

TOXICITY.   Progesterone should not be administered to patients in whom genital malignancy is suspected. Spotting and irregular bleeding, nausea and lethargy may occur when it is administered for short periods of time.

When the use of progesterone is prolonged, gastrointestinal disturbances, edema, weight gain, headache, dizziness, oligomenorrhea or amenorrhea, congestion of the breast and decreased libido may occur.

DOSE.   5 to 50 mg. I.M. (deep) daily.

ETHISTERONE, N.F., B.P. (LUTOCYLOL, PRANONE, PREGENINOLONE, PROGESTORAL).   This synthetic analog of progesterone is effective by oral administration, but it has only about one fifth the potency of intramuscularly administered progesterone.

The actions and side effects resemble those of progesterone.

DOSE.   40 to 80 mg. orally daily.

HYDROXYPROGESTERONE CAPROATE (DELALUTIN).   Hydroxyprogesterone caproate is a long-acting form of progesterone, having a duration of action of 7 to 14 days. It is usually indicated when long term therapy is desired.

DOSE.   125 to 250 mg. I.M. about 12 days before the menstrual period in the treatment of amenorrhea. 1 Gm. weekly is used in the treatment of habitual abortion.

MEDROXYPROGESTERONE ACETATE, U.S.P. (PROVERA). This synthetic progesterone is considerably more potent than ethisterone on a weight to weight basis when administered orally. Its ability to suppress ovulation in humans is doubtful. Because of its long duration of action when administered intramuscularly, it must be given orally for the treatment of amenorrhea, dysmenorrhea or functional uterine bleeding. It may be administered orally or intramuscularly to treat threatened abortion.

DOSE. 2.5 to 30 mg. orally daily. 50 mg. I.M. weekly for threatened abortion.

NORETHINDRONE (NORLUTIN); NORETHINDRONE ACETATE (NORLUTATE). Norethindrone acetate when given orally is about four times as potent as parenteral progesterone and about twice as potent as oral progesterone. When administered with estrogens, it is effective in suppressing ovulation, and both norethindrone and norethindrone acetate have been used in the prevention of conception.

Since masculinization of the female fetus has been reported following administration of norethindrone for threatened abortion, its use for this purpose is somewhat limited.

DOSE. 5 to 40 mg. orally daily.

ORAL CONTRACEPTIVES

At present an estimated seven million women are using accepted oral contraceptives. Although much publicity, both good and bad, has been given to these agents, no definite cause-and-effect relationship has been established between these agents and pathological changes in some women who have become ill while they were taking these drugs.

There are, however, disturbing gaps in the accurate scientific knowledge available concerning these hormonal preparations, which require extensive research before they may be deemed absolutely harmless for most women taking them for contraceptive purposes over a period of years.

Estrogens are the most potent agents known for the prevention of ovulation. When they are administered alone, however, unpleasant side effects occur, such as breakthrough bleeding and prolonged menses because of the development of a vascular, nonglandular endometrial lining. The use of an estrogen-progesterone combination minimizes these effects. Although the progestogen-estrogen combination in each tablet is used in most instances, newer preparations provide sequential therapy in the form of estrogen alone for the first 15 or 16 days of the cycle, followed by a combination tablet of estrogen and progestogen for the next five days. The sequential form of therapy has fewer side effects and does not significantly alter the uterine endometrium from that of a normal menstrual cycle in sharp contrast to the glandular atrophy of the endometrium that occurs in patients on progestogens alone or the combination tablets. This may be a mixed advantage, however, since if breakthrough ovulation and fertilization should occur during the cycle, implantation of the fertilized ovum in the endometrium is possible; pregnancies occur slightly more often with this form, particularly if a tablet or two is not taken. The sequential contraceptives have proven reliable, however, and pregnancies are rare among women who have followed the daily regimen of taking these drugs.

The oral contraceptives suppress or inhibit the secretion of pituitary gonadotropins by maintaining high blood levels of estrogen and progestogen. Since these sex hormones cause reciprocal inhibition of pituitary FSH, the ovarian follicles cannot mature, and ovulation does not take place during the cycle.

Upon withdrawal of the drug after 20 or 21 days of therapy, uterine bleeding occurs as the thickened uterine endometrium produced by the progesterone is sloughed off, simulating a normal menstrual flow. Following a five day recess the cycle is repeated.

In addition to their use as contraceptive compounds, progestogens have also been used in the treatment of menstrual cycle aberrations, dysmenorrhea, menorrhagia and endometriosis. Unfortunately, reports concerning their effectiveness in these conditions are quite conflicting. In many cases the original complaint recurs when treatment is discontinued.

Patients should be told the importance of keeping these drugs out of the reach of children. They are attractively packaged and many cases of children swallowing a month's supply have been reported.

TOXICITY

Oral contraceptives are contraindicated in patients with a history of breast or genital cancer, preexisting liver, renal or cardiac disorders or exacerbation of attacks of epilepsy. They should be administered with caution to patients with a predisposition toward migraine headaches or asthmatic attacks because of the possibility of fluid retention. Pretreatment examination should specifically include the breasts, pelvic organs and a Papanicolaou smear. Preexisting uterine fibroids may enlarge under the influence of these preparations. Although oral contraceptives are not carcinogenic, they accelerate the growth of preexisting breast and uterine carcinomas.

Side effects may include nausea, vomiting, gastrointestinal disorders, fluid retention, chloasma, breast enlargement, breakthrough bleeding, breast changes, loss of scalp hair, weight change, changes in cervical erosion and secretions, suppression of lactation when given immediately post-partum, dermatoses, headache, nervousness and mental depression.

Thrombophlebitis, pulmonary embolism and neuro-ocular lesions have occurred, although a cause-and-effect relationship has not been established.

COMBINATION PROGESTOGEN-ESTROGEN PREPARATIONS. The doses given are those contained in each tablet. The usual dose is one tablet daily for 20 or 21 days with a five day recess between cycles.

Enovid
Two strengths are available: (10. mg. size) (5 mg. size)
Norethynodrel 9.85 mg. 5.0 mg.
Mestranol 0.15 mg. 0.075 mg.
Enovid-E
Norethynodrel 2.5 mg.
Mestranol 0.1 mg.
Ortho-Novum
Three strengths are available: (10 mg.) (2 mg.) (1 mg.)

Norethindrone 10 mg. 2 mg. 1 mg.
Mestranol 0.06 mg. 0.1 mg. 0.05 mg.
Norinyl
Two strengths are available: (2 mg.) (1 mg.)
Norethindrone 2 mg. 1 mg.
Mestranol 0.1mg. 0.05 mg.
Ovulen
Ethynodiol diacetate 1 mg.
Mestranol 0.1 mg.
Norlestrin
Norethindrone acetate 2.5 mg.
Ethinyl estradiol 0.05 mg.
Provest
Medroxyprogesterone 10 mg.
Ethinyl estradiol 0.05 mg.

SEQUENTIAL COMBINATIONS

C-Quens
15 tablets contain only: Mestranol 80 mcg.
5 tablets contain: Mestranol 80 mcg.
Chlormadinone acetate 2 mg.
Oracon
16 tablets contain only: Ethinyl estradiol 0.1 mg.
5 tablets contain: Ethinyl estradiol 0.1 mg.
Dimethisterone 25 mg.
Ortho-Novum SQ
14 tablets contain only: Mestranol 80 mcg.
6 tablets contain: Mestranol 80 mcg.
Norethindrone 2 mg.

OVULATORY AGENTS

Concurrent with the need to control ovulation and to prevent pregnancy, there is also a need for drugs to enhance fertility and increase the chances of pregnancy in anovulatory women. The use of these drugs must be supervised only by those experienced in the field, and generally is restricted to appropriately selected patients.

CLOMIPHENE CITRATE (CLOMID). This orally administered nonsteroidal drug appears to increase the output of pituitary gonadotropins, which in turn stimulate the maturation and endocrine activity of the ovarian follicle and the subsequent development and function of the corpus luteum.

Clomiphene is contraindicated in the presence of an ovarian cyst since further enlargement of the ovary may occur. The basal body temperature should be recorded throughout all treatment cycles, and the patient should be carefully observed to determine whether ovulation occurs, because this drug is contraindicated in pregnancy. Clinical evaluation of liver function should always precede therapy, and the drug should be withheld if there is evidence of liver damage or malfunction.

The incidence of multiple pregnancies (including triplets, quadruplets and quintuplets) has increased to tenfold when conception takes place during a cycle in which clomiphene is administered.

TOXICITY. Patients should be advised that blurring and other visual symptoms may occasionally occur during therapy. This may render activities such as driving a car or operating machinery more hazardous than usual, particularly under conditions of variable lighting. Other symptoms may include hot flashes, abdominal or pelvic discomfort, nausea and vomiting, breast discomfort, increased nervous tension, headache, dizziness, heavier menses, allergic dermatitis, weight gain and reversible hair loss.

DOSE. 50 mg. orally daily for five days. Therapy may be started at any time in the patient who has had no recent uterine bleeding. If spontaneous uterine bleeding occurs prior to therapy, the five day regimen should be started on or about the fifth day of the cycle.

If ovulation appears not to have occurred after the first course of therapy, a second course of 100 mg. daily for five days should be given. This may be started as early as 30 days after the previous course of therapy. Increasing the dosage or duration of therapy beyond 100 mg. daily for five days should never be undertaken.

MENOTROPINS (PERGONAL). Menotropins is an extract of the gonadotropic hormones containing both follicle stimulating hormone (FSH) and luteinizing hormone (LH). The urine of postmenopausal women is the usual commercial source of the hormones, since without the feedback inhibition of active ovarian function the gonadotropins are secreted continuously from the pituitary and are excreted unchanged in the urine. The hormones are extracted, purified and standardized for commercial use.

Gonadotropins are used therapeutically to induce growth and maturation of the graafian follicle in women with primary ovarian failure. Following a daily dose of menotropins for 9 to 12 successive days, follicle maturation usually occurs. It can be assessed indirectly by the appearance of cells from vaginal mucosa, the appearance of cervical mucus or by measurement of the urine estrogen level. The course of therapy is then followed, one day after the last dose of menotropins, by a single dose of 10,000 units of chorionic gonadotropin.

Multiple births, including up to nine fetuses, have been reported in about 20% of pregnancies induced in this manner. There is a high risk of premature births and neonatal morbidity and mortality in multiple pregnancies of this sort, and frequently none of the fetuses survive.

TOXICITY. Mild to moderate ovarian enlargement occurs which may be accompanied by abdominal distension and/or pain. This generally decreases in 2 to 3 weeks without treatment, however. Infrequently, sudden ovarian enlargement may occur with ovarian hyperstimulation, accompanied by ascites and hemoconcentration associated with fluid loss into the abdominal cavity. The hyperstimulation occurs within two weeks of therapy and develops rapidly over a 3 to 4 day period; thus, frequent examinations should be carried out within this two week period, and if hyperstimulation is found to occur, the patient should be hospitalized. Menotropins should not be administered if there are signs of abnormal ovarian enlargement, or if patients have thyroid or adrenal dysfunction.

DOSE. 75 units each FSH or LH I.M. daily for 9 to 12 days until there is evidence of follicle maturation.

CHORIONIC GONADOTROPIN (A.P.L., FOLLUTEIN). This purified hormonal extract is obtained commercially from the urine of pregnant women. It is used in females to stimulate ovulation, and it may be used in males to stimulate the interstitial testicular cells to produce increased amounts of androgen. In addition, it has been employed to aid in the descent of the testes in cryptorchidism, in hypogonadism secondary to pituitary deficiency and in dwarfism associated with hypogonadism.

TOXICITY. Males — The development of sexual precociousness necessitates withdrawal of the drug. Peripheral edema may occur as a result of hormone induced salt and water retention and requires decreased dosage.
Females — Hypersensitivity reactions occur occasionally. Single dose injections do not cause problems associated with long term therapy in males.

DOSE. Males (cryptorchidism) — 4000 units I.M. three times weekly for 2 to 3 weeks.
Females (infertility) — 10,000 units in one dose I.M. one day after completion of course of menotropins therapy.

MALE REPRODUCTIVE SYSTEM

In the human male the reproductive processes are much simpler than in the female. FSH from the anterior pituitary causes production of the spermatozoa, whereas LH (also called ICSH, or interstitial cell stimulating hormone), causes development of the interstitial cells that produce testosterone.

Testosterone is responsible for normal development of the male reproductive tract and maintains the secondary sex characteristics. It is involved in the development of the penis, the seminal vesicles and the prostate gland and the descent of the testes from the abdominal cavity. The secondary sex characteristics that are affected by testosterone are the depth of the voice, the distribution of facial and body hair and the development of the masculine skeletal muscles and muscular strength and endurance. Testosterone confers a sense of well-being, restores mental equilibrium and energy and can also increase the resistance of the central nervous system to fatigue.

MALE HORMONE THERAPY

Androgens (natural and synthetic male hormones) may be used therapeutically to treat the following conditions:

1. Sexual infantilism. Replacement of the male hormone allows normal development of the sexually immature individual.

2. Relief of male climacteric symptoms.

3. In females, to treat certain ovarian dysfunctions, such as menorrhagia and dysmenorrhea.

4. To treat breast engorgement and to suppress lactation by counteracting the effect of estrogen.

5. As an anabolic agent to promote muscular growth and weight gain. The newer synthetic forms only slightly affect the development of the secondary characteristics, but aid in the development of muscular tissue, improve appetite and convey the sense of well-being typical of testosterone. These agents are used mostly in elderly, debilitated patients.

TESTOSTERONE, N.F., B.P. (ANDROLIN, ORETON-F, SYNANDROL F). Testosterone is available in intramuscular pellets, as an aqueous injectable suspension and in tablets for oral and sublingual administration. It is used for

testosterone

relief of symptoms of breast cancer and for maintenance doses of male hormone.

DOSE. 5 to 25 mg. orally or I.M. daily.

TESTOSTERONE PROPIONATE, U.S.P., B.P. (NEOHOMBREOL, ORETON, PERANDREN, SYNANDROL). Testosterone propionate is synthesized from cholesterol or extracted from bulls' testes. It is available as buccal tablets or as a solution for intramuscular use. Since this preparation provides a longer effective blood level, through the formation of an insoluble depot in the muscle, the dosage frequency may be reduced.

DOSE.   100 mg. I.M. three times weekly. 10 mg. buccally daily

Testosterone enanthate, U.S.P., N.F. (Dela-testryl).   This oil soluble form of testosterone is administered as a repository form of the hormone. Its effects may last three weeks or more.

DOSE.   100 to 400 mg. intramuscularly every four to six weeks.

Methyltestosterone, U.S.P., B.P. (Metandren, Neo-Hombreol-M, Oreton-M, Testora).   Methyltestosterone can be administered orally, buccally or sublingually because it is readily absorbed from the oral mucous membranes. It may be administered for general male hormone therapy or to suppress lactation.

DOSE.   10 to 40 mg. daily orally, buccally or sublingually.

Fluoxymesterone, B.P. (Halotestin, Ora-Testryl, Ultandren).   Fluoxymesterone, a halogenated derivative of methyltestosterone, is about five times as potent as methyltestosterone when administered orally. It is used primarily in the treatment of the androgen-deficient male to promote the development of secondary sex characteristics. It has been used for primary hypogonadism, testicular hypofunction, eunuchism, Klinefelter's syndrome, male climacteric and cryptorchidism. In the treatment of cryptorchidism, fluoxymesterone should be used only if therapy with chorionic gonadotropin has proved unsuccessful since variable results are obtained with this agent.

Fluoxymesterone is used in the female to treat menorrhagia, metrorrhagia, premenstrual tension, functional dysmenorrhea, menopausal symptoms, endometriosis and inoperable mammary carcinoma.

It may be used as an anabolic agent in both males and females and is of some value in the treatment of osteoporosis.

TOXICITY.   Prolonged administration in the male may inhibit testicular function, resulting in decreased sperm production and hormone secretion. Priapism occurs occasionally. It is contraindicated in prostatic carcinoma because the carcinoma will grow more rapidly and should be used with caution in young males, since precocious sexual development and premature epiphyseal closure occur on continued therapy.

In the female, large doses or prolonged administration may produce virilizing effects.

Retention of sodium, potassium and water may occur. Jaundice has been occasionally observed.

DOSE.   2.5 to 10 mg. orally daily.

Stanolone   (Androlone,   Neodrol).   Stanolone is used for its androgenic and anabolic effects. Perhaps its chief clinical application is in the treatment of inoperable or metastatic mammary carcinoma.

DOSE.   10 to 50 mg. orally daily.

Methandriol   (Stenediol,   Crestabolic).   Like the other androgenic hormones, methandriol increases nitrogen, potassium and phosphorus retention and decreases protein catabolism.

It is useful in instances in which a positive nitrogen balance is desired, and it is used as adjunctive therapy preoperatively and postoperatively. A high protein diet greatly enhances the activity of this drug, since the anabolic process depends ultimately upon the nutritional state of the patient.

Methandriol has been used in children with retarded bone growth and development, but it causes bone maturation and early epiphyseal closure as well as increased linear growth.

DOSE.   7.5 to 25 mg. orally daily.

Methandrostenolone (Dianabol).   Methandrostenolone is primarily used to promote nitrogen retention and protein anabolism, but it may also be used to reverse the excessive excretion of calcium and nitrogen accompanying corticosteroid therapy.

DOSE.   5 to 10 mg. orally daily.

NANDROLONE PHENPROPIONATE (DURABOLIN), NANDROLONE DECANOATE (DECA-DURABOLIN). Nandrolone is seldom used for replacement male hormone therapy since its androgenic effects are considerably less than those of other available testosterone derivatives. It has a protein anabolic effect equal to or slightly greater than that of testosterone propionate; it is often administered intramuscularly for this purpose. Like testosterone, it promotes nitrogen, potassium and phosphorus retention, weight gain and a feeling of well-being.

A high protein diet greatly enhances therapy with nandrolone.

DOSE. Nandrolone phenpropionate— 25 to 50 mg. I.M. weekly initially, then 25 mg. weekly. Nandrolone decanoate —50 to 100 mg. I.M. monthly for four months. Following a resting period of six to eight weeks, another course of treatment may be given if necessary.

NORETHANDROLONE, B.P. (NILEVAR). Norethandrolone is administered for its protein anabolic effects, which are equivalent to those of testosterone.

DOSE. 30 mg. orally or I.M. daily in divided doses.

STANOZOLOL (WINSTROL). Although the anabolic effects of stanozolol are favorable, it has few androgenic effects when administered. Children are especially sensitive to the androgenic effects, however, and it may cause masculinization in females and early epiphyseal closure in males.

DOSE. 2 mg. orally three times daily.

OXYMETHOLONE (ADROYD, ANADROL). Like stanozolol, oxymetholone is administered for its protein anabolic effects.

DOSE. 7.5 to 15 mg. orally daily.

OXANDROLONE (ANAVAR). Oxandrolone is administered for its protein anabolic effects. Its actions and side effects are similar to those of the other synthetic anabolic agents.

DOSE. 2.5 mg. orally three times daily.

GUIDE FOR THE NURSING ASSESSMENT OF A PATIENT RECEIVING INSULIN

I.   Why is this patient receiving insulin? Does he require insulin routinely or is it needed presently because of infection or other pathologic condition? How long has the patient been a diabetic? What is his attitude toward diabetes and insulin therapy?

II.   What type of insulin is this patient receiving? When is its onset of action? When is the peak of action likely to occur? What is the duration of action of this type of insulin?

III.   Is the insulin being administered correctly? Is it kept refrigerated? Is the patient receiving the correct dosage and type of insulin? Are the sites for subcutaneous injection being rotated routinely and according to plan? Is the correct technique for subcutaneous injection of insulin being used? If the patient is on a sliding scale for insulin dosage, are the urine specimens obtained correctly, i.e., is the specimen collected after the bladder has been emptied completely? Is this patient receiving other drugs which may interfere with the accuracy of tests for glycosuria?

IV.   Is the insulin therapy producing the desired effect? Has the patient's blood sugar level decreased? Do the results of urine tests for glycosuria and acetone indicate that the diabetes is under control? Have the signs and symptoms of diabetes mellitus receded, i.e., polyuria, polydipsia, polyphagia, fatigue, etc.? Does the patient exhibit any symptoms of hyperglycemia or diabetic coma? If so, what has been the patient's dietary intake? Does the patient have any signs of infection? Is this patient receiving any drugs which may cause or contribute to the development of hyperglycemia?

V.   Does this patient have any side effects of insulin therapy? Has the patient had signs and symptoms of hypoglycemia or insulin shock? If so, when do they occur? Has the patient's dietary intake decreased? Has the patient had more physical activity and exercise than usual? Is the patient receiving other drugs which may cause or contribute to the development of hypoglycemia? Does the patient have any indications of local tissue reaction and subcutaneous tissue degeneration at the sites of insulin injection?

VI.   What are the patient's (and family's) learning needs? Does the patient understand the reason why insulin is needed and the necessity of his receiving it? Does he understand insulin therapy and its relationship to his diet and degree of exercise? Does he understand other aspects of his care involving the prevention of the complications of diabetes (e.g., foot care, prevention of infection, etc.)? Does the patient and his family know the signs and symptoms, causes and immediate treatment for diabetic coma and insulin shock? Does the patient carry an identification card indicating that he is a diabetic, and other information related to his condition and treatment? Do the patient and his family understand how to administer insulin correctly? (See all of the items under III.) Do they understand the techniques involved in maintaining asepsis? Is the patient's eyesight sufficient to permit him to measure his insulin correctly? Does the patient understand the need for continual medical supervision and follow-up care?

GUIDE FOR THE NURSING ASSESSMENT OF A PATIENT RECEIVING A GLUCOCORTICOID

I.   Why is this patient receiving a glucocorticoid? For replacement therapy in adrenal insufficiency or for a therapeutic effect? How long has the patient been receiving glucocorticoids?

II.   Is the drug being administered correctly? Are oral doses given with or after meals to decrease the possibility of gastric irritation? If given for replacement therapy, does the scheduling of dosage provide a sufficiently constant effect in this patient during his daily activities? Are precautions taken to insure that a dose is not omitted inadvertently?

III.   Is the drug producing the intended effect? If given for adrenal insufficiency, are there indications of Addisonian crisis, such as a decrease in blood pressure, nausea, vomiting, anorexia, fatigue and muscle weakness? If given for a therapeutic effect, have signs and symptoms of inflammation or allergic reaction decreased? Is there a decrease in the symptoms of the condition for which this drug was prescribed?

IV.   Does the patient have any indications of increased glucocorticoid effect? Has the patient shown a gain in weight? Is there evidence of edema or fluid retention? Are there indications of fluid and electrolyte imbalance? Does the patient have the appearance of a person with Cushing's syndrome? Does the patient have hirsutism or acne? Has the patient's blood sugar level risen? Does the patient have glycosuria? Does the patient have any symptoms of hyperglycemia? Is the patient observed carefully for any indication of an infectious process or delayed wound healing? Is the patient protected from sources of infection? Does the patient have any signs and symptoms which may indicate the development of a peptic ulcer? Does the patient have any petechiae or ecchymotic areas that might indicate a bleeding tendency? Has there been a change in the patient's personality or behavior?

V.   What are the learning needs of the patient and his family? If the patient has Addison's disease, or has had any adrenalectomy or hypophysectomy: Does he understand his condition and the need for life-long drug therapy? Does he understand the role of stress in his condition and its relationship to drug dosage and scheduling? Do the patient and his family know the symptoms of Addisonian crisis and the actions which should be taken? If the patient is receiving large doses of glucocorticoids for therapeutic reasons over an extended period of time: Is the patient aware of the side effects which he should report? Does he understand the need for sodium restriction and other measures if these are prescribed? Does the patient understand the need to take the dosage as prescribed and not to omit a dose or stop taking the drug without his physician's consent? Has the patient been advised that, in the event of future serious illnesses or surgery, he should inform medical personnel that he has had glucocorticoid therapy in the past?

QUESTIONS FOR DISCUSSION AND REVIEW

1.   Review and explain the feedback mechanisms involved in hormone regulation.

2.   Explain how a large daily dose of dexamethasone affects the body's endocrine system.

3.   What symptoms would you expect in a patient with a tumor of the anterior pituitary?

4. Which types of diabetics are usually helped with oral hypoglycemia agents? Why?

5. List the various disorders that result from thyroid dysfunction. What are the nursing implications?

6. How would you, as a nurse, help a patient adjust to diabetes? What would you include in a teaching plan?

7. What observations would you make and what actions should you take if you found a diabetic patient unconscious?

8. Why would a patient who has received glucocorticoids in the past require a glucocorticoid when he is undergoing surgery?

9. Outline a teaching plan for a patient with Addison's disease or for a patient who has had an adrenalectomy or hypophysectomy.

BIBLIOGRAPHY

AMA Drug Evaluations. Chicago, American Medical Association, 1971.

Aurbach, G. D. and Potts, J. T., Jr.: Parathyroid hormone. *Amer. J. Med., 42*:1, 1967.

Best, C. H. and Taylor, N. B.: *The Physiological Basis of Medical Practice.* 6th Ed. Baltimore, The Williams and Wilkins Co., 1965.

Bond, V. P. (moderator): Symposium on insulin. *Amer. J. Med., 40*:651, 1966.

Bradley, R. F.: Treatment of ketoacidosis and coma. *Med. Clin. N. Amer., 49*:961, 1965.

Coates, F. C. and Fabrykant, M.: Insulin injection technique for preventing skin reactions. *Amer. J. Nurs., 65*:127, (February) 1965.

The complications of corticosteroids. *J.A.M.A., 195*:52, 1966.

Connell, E. B.: The pill and the problems. *Amer. J. Nurs., 71*:326, (February) 1971.

Davis, M. E., Strandjord, N. M. and Lanze, L. H.: Estrogens and the aging process. *J.A.M.A., 196*:219, 1966.

DeGroot, L. J.: Therapy of thyrotoxicosis. *Mod. Treatm., 1*:176, 1964.

Derr, S. D.: Testing for glycosuria. *Amer. J. Nurs., 70*:1513, (July) 1970.

DiPalma, J. R. (ed.): *Drill's Pharmacology in Medicine.* 4th Ed. New York, McGraw-Hill Book Co., 1971.

DiPalma, J. R.: Drugs for diabetes mellitus. *R.N., 30*:71, (October) 1967.

Ellis, M.: Assessment of thyroid function. *Canad. Nurs., 61*:881, 1965.

Frohman, L. P.: The adrenocorticosteroids. *Amer. J. Nurs., 64*:120, (November) 1964.

Fruehan, A. E. and Frawley, T. H.: Current status of anabolic steroids. *J.A.M.A., 184*:527, 1963.

Goodman, L. S. and Gilman, A.: *Pharmacological Basis of Therapeutics.* 4th Ed. New York, Macmillan Co., 1970.

Gorman, C. K.: Hypoglycemia, a brief review. *Med. Clin. N. Amer., 49*:947, 1965.

Goth, A.: *Medical Pharmacology.* 3rd Ed. St. Louis, C. V. Mosby Co., 1968.

Govoni, L. E. and Hayes, J. E.: *Drugs and Nursing Implications.* 2nd Ed. New York, Appleton-Century-Crofts, 1971.

Greenblatt, R. B., et al.: Addison's disease and nursing care of the patient with Addison's disease. *Amer. J. Nurs., 60*:1249, (September) 1960.

Hilf, R.: Mechanism of action of ACTH. *New Eng. J. Med., 273*:798, 1965.

Hornback, M.: Diabetes mellitus — the nurse's role. *Nurs. Clin. N. Amer., 5*:3, (March) 1970.

Keele, C. A. and Neil, E.: *Samson Wright's Applied Physiology.* 11th Ed. London, Oxford University Press, 1965.

Kelly, M.: Steroids: drugs of addiction to patient and doctor. *J. Chronic Dis., 17*:461, 1964.

Lammert, A.: The menopause: a physiologic process. *Amer. J. Nurs., 62*: 56, 1962.

Lerman, J.: Treatment of hypothyroidism. *Mod. Treatm., 1*:146, 1964.

Liddle, G. W.: Clinical pharmacology of the anti-inflammatory steroids. *Clin. Pharmacol. Ther., 2*:615, 1961.

London, D. R.: The corticosteroids. *Practitioner, 200*:113, 1968.

Lukens, F. D. W.: Insulin and protein metabolism. *Diabetes, 13*:451, 1964.

Lukens, F. D. W.: The rediscovery of regular insulin. *New Eng. J. Med., 272*:130, 1965.

Main, R. J. and Richardson, A. W.: *Physiology.* 2nd Ed. St. Louis, C. V. Mosby Co., 1953.

Martin, M.: Diabetes mellitus: current concepts. *Amer. J. Nurs., 66*:510, (March) 1966.

Martin, M.: Insulin reaction. *Amer. J. Nurs., 67*:328, (February) 1967.

Martin, M.: The unconscious diabetic patient. *Amer. J. Nurs., 61*:92, 1961.

Miale, J. E. and Plotz, C. M.: Nursing care of patients with rheumatoid arthritis during therapy with cortisone. *Amer. J. Nurs., 53*:290, 1953.

Nelson, D. H. (ed.): Treatment of adrenal disorders. *Mod. Treatm., 3*: 1328, (November) 1966.

Ormerod, T. P., et al.: The treatment of diabetes. 3. Insulin and oral hypoglycemia drugs. *Nurs. Times, 65*:750, (June 12) 1969.

Pansky, B. and House, E. L.: *Review of Gross Anatomy.* New York, Macmillan Co., 1964.

Pearson, O. H. and Lubic, R. W.: Adrenalectomy and hypophysectomy and nursing care after adrenalectomy and hypophysectomy. *Amer. J. Nurs., 62*:80, (April) 1962.

Randall, R. V.: Treatment of diabetes insipidus. *Mod. Treatm., 3*:180, (January) 1966.

Reich, B. and Hwalt, L. P.: Nursing care of the patient with Addison's disease. *Amer. J. Nurs., 60*:1252, (September) 1960.

Reveno, W. S. and Rosenbaum, H.: Observations on the use of anti-thyroid drugs. *Ann. Intern. Med., 60*:982, 1964.

Rodman, M. J.: The corticosteroids. *R.N., 32*:32, (September) 1969.

Rodman, M. J.: The female sex hormones. *R.N., 31*:41, (May) 1968.

Rodman, M. J.: The male sex hormones and anabolic steroids. *R.N., 30*: 41, (May) 1967.

Rodman, M. J.: The oral contraceptives. *R.N., 29*:51 (March) 1966.

Rodman, M. J.: The thyroid and antithyroid drugs. *R.N., 31*:55, (February) 1968.

Rosenbloom, A. L.: Growth hormone replacement therapy. *J.A.M.A., 198*:364, 1966.

St. James, P.: Insulin injection — a new technique. *Canad. Nurs., 65*:32, (July 3) 1969.

Sharp, G. W. G. and Leaf, A.: Mechanism of action of aldosterone. *Physiol. Rev., 46*:593, 1966.

Shea, K. M., et al.: Teaching a patient to live with adrenal insufficiency. *Amer. J. Nurs., 65*:80, 1965.

Shuman, C. R. (ed.): Symposium on treatment of complications of diabetes. *Mod. Treatm., 4*:13, (January) 1967.

Sparbeg, M. and Kirsuer, J. B.: Steroid therapy and infections. *J.A.M.A., 188*:680, 1964.

Tepperman, J.: *Metabolic and Endocrine Physiology.* Chicago, Year Book Medical Publishers, Inc., 1962.

Thorm, G. W.: Clinical considerations in the use of corticosteroids. *New Eng. J. Med., 274*:775, 1966.

Wallace, C. M.: Modified insulin and the nurse. *Nurs. Mirror, 128*:38, (February) 1969.

Watkins, J., et al.: Observation of medication errors made by diabetic patient in the home. *Diabetes, 16*:882, (December) 1967.

Watkins, J. D. and Moss, F. T.: Confusion in the management of diabetes. *Amer. J. Nurs., 69*:521, (March) 1969.

Weller, C.: Oral hypoglycemic agents. *Amer. J. Nurs., 64*:90, 1964.

Wintrobe, M. M., et al. (eds.): *Harrison's Principles of Internal Medicine.* 6th Ed. New York, McGraw-Hill Book Co., 1970.

Youmans, W. B.: *Fundamentals of Human Physiology.* 2nd Ed. Chicago, Year Book Medical Publishers, Inc., 1962.

Chapter 16 Drugs that Affect the Respiratory Tract

Important Concepts Discussed

1. *Respiration is ultimately controlled by the respiratory center in the medulla.*

2. *Respiration can be stimulated by appropriate pharmacologic agents.*

3. *Antitussives and expectorants are useful adjuncts in the management of respiratory infections.*

4. *Asthma is a respiratory disorder that is produced by an allergic reaction and may be treated by antihistamines and smooth muscle relaxants.*

5. *Nursing measures should promote the removal of respiratory secretions and the maintenance of a patent airway.*

Respiration, the exchange of gases between the organism and its environment, must be carried on continually and with at least moderate efficiency for life to be maintained. A continual supply of oxygen is necessary at the cellular level for many enzymatic processes. Oxygen is necessary for utilization of food and water taken into the body; in addition it is essential for the action of the central nervous system and the heart as well as skeletal muscle contraction and elimination of body wastes. Almost every energy-expending activity of the body is performed by using ATP, a high energy phosphate that may be formed only by a series of enzymatic reactions dependent on oxygen.

In addition to supplying the body with oxygen, the respiratory tract removes carbon dioxide, one of the chief by-products of body metabolism. If carbon dioxide is not removed as it is formed, the acid-base balance of the body is disturbed, respiration increases and urinary bicarbonate secretion is decreased to preserve homeostasis. In some cases of chronic lung disease in which the carbon dioxide level is always higher than normal, the respiratory center becomes less sensitive to carbon dioxide, and respiration depends more completely on the lowered oxygen level in the blood. Persons with chronic lung disease should never be given pure oxygen inhalation for this reason, since the rapid rise in oxygen saturation of the blood causes decreased activity of the oxygen receptors, and a prolonged period of apnea may result regardless of the concurrent carbon dioxide level in the blood. If these patients do receive oxygen, it is administered in low concentrations by using a

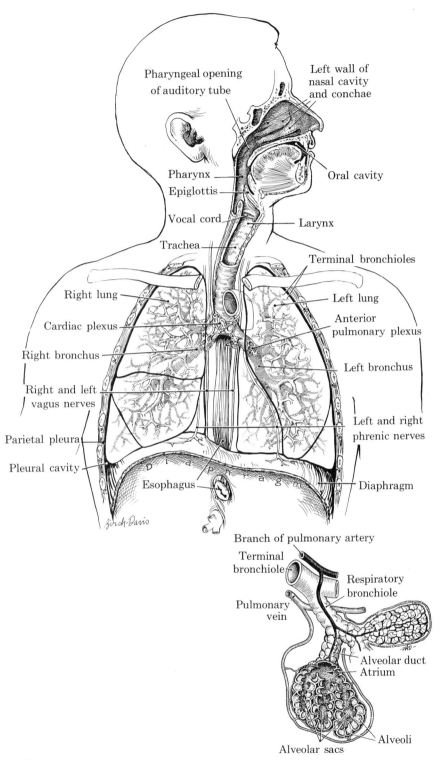

FIGURE 48. The respiratory tract. (*Dorland's Illustrated Medical Dictionary.* Ed. 24. W. B. Saunders Co., Philadelphia, 1965.)

low liter flow and special masks that provide low concentrates of oxygen to the patient.

The capillaries surrounding the lung alveoli are in constant contact with inspired air. The thin walls of the alveoli and capillaries readily permit the blood to receive oxygen and release carbon dioxide, the process referred to as pulmonary or external respiration; the blood's exchange of oxygen for carbon dioxide at the cellular level is referred to as internal respiration.

Regulation of breathing has two aspects:

1. Automatic control of the amplitude and duration of the cycle. Slow, deep breathing may accomplish the same oxygen–carbon dioxide exchange as rapid, shallow breathing. Adjustments are made by the body to develop a pattern that requires the least energy. The depth and rate are largely determined by the compliance (or elasticity) of the lung, the diameter of the airway, and the mechanical resistance (i.e., due to fibrosis) in the lung. These factors may often be altered or the progressive changes of chronic lung disease slowed by drug therapy.

2. Regulation of total alveolar ventilation. All alveoli do not function in gaseous exchange with each inspiration. The total ventilation of the lung varies greatly with the rate of body metabolism and of carbon dioxide production.

Development of rhythmic respiration depends on the neural organization of the respiratory system and involves "inhibitory loops," which are feedback mechanisms. These inhibitory loops are not located entirely in or around the medullary respiratory center; rather external influences are very important in regulating respiration.

The various centers and inhibitory loops may be considered as shown on the accompanying diagram.

The inspiratory center and the expiratory center are located in the medulla and are mutually inhibitive; that is, when one is actively stimulating the muscles of respiration the other is being inhibited. The expiratory center also inhibits the apneustic center, a small area in the pons that stimulates the inspiratory center and brings about a strong inspiratory effort. The pneu-

motaxic center and the apneustic center form an additional inhibitory loop system that aids smooth respiration. If this second inhibitory loop is removed from control, as

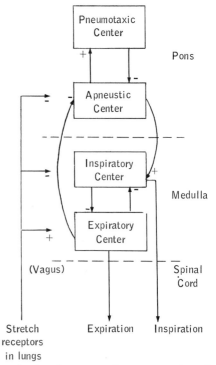

by sectioning between the pons and medulla, respiration proceeds, but breathing is gaspy and irregular.

The vagal afferent fibers with sensory endings in the stretch receptors in the lungs stimulate the expiratory center when the lungs are stretched at the end of inspiration. By simultaneously inhibiting the inspiratory center and the apneustic center, expiration is allowed to proceed at once. When the vagi are cut, respiration continues, but it is slower and deeper.

Chemoreceptors located at various places in the body are also effective in controlling the rate and depth of respiration. There is believed to be a chemoreceptor in the medulla that is very sensitive to changes in carbon dioxide and hydrogen ion concentrations in the cerebrospinal fluid. In addition, chemoreceptors in the carotid and aortic bodies are sensitive to a decrease in the oxygen level of the blood. These receptors are much less sensitive to an increase in carbon dioxide than are the medullary receptors, and they are the centers that control respiration in chronic obstructive lung disease.

DRUGS AFFECTING THE RESPIRATORY CENTER

RESPIRATORY STIMULANTS

Many central nervous system stimulants are also respiratory stimulants because they accelerate the activity of the centrally located respiratory centers. The stimulating effects of many of these drugs have been discussed in the chapter dealing with the central nervous system; they will be discussed in this section only with reference to their effects on the respiratory system.

BEMEGRIDE, U.S.P., B.P. (MEGIMIDE). The exact mode of action of bemegride is unknown, but it is somewhat more specific in its action upon the respiratory center than are other central stimulants. Its chief use as a respiratory stimulant is in the treatment of barbiturate and glutethimide intoxication, but its effectiveness as a barbiturate antagonist is questionable.

> **TOXICITY.** Overdosage may cause convulsions. Sodium thiopental may be administered intravenously as an antidote.

> **DOSE.** 50 to 200 mg. intravenously, in intermittent doses of 50 mg. every 3 to 5 minutes until muscle tone and pharyngeal and laryngeal reflexes return.

CAFFEINE AND SODIUM BENZOATE, U.S.P. Caffeine is a descending central nervous system stimulant, which exerts its primary effect on the higher cerebral centers. It may be used as a mild respiratory stimulant, particularly in the newborn. Tolerance to the stimulant effects of caffeine is observed in adults who consume large amounts of caffeine-containing beverages. It is therefore not routinely employed for adult therapy.

> **DOSE.** 0.5 to 1 Gm. I.M. or I.V.

ETHAMIVAN (EMIVAN). Ethamivan exerts its primary effect upon the respiratory center in the medulla to increase both the depth and rate of respiration. In addition it induces mild vasoconstriction and a rise in peripheral blood pressure, but it has no effects on cardiac rate or rhythm. Respiratory stimulation may be noted within one minute after intravenous administration and lasts about 10 minutes.

> **USES.** Ethamivan is used intravenously to treat overdosage with barbiturates or as an adjunct to recovery from general anesthesia. It is of some benefit in the treatment of chronic obstructive lung diseases with increased carbon dioxide retention. The inconvenience of intravenous administration and the short duration of action make it impractical, however. Although ethamivan is considerably less effective orally, some increase in the rate and depth of respiration may be noted for three or four hours following administration.

> **TOXICITY.** Coughing, sneezing, laryngospasm or convulsions may be observed during intravenous administration. Dermatoses, dizziness and flushing have been noted upon oral administration.

> **DOSE.** I.V.—single dose of 1 or 2 mg./ kg. of body weight over a 30 to 90 second period. Oral—20 to 60 mg. two to four times daily.

NIKETHAMIDE INJECTION, N.F., B.P. (CORAMINE). Nikethamide is a central stimulant that acts chiefly on the respiratory centers in the medulla to increase the rate and depth of respiration. It is also believed to influence the carotid sinus to elevate systemic blood pressure.

> **USES.** Nikethamide is used to counteract the respiratory depression resulting from overdoses of opiates, alcohol, carbon monoxide and nonbarbiturate sedatives, but it has little or no effectiveness in the treatment of barbiturate intoxication. It has moderate effectiveness in treatment of chronic obstructive lung disease, and it has been used to

counteract the apnea resulting from oxygen administration to these patients.

TOXICITY. Toxic reactions are the result of excessive central stimulation. Convulsions may occur if an overdose is administered.

DOSE. 5 to 10 ml. of a 25% solution I.V., followed by 5 ml. every 5 minutes for the first hour. No more than 5 ml. should be administered each hour thereafter until response is obtained.

PENTYLENETETRAZOL INJECTION, N.F. (METRAZOL). Pentylenetetrazol is a central stimulant that acts primarily on the respiratory, circulatory and vagal centers in the medulla to increase circulation and respiration. It is more effective on the respiratory center when this center is depressed than when it is functioning normally.

USES. Pentylenetetrazol has been used in the treatment of barbiturate, opiate, paraldehyde and nonbarbiturate sedative toxicity. In addition it is recommended for geriatric use as an oral analeptic agent.

TOXICITY. Excessive central stimulation and convulsions. It is contraindicated for resuscitation of the newborn and for the treatment of patients with convulsive disorders.

DOSE. I.V.—5 ml. of a 10% solution, then 10 ml. after 30 minutes. A third dose of 20 ml. may be given and repeated at 30 minute intervals until response is obtained. Oral—200 mg. three times daily.

AROMATIC AMMONIA SPIRIT. This hydroalcoholic, scented solution contains approximately 4 per cent ammonium carbonate. It is the chief ingredient of smelling salts. Because of the irritant effect ammonia has on the sensory receptors in the nasal mucous membrane, reflex respiratory stimulation is accomplished.

TOXICITY. Irritation may be quite uncomfortable if excessive amounts are inhaled. This is accompanied by lacrimation, coryza and coughing.

DOSE. Inhaled as needed.

CARBON DIOXIDE, U.S.P., B.P. Carbon dioxide, an odorless, colorless, tasteless gas, is one of the principal by-products of body metabolism. Under ordinary circumstances it is the natural respiratory stimulant because of its effects on the chemoreceptors in the medulla, carotid body and aortic arch. The extremely rich blood supply to these chemoreceptors enables detection of even slight changes in the carbon dioxide level. The medullary receptors are much more receptive to these changes than are the carotid and aortic receptors.

USES. Carbon dioxide is often combined with oxygen for inhalation to prevent respiratory depression from hyperventilation or apnea in patients whose respiration is induced by decreased oxygen levels rather than elevated carbon dioxide levels. It may be used to stimulate respiration during or after general anesthesia, but it is not potent enough to be used alone for the treatment of drug-induced respiratory depression.

Carbon dioxide may be administered by inhalation for four minute periods to relieve hiccoughs. Its value here is questionable, however, The home remedy of breathing into a paper bag as a cure for hiccoughs works on this principle, since with repeated expiration into the bag, the carbon dioxide level naturally increases.

TOXICITY. Prolonged inhalation of high levels of carbon dioxide may cause dyspnea, dizziness, nausea, elevated blood pressure because of central action on the vasoconstrictor center, malaise and a feeling of suffocating.

DOSE. 5% concentration with 95% oxygen. Inhalation as needed.

ATROPINE SULFATE, U.S.P., B.P. Atropine, an anticholinergic agent, is often prescribed with morphine as a preoperative medication because it stimulates respiration and inhibits secretions of the respiratory tract. Because of its anticholinergic effect, it inhibits the slowing effect of the vagus on the heart and thus increases the heart rate, an additional useful effect when atropine is prescribed with the depressant morphine.

Although it increases the rate and depth of respiration, it is not powerful enough to stimulate respiration when toxic doses of depressants have been administered.

DOSE. 0.5 mg. s.c. or I.M.

RESPIRATORY DEPRESSANTS

Narcotic analgesics, barbiturates and many tranquilizers and nonbarbiturate sedatives produce respiratory depression, which in most instances is considered to be their most serious side effect. It is the first symptom specifically treated in poisoning with these agents. In rare instances in which coughing is extremely painful or harmful, however, these drugs are administered to decrease the rate of respiration and to depress the cough reflex.

DRUGS AFFECTING THE COUGH CENTER AND RESPIRATORY TRACT

Antitussives

Antitussives, drugs that inhibit the cough reflex, act primarily upon the cough center in the central nervous system. The most powerful antitussives are the narcotic agents, but a few non-narcotic agents have proved powerful enough to have gained extensive popularity. The antitussives are often combined in cough preparations with demulcents and expectorants for optimal treatment of the cough. Antitussives should not be employed in respiratory conditions such as tuberculosis in which a productive cough is desired to expel the pulmonary exudate.

The nurse should appreciate that a cough is essentially a protective mechanism to expel material from the respiratory tract. It may also be an important warning signal for chronic respiratory disease or pulmonary carcinoma. Persons should be educated on the dangers of self-medication for coughs and on the need to seek medical help for the treatment of persistent or recurring coughs. Antitussives are needed, however, if the cough is nonproductive and interferes with the patient's rest or sleep.

Nursing measures can assist in producing the intended effect of antitussive drugs. An adequate fluid intake is necessary to aid in liquefying mucous secretions. Beverages and hard candy or lozenges may help to provide a soothing effect on the pharyngeal mucosa. Liquid cough preparations that are intended to have a soothing effect on the pharyngeal mucosa should be administered undiluted and should not be followed by water or other liquid.

Since coughing is usually reduced when the patient is in an upright position, elevation of the head of the bed or the use of pillows may be helpful. The nurse should assist the patient during coughing episodes by providing tissues, helping the patient to an upright position, and by providing support to the incision in a postoperative patient.

CODEINE PHOSPHATE, U.S.P., B.P. (METHYL-MORPHINE). Codeine, an extract of the opium poppy, in addition to its analgesic effect is quite useful in the treatment of coughs produced by irritation of the bronchi and trachea. When combined in cough preparations in not more than one grain (60 mg.) per ounce, the preparations are termed "exempt narcotics" and may be purchased without a prescription. When codeine is present in higher concentrations, a narcotic prescription is required

> **TOXICITY.** Central depression. Somewhat addicting, although not as seriously as morphine.

> **DOSE.** 8 mg. orally every 3 or 4 hours.

DIHYDROCODEINONE BITARTRATE, N.F. (DICODID, HYCODAN, MERCODINONE). Dihydrocodeinone is a synthetic analog of codeine, and it is more potent in its addiction liabilities and in its cough depressant effect. It has a marked sedative effect in some patients, and they should be warned about driving and operating machinery when taking preparations containing this drug. A narcotic prescription is required.

TABLE 12   Examples of Over-the-Counter Antitussives†

product	manufacturer	narcotic	non-narcotic	sympatho-mimetic	anti-histamine	expectorant	other
Adulton	Bristol Myers	—	dextromethorphan HBr 30 mg	phenylephrine HCl 10 mg	chlorpheniramine maleate 2 mg	terpin hydrate 100 mg	acetaminophen 330 mg alcohol 30%
Anahist Cough Medicine	Warner-Lambert	—	dextromethorphan HBr 15 mg/5 cc	phenylpropanolamine HCl 10 mg	thonzylamine HCl 6.25 mg	ammonium chloride 50 mg sod. citrate 135 mg	alcohol 0.5% ascorbic acid 10 mg
Anahist Cough Syrup	Warner-Lambert	—	dextromethorphan HBr 10 mg/10 ml	—	thonzylamine HCl 12.5 mg	ammonium chloride 100 mg sod. citrate 270 mg	alcohol 0.5%
Arrestin	Johnson & Johnson	—	dextromethorphan HBr 10 mg/5 cc	—	—	glyceryl guaiacolate 25 mg sod. citrate 50 mg chloroform 29.5 mg	sod. benzoate 0.1% alcohol 10%
Bristalin Cough Syrup	Bristol	—	—	—	phenyltoloxamine citrate 75 mg/fl oz	ammonium chloride 0.347 gm ipecac fl ext. 0.06 ml menthol 0.003 gm sod. citrate 0.322 gm	—
Cheracol	Upjohn	codeine phosphate 1 gr/fl oz	—	—	—	ammonium chloride 8 gr antimony pot. tartrate $\frac{1}{12}$ gr chloroform 2 gr pot. guaiacol-sulfonate 8 gr white pine	alcohol 3% wild cherry bark
Cheracol D	Upjohn	—	dextromethorphan HBr 60 mg/fl oz	—	—	chloroform 2 gr glyceryl guaiacolate $1\frac{2}{3}$ gr ammonium chloride 8 gr antimony pot. tartrate $\frac{1}{12}$ gr white pine	alcohol 3% wild cherry bark
Colban	Mentholatum	—	—	—	pyrilamine maleate 75 mg/fl oz	ammonium chloride 300 mg glyceryl guaiacolate 350 mg chloroform 2 min sod. citrate*	ascorbic acid* sod. salicylate 129 mg sod. benzoate
Coldene Adult	WTS-Pharmacraft	—	—	phenylpropanolamine HCl 18 mg/5 cc	chlorpheniramine maleate 1 mg	chloroform 0.5% glyceryl guaiacolate 30 mg sod. citrate 108 mg	alcohol 6% sod. salicylate 216 mg
Conar	Massengill	—	noscapine 10 mg/5 cc	phenylephrine HCl 5 mg	pheniramine maleate 10 mg	chloroform 12 mg menthol 0.2 mg	—
Conar Expectorant	Massengill	—	noscapine 10 mg/5 cc	phenylephrine HCl 5 mg	pheniramine maleate 10 mg	chloroform 12 mg glyceryl guaiacolate 100 mg menthol 0.2 mg	—
Contac Cough Control	Menley & James	—	dextromethorphan HBr 15 mg/5 cc	phenylpropanolamine HCl 12.5 mg	chlorpheniramine maleate 1 mg	chloroform 0.2%	alcohol 8%
Coricidin Cough Formula	Schering	—	—	phenylpropanolamine HCl 12.5 mg/15 cc	chlorpheniramine maleate 2 mg	ammonium chloride 100 mg chloroform 0.25% glyceryl guaiacolate 50 mg	
Coryban-D	Roerig	—	dextromethorphan HBr 7.5 mg/5 cc	phenylephrine HCl 5 mg	chlorpheniramine maleate 1 mg	chloroform 0.5% glyceryl guaiacolate 50 mg	alcohol 7.5% acetaminophen 120 mg ascorbic acid 12.5 mg
Cosadein	Parke, Davis	codeine phosphate 1 gr/fl oz	—	—	—	chloroform 2 gr eriodictyon 16 gr poplar bud 4 gr white pine 32 gr	alcohol 20% wild cherry 32 gr glycerin 120 min
Cosanyl	Parke, Davis	codeine phosphate 1 gr/fl oz	—	—	—	squill 24 min menthol $\frac{3}{25}$ gr	alcohol 6% euphorbia 120 min cascara ext. 8 gr cocillana 40 min wild lettuce 120 min
Covan-amine Ex-pectorant	Mallinckrodt	—	—	phenylephrine HCl 3.75 mg/5 cc phenylpropanolamine HCl 6.25 mg	chlorpheniramine maleate 1 mg pyrilamine maleate 6.25 mg	glyceryl guaiacolate 100 mg	—

*Quantitative statement not provided.
†From Penna, Darlington, and Chalmers: *Handbook of Non-Prescription Drugs.* Washington, D.C., American Pharmaceutical Association, 1968, p. 23.

Table 12 *continued on opposite page.*

TABLE 12 Examples of Over-the-Counter Antitussives (*Continued*)

product	manufacturer	narcotic	non-narcotic	sympatho-mimetic	anti-histamine	expectorant	other
Creomulsion Cough Medicine	Creomulsion Co.	—	—	—	—	beechwood creosote* white pine ipecac* menthol*	cascara* wild cherry alcohol 1%
Creo-Terpin	Denver Chemical	—	—	—	—	creosote 2 min/fl oz sod. glycero-phosphate 4 gr chloroform 1 min terpin hydrate 2 gr	alcohol 25%
DeWitt's Cough Control Medicine	DeWitt Co.	—	dextrome-thorphan HBr 8 mg/5 cc	—	—	ammonium chloride 80 mg pot. guaiacol sulfonate 75 mg chloroform 20 mg	glycerin alcohol 3%
Dristan Cough Formula	Whitehall	—	dextrome-thorphan HBr 10 mg/5 cc	phenylephrine HCl 5 mg	chlorphenira-mine maleate 1 mg	sod. citrate* glyceryl guaiacolate* chloroform*	alcohol 12%
Endo-tussin-C	Endo	codeine phosphate 10 mg/5 cc	—	—	pyrilamine maleate 12.5 mg	ammonium chloride 60 mg sodium citrate 85 mg	homatropine methylbromide 0.5 mg
Endo-tussin-NN	Endo	—	dextrome-thorphan HBr 10 mg/5 cc	—	pyrilamine maleate 7.5 mg	ammonium chloride 40 mg sodium citrate 60 mg	homatropine methyl bromide 0.25 mg
Fletcher's Children's Cough Syrup	Glenbrook	—	dextromethor-phan HBr 5 mg/5 cc	phenyleph-rine HCl 2.5 mg	chlorphenira-mine maleate 1 mg	chloroform 0.04 cc pot. guaiacol-sulfonate 12.5 mg antimony pot. tartrate 1.25 mg	alcohol 10% cherry flavor
Histadyl EC	Lilly	codeine phosphate 1 gr/30 cc	—	ephedrine HCl 30 mg	methapyrilene fumarate 81 mg	ammonium chloride 660 mg chloroform 0.06 cc menthol	alcohol 0.5%
Ipsatol Cough Troches	Davies Rose Hoyt	—	—	—	—	ipecac* ammonium chloride* eucalyptus* squill*	tolu balsam*
Naldetuss	Bristol	—	dextrome-thorphan HBr 15 mg/5 cc	phenylpro-panolamine HCl 17.5 mg	phenyltoloxa-mine citrate 7.5 mg	—	acetaminophen 162 mg
Pertussin 8-Hour	Chesebrough-Ponds	—	dextrome-thorphan HBr 7.5 mg/5 cc	—	—	ammonium chloride* chloroform 0.3% sodium citrate*	alcohol 9.5%
Pinex Regular	Pinex Co.	—	—	—	—	chloroform 3 min/fl oz pot. guaiacolsulfo-nate* oil of pine* oil of eucalyptus* ext grindelia*	alcohol 3% glycerine
Quelidrine	Abbott	—	dextrome-thorphan HBr 10 mg/5 cc	ephedrine HCl 5 mg phenyl-ephrine HCl 5 mg	chlorphenira-mine maleate 2 mg	ammonium chloride 40 mg ipecac fl ext 0.005 ml	alcohol 2%
Rem	Maryland Pharm.	—	—	—	—	chloroform 0.7% squill* ipecac* tar* tolu* menthol* ammonium chloride* lobelia* horehound* white pine* sanguinaria	alcohol 1.2% wild cherry
Robitussin	Robins	—	—	—	—	glyceryl guaiacolate 100 mg	alcohol 3.5%
Robitussin AC	Robins	codeine phosphate 10 mg/5 cc	—	—	pheniramine maleate 7.5 mg	glyceryl guaiacolate 100 mg	alcohol 3.5%
Robitussin DM	Robins	—	dextrome-thorphan HBr 15 mg/5 cc	—	—	glyceryl guaiacolate 100 mg/5 cc	alcohol 1.4%
Romilar CF	Sauter	—	dextrome-thorphan HBr 15 mg/5 cc	phenyl-ephrine HCl 5 mg	chlorphenira-mine maleate 1 mg	chloroform 12.5 mg	acetamino-phen 120 mg. alcohol 10%
Romilar Cough Lozenges	Sauter	—	dextrome-thorphan HBr 5 mg	—	—	—	benzyl alcohol 0.5%

* Quantitative statement not provided.

Table 12 *continued on following page.*

TABLE 12   Examples of Over-the-Counter Antitussives (*Continued*)

product	manufacturer	narcotic	non-narcotic	sympatho-mimetic	anti-histamine	expectorant	other
St. Joseph's Cough Syrup for Children	Plough	—	dextrome-thorphan HBr 7.5 mg/5cc	—	—	ipecac* sod. citrate* menthol*	—
Sedatole	MSD	codeine sulfate 30 mg/fl oz	—	—	—	squill* menthol* sanguinaria* poplar bud	alcohol 6% wild cherry bark* phosphoric acid*
Thorexin	Isodine	—	dextrome-thorphan HBr 5 mg/5 cc	—	—	ammonium chloride 90 mg chloroform 20 mg potassium guaiacolsulfonate 90 mg antimony pot. tartrate 0.9 mg	alcohol 3%
Trimetose	Schering	—	—	—	prophenpyrid-amine maleate 7.5 mg/4 cc	ammonium chloride 104.8 mg sod. citrate 43 mg chloroform 17.5 mg	alcohol 7%
Trind	Mead Johnson	—	—	phenyl-ephrine HCl 2.5 mg/5 cc	—	glyceryl guaiacolate 50 mg	acetamino-phen 150 mg alcohol 15%
Triaminic Expect-orant	Dorsey	—	—	phenylpro-panolamine HCl 12.5 mg	pheniramine maleate 6.25 mg pyrilamine maleate 6.25 mg	glyceryl guaiacolate 100 mg	alcohol 5%
Triaminicol	Dorsey	—	dextrome-thorphan HBr 15 mg/5 ml	phenylpro-panolamine HCl 12.5 mg	pheniramine maleate 6.25 mg pyrilamine maleate 6.25 mg	ammonium chloride 90 mg	nonalcoholic
Vick's Cough Syrup	Vick	—	dextrome-thorphan HBr*	—	—	ammonium chloride* camphor* menthol* sod. citrate* eucalyptus*	cetyl pyridium chloride*
Vick's Formula 44 Cough Mixture	Vick	—	dextrome-thorphan HBr*	—	doxylamine succinate*	chloroform 0.5% sod. citrate*	cetyl pyridium chloride* alcohol 10%
Vick's Formula 44 Cough Discs	Vick	—	dextrome-thorphan HBr*	—	—	menthol* peppermint*	benzocaine* cetyl pyridium chloride*

* Quantitative statement not provided.

It is supplied as a syrup and tablets containing 5 mg. of dihydrocodeinone and 1.5 mg. of homatropine methylbromide per teaspoonful or tablet. The combination quite effectively dries excessive respiratory secretions and depresses the cough reflex.

DOSE.   5 to 10 mg. orally three or four times daily.

METHADONE HYDROCHLORIDE, U.S.P., B.P. (ADANON, AMIDON, DOLOPHINE). Methadone is the most potent narcotic used as a cough depressant. It is not commonly employed in cough suppressants unless other less depressant and less addicting drugs have failed. A narcotic prescription is always required to obtain this drug.

DOSE.   1.5 to 2 mg. orally every 2 to 3 hours.

DEXTROMETHORPHAN HYDROBROMIDE, N.F. (ROMILAR). Dextromethorphan is structurally similar to levorphanol (Levo-Dromoran) but does not have the addicting, analgesic and depressant effects of narcotic analgesics. Consequently, it is not subject to the federal narcotic laws. Its antitussive action is equivalent to that of codeine and, like codeine, it has no expectorant action. It is most effective in the palliation of the chronic, nonproductive cough produced by irritation of the tracheobronchial tree.

TOXICITY.   Nausea, dizziness and drowsiness in susceptible persons.

DOSE.   10 to 20 mg. orally two to four times daily.

LEVOPROPOXYPHENE NAPSYLATE, U.S.P. (NOV-RAD).   This drug is the levo isomer of the analgesic dextropropoxyphene (Darvon), but it has no analgesic properties. It is used as a central antitussive, but its value is highly questionable. It is not used as extensively as the other antitussive compounds.

The main advantage of this compound is that it can be administered in the form of capsules rather than in liquid preparations.

TOXICITY. Nausea, dizziness, drowsiness and dermatoses have been noted.

DOSE. 50 to 100 mg. orally every 4 hours.

EXPECTORANTS

An expectorant is a drug that either increases or liquefies the mucous secretions of the respiratory tract and thus aids in their expulsion while coughing. As noted previously, expectorants and antitussives are often prescribed together; the antitussive agents depress the irritating, nonproductive cough, and the expectorants liquefy secretions, thus enabling their expulsion when coughing does occur. Although this perhaps seems contradictory, it is not, because antitussives can rarely suppress coughing entirely.

Adequate fluid intake of the patient taking an expectorant is essential unless contraindicated. Other nursing measures, such as turning the patient frequently and encouraging him to take deep breaths and cough, should be used to aid in expulsion of mucous secretions.

GLYCERYL GUAIACOLATE (INCORPORATED IN ROBITUSSIN). Glyceryl guaiacolate increases the flow of secretions from the lining of the respiratory tract, reducing the viscosity of the inflammatory exudate that often lines the tracheobronchial tree during respiratory infections. It is quite effective as an expectorant.

This drug is often used in preparations for tuberculous patients in whom codeine or its derivatives would be undesirable because coughing is desired here. It is effective in productive and nonproductive coughs, especially in instances in which dry, nonproductive coughing has irritated the mucous membrane linings of the air passages.

DOSE. 100 to 200 mg. (1 to 2 teaspoonfuls) orally three or four times daily.

HYDRIODIC ACID, U.S.P., B.P. Hydriodic acid syrup contains 1.4 per cent of hydrogen iodide in a palatable syrup. The iodides are expectorants because the iodide ion is excreted in part by the bronchial glands and tends to liquefy viscous sputum. It is used for the treatment of chronic bronchitis and bronchial asthma.

TOXICITY. Iodides are contraindicated in the treatment of tuberculous patients since they may cause irritant reactions and may even reactivate dormant lesions. The syrup is quite acidic; it should be taken with a straw to preserve tooth enamel. Other side effects are due to the iodine content and include gastrointestinal disturbances, skin lesions, iodism, fever and depression.

DOSE. 5 ml. of 1.4% solution orally three times daily.

POTASSIUM IODIDE, U.S.P. As in hydriodic acid, the iodide in this preparation is excreted by the bronchi, thus increasing and liquefying bronchial secretions. It is often administered to promote coughing by its irritant and nauseant effects in the stomach. It is used quite often in asthmatic children who have trouble expelling sputum.

TOXICITY. Contraindicated in tuberculosis. Symptoms of iodism (burning sensation in the mouth, soreness of gums, increased salivation, coryza and sneezing) and dermatoses are observed when the drug is taken over an extended period of time. The solution should not be used when a brown coloration is noted, because this signifies deterioration or oxidation of the solution.

DOSE. 15 to 20 drops of the saturated solution (SSKI) orally every 2 to 4 hours. It should be diluted in juice because of its unpleasant taste and because of the small volume of the drug.

AMMONIUM CHLORIDE, U.S.P. This acid-forming salt is used as an expectorant because it increases secretions of the bronchi and thus soothes inflamed membranes. It is often incorporated in cough mixtures. When administered over a long period of time, however, systemic acidosis may occur. It has a diuretic effect on the kidneys; however, if kidney damage is present, the systemic acidosis may become a therapeutic problem.

> **TOXICITY.** Acidosis, nausea, vomiting and gastrointestinal irritation. Liquid preparations should be given with a full glass of water to reduce the gastric irritation.
> Contraindicated in renal insufficiency.
>
> **DOSE.** 250 to 500 mg. orally every 2 to 4 hours.

IPECAC SYRUP, U.S.P. Ipecac is prepared from the dried rhizomes and roots of *Cephaëlis* ipecacuanha. The crude extract contains several alkaloids of which emetine is the most widely used for medicinal purposes. Ipecac syrup should not be interchanged with the more potent fluid extract.

When taken orally, ipecac is a nauseant expectorant to stimulate bronchial secretions that soothe the irritated mucous membrane linings of the respiratory tract.

In larger doses the syrup is used as an emetic. The syrup was recently removed from the category of drugs that may be sold by prescription only; it is readily available for use in the home should accidental poisoning of children occur. The syrup, when given orally for this purpose, should always be followed by one-half to one glassful of water, since emesis sometimes does not occur with the small volume of syrup administered.

> **DOSE.** Expectorant—1 to 2 ml. orally three times daily. Emetic—8 to 15 ml. orally in one dose, followed by water.

TERPIN HYDRATE, N.F. Terpin hydrate is quite useful as an expectorant to lessen the abundant sputum produced in chronic lung diseases. It is usually administered as an elixir that has a high alcoholic content, and thus should not be given to patients taking disulfiram. The elixir is supplied both with and without codeine.

> **DOSE.** 5 to 10 ml. of elixir (0.08 to 0.17 Gm.) orally three times daily.

ACETYLCYSTEINE (MUCOMYST). Acetylcysteine is a derivative of the amino acid cysteine, and it is effective in liquefying mucus and DNA (the component of pus that is responsible for its viscosity). It has no action on fibrin or living tissue and does not depolymerize proteins; unlike enzymatic agents, it is of no value in debriding wounds.

When administered by inhalation in a nebulizer or apparatus to assist breathing, acetylcysteine reduces the viscosity of pulmonary secretions, thus facilitating their removal by coughing or postural drainage. The loosened secretions must be removed by coughing, postural drainage or suctioning in some instances. It has also been used following surgery or chest trauma and as an adjunct in the treatment of chronic bronchopulmonary diseases and cystic fibrosis.

Vials of acetylcysteine which have been opened should be refrigerated and not used after 96 hours. The inhalation equipment used should not have metal or rubber on its interior surface, since this drug reacts with these substances.

> **TOXICITY.** Toxic reactions are infrequent, but stomatitis, nausea and occasional rhinorrhea have been reported.
>
> **DOSE.** 3 to 5 ml. of a 10 to 20% solution three or four times daily by inhalation.

TERGEMIST. Tergemist is a mucolytic detergent that contains 0.125 per cent 2-ethylhexyl sulfate sodium (detergent) and 0.1 per cent potassium iodide. Because of its ability to lower surface tension and viscosity of bronchial secretions, it is used as an aerosol adjunct in the treatment of conditions that are characterized by thick, tenacious sputum, such as bronchitis, atelectasis, pulmonary abscess and bronchiectasis. Like acetylcysteine, this compound is not effective in depolymerizing proteinaceous material.

TOXICITY. The iodide component of this product prohibits its use in thyroid dysfunctions except in select cases under the close supervision of a physician. Allergic reactions may develop to both the detergent and the iodide.

DOSE. 3 to 5 ml. by inhalation four times daily for periods of 30 minutes each.

ALEVAIRE. Alevaire, a mucolytic detergent for aerosol administration, contains 0.125 per cent tyloxapol (detergent), 2 per cent sodium bicarbonate and 5 per cent glycerin.

It is indicated for use in the treatment of bronchiectasis, lung abscesses and other infectious disorders accompanied by thick mucous secretions, and following intrathoracic surgery when the coughing mechanism is somewhat compromised. It should be administered undiluted by an aerosol nebulizer that delivers a fine mist without large droplets.

Since the liquid contains no preservative, the unused portion of an opened container should be discarded after two or three days or sooner if the contents become cloudy. Refrigeration delays deterioration of the product.

TOXICITY. Pulmonary edema could occur if too great an amount of moisture is administered too rapidly.

DOSE. May be used for continuous aerosol therapy in a dose not exceeding 500 ml. every 12 to 24 hours.

ADMINISTRATION OF DRUGS BY INHALATION

Certain drugs may be administered by inhalation for local effects on the respiratory tract. These drugs may be given to relieve spasm or constriction of the bronchi or to promote the expulsion of mucus by liquefying or loosening the secretions of the respiratory tract. Although they primarily have a local action and effect, systemic absorption

from the respiratory tract is possible; patients should be observed carefully for systemic effects. For example, Isuprel is given by inhalation for its local effect as a bronchodilator but systemic absorption can occur resulting in a stimulating effect on the heart which can be undesirable in patients with cardiac disease.

Inhalation of drugs is usually accomplished by the use of a hand nebulizer or by the use of an intermittent positive pressure breathing (IPPB) machine which provides greater depth and distribution of the drug into the respiratory tree by providing pressurized flow. The drug is placed into a nebulizer where the flow of air results in aerosol form of the drug.

When an IPPB machine is used, the patient should be in a upright position if possible, in order to reduce the possibility of the air being forced into the stomach. The patient needs to be carefully instructed in using the machine. After oxygen flow has been initiated his lips should be closed tightly around the mouthpiece and he should breathe only through the mouthpiece. It may be necessary to have the patient hold his nose or use a noseclip. If a mask is used, it should be applied firmly over the mouth and nose in order to prevent leakage of air.

The patient should be told to breathe slowly and at his own rate. The patient should be closely observed during the treatment since he may experience nausea, vomiting and dizziness from the effects of increased intrathoracic pressure on the circulatory response of the heart. If a mask is used, the possibility of the patient vomiting presents the danger of aspiration of vomitus into the lungs.

The use of intermittent positive pressure breathing machines without nebulization results in the excessive drying of respiratory tract secretions, which defeats the purpose of the treatment. Therefore, care should be taken that there is a sufficient volume of the drug or prescribed solution to last for the duration of the treatment. The nebulizer should be thoroughly washed and dried after each treatment in order to prevent obstruction of the nebulizer and to reduce the possibility of bacterial growth.

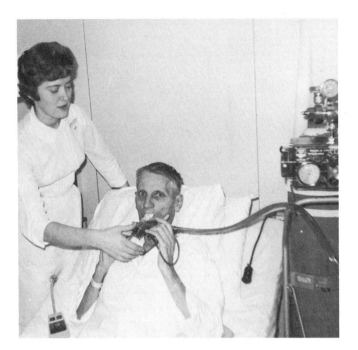

FIGURE 49. Patient receiving medication via an IPPB apparatus.

The settings regulating the pressure to be exerted on inspiration (usually 15 to 20 cm. of water), the sensitivity of the machine and other settings are usually determined by the physician based on the condition of the patient, the purpose of the treatment and the recommendations of the anesthesiologist or inhalation therapist. Depending on the individual institution, these treatments may be done by the nursing staff or by the inhalation therapy department.

Patients should be observed for the effectiveness of the treatment. Such observations would include easier breathing, decreased wheezing and increased production of sputum with productive cough. The nature, amount and odor of the sputum should be noted. Postural drainage may be ordered after these treatments.

ANTIASTHMATIC DRUGS

Bronchial asthma is a chronic, progressive, obstructive lung disease that is characterized by recurrent paroxysms of wheezing and expiratory difficulty due to constriction of the lumen of the smaller respiratory passages.

Although an allergy is often the cause of asthma, emotional factors are highly significant. Attacks may be precipitated, exacerbated or relieved by changes in the emotional environment of susceptible persons.

Most antiasthmatic drugs provide symptomatic relief of attacks by relaxing the smooth muscle of the bronchioles. Sedatives are a useful adjunct to therapy.

EPINEPHRINE INJECTION, U.S.P., B.P. (ADREN-ALIN). This adrenergic hormone is the most effective drug available to combat the acute bronchoconstriction of asthmatic attacks, but it is so potent that it is accompanied by a variety of side effects, and is restricted to use in emergency situation.

The peak effect is observed one half hour after injection, and the duration of action is only one to two hours.

TOXICITY. Epinephrine should be used with caution in patients with severe hypertension, hyperthyroidism or occlusive heart disease because of its cardiac accelerator and vasoconstricting effects.

DOSE. 0.3 to 0.5 ml. of a 1:1000 solution s.c.

THEOPHYLLINE ETHYLENEDIAMINE, U.S.P. (AMINOPHYLLINE). Theophylline, a xanthine alkaloid, is effective but not as powerful as epinephrine in relaxing spasms of the bronchioles. It is useful as a prophylactic oral medication in the treatment of asthma and may be administered in suppository or retention enema form for the treatment of asthmatic attacks. When administered intravenously, a 500 mg. dose should not be given over a shorter period than 20 minutes since serious cardiovascular reactions may be precipitated.

> **TOXICITY.** It may be irritating to the gastrointestinal mucosa on oral administration, producing nausea, vomiting and gastric discomfort. These symptoms are minimized by the use of enteric coated tablets. Headache, palpitation, dizziness and hypotension occur upon rapid intravenous administration.

> **DOSE.** Oral—300 to 600 mg. two or three times daily. Rectal—0.25 to 0.5 Gm. two or three times daily. I.V.—500 mg. over a 20 minute period.

ISOPROTERENOL HYDROCHLORIDE, U.S.P. (ISU-PREL). Isoproterenol effectively relaxes bronchospasm when administered by oral inhalation. It is supplied for this purpose in dosage forms called Mistometers or Medihalers, which deliver measured doses of isoproterenol for deep inhalation.

This drug is not used for prophylactic asthmatic therapy, but it is quite useful in the treatment of acute attacks.

> **TOXICITY.** Increased cardiac output, palpitations, anginal pain, headache, nausea, nervousness, tremor, weakness, sweating and central excitation may occur upon continued use.

> **DOSE.** 0.1 to 0.25 mg./kg. of body weight by oral inhalation as necessary.

EPHEDRINE SULFATE, U.S.P. Ephedrine is a synthetic adrenergic compound that, like epinephrine, relaxes constricted bronchial muscles. It is not as effective as epinephrine for this purpose, but two advantages are that it can be administered orally and it has fewer cardiovascular effects. It does cause central excitation, however.

Ephedrine may be used for routine or prophylactic asthmatic therapy.

> **TOXICITY.** Central stimulation, nervousness, delayed emptying time of the stomach and urinary retention.

> **DOSE.** 25 to 50 mg. orally three times daily.

CORTICOSTEROIDS. The administration of ACTH or hydrocortisone can provide dramatic relief of severe bronchial asthma. Prolonged therapy is reserved for patients who are not responsive to other antiasthmatic drugs, since fluid and electrolyte retention, altered fat deposition and elevated blood sugar levels may occur upon prolonged administration.

SEDATIVES. Sedatives are valuable in allaying the anxiety brought on by asthmatic attacks. Morphine is contraindicated, however, since respiratory depression is definitely to be avoided in chronic obstructive lung disease.

Phenobarbital is quite useful, as are pentobarbital, glutethimide, meprobamate and hydroxyzine.

ANTIHISTAMINES. Antihistamines are generally disappointing in the treatment of asthma, which is remarkable in light of the accepted hypothesis of allergic disorders being the basis for asthmatic attacks. Approximately 30 to 50 per cent of asthmatics are benefited by antihistamine therapy, but invariably these are mild cases that would also respond to almost any asthmatic drug. Antihistamines may be used for prophylactic therapy, but they are of no value in the treatment of acute attacks.

NURSING IMPLICATIONS IN ASTHMATIC ATTACKS

The patient experiencing an asthmatic attack is usually quite anxious; nursing measures should be directed toward alleviating the physical and psychological stress. Patients should be supported in the position providing the greatest ease in breathing.

Usually patients find some relief from dyspnea by sitting upright or bending forward and leaning on an over-the-bed table. Oxygen may be administered if cyanosis is present, but it is given cautiously in order to avoid apnea resulting from suddenly decreasing the carbon dioxide level in patients with chronic lung disease.

Sedation is usually provided, but opiates are usually avoided since they tend to produce bronchial constriction. A quiet environment is essential and it may be necessary to restrict visitors. Reassuring both the patient and family is important.

Measures should be taken after the acute attack to determine the cause of the asthma. Tests for allergens should be done, and the source of the psychological stress, if any, which precipitated the attack should be determined.

QUESTIONS FOR DISCUSSION AND REVIEW

1. Is there a valid medical basis for the use of smelling salts? Why?
2. What is the most dangerous effect of an overdose of morphine? How may this be treated?
3. How do expectorants act? Of what value is this effect in respiratory disorders? What nursing measures may help?
4. Why is epinephrine effective in acute asthmatic attacks? Would any sympathomimetic drug have this effect?
5. Why is it advisable to control anxiety symptoms when an individual is experiencing respiratory distress?
6. Review the principles and techniques of postural drainage.
7. What nursing measures can be used to decrease the coughing of a patient?
8. Visit the inhalation therapy department to become familiar with the types of intermittent positive pressure machines commonly used.
9. What observations should be made while the patient is receiving drugs by inhalation? What observations should be made afterwards?

BIBLIOGRAPHY

Adriani, J.: The use of respiratory stimulants. *Postgrad. Med., 27*:723, 1960.
AMA Drug Evaluations. Chicago, American Medical Association, 1971.
Balagot, R. C. and Bandelin, V. R.: Preoperative and postoperative inhalation therapy. *Surg. Clin. N. Amer., 48*:29–36, (February) 1968.
Bickmerman, H. A.: Clinical pharmacology of antitussive agents. *Clin. Pharmacol. Ther., 3*:353, 1962.
Blaug, S. M. and Karig, A. W.: Oral inhalation aerosols. *Amer. J. Hosp. Pharm., 24*:602, 1967.
Brunner, L. S. et al.: *Textbook of Medical-Surgical Nursing.* 2nd Ed. Philadelphia, J. B. Lippincott Co., 1970.

Caplin, I. and Haynes, J. T.: Complications of aerosol therapy in asthma. *Ann. Allergy, 27*:65, 1969.

Chodosh, S.: Newer drugs in the treatment of chronic bronchitis. *Med. Clin. N. Amer., 51*:1169, 1967.

Comroe, J. H.: *Physiology of Respiration.* Chicago, Year Book Medical Publishers, Inc., 1965.

DeMeyer, J.: Emphysema: effective positive pressure therapy. *R.N., 31*:44, (January) 1968.

Flatter, P.: Hazards of oxygen therapy. *Amer. J. Nurs., 68*:80, 1968.

Goss, C. M. (ed.): *Gray's Anatomy of the Human Body.* 28th Ed. Philadelphia, Lea and Febiger, 1966.

Govoni, L. E. and Hayes, J. E.: *Drugs and Nursing Implications.* 2nd Ed. New York, Appleton-Century-Crofts, 1971.

Graham, J. D. P.: Cough suppressants. *Practitioner, 183*:344, 1959.

Harris, R. L. and Riley, H. D., Jr.: Reactions to aerosol medications in infants and children. *J.A.M.A., 201*:953, 1967.

Johnson, M. E. and Fassett, B. A.: Bronchopulmonary hygiene in cystic fibrosis. *Amer. J. Nurs., 69*:320, (February) 1969.

Keele, C. A. and Neil, E.: *Samson Wright's Applied Physiology.* 11th Ed. London, Oxford University Press, 1965.

Levine, E. P.: Inhalation therapy—aerosols and intermittent positive pressure breathing. *Med. Clin. N. Amer., 51*:307, 1967.

Lovejoy, F. W. and Morrow, P. E.: Aerosols, bronchodilators and mucolytic agents. *Anesthesiology, 23*:460, 1962.

Main, R. J. and Richardson, A. W.: *Physiology.* 2nd Ed. St. Louis, C. V. Mosby Co., 1953.

McArdle, K. H.: The patient and the Bennett. *Nurs. Clin. N. Amer., 1*: 143, (March) 1966.

Pansky, B. and House, E. L.: *Review of Gross Anatomy.* New York, Macmillan Co., 1964.

Rodman, M. J.: The central nervous system stimulants, *R.N., 30*:85, (September) 1967.

Rodman, M. J.: Drugs for relief of asthma. *R.N., 30*:35, (March) 1967.

Rodman, M. J.: Drugs for treating coughs and colds. *R.N., 27*:85, (March) 1964.

Segal, M. S.: The use of therapeutic aerosols, *G.P., 26*:108, (September) 1962.

Siegal, S.: The asthma-suppressive reaction of potassium iodide. *J. of Allergy, 35*:252, 1964.

Stephen, P.: Nebulization under intermittent positive pressure. *Amer. J. Nurs., 57*:1158, (September) 1957.

Symposium on inhalation therapy. *Anesthesiology, 23*:407, 1962.

Vaughn, V. C. III: The place of drug therapy in childhood asthma. *Amer. J. Nurs., 66*:1049, (May) 1966.

Wintrobe, M. M., et al.: *Harrison's Principle of Internal Medicine.* 6th Ed. New York, McGraw-Hill Book Co., 1970.

Youmans, W. B.: *Fundamentals of Human Physiology.* 2nd Ed. Chicago, Year Book Medical Publishers, Inc., 1962.

Chapter 17 Drugs that Affect the Gastrointestinal Tract

Important Concepts Discussed

1. *The process of digestion has many phases and utilizes numerous secretions from the mouth, stomach, pancreas, liver and small intestine.*

2. *Gastrointestinal symptoms are often a valuable diagnostic aid in determining a pathological condition.*

3. *Many gastrointestinal disorders are merely symptoms of various diseases, and drug therapy, to be effective, must be directed toward the causes of the disorder and not merely toward the symptoms themselves.*

4. *Other physiological disorders must often be taken into account when gastrointestinal drugs, such as laxatives, are ordered for a patient.*

The gastrointestinal tract is composed of hollow, tubular structures and associated secretory glands that enable food to be ingested, digested and absorbed into the blood in a form that is readily usable by the body. Optimal digestion and absorption are dependent on many factors: adequate mechanical breakdown of the food particles in the mouth, systematic movement of the food through the tract by peristalsis, secretion of digestive juices and enzymes in the proper amount and in response to the presence of various food components, and an intact gastrointestinal lining that is able to transport the food nutrients across the mucous membrane into the blood.

In the mouth, food is cut and ground by the teeth and, if the eating process is not too rapid, the food is thoroughly mixed with saliva. In man, the salivary glands (parotid, sublingual and submaxillary) secrete 1 to 2 liters of saliva daily. Saliva, a mixture of water, mucin and the enzyme ptyalin, softens food particles and enables them to be tasted, protects and lubricates the structures and membranes of the mouth and begins the digestion of carbohydrates. This phase of the digestive process is very important, and discomfort or even pain may be experienced when inadequately chewed food is swallowed.

In the stomach, secretory glands produce hydrochloric acid, mucin and the digestive enzymes rennin, pepsin and lipase. Rennin produces a flocculent mass (curd) and a watery fluid (whey) from milk. Pepsin, the enzyme that breaks down proteins, depends greatly on the hydrochloric acid secretion to

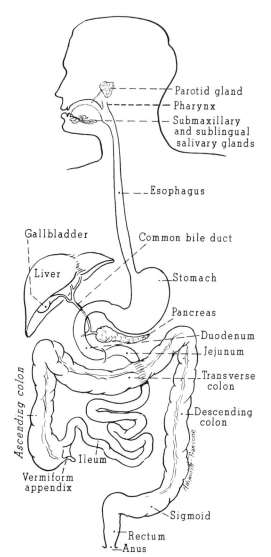

FIGURE 50. Diagram of the gastrointestinal tract. (Jacob and Francone: *Structure and Function in Man.* Ed. 2. W. B. Saunders Co., Philadelphia, 1970).

provide an acid medium. In achlorhydria, the action of pepsin may be minimal or absent. Lipase is present in small amounts in the gastric secretion, but the digestion of fats largely depends upon pancreatic enzymes, which are secreted into the duodenum. In addition to providing an acid medium for the action of pepsin, hydrochloric acid also kills or inhibits many microorganisms that find their way into the stomach via food or other ingested materials. Mucin is largely responsible for protecting the gastric mucosa

from the eroding and digesting effects of the acid and enzymes in the stomach.

Additional enzymes are secreted by the cells of the intestinal mucosa: erepsin, which converts peptones to amino acids; enterokinase, which converts the inactive pancreatic trypsinogen into active trypsin; invertase, which changes sucrose to glucose and fructose; maltase, which splits maltose into two glucose molecules; lactase, which splits lactose into glucose and galactose; and lipase, which breaks down lipids. When the acidified food particles reach the intestine, stimulation of the intestinal mucosa causes release of two hormones, secretin and pancreozymin, which are carried by the blood to the pancreas and stimulate release of pancreatic juices.

Stimulation of the pancreas causes the following enzymes to be released into the intestinal tract: amylase, which converts starch to maltose; maltase, which converts maltose to glucose; steapsin, which hydrolyzes triglyceride fats into fatty acids and glycerin; trypsin, which splits proteins into amino acids (following its activation by enterokinase); chymotrypsin, which also digests protein (following its conversion from inactive chymotrypsinogen by trypsin); and carboxypeptidase, which aids in the digestion of protein by splitting terminal amino acids from the amino acid chains.

The sodium bicarbonate secreted by the pancreas neutralizes the partially digested acidic food as it enters the intestine, but perhaps more importantly, it provides an optimal pH for steapsin, which cannot act effectively in an acid medium. The pH in various portions of the gastrointestinal tract varies greatly from individual to individual. Many enteric-coated tablets depend on the alkalinity of the small intestine for the coatings to be dissolved. Because of the possible range of pH, however, the tablets may pass through the entire tract without being dissolved.

Secretions from the bile duct are also liberated into the intestine following the ingestion of fatty foods. Fats in contact with the mucosa of the duodenum cause the release of another hormone, cholecystokinin, which is carried in the blood and causes contraction of the gallbladder. The bile salts emulsify or break fat droplets into small particles, called micelles, which may readily be attacked and broken down by lipase. Obstruction of the bile duct by stones or strictures greatly interferes with the digestion of fats, and it is the cause of much discomfort and flatus following the ingestion of fatty foods.

DRUGS THAT AFFECT THE MOUTH

GARGLES AND MOUTHWASHES. These liquids, sometimes called collutoria, are pleasantly flavored, aromatic, aqueous or hydroalcoholic solutions intended to exert an antiseptic, deodorant or astringent effect in the oral cavity. These solutions are often highly overrated in advertisements, however; they are usually only weakly medicated and cannot be depended upon to correct bad breath, heal mouth lesions, cure sore throats or perform the many other health-preserving effects for which they are promoted. Malodorous breath may be caused by decaying teeth, poor oral hygiene, pyorrhea or infected tonsils; mouth lesions or canker sores may be caused by various internal conditions or infectious processes. Although a sore throat may be caused by smoke inhalation or excessive shouting, it is more often produced by infectious processes over which the weakly antiseptic mouthwashes have no curative powers. In short, these agents should be employed for their refreshing properties as an adjunct to, but not as a replacement for, proper oral hygiene and dental care.

Alkaline solutions, such as compound sodium borate solution (Dobell's solution), and alkaline aromatic solutions have a solvent action on mucous and saliva and are usually less astringent than other types. Astringent mouthwashes precipitate the surface protein of the oral mucous membranes, thus giving the tingling or refreshing feeling. Ferric chloride and tannic acid are often employed as astringent ingredients.

Perborates, potassium chlorate and hydrogen peroxide liberate oxygen; thus they are weakly antiseptic. Phenolic compounds, such as menthol, thymol, cresol and chloramine-T, are also incorporated for antiseptic purposes. Antibiotic and other chemotherapeutic agents may occasionally be used as mouthwashes and gargles. Nystatin suspension or gentian violet solution is often swabbed in the oral cavity to treat fungal infections such as thrush. In this case the mouthwash is therapeutic because topical application is a very effective method of combating fungal infections in the mouth.

HEMOSTATS, ASTRINGENTS AND STYPTICS. Astringents may be applied in the mouth to arrest capillary bleeding or to precipitate surface protein. These agents, such as epinephrine, aluminum compounds, iron preparations, tannic acid and zinc chloride, may be used in the practice of dentistry or medicine to relieve oral irritation or bleeding. They are ordinarily not for self-treatment.

PREPARATION FOR HYPERSENSITIVE DENTIN. Dentin, which may be exposed on the tooth surface following gum retraction, is often highly sensitive to temperature changes and food. Dentists may paint substances, such as ammoniacal silver nitrate solution, formalin or liquefied phenol, on the tooth for relief of the pain.

DENTURE ADHESIVES. Denture adhesives are composed of carbohydrate gums, such as karaya, tragacanth or acacia. They are of limited benefit in preventing the slipping of dentures, and they are of little or no value if the problem is due to ill-fitting plates.

DRUGS THAT AFFECT THE STOMACH

Many drugs may be taken by mouth for their effects on the stomach and digestion. Some agents, such as digestants, are intended for replacement therapy, whereas others, such as antacids, emetics and antiemetics, modify, alter or improve gastric function and the milieu of the gastrointestinal tract.

PEPTIC ULCER

Peptic ulcers may be located in either the stomach or the duodenum. Although duodenal ulcers occur most commonly when there is excessive secretion of gastric hydrochloric acid, gastric ulcers often occur in individuals with normal or even decreased gastric acidity. It has been postulated that gastric ulcers occur, not because of increased stomach acidity, but because of a decrease in the amount or protective ability of mucin. In addition, gastric ulcers often undergo malignant degeneration, whereas this is uncommon with duodenal ulcers. Stress may precede the formation of duodenal ulcers, whereas gastric ulcers are more common in individuals who habitually eat rough or excessively spicy foods.

Antacid therapy is used in the treatment of ulcers. Although healing of the ulcerations as shown by X-ray examination is not appreciably more rapid when antacids are administered, their protective qualities nevertheless contribute greatly to the relief of pain and discomfort during the healing process. Surgical intervention is often necessary if noticeable healing of the ulcer does not occur in a short period of time, in the case of gastric ulcers, because malignant degeneration may be the reason for the slowness or lack of healing.

ANTACIDS

Antacids are substances that react with hydrochloric acid to decrease the acidity of the gastric secretions. Antacids used in therapy may be divided into two classes: systemic antacids, which are absorbed and affect the acid-base mechanisms of the body, and nonsystemic antacids, which because of their insolubility are not absorbed and influence only the acidity within the gastrointestinal tract.

Some antacids tend to cause constipation, whereas others may cause diarrhea. The nurse should check the patient's bowel habits regularly so that these side effects may be detected early and treated. The absorption of certain drugs, such as antibiotics and coumarin anticoagulants, may be impeded by the concurrent administration of antacids.

In the early stages of treatment of a pep-

tic ulcer or after gastric bleeding, antacids may be ordered to be given alternately with milk every 30 minutes. Antacids may be left at the bedside for frequent self-administration by the patient if he is capable of doing so. Antacids may also be diluted and given via a nasogastric tube. If antacids are in liquid form, sufficient water must be given along with them to insure their passage into the stomach.

SODIUM BICARBONATE, U.S.P., B.P. (BAKING SODA). Sodium bicarbonate is a readily accessible and common home remedy for gastric hyperacidity, upset stomach and heartburn. It is greatly overused, however, and continued administration may have many undesirable effects. Because sodium bicarbonate is very soluble in water, it rapidly neutralizes all the free acid in the stomach. Frequently the body employs its defense mechanism, an "acid rebound," whereby an even larger amount of acid is secreted following the rapid neutralization and alkalination of the stomach. For this reason, considerable distress is often experienced shortly after taking sodium bicarbonate. To treat this, another dose is often self-prescribed, and the cycle is repeated.

If excessive sodium bicarbonate is ingested, it passes into the intestine and is absorbed. Serious systemic alkalosis may be produced and results in renal stress as the body attempts to regain a stable acid-base balance in body fluids by excretion of large amounts of sodium bicarbonate in the urine. Renal failure may occur if the disturbance is prolonged. Another disadvantage is the production of gas in the stomach as a result of the neutralization reaction:

$$HCl + NaHCO_3 \longrightarrow NaCl + H_2O + CO_2\uparrow$$

The carbon dioxide thus produced causes uncomfortable distention of the stomach, and the pressure may be sufficient to perforate a gastric ulcer, resulting in severe and even fatal complications.

TOXICITY. Alkalosis, gas formation and impairment of pepsin's activity.

DOSE. 2 Gm. orally three times daily.

NONSYSTEMIC ANTACIDS

ALUMINUM HYDROXIDE GEL, U.S.P., B.P. (CREAMALIN, AMPHOJEL). Aluminum hydroxide gel, formed when dry aluminum oxide is added to water, is a colloidal suspension that may be flavored with peppermint, sucrose, saccharin or similar substances. Because of its insolubility in water, it adheres to the surface mucosa of the stomach and coats and protects irritated mucosa and ulcers. The aluminum chloride formed upon reaction of aluminum hydroxide and hydrochloric acid is an astringent, again protecting denuded mucosa. In contrast to sodium bicarbonate, which effects almost instant neutralization of the acid, aluminum hydroxide requires 5 to 15 minutes for this action. Because of the slower rate of neutralization and the slower emptying rate associated with use of this antacid, there is no acid rebound. The discomfort of distention is also eliminated, since no gas is formed as a result of the neutralization process. It is practically inabsorbable from the gastrointestinal tract; there is therefore, no interference with systemic acid-base balance.

Aluminum hydroxide gel is employed almost exclusively in the treatment of peptic ulcer and may be alternated hourly with small amounts of milk or cream.

TOXICITY. Constipation and even bowel impaction may occur when large amounts of insoluble aluminum hydroxide are present in the lower gastrointestinal tract. The aluminum ion interferes with the enzymatic action of pepsin and with the absorption of phosphates from the gastrointestinal tract.

DOSE. 8 ml. orally every 2 to 4 hours.

MAGNESIUM TRISILICATE, U.S.P., B.P. (INCORPORATED IN GELUSIL, TRI-CREAMALATE). Magnesium trisilicate, a white, insoluble powder that forms a gelatinous suspension in water adsorbs and neutralizes gastric hydrochloric acid. The gelatinous consistency of the suspension causes it to adhere closely to the surface of ulcers. No gas formation accompanies neutralization, and because of its insolubility, there is no interference with systemic acid-base balance.

TOXICITY. When magnesium salts are administered alone they produce diarrhea. This antacid is therefore often commercially combined with aluminum hydroxide gel to produce an effective and efficient antacid combination that is marketed as Gelusil and Tri-Creamalate.

DOSE. 1 Gm. orally four times daily. Tablets should be chewed and taken with water.

PRECIPITATED CALCIUM CARBONATE, U.S.P., B.P. (PRECIPITATED CHALK). Precipitated calcium carbonate is an insoluble, tasteless white powder of fine particle size that may be stirred into liquid immediately before administration. The obvious advantage of this form of administration is the convenience and ready accessibility of the powders when medication must be taken many times throughout the day.

Calcium carbonate may be incorporated in commercial preparations with other antacids, such as magnesium carbonate, magnesium trisilicate or aluminum hydroxide. Marblen liquid, an example of such a combination, consists of calcium carbonate, magnesium carbonate, magnesium trisilicate, magnesium phosphate and aluminum hydroxide. Although there is no advantage to this particular combination of antacids, this preparation is available in peach and apricot flavors and is often a welcome change from the standard peppermint flavor of most commercial antacid preparations.

TOXICITY. Calcium preparations should be administered with caution to patients with kidney disorders, since inefficient excretion of even the small amounts of calcium absorbed may elevate the blood calcium level. They should not be administered to patients with hyperparathyroidism. Absorbed calcium salts may increase the production of gastric hydrochloric acid, thus defeating their own purposes in some instances.

DOSE. 1 Gm. orally four times daily.

MAGNESIUM OXIDE, U.S.P., B.P. Magnesium oxide, like calcium carbonate, is an antacid that is available in powdered dosage forms. When magnesium oxide is placed in water, magnesium hydroxide is formed, and this colloidal suspension (milk of magnesia) may also be administered as an antacid.

> **TOXICITY.** Continued use causes diarrhea.

> **DOSE.** 250 mg. orally three or four times daily.

DIHYDROXYALUMINUM AMINOACETATE (ALZINOX, ROBALATE). This aluminum salt of the amino acid glycine is slightly soluble in water, but its hydroxylated form readily forms a colloidal gel. It is an effective antacid and protective agent for irritated or ulcerated gastric mucosa. It is used principally in the treatment of peptic ulcer.

> **TOXICITY.** Constipation may occur upon prolonged or frequent use. It may be necessary to alternate this antacid and a magnesium salt to maintain satisfactory bowel elimination.

> **DOSE.** 0.5 to 1 Gm. orally after meals and at bedtime.

MAGALDRATE (HYDRATED MAGNESIUM ALUMINATE, RIOPAN). This chemical combination of magnesium and aluminum hydroxides is an effective antacid that is used primarily in the treatment of peptic ulcer.

> **TOXICITY.** Mild constipation.

> **DOSE.** 800 mg. orally four times daily, between meals and at bedtime.

DIGESTANTS

Digestants are drugs or combinations of drugs that replace deficient enzymes or digestive juices in the gastrointestinal tract. These drugs are of limited usefulness, because it is difficult to obtain the proper concentration of enzymes and other digestive secretions in the proper areas of the tract. These compounds are occasionally prescribed as placebo medications.

HYDROCHLORIC ACID DILUTED, N.F.; DILUTE HYDROCHLORIC ACID, B.P. A deficiency or absence of gastric hydrochloric acid may result from many conditions, such as inadequate secretion of the acid, excessive secretion of mucus, which neutralizes the acid, regurgitation of alkaline intestinal substances, pernicious anemia and carcinoma of the stomach.

Hypochlorhydria is a deficient secretion of hydrochloric acid in the stomach. *Achlorhydria*, an absence of hydrochloric acid secretion, occurs typically in pernicious anemia and carcinoma of the stomach, occasionally in infectious conditions, renal diseases and diabetes and, rarely, in otherwise healthy individuals. Hydrochloric acid has been given orally in the past in an attempt to correct these two conditions; however, it is almost impossible to administer the acid in quantities sufficient to produce the necessary acidity in the stomach to effect this end.

The acid is taken diluted in water, and a glass straw placed in back of the teeth is used to protect dental enamel.

> **DOSE.** 4 to 8 ml. (of the dilute acid) orally three times daily with meals.

GLUTAMIC ACID HYDROCHLORIDE, N.F. (ACIDULIN). Glutamic acid hydrochloride is the result of chemical combination of hydrochloric acid with glutamic acid. The resultant compound is a dry powder that can easily be dispensed in capsule form, which is usually more convenient and agreeable to the patient. Upon dissolution of the capsule in the stomach, free hydrochloric acid is released.

This preparation is used in the treatment of achlorhydria and hypochlorhydria, but each capsule (340 mg. glutamic acid hydrochloride) releases the equivalent of only 10 minims of dilute hydrochloric acid, which makes it less beneficial than the liquid form.

> **TOXICITY.** Systemic acidosis if the drug is given in excessive amounts or in the presence of renal failure.

> **DOSE.** 1 to 3 capsules orally three times daily with meals.

TABLE 13 Examples of Over-the-Counter Antacids†

Product	Dosage form	Manu-facturer	Sodium bicar-bonate	Calcium car-bonate	Aluminum hydroxide	Magne-sium oxide or hydroxide	Magne-sium tri-silicate	Dihydroxy-aluminum amino-acetate	Other ingredients	So-dium[a]
Alglyn	tablet or magma	Brayten	—	—	—	—	—	0.5 Gm/tab 0.25 Gm/5 cc	—	—
Alka Seltzer	tablet	Miles	—	—	—	—	—	—	aspirin* calcium phosphate citric acid	—
Alkets	tablet	Upjohn	—	0.8 Gm (12 gr)	—	0.065 Gm (1 gr)	—	—	mag. carb. 0.13 Gm (2 gr)	—
Aludrox	tablet and suspen-sion	Wyeth	—	—	0.5 Gm/tab 0.5 Gm/5cc	***	—	—	—	13.5 mg/15 cc
Alzinox	tablet and magma	Smith, Miller and Patch	—	—	—	—	—	0.5 Gm/tab or 5 cc	—	—
Amitone	tablet	Norex	—	*	—	—	—	—	glycine* mint flavor	—
Amphojel	tablet and suspen-sion	Wyeth	—	—	0.32 Gm/tab; 0.60 Gm/tab	—	—	—	—	24.6 mg/15 cc
A.M.T.	tablet and suspen-sion	—	—	—	0.15 Gm/tab	—	0.25 Gm/tab 0.65 Gm/5 cc	—		25.5 mg/15 cc
Andercid	tablet	Ander-son	—	0.5 Gm/tab	—	—	0.5 Gm/tab	—	—	—
Bellans	tablet	Bell & Co.	4.08 gr	—	—	—	—	—	willow charcoal 0.06 gr Gingerine 0.005 minim	—
BiSoDol	tablet and powder	White-hall	—	*	—	*	*	—	peppermint	471 mg/3 Gm of pow-der
Calcium Carbonate & Soda	tablet	Lilly	1.95 Gm	—	—	—	—	—	—	—
Caltase	tablet	Parke, Davis	—	0.66 Gm (10 gr)	—	—	—	—	pepsin 1 gr takadiastase 1/2 gr	—
Chooz	mint	Phar-maco	—	*	—	—	*	—	peppermint oil	—
Creamalin	capsule tablet and magma	Win-throp	—	—	0.32 Gm/tab or /5 cc	—	0.75 Gm/tab or 5 /cc	—	mint flavored magma	9 mg/15 cc
Cremo Carbonates	magma	Merck Sharp and Dohme	—	0.1 Gm/5 cc	—	—	—	—	chloroform 10 mg bis. subcarb. 0.2 Gm mag. carb. 0.2 Gm	—
Dicarbosil	tablet	Arch	—	0.489 Gm	—	—	0.006 Gm	—	mag. carb. 0.011 Gm oil of pepper-mint	2.7 mg/tab
Di-Gel	tablet	Plough	—	—	*	*	—	—	mag. carb.* methyl poly-siloxane 25 mg	—
Gelusil	liquid and tablet	Warner-Chilcott	—	—	0.25 Gm/tab or /5 cc	—	0.5 Gm/tab or /5 cc	—	mint flavor	19.5 mg or /15 cc
Gelusil-Lac	powder	Warner-Chilcott	—	—	1 Gm/pack	—	2 Gm/pack	—	high protein, low fat milk solids	6.5 mg/15 cc pack
Krem	tablet	Neisler	—	0.4 Gm	—	—	—	—	mag. carb. 0.2 Gm cream & milk powder 0.5 Gm mint or cherry flavor	—

* Quantitative statement not provided.
*** Amounts in one teaspoonful or one tablet equivalent to 1/4 teaspoonful milk of magnesia.
(a) Amounts determined from the literature; if amounts are not given, it does not necessarily mean that sodium content is absent.

† From Penna, Darlington, and Chalmers: *Handbook of Non-Prescription Drugs.* Washington, D.C., American Pharmaceutical Association, 1968, p. 10.

Table 13 *continued on opposite page.*

TABLE 13 Examples of Over-the-Counter Antacids (*Continued*)

Product	Dosage form	Manu-facturer	Sodium bicar-bonate	Calcium car-bonate	Aluminum hydroxide	Magne-sium oxide or hydroxide	Magne-sium tri-silicate	Dihydroxy-aluminum amino-acetate	Other ingredients	So-dium(a)
Maalox	suspen-sion	Rorer	—	—	*	*	—	—	—	—
Maalox #1	tablet	Rorer	—	—	†	†	—	—	—	14 mg/15 cc
Maalox #2	tablet	Rorer	—	—	**	**	—	—	—	28 mg/15 cc
Malcogel	suspen-sion	Upjohn	—	—	0.33 Gm/5 cc	—	0.66 Gm/5 cc	—	—	—
Milk of Trinesium	suspen-sion	Abbott	—	—	0.108 Gm/5 cc	—	0.65 Gm/5 cc	—	—	18 mg/15 cc
Mucotin	tablet	Warner-Chilcott	—	—	0.25 Gm	0.65 Gm	0.45 Gm	—	gastric mucin 0.065 Gm	—
Mylanta	tablet and liquid	Stuart	—	—	0.2 Gm	0.2 Gm	—	—	simethicone 20 mg	75 mg/15 cc
Phosphaljel	suspen-sion	Wyeth	—	—	—	—	—	—	aluminum phosphate gel (4% est.)	39 mg/15 cc
Riopan	tablet or suspen-sion	Ayerst	—	—	—	—	—	—	hydrated magnesium aluminate 0.4 Gm/tab or /5 cc	2.1 mg/15 cc
Rolaids	tablet	Amer. Chicle	—	—	—	—	—	—	dihydroxy aluminum sodium carbonate 330 mg	53 mg/tab
Robalate	tablet and suspen-sion	Robins	—	—	—	—	—	0.5 Gm/tab or /5 cc	—	28 mg/15 cc
Soda Mint	tablet	Lilly	0.33 Gm	—	—	—	—	—	oil of peppermint	44 mg/tab
Syntrogel	tablet	Sauter	—	0.071 Gm	0.144 Gm	—	—	—	mag. peroxide 0.086 Gm	—
Titralac	tablet and suspen-sion	Riker	—	0.42 Gm/tab 1 Gm/5 cc	—	—	—	—	glycine 0.18 Gm /tab 0.3 Gm/5 cc	37 mg/15 cc
Trangest	tablet	Colfax	—	0.050 Gm/tab	0.125 Gm	0.125 Gm	—	—	scopolamine aminoxide 0.05 mg chlorpheni-ramine maleate 1 mg caffeine 7.5 mg amylase	—
Trevidal	tablet and suspen-sion	Organon	—	0.105 Gm/tab or /5 cc	0.09 Gm/tab or /5 cc	—	0.15 Gm/tab or /5 cc	—	protein binder from oat cyamopsis tetragono-laba gum	5 mg/15 cc
Tricreama-late	tablet and suspen-sion	Winthrop	—	—	0.3 Gm/5 cc 0.324/tab	—	0.6 Gm/5 cc 0.162/tab	—	—	123mg/15 cc
Trisogel	capsule	Lilly	—	—	0.1 Gm (1 1/2 gr)	—	0.3 Gm (4 1/2 gr)	—	—	48 mg/15 cc (in suspen-sion)
Trisomin	tablet	Lilly	—	—	—	—	0.5 Gm	—	—	—
Tums	tablet	Lewis-Howe	—	—	*	—	*	—	mag. carb. oil of peppermint	2.7 mg/tab
Wingel	tablet and liquid	Winthrop	—	—	††	††	—	—	—	16 mg/65 cc

* Quantitative statement not provided.
† Amounts listed as 0.4 Gm combined hydroxides of magnesium and aluminum. Individual concentrations are not listed.
** Amounts listed as 0.8 Gm combined hydroxides of magnesium and aluminum. Individual concentrations are not listed.
†† Amounts listed as 410 mg combined hydroxides of magnesium and aluminum, per tablet or /5 cc liquid. Manufacturer states 20% of each ingredient.
(a) Amounts determined from the literature; if amounts are not given, it does not necessarily mean that sodium content is absent.

MALT SOUP EXTRACT (MALTSUPEX). Malt soup extract, prepared from germinated barley, is a mixture of dextrin, amolytic enzymes, maltose and glucose, the products of the hydrolysis of malt. It increases peristalsis and growth of intestinal flora and is used as a mild laxative. It may be taken prophylactically for this purpose to keep stools soft.

DOSE. 30 ml. orally two or three times daily.

ELIXIR OF LACTATED PEPSIN, N.F. The pepsin component of this digestant elixir is obtained from the glandular layer of the hog's stomach. The lactate component renders the compound slightly acidic to maintain activity of the enzyme. It is of palliative benefit only as a digestant, but it is often used as a pleasant-tasting vehicle for other drugs administered in liquid form, such as antispasmodics.

DOSE. 8 ml. orally three times daily.

PANCREATIN, N.F., B.P. (PANTERIC GRANULES, VIOKASE). Pancreatin is prepared commercially from the whole pancreas of hogs and oxen. It contains amylase, lipase, trypsin, esterases, nucleases and elastase. A dose of pancreatin can lyse 25 times its own weight of starch and casein into absorbable carbohydrates and proteoses.

Pancreatin is used for replacement therapy for pancreatic insufficiency in conditions such as pancreatitis and the malabsorption syndromes, after gastrectomy and in the treatment of cystic fibrosis.

DOSE. 500 mg. orally three times daily with meals.

PANCRELIPASE (COTAZYM). Pancrelipase is a standardized pancreatic replacement, which is obtained from hog pancreas. On a weight to weight basis it has 12 times the lipolytic activity and four times the trypsin and amylase content of pancreatin.

It is used for replacement therapy in pancreatic insufficiency and unrelated functional digestive disorders.

Because of the increased potency, pancrelipase can be dispensed in capsule form, which is considerably more convenient than the bulk powder form of pancreatin.

DOSE. 900 mg. orally with each meal and 300 mg. with each snack.

OX BILE EXTRACT, N.F. Ox bile extract that is used commercially is an alcoholic extract of ox bile. It is used for replacement therapy when there is an absence or deficiency of natural bile in the intestine, and it is an adjunct to fat digestion. When absorbed, the bile acids increase secretion of natural bile.

TOXICITY. Ox bile should be used with caution in patients with obstructive jaundice since toxic levels of the bile acids may result when the additional bile salts are added to the already elevated level in the blood. The dose should be decreased if symptoms of loose stools and cramps occur.

DOSE. 300 mg. orally three times daily after meals.

DEHYDROCHOLIC ACID, N.F. (DECHOLIN). Dehydrocholic acid, one of the constituents of natural bile, may be administered orally to replace natural bile acids and to increase the flow of bile in conditions such as biliary stasis or dyskinesia. It may be used following surgery on the biliary tract and as an adjunct in the treatment of cholecystitis and cholangitis. Its use as a diagnostic agent is discussed in Chapter 23.

TOXICITY. This compound is contraindicated in complete biliary obstruction or jaundice because of possible increased and toxic levels of bile salts in the blood.

DOSE. 250 to 500 mg. orally three times daily after meals.

KETOCHOLANIC ACIDS (KETOCHOL). This preparation is a combination of four natural bile acids: cholic, desoxycholic, chenodesoxycholic and lithocholic. It is used to promote the production and flow of natural bile and as replacement therapy in biliary obstruction, cholecystitis and cholangitis.

TOXICITY. Contraindicated in jaundice and complete obstruction of the bile duct.

DOSE. 250 to 500 mg. orally three times daily with meals.

FLORANTYRONE (ZANCHOL). Florantyrone, a synthetic cholerectic, is at least as effective as dehydrocholic acid. It is used both for replacement therapy and to increase the flow of natural bile in stasis and inflammatory conditions.

TOXICITY. Contraindicated in jaundice and total biliary obstruction.

DOSE. 250 mg. orally three or four times daily with or immediately after meals.

TOCAMPHYL (GALLOGEN, SYNCUMA). The curcuma plant has been used for many years by the natives of the Dutch East Indies for the treatment of digestive problems. The active component of this plant is now synthesized commercially as tocamphyl. It is not a bile salt, but it acts directly on the liver to stimulate the secretion of natural bile.

Tocamphyl may be used in functional disturbances of the liver and biliary tract and is a useful adjunct to therapy in the treatment of chronic cholecystitis, cholelithiasis and following cholecystectomy.

TOXICITY. Contraindicated in jaundice and complete biliary obstruction.

DOSE. 75 mg. orally three times daily.

EMETICS

Emetics are drugs that induce vomiting either by irritating the stomach mucous membranes or by stimulating the vomiting center. Various emetics, such as tepid water, warm salt water, mustard in lukewarm water or a mild soapsuds solution, may be used in the home.

Emetics should never be administered following the ingestion of petroleum products, such as gasoline or turpentine, or corrosives, such as lye or strong acids, since more damage would be caused by their repeated contact with the esophagus.

APOMORPHINE HYDROCHLORIDE, N.F., B.P. For many years apomorphine was subject to the federal narcotic laws because it is pre-

pared synthetically from morphine and retains many of the addicting properties of the parent compound. The addicting potentiality of this compound is largely theoretical, however, since the vomiting produced by the central stimulation of the vomiting center largely eliminates this drug from the addict's list of preferences.

Apomorphine is of little value when administered orally, but it may produce vomiting within 10 or 15 minutes following subcutaneous injection.

TOXICITY. Central depression occurs with this drug; it should not be used in the presence of shock or when the patient is under the influence of other central depressants, such as barbiturates, opiates or alcohol, since an additive effect occurs. For the same reason, repeated doses of this compound should not be administered if vomiting does not occur with the first dose. Levallorphan or nalorphine should be available as antidotes.

DOSE. 5 to 10 mg. subcutaneously.

apomorphine hydrochloride

IPECAC SYRUP, U.S.P. The active ingredient of ipecac syrup, emetine, is a potent emetic that causes vomiting within 30 to 60 minutes following oral administration. A glass of water should always be given following the administration of the syrup to hasten dissolution of the emetine.

Ipecac syrup may also be employed as a nauseant expectorant in the treatment of asthma and chronic bronchitis because of the forceful vomiting contractions and regurgitant effects it has on the secretions of the bronchial tree.

Ipecac syrup should not be confused with fluid extract of Ipecac.

DOSE. 8 to 15 ml. orally as an emetic. 1 to 2 ml. orally as an expectorant.

CUPRIC SULFATE, U.S.P., B.P. Copper sulfate, although it has fallen into disuse, rapidly induces emesis before extensive or serious irritation of the gastric mucosa occurs. If vomiting does not occur, however, this substance must be removed by gastric lavage.

Cupric sulfate is useful in the treatment of phosphorus toxicity, since metallic copper is precipitated in preference to the unabsorbed phosphorus, thus preventing its entry into the blood.

TOXICITY. Excessive gastric irritation and copper toxicity if absorbed.

DOSE. 250 to 500 mg. orally in 100 ml. warm water.

BLACK MUSTARD, N.F. (BROWN MUSTARD). The seed of the black mustard plant, *Brassica nigra,* produces vomiting because of its irritant volatile oil, allyl isothiocyanate. It is a rapidly acting, although quite unpleasant emetic that can be quite irritating to the gastric mucous membrane.

Black mustard is still employed occasionally as a rubefacient mustard plaster, a home remedy of questionable value for respiratory infections. When applied locally to the chest, it does provide palliative relief of deeper pain and discomfort by creating a sensation of warmth on the skin. If applied for prolonged periods, serious irritation and even blistering of the skin may occur.

DOSE. 10 Gm. orally in a glass of tepid water.

ANTIEMETICS

Antiemetics, or antinauseants, are agents to relieve nausea and vomiting. They may exert this effect via local relief of intestinal hypermotility, by central action on the medullary vomiting center, or by mild sedation when nausea is produced by emotional disorders. Oral forms of these drugs must be given before vomiting occurs since it is likely that, after vomiting has started, they will not be absorbed before they are vomited. Parenteral routes of appropriate medication are usually necessary once vomiting has begun.

Hot tea, carbonated drinks or undiluted Coca-Cola syrup in cracked ice are readily available home remedies for nausea. Sodium bicarbonate and other alkalizers, such as Bromo-Seltzer or Alka-Seltzer, may be used, but they may have serious systemic effects if used inordinately. More potent antinauseants may be obtained only with a prescription. Antinauseants should be used very cautiously for morning sickness of early pregnancy because of the possible effects on the fetus.

PHENOTHIAZINES. Phenothiazines, e.g., chlorpromazine, prochlorperazine and trifluoperazine, may be prescribed for the relief of severe nausea and vomiting. In addition to providing a tranquilizing effect on the central nervous system, these agents also effectively depress the vomiting center in the medulla. The side effects of these compounds prohibit their continued use as antinauseants, but they are often the agents of choice in the treatment of postsurgical vomiting or following the administration of nausea-producing pharmacologic agents such as the antineoplastic drugs.

PIPAMAZINE (MORNIDINE). Although pipamazine is a phenothiazine derivative, it produces few if any tranquilizing effects in recommended therapeutic doses. It has been prescribed for the relief of nausea and vomiting in early pregnancy, but publicity regarding the possible teratogenic effects of many drugs during the early months of pregnancy has decreased its use considerably.

TOXICITY. Drowsiness is observed following administration, particularly in large doses.

DOSE. 5 mg. orally every 4 to 6 hours.

THIETHYLPERAZINE MALEATE (TORECAN). Also a phenothiazine derivative, this agent is effective in the control of nausea and vomiting because of its action on both the cerebral chemoreceptor trigger zone and the vomiting center.

It is available in oral, injectable and suppository forms for the treatment of postoperative nausea, following radiation therapy and treatment with antineoplastic drugs and for the nausea and vomiting associated with middle ear disturbances.

TOXICITY. Contraindicated in pregnancy. Drowsiness, dryness of the oral and nasal mucous membranes, depression, restlessness, hypotension and extrapyramidal effects have been observed.

DOSE. 10 mg. orally, rectally or I.M. (usually used as the initial dose only) one to three times daily.

TRIMETHOBENZAMIDE HYDROCHLORIDE, N.F. (TIGAN). Although this agent is chemically closely related to the antihistamines, its pharmacologic properties resemble those of the phenothiazines. Like the phenothiazines, trimethobenzamide acts via the chemoreceptor trigger zone and the vomiting center to decrease nausea and vomiting.

It is cautiously recommended for use during pregnancy to control nausea and vomiting, and it may be used to treat the nausea and vomiting associated with radiation therapy, antineoplastic drugs, middle ear infections and nonspecific gastritis.

TOXICITY. Drowsiness and allergic reactions have been observed.

DOSE. 100 to 250 mg. orally, I.M. or rectally one to four times daily.

DIMENHYDRINATE, U.S.P., B.P. (DRAMAMINE). Dimenhydrinate, already discussed under the antihistamines, relieves motion sickness and controls the nausea, vomiting and vertigo associated with other conditions, such as radiation sickness, hypertension, electroshock therapy and mild emotional disorders.

TOXICITY. Drowsiness.

DOSE. 50 mg. orally 30 minutes before departure (for motion sickness). 50 mg. orally, rectally or I.M. one to three times daily for control of other conditions associated with nausea and vomiting.

dimenhydrinate

MECLIZINE HYDROCHLORIDE, U.S.P. (BONINE). Meclizine is similar to dimenhydrinate in action and effects. It is cautiously recommended for control of the nausea and vomiting in the early months of pregnancy and in other conditions.

TOXICITY. Drowsiness.

DOSE. 25 mg. orally three times daily.

CYCLIZINE HYDROCHLORIDE, U.S.P. (MAREZINE). Also an antihistamine, cyclizine is cautiously recommended for the control of nausea and vomiting in the early months of pregnancy and may be used for motion sickness or other conditions accompanied by mild nausea and vomiting.

TOXICITY. Drowsiness.

DOSE. Oral: 50 mg. three times daily. I.M.: 50 mg. three or four times daily. Rectal: 100 mg. every four to six hours.

CARMINATIVES

Carminatives are weakly medicated substances that are administered orally to relieve gaseous distention of the stomach and intestines by stimulating peristalsis. Candy mints taken after meals serve the same purpose, as do various after dinner drinks or whiskey or brandy in hot water. These agents are of questionable therapeutic benefit, but serve a palliative purpose. Carminative solutions are occasionally used as pleasant-tasting vehicles for drugs administered in liquid form.

Peppermint Spirit (Essence of Peppermint). Dose—1 ml. orally in water after meals.

Peppermint Water, U.S.P.; Concentrated Peppermint Water, B.P. Dose—1 to 4 ml. orally after meals.

Rhubarb and Soda Mixture, N.F. Dose—4 to 8 ml. orally after meals.

DEFOAMING AND ANTIFLATULENT AGENTS

Gas bubbles may become trapped in the gastrointestinal tract as a secondary effect of peptic ulcer, spastic colon, enteritis, gastritis, duodenitis and other nonspecific disorders. In many cases, patients are unable to obtain relief from this gas by the use of antacids and anticholinergic drugs. Defoaming agents mechanically reduce the surface tension of gas bubbles, allowing them to coalesce and be more easily expelled from the gastrointestinal tract.

SIMETHICONE (METHYLPOLYSILOXANE, MYLICON). Simethicone is a surface-active agent that acts mechanically, similar to a detergent, to reduce the surface tension of gas bubbles in the gastrointestinal tract and aid in their expulsion. Gas retention is considerably reduced throughout the entire gastrointestinal tract, and clinical relief has been obtained in many instances. Simethicone-containing preparations may also be administered prior to diagnostic X-ray examinations to enhance visibility of internal structures that may be occluded in the presence of large amounts of gas in the gastrointestinal tract.

DOSE. 40 mg. orally four times daily after meals and at bedtime.

Simethicone may also be combined with other pharmacologic agents:

Mylanta (following doses are incorporated in 5 ml. liquid or one tablet):
20 mg. simethicone
200 mg. magnesium hydroxide
200 mg. aluminum hydroxide gel
Dose—one to two tablets (5 to 10 ml. liquid) orally three or four times daily.

Silain-Gel (following doses are incorporated in 5 ml. liquid or one tablet):
25 mg. simethicone
85 mg. magnesium hydroxide
282 mg. co-precipitated magnesium carbonate and aluminum hydroxide
Dose—two tablets (10 ml. liquid) orally three or four times daily.

Phazyme (following doses in one tablet):
20 mg. simethicone ⎫
100 mg. pepsin ⎬ in outer layer
25 mg. diastase ⎭
40 mg. simethicone ⎫ in core for release in
240 mg. pancreatin ⎭ the duodenum
Dose—one tablet orally four times daily.

DRUGS THAT AFFECT THE INTESTINES

ADSORBENTS

Adsorbents are agents that cause particles to adhere to their surface by physical rather than chemical means. Although adsorbents are intended primarily for the adsorption of noxious substances, such as gases, toxins, bacteria and products of bacterial metabolism, these agents are unfortunately nonspecific in regard to the materials adsorbed; nutrients, enzymes and other beneficial substances may be carried from the gastrointestinal tract by these compounds.

Adsorbents are used in the treatment of diarrhea, dysentery, chronic ulcerative colitis and related conditions. Except for activated charcoal, which is used specifically as an adsorbent, other agents with this therapeutic effect will be discussed under antidiarrheal medications.

ACTIVATED CHARCOAL, U.S.P. (MEDICINAL CHARCOAL). Activated charcoal is the product of the destructive distillation of various organic materials that has been treated with substances such as carbon dioxide, zinc chloride or steam to activate the finely subdivided particles by removing substances previously adsorbed on them.

Although formerly used for the treatment of flatulence and diarrhea, it is of doubtful benefit in these conditions. The almost exclusive use of this substance at present is in universal antidote, which also contains magnesium oxide and tannic acid and is used as a nonspecific and emergency measure to slow absorption of ingested poisons until gastric lavage can be performed.

DOSE. 4 to 8 Gm. orally in water.

DEMULCENTS

Demulcents are agents that symptomatically sooth the irritated mucous membranes of the gastrointestinal tract and may simultaneously act as adsorbents or antacids. Demulcents discussed under other headings in this text include calcium carbonate, magnesium oxide, pectin and glycerin.

CATHARTICS

Cathartics are drugs that relieve constipation and speed the passage of fecal material from the gastrointestinal tract.

Constipation does not exist merely when bowel elimination does not occur regularly every 24 hours, but rather it may be presumed to occur when the fecal volume is too small and a significant amount of feces remains in the rectum after defecation, and when the feces are too hard so that the patient experiences difficulty and pain in passing them.

Although cathartics are useful in the treatment of these conditions, one should first try to relieve the constipation by correction of contributory habits or patterns of living. Factors that may contribute to constipation are incorrect bowel habits or failure to obey the defecation impulse, a diet deficient in salads, fruits, vegetables and cereals, insufficient fluid intake, insufficient exercise and emotional disorders.

It is important to remember that there is no set time limit between bowel movements. Many parents become extremely upset if a child does not develop regular every-twenty-four-hour bowel habits, and it is possible to create an emotional problem as well as constipation in the child by continually expounding on this point. As long as the stool is of normal consistency and there is no discomfort due to distention following elimination, there is no constipation. Some perfectly healthy individuals may have normal eliminations no more often than every two or three days.

In general, the administration of laxatives or cathartics must be absolutely avoided in the presence of abdominal pain, nausea, vomiting and similar symptoms that may indicate the presence of appendicitis, and they must be administered cautiously in the third trimester of pregnancy.

NURSE'S ROLE IN PREVENTING AND TREATING CONSTIPATION

The nurse has a very important role in, and frequent opportunities for, education of patients and the public in the use of laxatives and the prevention and treatment of constipation. Regularity of bowel habits should be emphasized as being of more importance than a specific frequency.

The use of laxatives over extended periods of time should be discouraged because the colon eventually becomes dependent upon the laxative for stimulation of the defecation reflex and no longer responds to normal stimuli.

Measures to promote normal bowel habits include adequate hydration (eight glasses of liquid a day), adequate bulk in the diet and a sufficient amount of exercise. Setting aside sufficient time at a relaxed time of day helps a person to gain or maintain regular bowel habits. Since peristalsis of the entire gastrointestinal tract is stimulated by the ingestion of food, a time immediately after meals would be more likely to produce results.

Because hospitalized patients usually have a reduced amount of exercise, especially if on bedrest, they are more prone to develop constipation. The psychological dislike and inconvenience of using a bedpan is another factor. Certain drugs that decrease peristalsis, such as morphine, also may make a patient more prone to constipation.

Constipation and the resulting straining is particularly dangerous for the patient with cardiac disease. The forced expiration against the closed glottis, which occurs during straining, is called the Valsalva maneuver. This causes an increase in thoracic pressure which impedes the return of venous blood to the right atrium. When the breath is released, the resulting rapid flow of blood into the heart produces a tachycardia. The tachycardia is then reflexly lowered into a bradycardia which may be fatal in a patient with a diseased heart.

Several measures should be initiated by

the nurse to prevent and detect constipation in hospitalized patients. One measure is assuring adequate fluid and bulk in the diet unless contraindicated. Offering the bedpan frequently to bedridden patients is important, and adequate screening and privacy are essential.

Most nursing units have a method by which the patient's bowel habits are checked each day, usually when vital signs are checked in the entire unit. A list is then made of patients who should receive laxatives that evening. It may be necessary to obtain a doctor's order if a p.r.n. laxative has not been ordered previously.

Laxative orders may be written to be given either p.r.n. or daily. The physician often leaves the patient the choice of which laxative he prefers. The nurse should guide the patient in his choice, especially in relation to the time span before the laxative exerts its action; e.g., a short-acting one given at bedtime would require the patient to be up during the night.

It may be necessary for the nurse to bring to the doctor's attention that the patient may need an enema or suppository.

BULK-INCREASING LAXATIVES

The bulk-increasers exert their laxative or cathartic effect by swelling in the presence of water and thus mechanically stimulating the intestine to contract reflexly because of the increased volume. Bulk-increasing laxatives are used when it is desirable to keep the stool soft, and they may be taken frequently by elderly patients, who, perhaps because of a faulty diet or decreased peristalsis, need the added stimulus of increased bulk for normal bowel movements. They are safe to administer to children, but they are not usually the agents of choice following gastric surgical procedure or trauma, since additional bulk is undesirable in these instances. Ordinarily 24 to 48 hours is required for a laxative effect.

Bulk-increasing laxatives can be mixed with food or liquid just before administration. It is important that tablets not be chewed and that sufficient fluid is given immediately afterward so that the drug does not swell in the esophagus and cause obstruction.

AGAR, U.S.P. (INCORPORATED IN AGORAL, PETROGALAR). Agar is obtained commercially from seaweed and is composed chiefly of colloidal substances that swell in water to form a mucilaginous suspension. The colloidal particles are too large to be absorbed from the gastrointestinal tract. They therefore increase the bulk of the fecal material by holding water in the tract and preventing excessive resorption of water and hardening of the feces.

DOSE.   4 Gm. orally once or twice daily.

PSYLLIUM SEED, N.F. (PLANTAGO SEED, METAMUCIL, CASYLLIUM). Psyllium seeds upon processing yield a hydrophilic colloid that swells in water to form a gel. Like agar, psyllium seed extracts hold water in the gastrointestinal tract and soften the fecal material. It is not ordinarily considered habit-forming, and it is not irritating to the bowel mucosa.

DOSE.   Four to eight Gm. orally one to three times daily. Take with fluids.

METHYLCELLULOSE, U.S.P. (CELLOTHYL, COLOGEL, HYDROLOSE). Methylcellulose is prepared synthetically by the methylation of natural cellulose. In water it forms a tasteless, hydrophilic gel, and it may be taken in tablet or liquid form, alone or in combination with other laxatives for the relief of constipation.

DOSE.   1 Gm. orally two to four times daily.

LUBRICANT LAXATIVES

Lubricant laxatives exert their effect by mechanically mixing with and softening fecal material, but they do so without increasing the bulk of the intestinal contents. From 12 to 18 hours is required for effect.

The unpleasant taste of these oily preparations may be alleviated by several nursing measures. Refrigeration of the oils will decrease the volatility and the accompanying odor which contribute to the taste sensation. They may be given with fruit juice; ice chips and mouth wash may be used before and after administration.

LIQUID PETROLATUM, U.S.P.; LIQUID PARAFFIN, B.P. (MINERAL OIL). Liquid petrolatum is a mixture of hydrocarbons obtained commercially from petroleum. It is completely indigestible and is not absorbed from the gastrointestinal tract. It should not be taken with food or immediately after a meal since mineral oil tends to delay gastric emptying. When taken orally, it is an effective lubricant laxative, but it occasionally leaks from the rectum, soiling clothing and bed linen.

Continued administration of liquid petrolatum may create a deficiency in oil-soluble vitamins since they may be carried through the gastrointestinal tract with petrolatum without being absorbed.

Care should be taken that the patient does not aspirate the preparation into his lungs because it can lead to lipid pneumonia. Only water-soluble lubricants, never mineral oil, should be used around the mouth or nose.

DOSE.   15 ml. orally once or twice daily.

OLIVE OIL, U.S.P., B.P.   Olive oil is a bland oil that is usually digested in and absorbed from the gastrointestinal tract. When large or frequent doses are administered, however, some oil is retained in the triglyceride form in the intestines and acts as a bulk lubricant. Because of the unpredictability of the absorption of this oil, it is not as an effective a lubricant laxative as mineral oil.

DOSE.   15 ml. orally once or twice daily.

CORN OIL, U.S.P.   Like olive oil, corn oil is a digestible oil that is somewhat effective as a lubricant laxative when administered in large does. Physicians do not prescribe it as a laxative, but it is employed occasionally as a home remedy.

DOSE.   15 ml. orally once or twice daily.

SALINE CATHARTICS

Saline cathartics are highly water soluble yet not absorbed from the gastrointestinal tract when administered orally. Because of the high osmotic pressure exerted within the tract by these substances, ingested water is not only retained, but additional water is pulled into the gastrointestinal tract from surrounding tissues to contribute to the fecal mass. These drugs should therefore never be given to patients with fluid and electrolyte imbalance. The sudden and sometimes excessive stretching and irritation of the intestine produces rapid contraction of the smooth muscle and vigorous peristaltic movements that result in expulsion of watery feces. Before more suitable drugs were known, saline cathartics were employed to reduce edema through its osmotic activity.

Because saline cathartics act in one to four hours after oral administration, they are used when rapid evacuation is desired, such as following the ingestion of poisons or for elimination of intestinal parasites following the administration of anthelmintic medications. Considerable discomfort and intestinal griping may be produced following administration of the saline cathartics. With the exception of milk of magnesia, they are not suitable for administration to children.

MAGNESIUM HYDROXIDE MAGMA, U.S.P.; MAGNESIUM HYDROXIDE MIXTURE, B.P. (MILK OF MAGNESIA).   Because it is insoluble in the gastrointestinal tract, magnesium hydroxide magma is slower acting and more gentle than other saline cathartics. It is an effective antacid in smaller doses, and it produces a laxative effect approximately 8 to 12 hours after administration of larger doses. It may be used for children.

DOSE.   4 ml. orally three or four times daily with 1 oz. of water (antacid). 15 ml. orally with a glass of water (cathartic).

MAGNESIUM SULFATE, U.S.P., B.P. (EPSOM SALT).   Magnesium sulfate is a very potent saline cathartic that produces rapid intestinal evacuation accompanied by discomfort and griping. It is usually the agent of choice following ingestion of poisons or anthelmintic medications.

TOXICITY.   Magnesium sulfate should not be administered when renal function is decreased because of the danger of increased levels of magnesium. Early signs of magnesium toxicity include thirst and a feeling of warmth throughout the body. One Gm. of calcium gluconate should be administered intravenously as an antidote.

DOSE.   15 Gm. orally followed by one or two glassfuls of water.

MAGNESIUM CITRATE SOLUTION, N.F. (CITRATE OF MAGNESIA).   Magnesium citrate solution is a rapidly acting saline cathartic administered in liquid form. Since the solution contains a considerable amount of sugar, it should not be administered to diabetic patients unless the carbohydrate content is taken into consideration in the diet.

DOSE.   6 to 12 oz. orally in one dose.

IRRITANT CATHARTICS

The irritant cathartics produce reflex peristaltic movements and hasten fecal elimination by local irritation of the intestinal mucosa. They are usually effective in producing semifluid stools within six to eight hours after administration. The chronic use of these cathartics can cause fluid and electrolyte disturbances.

CASTOR OIL, U.S.P., B.P.   In the intestine, castor oil is hydrolyzed by lipases into glycerin and ricinoleic acid. The ricinoleic component is a local irritant and therefore produces the cathartic effect. This oil should be administered in larger doses than needed for the laxative effect, since unhydrolyzed oil remaining in the fecal mass lubricates and soothes the intestinal mucosa as the mass moves along the intestinal tract.

Castor oil is often administered following barium sulfate administration for roentgenographic examination of the gastrointestinal tract to hasten the elimination of the barium.

The oil is best tolerated if given cool or in fruit juice.

DOSE.   15 ml. orally.

AROMATIC CASCARA SAGRADA FLUIDEXTRACT, U.S.P.; CASCARA ELIXIR, B.P.; CASCARA TABLETS, N.F., B.P. (HINKLE'S PILLS, CASCARA TABLETS).   Cascara sagrada is perhaps the most commonly used irritant cathartic. It is effective,

yet it does not produce extensive gastrointestinal irritation unless used continuously. It is less likely to produce intestinal griping than are many other irritant cathartics.

DOSE.   325 mg. orally daily (tablet). 1 to 4 ml. orally daily (fluidextract).

PHENOLPHTHALEIN TABLETS, N.F., B.P. (INCORPORATED IN FEEN-A-MINT GUM, EX-LAX).   Phenolphthalein is an odorless, tasteless compound that lends itself readily to incorporation in the candy and gum laxatives. It is moderately effective in this form and is not usually accompanied by griping.

Although flavored laxative candy facilitates administration of laxatives to children, serious poisonings have resulted by accidental ingestion of overdoses by children thinking they are candy. Special precautions should be taken to keep these compounds out of the reach of children.

TOXICITY.   Nausea, skin reactions, hypotension and cardiovascular collapse in overdose.

DOSE.   60 mg. orally daily.

BISACODYL (DULCOLAX).   Bisacodyl exerts its laxative effect in the colon through a reflex action upon physical contact with the nerve plexi in the intestinal mucosa. Stimulation occurs locally at first, but it is followed by contractions of the entire colon. It is not absorbed systemically.

Bisacodyl may be administered to cleanse the colon prior to surgical procedures, radiological examinations, barium enemas and proctoscopic examinations as well as to treat constipation.

The patient should be instructed not to chew the tablet. Antacids or milk should not be given within one hour of administration. Evacuation occurs within one half hour when administered in suppository form, and within 6 to 12 hours after oral administration.

TOXICITY.   Mild abdominal cramps and, rarely, diarrhea.

The suppositories may be locally irritating in the rectum.

DOSE. 5 to 15 mg. orally. 10 mg. rectally.

DANTHRON, N.F. (CHRYSAZIN, DORBANE). Danthron is a synthetic drug that structurally resembles the anthraquinones. When taken orally, it stimulates peristalsis in the large intestine and increases water retention in the large intestine.

TOXICITY. Diarrhea and hypokalemia occur with continued administration. It is secreted in the milk of nursing mothers, producing diarrhea in the infant.

DOSE. 75 to 150 mg. orally daily.

FECAL SOFTENERS

Fecal softeners are the newest cathartic drugs. They are largely surface active or wetting agents, which by virtue of their detergent properties, mix with the fecal material, emulsify it and soften it for easier elimination.

These agents are nontoxic, inert, do not increase the bulk in the intestine and do not irritate the intestinal mucosa. For these reasons they are the agents of choice for cardiac patients, who must not be allowed to strain when defecating, for the elderly, for infants and young children and for other patients when rapid elimination is not necessary but prophylactic medication is desired to retain soft stools. Ordinarily one to three days is required for a laxative effect.

DIOCTYL CALCIUM SULFOSUCCINATE (SURFAK). When administered orally, dioctyl calcium sulfosuccinate lowers the surface tension in the gastrointestinal tract, permitting water to penetrate and soften the fecal material.

No digestion or absorption of this compound occurs, and it is excreted from the colon unchanged. It may be used for prophylactic fecal mass softening in cardiac patients and in patients with anal fissures, megacolon and related conditions.

DOSE. 240 mg. orally daily.

DIOCTYL SODIUM SULFOSUCCINATE, N.F. (COLACE, DOXINATE). There is no therapeutic or pharmacologic difference between the sodium and calcium salts of this detergent. The sodium salt is often combined with other laxative agents, such as the irritant cathartics and bulk-increasing laxatives.

DOSE. 50 to 200 mg. orally daily.

Combinations of dioctyl sodium sulfosuccinate are found in the following commercial preparations:*

> *Dorbantyl*
> Dioctyl sodium sulfosuccinate 50 mg.
> Danthron 25 mg.
> Dose—1 or 2 capsules orally daily.
> *Dorbantyl Forte*
> Dioctyl sodium sulfosuccinate 100 mg.
> Danthron 50 mg.
> Dose—1 or 2 capsules orally daily.
> *Peri-Colace*
> Dioctyl sodium sulfosuccinate 100 mg.
> Casanthranol 30 mg.
> Dose—1 or 2 capsules orally daily.
> *Senokap*
> Dioctyl sodium sulfosuccinate 50 mg.
> Senna extract 225 mg.
> Dose—1 capsule orally daily.
> *Dialose*
> Dioctyl sodium sulfosuccinate 100 mg.
> Sodium carboxymethylcellulose 400 mg.
> Dose—1 or 2 capsules orally daily.
> *Dialose Plus*
> Dioctyl sodium sulfosuccinate 100 mg.
> Sodium carboxymethylcellulose 400 mg.
> Di(acetylhydroxyphenyl)isatin 3 mg.
> Dose—1 or 2 capsules orally daily.
> *Doxan*
> Dioctyl sodium sulfosuccinate 60 mg.
> Danthron 50 mg.
> Dose—1 or 2 tablets orally daily.

POLOXALKOL (MAGCYL, POLYKOL). When administered orally, poloxalkol lowers surface tension of fecal material in a manner similar to the other fecal softeners.

DOSE. 400 to 800 mg. orally daily.

ANTIDIARRHETICS

Antidiarrhetics are agents that are used to treat diarrhea, a condition characterized by frequent, watery evacuations and griping

---

*All doses shown are the strength per capsule or tablet.

TABLE 14 Examples of Over-the-Counter Laxatives**

Product and site of action†	Dosage form	Manu-facturer	Stimulant	Saline	Bulk-forming	Emollient	Other ingredients
Agoral (2)	emulsion	Warner-Chilcott	phenolphthalein 20 gr/100 cc (not in plain)	—	—	mineral oil*	egg albumen agar gel tragacanth acacia glycerin
Alophen (2)	pill	Parke, Davis	aloin ¼ gr phenolphthalein ½ gr	—	—	—	belladonna extract ⅟₃₄ gr ipecac ⅟₁₅ gr
Aquatyl (2)	tablet	Neisler	—	—	—	dioctyl sod. sulfosuccinate 50 mg	cholic acid 100 mg
Bassoran (3)	granule	Merrell	cascara extract (not in plain) 390 mg/9 gm	—	karaya gum 87%	—	aluminum and magnesium hydroxide 360 mg of each (390 mg in plain)
Black Draught (2)	syrup, tablet, granule and powder	Chattanooga Medicine	senna* rhubarb* (rhubarb identified only in syrup)	—	—	—	anise peppermint cinnamon clove nutmeg (spices identified only in syrup)
Calotabs (3)	tablet	Calotabs	calomel 2 gr aloe* jalap*	—	—	—	peppermint extract of bitter apple oil of cloves orizaba
Caroid and Bile Salts with Phenolphthalein (2)	tablet	Breon	ext cascara sagrada 50 mg phenolphthalein 30 mg	—	—	—	papaya extract 75 mg capsicum 6 mg bile salts 70 mg
Carter's Little Pills (3)	pill	Carter	aloe 16 mg podophyllum 4.5 mg	—	—	—	
Casafru (2)	liquid	Davies, Rose-Hoyt	senna fruit extractives 30%	—	—	—	—
Cas-Evac (2)	liquid	Parke, Davis	cascara sagrada 200 mg/100 cc	—	—	—	alcohol 18%
Fletcher's Castoria (2)	syrup	Glenbrook	senna extract aqueous ⅔ v/v	—	—	—	
Casyllium (3)	powder	Upjohn	cascara fluid ext 230 min prune powder 85 gr/oz	—	psyllium husk 300 gr/oz	—	—
Cellothyl (3)	tablet	Warner-Chilcott	—	—	methylcellulose 0.5 Gm	—	—
Ceo-Two (2)	suppository	Beutlich	—	potassium bitartrate* sod. bicarbonate*	—	polyethylene glycol*	—
CMC (3)	capsule	Stuart	—	—	sod. carboxy-methylcellulose 0.575 Gm	—	—
Colace (2)	capsule, liquid and syrup	Mead Johnson	—	—	—	dioctyl sod. sulfosuccinate 50 and 100 mg/cap 1% solution 20 mg/5cc syrup	—
Doxan (2)	tablet	Lloyd	danthron 50 mg	—	—	dioctyl sod. sulfosuccinate 60 mg	—
Doxinate (2)	capsule and 5% solution	Lloyd	—	—	—	dioctyl sod. sulfosuccinate 60 and 240 mg	—
Dr. Edward's Olive Tablets (3)	tablet	Plough	aloin* cascara sagrada* podophyllin*	—	—	—	—
Dulcolax (2)	tablet	Geigy	bisacodyl 5 mg tab and 10 mg suppository	—	—	—	—
Effergel (3)	powder	Stuart	acetphenolisatin 5 mg/7 Gm	—	sod. carboxy-methylcellulose 2 Gm/7 Gm	—	—
Effersyl (3)	powder	Stuart	acetphenolisatin 3 mg/7 Gm	—	psyllium hydrocolloid 3 Gm/7 Gm	—	—
Effersyllium (3)	powder	Stuart	—	—	psyllium hydrocolloid 3 Gm/7 Gm	—	—
Emulserol (2)	emulsion	Upjohn	cascara fluid extract 3.1% (in Emulserol with Cascara)	—	—	mineral oil 80%	vitamin A 5,000 units
Espotabs (2)	tablet	Combe	yellow phenol-phthalein*	—	—	—	—

*Quantitative statement not provided.
†Site of action legend: 1 = small intestine 2 = colon; 3 = small and large intestine

**From Penna, Darlington, and Chalmers: *Handbook of Non-Prescription Drugs*. Washington, D.C., American Pharmaceutical Association, 1968, p. 44.

Table 14 *continued on opposite page.*

TABLE 14   Examples of Over-the-Counter Laxatives (*Continued*)

Product and site of action†	Dosage form	Manu-facturer	Stimulant	Saline	Bulk-forming	Emollient	Other ingredients
Evac-U-Gen (2)	tablet	Walker Corp.	yellow phenol-phthalein*	—	—	—	sod. salicyl-ate ¹/₄ gr bismuth sub-carbonate ¹/₃ gr bismuth sub-gallate ¹/₈ gr
Ex-Lax (2)	pill and chocolate	Ex-Lax	yellow phenol-phthalein 1¹/₂ gr	—	—	—	—
Feen-A-Mint (2)	chewing gum	Pharmaco	yellow phenol-phthalein*	—	—	—	—
Fleet Enema (2)	enema	Fleet	—	sod. phos-phate 6 Gm/100 ml sod. biphos-phate 16 Gm 100 ml	—	—	—
Fleet Enema Oil Retention (2)	enema	Fleet	—	—	—	mineral oil 127 ml	—
Gentlax (3)	granule and tablet	Purdue Frederick	senna concentrate 326 mg	—	guar gum 1 gm	—	polygalacturonic acid 100 mg
Glysennid (2)	tablet	Sandoz	senna glycosides (sennosides A and B as calcium salt) 12 mg	—	—	—	—
Haley's M-O (3)	emulsion	Glenbrook	—	milk of magnesia	—	mineral oil	—
Hydrolose (3)	syrup	Upjohn	(in Fortified only) acetphenolisatin 15 mg/fl oz prune powder 1.48 Gm	—	methylcellulose 5.91 Gm/fl. oz	—	—
Imbicoll (3)	granule	Upjohn	(in Imbicoll with Cascara) cascara sagrada fl ext 15 min	—	karaya gum 86%	—	(in Imbicoll with Vitamin B₁) thiamine HCl 1 mg
Innerclean Herbal (3)	powder	Innerclean	senna* frangula*	—	agar* psyllium*	—	—
Isocrin (2)	tablet	Warner-Chilcott	acetphenolisatin 5 mg	—	—	—	—
Kondremul (2)	emulsion	Smith, Miller and Patch	(in Kondremul with Cascara only) ext cascara* (in Kondremul with Phenolph-thalein only) phenolphthalein 2.2 gr/tbsp	—	—	mineral oil 55%	chondrus as emulsifier
Konsyl (3)	powder	Burton, Parsons	—	—	psyllium 100%	—	—
L. A. Formula (3)	powder	Burton, Parsons	—	—	psyllium 50%	—	dextrose and lactose 50%
Lapatic (2)	pill	Quinton	aloin 15 mg	—	—	—	belladonna ext 5 mg ipecac 4 mg
Lavema (2)	enema	Winthrop	phenolisatin 20 mg/180 ml	—	—	propylene glycol 9 ml tyloxapol 135 mg/180 ml	—
Metamucil (3)	powder	Searle	—	—	psyllium 50%	—	dextrose 50%
Metamucil Instant Mix (3)	powder	Searle	—	—	psyllium 3.7 Gm	—	citric acid sod. bicarbo-nate (equiva-lent to 0.25 Gm sodium)
Milkinol (2)	liquid	Kremers-Urban	—	—	—	mineral oil 4.75 cc dioctyl sod. sulfosuccinate 3.3 mg/5 cc	—
Modane (2)	liquid and tablet	Warren-Teed	danthron 75 mg/tab or/10 cc	—	—	—	d-calcium pantothenate 25 mg/tab or/10 cc
Mucara (3)	granule	Ives	—	—	karaya gum 80%	—	—
Mucilose (3)	flakes and powder	Winthrop	—	—	psyllium 50%	tyloxapol 50 mg/5 Gm	dextrose 50% in powder
Mucilose Compound (3)	tablet	Winthrop	—	—	psyllium 15.4% methylcellulose 58%	—	—
Nature's Remedy (2)	tablet	Lewis-Howe	aloe* cascara sagrada*	—	—	—	—
Neo-Kondremul (2)	emulsion	Smith, Miller and Patch	casanthranol (cascara sagrada fraction) 30 mg/15 ml	—	—	mineral oil	chondrus

Table 14 *continued on following page.*

TABLE 14 Examples of Over-the-Counter Laxatives (*Continued*)

Product and site of action†	Dosage form	Manu-facturer	Stimulant	Saline	Bulk-forming	Emollient	Other ingredients
Neoloid (1)	emulsion	Lederle	castor oil 36.4%	—	—	—	—
Peri-Colace (2)	capsule	Mead Johnson	casanthranol 30 mg	—	—	dioctyl sod. sulfosuccinate 100 mg	—
Petrogalar (2–3)	aqueous suspension	Wyeth	(in Cascara Petrogalar) ext cascara sagrada 13.2% (in Phenolphthalein Petrogalar) phenolphthalein 0.3%	(in Alkaline Petrogalar) magnesium hydroxide 8%	—	mineral oil 65%	—
Phenolax (2)	wafer	Upjohn	phenolphthalein 1 gr	—	—	—	sugar aromatics
Phospho-Soda (3)	liquid	Fleet	—	sod. phosphate 18 Gm/100 ml sod. biphosphate 48 Gm/100 ml	—	—	(also comes in ginger-lemon flavor)
Plova (3)	powder	Washington Ethical	—	—	psyllium 100%	—	(flavored form 50% psyllium)
Polykol (2)	capsule and liquid	Upjohn	—	—	—	polyoxakol 250 mg cap and 200 mg/cc	—
Prulose Complex (3)	tablet	Warner-Chilcott	acetphenolisatin 1 mg prune concentrate 130 mg	—	methylcellulose 389 mg	—	—
Rectalad (2)	enema	Wampole	—	—	—	glycerin 76% dioctyl pot. sulfosuccinate 5%	soft soap 10%
Regutol (2)	tablet	Pharmaco	—	—	—	dioctyl sod. sulfosuccinate 100 mg	cal. pantothenate 50 mg
Revac Sup-prettes (2)	suppository	Webster	—	—	—	dioctyl sod. sulfosuccinate 100 mg	Neocera base
Sal Hepatica (3)	powder	Bristol-Myers	—	sod. biphosphate 43%	—	—	sod. bicarbonate 38.? citric acid 5%
Saraka (3)	granule	Pharmaco	frangula*	—	karaya gum*	—	thiamine HCl 0.5 mg/6 Gm
Senokot (2)	granule	Purdue Frederick	senna concentrate 163 mg/gm	—	—	—	—
Senokap (2)	capsule	Purdue Frederick	senna concentrate 163 mg	—	—	dioctyl sod. sulfosuccinate 50 mg	—
Serutan (3)	powder and granule	JB Williams	—	—	psyllium* methylcellulose*	—	—
Siblin (3)	tablet and granule	Parke, Davis	—	—	psyllium 65% (in tablet only) karaya gum* agar* pectin*	—	thiamine HCl 0.5 mg/tab or 2 mg/4.5 Gms
Sigmol (2)	enema	Pharmaseal	—	—	—	dioctyl pot. sulfosuccinate 0.14 Gm/140 ml sorbitol 49.5 Gm	—
Surfak (2)	capsule	Lloyd	—	—	—	cal. dioctyl disulfosuccinate 50 mg	—
Swiss Kriss (2)	powder	Modern	senna leaves*	—	—	—	many spices
Syllamalt (3)	powder	Borcherdt	—	—	psyllium 50%	—	malt extract 50%
Turicum (3)	emulsion	Whittier	—	magnesium hydroxide 0.70 Gm/tbsp	sod. carboxymethylcellulose 0.36 Gm/tbsp	—	—
Urbalax (2)	tablet	Kremers-Urban	acetphenolisatin 2 mg	—	—	dioctyl sod. sulfosuccinate 60 mg	—
Vacuettes (2) Adult	suppository	Dorsey	—	sod. biphosphate* sod. acid pyrophosphate* sod. bicarbonate*	—	polyethylene glycols*	—
Veracolate (2)	tablet	Standard	phenolphthalein 0.50 gr cascara sagrada ext 1 gr	—	—	—	capsicum 0.05 min bile salts 1.07 gr

* Quantitative statement not provided.
† Site of action legend: 1 = small intestine; 2 = colon; 3 = small and large intestine.

caused by the too rapid passage of intestinal contents. They may adsorb noxious substances, kill infectious gastrointestinal microorganisms or merely soothe irritated bowel mucosa and reduce spasm.

The treatment of diarrhea depends upon the specific cause. If it is caused by food poisoning, the only effective cure is elimination of the offending material; in some cases a cathartic may even be beneficial, rather than an antidiarrhetic agent. If the diarrhea is produced by an intestinal infection, antibacterial therapy must be instituted.

The nurse should observe the patient carefully for signs or symptoms of fluid and electrolyte imbalance. The number and consistency of the stools should be observed and recorded. Hot or cold liquids taken orally should be avoided since these may further stimulate intestinal peristalsis.

KAOLIN, N.F., LIGHT KAOLIN, B.P. (INCORPORATED IN KAOPECTATE). Kaolin is a purified material consisting primarily of hydrated aluminum silicate obtained from clay. Its effectiveness is variable, but if administered in effective doses, it relieves simple diarrhea because of its adsorbing capacity. It is not effective in diarrhea produced by malignant changes or serious bowel disorders. The most commonly used form of kaolin is in Kaopectate, a commercial suspension that contains 2.4 Gm. of kaolin and 0.6 Gm. of pectin per 15 ml.

> **DOSE.** (Kaopectate) 15 to 100 ml. orally after each loose stool.

PECTIN, N.F. (INCORPORATED IN KAOPECTATE). Pectin is a purified carbohydrate obtained commercially from the inner portions of citrus rinds. It is the important component in the apple or banana diet for the treatment of diarrhea.

Although the mechanism of action in the treatment of diarrhea is not known, pectin has soothing and demulcent effects on irritated bowel mucosa.

> **DOSE.** (Kaopectate) 15 to 100 ml. orally after each loose stool.

NEOMYCIN SULFATE, U.S.P., B.P. Neomycin sulfate is a broad-spectrum antibiotic that effectively kills or inhibits harmful bacterial flora in the gastrointestinal tract. It is not absorbed when given orally and may be administered in the treatment of diarrhea without undue concern about possible systemic effects.

> **DOSE.** 500 mg. orally four times daily.

LACTOBACILLUS ACIDOPHILUS AND L. BULGARICUS (LACTINEX, BACID). *Lactobacillus acidophilus* and *L. bulgaricus* are commercially available as viable, mixed cultures with their naturally occurring enzymes. The preparation should be refrigerated to maintain viability.

The administration of lactobacilli in the treatment of diarrhea is limited largely to conditions in which diarrhea is due to antibiotic therapy, metabolic conditions or an imbalance of the gastrointestinal flora.

It is useful in the treatment of infectious diarrhea, colostomies with either diarrhea or constipation, constipation from certain drugs, mucous or spastic diarrhea, diverticulitis, ulcerative colitis, abnormal fermentation and related conditions.

Lactobacilli are supplied both in tablet form and in packets of granules, which may be stirred with milk, yogurt or similar substances before administration.

> **DOSE.** 3 or 4 tablets (or one packet) orally three or four times daily for three or four days. For maximal benefit, the dose should be accompanied by at least one half glassful of milk or milk product.

PAREGORIC, U.S.P.; CAMPHORATED OPIUM TINCTURE, B.P. This tincture, which is prepared commercially from crude opium, increases the muscular tone of both the small and large intestines as well as the related sphincters. It interferes with peristalsis, so that the movement of fecal material along the gastrointestinal tract is slowed considerably. It may cause constipation if administration is not stopped as soon as the diarrhea is controlled.

Paregoric is often administered in a 50:50 combination with Kaopectate so that the combined effects of muscle contraction, absorption and demulcent actions aid in the control of diarrhea.

Paregoric is a narcotic and is subject to federal narcotic and dangerous drug laws.

> **DOSE.** 5 to 10 ml. orally, with sufficient amount of water to insure its passage into the stomach, three or four times daily.

DIPHENOXYLATE HYDROCHLORIDE AND ATROPINE SULFATE (LOMOTIL). Diphenoxylate is structurally similar to meperidine, but although it does retain the smooth muscle contracting potentialities of the narcotic analgesics, it has little or no addicting liabilities. In many states it has recently been removed from the list of drugs that may be obtained only with a narcotic prescription.

It has been used in the treatment of functional diarrhea, ulcerative colitis, spastic colitis, following gastrectomy and in the treatment of drug-induced diarrhea and miscellaneous related conditions.

The atropine content of the Lomotil tablet potentiates the action of diphenoxylate by its antispasmodic or anticholinergic effect on the gastrointestinal tract.

> **TOXICITY.** Nausea, sedation, drowsiness, dizziness, vomiting, pruritus, restlessness or insomnia. It is contraindicated in patients with cirrhosis or advanced liver disease, since the drug must be metabolized by the liver. Potentiation may occur if administered simultaneously with central depressants such as barbiturates.

> **DOSE.** 15 to 20 mg. orally daily in three or four divided doses.

QUESTIONS FOR DISCUSSION AND REVIEW

1. How would you explain normal bowel function to a mother worried about her four year old child's "irregular habits"?

2. What antacid would you suggest for routine use in gastric hyperacidity? Why?

3. Why do some antacids have a constipating effect while others cause diarrhea?

4. What nursing techniques must always be used when administering oral hydrochloric acid?

5. What side effects would you expect when dimenhydrinate is taken for motion sickness?

6. How does the common mixture of Kaopectate and paregoric arrest diarrhea?

7. What is the "laxative habit"? How it is usually begun?

8. What laxative would you suggest for:
   a. rapid action
   b. a child of 3 years
   c. a cardiac patient
   d. a normal adult
   e. an elderly person
   f. prior to surgery

9. What measures can be taken by the nurse to help prevent constipation in hospitalized patients?

10. What nursing measures may help the patient experiencing diarrhea? What observations should the nurse make in caring for the patient with diarrhea?

BIBLIOGRAPHY

AMA Drug Evaluations. Chicago, American Medical Association, 1971.

Barnes, M. R.: Clean colons without enemas. *Amer. J. Nurs., 69*:2128, (October) 1969.

Best, C. H. and Taylor, N. B.: *The Physiological Basis of Medical Practice.* 6th Ed. Baltimore, The Williams and Wilkins Co., 1965.

Davenport, H. W.: *Physiology of the Digestive Tract.* 2nd Ed. Chicago, Year Book Medical Publishers, Inc., 1966.

DiPalma, J. R.: Drugs in the management of peptic ulcer. *R.N., 26*:71, (April) 1963.

Downs, H. S.: The control of vomiting. *Amer. J. Nurs., 66*:76, (January) 1966.

Goodman, L. S. and Gilman, A.: *Pharmacological Basis of Therapeutics.* 4th Ed. New York, Macmillan Co., 1970.

Goss, C. M. (ed.): *Gray's Anatomy of the Human Body.* 28th Ed. Philadelphia, Lea and Febiger, 1966.

Goth, A.: *Medical Pharmacology.* 2nd Ed. St. Louis, C. V. Mosby Co., 1964.

Govoni, L. E. and Hayes, J. E.: *Drugs and Nursing Implications.* 2nd Ed. New York, Appleton-Century-Crofts, 1971.

Keele, C. A. and Neil, E.: *Samson Wright's Applied Physiology.* 11th Ed. London, Oxford University Press, 1965.

Main, R. J. and Richardson, A. W.: *Physiology.* 2nd Ed. St. Louis, C. V. Mosby Co., 1953.

Morgan, J. W.: The harmful effects of mineral oil purgatives. *J.A.M.A., 117*:1335, 1941.

Pansky, B. and House, E. L.: *Review of Gross Anatomy.* New York, Macmillan Co., 1964.

Rodman, M. J.: Drugs for G.I. distress. *R.N., 28*:49, (June) 1965.

Steigman, F.: Are laxatives necessary? *Amer. J. Nurs., 62*:90, (October) 1962.

Wintrobe, M. M. et al. (ed.): *Harrison's Principles of Internal Medicine.* 6th Ed. New York, McGraw-Hill Book Co., 1970.

Youmans, W. B.: *Fundamentals of Human Physiology.* 2nd Ed. Chicago, Year Book Medical Publishers, Inc., 1962.

Ziter, F. M. H.: Cathartic colon. *New York J. Med., 67*:546, 1967.

Chapter 18 Drugs that Affect the Skin and Mucous Membrane

Important Concepts Discussed

1. *The skin is a protective covering and an organ of heat regulation, sensation, excretion and absorption.*

2. *Drugs applied to the skin may have a replacement or protective role, or they may be applied to exert a therapeutic effect.*

3. *Dermatologic conditions are often only symptoms of systemic disorders, and although topical agents allay the symptoms, additional therapy must be instituted as well to correct the underlying pathology.*

4. *Skin disorders usually cause patients to feel self-conscious and may contribute to psychological and emotional problems.*

The skin, far from being an inert covering, is an indispensable organ of the body with many important physiological functions, including the following:

1. Maintenance of fluid and electrolyte balance through perspiration.

2. Control of body temperature through evaporation of water from the surface and radiation of heat.

3. Protection of body tissues from invasion by microorganisms. The skin surface also provides an environment that is unfavorable for the growth of pathogenic organisms.

4. Excretion of waste products via sweat and sebaceous glands.

5. Sensory transmission to the central nervous system through stimulation of nerves in the skin.

6. Synthesis of vitamin D from ergosterol in the presence of ultraviolet radiation.

The thickness of the skin varies from one part of the body to another. For example, it is extremely thick and keratinized on the palms of the hands and the soles of the feet, but it is very thin on the eyelids and scrotum.

Some areas of the body, such as the lips, mouth, nares and body canals, are lined with mucous membranes. In contrast to the skin, which has an oily or sebaceous secretion, the mucous membranes secrete an aqueous solution that contains mucin, a glycoprotein that lubricates and protects the surfaces of the mucous membranes from irritation by ingested food, secretions and waste material. Because of this difference between skin and mucous membranes, different bases and modes of administration must be used if drug absorption is to occur from their surfaces.

Since skin has an oily secretion, optimal absorption occurs from the surface if drugs are suspended or dissolved in oily media. Less absorption occurs with inorganic ointment bases, such as petrolatum, than with synthetic ointment bases that more closely resemble sebaceous secretions. Particle size is extremely important in surface absorption; little or no absorption occurs with large, insoluble particles, such as those in zinc oxide ointment, whereas a great deal of absorption occurs with a solution of oil of wintergreen (methyl salicylate) in olive oil or a lanolin base. Rubbing or massaging the skin increases absorption, since the warmth induced by this action dilates surface blood vessels and increases pore size, enabling the medication to penetrate deeper into skin.

In order for drugs to be optimally absorbed from mucous membrane surfaces, they should be applied in water-soluble or water-miscible bases. Suppository bases often contain theobroma oil (cocoa butter), which readily melts at body temperatures, allowing intimate contact of the drug with mucous membrane surfaces. Aminophyllin, aspirin, barbiturates and antinauseants are often administered rectally in suppository form. Absorption is somewhat less predictable from the rectal route, but it produces acceptable systemic blood levels of the drug. Oral mucous membranes are the site of absorption of a few drugs, e.g., nitroglycerin, testosterone and some enzymes. Absorption of these agents is often more efficient than if the tablets are swallowed.

These distinctions do not apply in instances in which the skin is broken, because absorption of all drugs is much more rapid when blood vessels and water-permeable cells of the deeper skin layers are exposed. Potentially toxic drugs should never be applied to denuded surfaces for this reason.

Many dermatologic preparations are not intended for systemic absorption; they are applied for their physical, rather than chemical or pharmacologic effects. These agents may act as protectives, adsorbents, demulcents, emollients or cleansing agents, and they may contain potentially active drugs or consist merely of inert substances. Most astringents, irritants, rubefacients, vesicants, sclerosing agents and keratolytics produce chemical changes in the skin surfaces for effect.

APPLYING DRUGS TO SKIN

In caring for patients with a condition affecting the skin the nurse should use certain guidelines and principles.

Gentle handling of skin lesions is important to prevent irritation; the danger of overtreating a lesion should also be kept in mind. The previously applied medication is usually, but not always, removed before a new application; the physician should be consulted. Excessive amounts should not be used since this is wasteful and may also allow the excess to come in contact with unaffected areas. The nurse should understand the nature of the lesion involved so that precautionary measures or aseptic technique may be used if the lesion is infectious or susceptible to infection.

Ointments should be rubbed onto the skin using a tongue depressor, finger or gauze pad. Lotions and liniments should be applied with gauze using a firm, gentle pressure. Powders should be applied to skin which has been thoroughly dried in order to prevent caking of the powder.

Conditions of the skin are often accompanied by feelings of rejection, disfigurement and a poor self-image. Emotional support of the patient is important, especially since many dermatologic conditions are chronic and discouraging to the patient. The nurse should be careful to avoid showing any sign of rejecting a patient with a skin condition, or reacting to the skin lesions or the treatment involved.

Education of the patient and the public concerning the dangers of self-treatment of skin lesions is an important nursing role. Consumer education is needed in order for the advertisements of mass media to be evaluated intelligently.

PROTECTIVES AND ADSORBENTS

Protective agents are applied to the skin to protect denuded or irritated surfaces from excessive drying, external irritants, secretions or other noxious substances. Many protectives are also adsorbents and tend to cause irritating particulate material and fluids to adhere to their surfaces.

DUSTING POWDERS

Many inert and insoluble substances are employed for their protective properties on skin and mucous membrane surfaces. These finely divided powders absorb moisture, decreasing friction and discouraging bacterial growth. If these substances are applied to denuded and oozing surfaces, however, the formation of moist, adherent cakes sometimes encourages bacterial growth.

BORIC ACID, U.S.P., B.P. (BORACIC ACID). Boric acid is obtained commercially from volcanic residue. It is applied topically in the form of dusting powders and may also be incorporated into topical and ophthalmic ointments as well as lotions.

The use of boric acid as a topical antiseptic and protective agent has decreased considerably because of an appreciable incidence of fatal poisoning, particularly in infants, following its use on abraded skin. Although it is effective and relatively innocuous in adults, it should not be applied to large, denuded areas, and its use should not be continued over a long period of time.

CALCIUM CARBONATE, U.S.P., B.P. (PREPARED CHALK, DROP CHALK). Although calcium carbonate theoretically could be used in topical powders, it is not used to any great extent at present primarily because it has no noticeable advantages over other commonly used topical powders. It is a frequent component of paste and powder dentifrices, however.

The oral use of calcium carbonate is discussed in Chapter 16.

ZINC STEARATE, U.S.P. Zinc stearate is used frequently in topical preparations, either alone or in combination with other substances. It is water repellent, adheres well to the skin and has antipruritic properties. Many dusting powders for infants contain zinc stearate as their chief active ingredient.

TALC, U.S.P. (PURIFIED TALC, TALCUM). When used as a dusting powder, talc is a useful protective for skin irritations, such as prickly heat and diaper rash. Since it is lubricating and does not cake on moist skin because of its low absorbability, it is useful for application to surfaces that are rubbed.

Talc is not used extensively to dust surgical gloves since it is not absorbed and is irritating to body cavities. It has largely been replaced by absorbable powders for this purpose.

ABSORBABLE DUSTING POWDER (BIO-SORB). This combination of cornstarch and magnesium sulfate is better than talc as a surgical dusting powder. It is absorbed from body cavities and does not cause the irritation or granuloma formation that occurs when talc is used for this purpose.

MECHANICAL PROTECTIVES

Mechanical protectives are applied to the skin to form a coating that protects the skin from moisture, bacteria and other environmental elements. There has been some discussion that anaerobic bacteria may be able to multiply under these occlusive coats, however; they are not used extensively at present.

COLLODION, U.S.P. This preparation contains 4 per cent pyroxylin in a solution of ether and alcohol. When collodion is applied to a dry surface, the volatile solvents evaporate and leave a film of pyroxylin on the skin. It is used topically to provide mechanical protection, to hold together the edges of incised wounds, to keep dressings in place and, in a few instances, to hold medications against the skin.

Although collodion protects the underlying tissues from external contamination, by the same mechanism it prevents proper drainage of exudate and may induce secondary infection.

FLEXIBLE COLLODION, U.S.P., B.P. Castor oil, when added to collodion, imparts more flexibility to the residue left on the skin following evaporation of the volatile solvents. Its action and uses are otherwise similar to those of collodion.

ZINC GELATIN, U.S.P. (UNNA'S BOOT, ZINC GELATIN BOOT). Zinc gelatin, a combination of gelatin, glycerin and zinc oxide, is applied in the molten state between gauze bandages for prolonged protective action.

It is used chiefly on the foot and lower part of the leg and has been referred to as a "boot." The circulation in the toes should be checked after the initial application and after it has dried. The impregnated bandage is left in position for several days to two weeks. It is a useful adjunct in the management of varicosities, eczema and leg ulcers.

The dressings may be removed by soaking in water that is about 98° F.

SOOTHING PREPARATIONS

EMOLLIENTS

Emollients are bland, fatty or oily substances that may be applied to the skin and mucous membranes to protect the tissues and to render them more pliable by penetrating the skin. These substances should be rubbed into the skin because the resulting increased blood flow aids in treatment of skin conditions. Water-soluble irritants, air and air-borne bacteria are excluded by the emollient; however, the retention of moisture under these agents and the exclusion of air encourage the growth of anaerobic bacteria. In addition, rubbing during application aids in the spread of cutaneous bacteria.

Emollients may be used as vehicles for lipid-soluble drugs, as ointment bases or as creams.

FIXED OILS. Fixed or nonvolatile oils frequently used as emollients include expressed almond oil, castor oil, corn oil, cottonseed oil, olive oil, peanut oil and sesame oil.

LANOLIN, U.S.P.; HYDROUS WOOL FAT, B.P. Lanolin, an extract of sheepswool combined with 25 to 30 per cent water, is often added to oily ointment bases. Although it is insoluble in water, lanolin takes up about twice its own weight of water. Water-soluble drugs may be dissolved and easily incorporated into lanolin before they are added to an oily ointment base. Lanolin also aids in the absorption of the medicament from the base, since it more closely approximates human skin fat and more readily mixes with sebaceous secretions.

Because of its tenacious properties, wool fat is not used alone but is always combined with other ointment bases.

Since this preparation does exhibit some sensitizing properties, some physicians are apprehensive about its continued application to the skin. When allergic reactions do occur, however, they are usually mild and of short duration.

GLYCERIN, U.S.P., B.P. (GLYCEROL). Glycerin is a clear, colorless liquid with a characteristic sweet taste and odor. It is one of the most valuable solvents and emollients known. When incorporated into lotions and solutions, it is useful as a humectant in keeping the surface moist, and it has value as an emollient in many skin diseases. Its hygroscopic properties tend to cause drying of skin when it is applied in the pure form.

Some ice collars and ice bags contain glycerin and water hermetically sealed within vulcanized rubber bags. The rubber bag may be sterilized by dipping in a germicidal solution and may be stored in the refrigerator until used.

LIGHT LIQUID PETROLATUM, N.F. (MINERAL OIL). Light liquid petrolatum is a mixture of the short carbon-chain liquid hydrocarbons obtained from petroleum. It is useful as a vehicle, especially for drugs to be applied to the nasal mucous membranes, or it may be incorporated into ointment bases to decrease their viscosity.

The application of mineral oil to the nasal mucous membranes is not as harmless as it was once supposed to be. The oil may be aspirated into the lungs after application, and, since it is not absorbed, may cause lipid pneumonias of varying severity. For this reason, nurses should use only water-soluble lubricants in giving mouth care or inserting catheters into the nose or mouth.

PETROLATUM, N.F.; SOFT PARAFFIN, B.P. (PETROLEUM JELLY, VASELINE). Petrolatum is a mixture of the heavier, semisolid hydrocarbons from petroleum. The natural preparation is yellow, but a bleached form, white petrolatum, is often preferred because it is odorless.

Petrolatum is frequently used as an ointment base. Medications are not readily absorbed from it, however. When applied alone, it is useful as an emollient and protective.

ROSE WATER OINTMENT, N.F. (COLD CREAM TYPE). This preparation was originated by Galen, the famous Roman physician of the second century, and its ingredients and preparation have changed very little.

It is a water-in-oil emulsion and contains spermaceti, white wax, almond oil, sodium borate, rose water and rose oil. The perfumed form is often preferred as an emollient on intact skin; the nonperfumed form is used more frequently as an ointment base for application to abraded areas since the perfume may cause sensitivity reactions.

HYDROPHILIC PETROLATUM, U.S.P. This mixture of cholesterol, stearyl alcohol, white wax and white petrolatum differs from rose water ointment in that it is an oil-in-water emulsion and is more easily rubbed into the skin. The wetting agent in the external water phase allows drugs to penetrate the oily secretions on the skin.

Hydrophilic petrolatum is typical of the vanishing cream preparations. It is not greasy and is readily washed off the skin.

THEOBROMA OIL, U.S.P., B.P. (COCOA BUTTER). Theobroma oil is the fat from the roasted seed of *Theobroma cacao*. Since it melts readily at skin temperatures, this compound is frequently employed as a suppository base. In addition, it is often used as a lubricant for application to sunburned areas and as a soothing agent for sore nipples.

Since this oil is the fatty constituent of chocolate and is chiefly what is left when the powdered cocoa is extracted, it has a faint odor resembling chocolate and a bland taste.

VITAMIN A AND D OINTMENT. Commercial vitamin A and D ointment contains these oil-soluble vitamins in a petrolatum base. It may be used as a protective and emollient for chapped skin and for the prevention and treatment of diaper rash.

DEMULCENTS

Demulcents are used chiefly to relieve irritation of mucous membranes and abraded skin. They are usually applied as viscid liquid preparations that readily cover the skin. These preparations are used to relieve the irritation, pain, catarrh and drying that may be caused by chemical, bacterial or mechanical agents. When demulcents are applied in the solid form as in lozenges or powders, the liquid is provided by secreted or exuded fluids.

The hydrophilic properties of demulcents make them useful as emulsifiers and suspending agents in lotions and ointments.

Many chemical substances have demulcent properties. These include the mucilages, gums, starches, certain sugars and glycols. They may be given orally for their soothing effect following the ingestion of a corrosive poison or they may be applied topically for the same effect.

BENZOIN, U.S.P. (GUM BENZOIN). Benzoin is a balsamic resin obtained from *Styrax benzoin* Dryander. It contains the benzoic and cinnamic acid esters of benzoresinol, free benzoic and cinnamic acids, styrol, cinnamyl cinnamate, vanillin, benzaldehyde and the alcohol *d*-sumaresinol.

This preparation may be used topically as an antiseptic and as a protective before tape is applied; it may also be added to boiling water and inhaled for its expectorant effect.

COMPOUND TINCTURE OF BENZOIN, U.S.P. (TURLINGTON'S DROPS). Compound tincture of benzoin has been used as a nostrum and has appeared in pharmacopoeias for the past 300 years. It has about 30 different names.

It contains, in addition to benzoin, specified amounts of aloe, storax and tolu balsam. When added to hot water it is valuable as an inhalant in the treatment of acute laryngitis and croup. It is occasionally administered on sugar for throat and bronchial inflammation.

When mixed with glycerin and water it may be used topically for ulcers, bedsores, cracked nipples and fissures of the lips and anus. When used in the care of bedsores, the compound should not be applied directly to an open area. It is applied around broken skin or where bedsores are developing to prevent the skin from breaking down. It should be allowed to dry completely before it comes in contact with clothing or linen, to prevent the cloth from adhering to the skin.

ACACIA, U.S.P., B.P. (GUM ARABIC). Acacia is the dried exudate from the stems and branches of *Acacia senegal* (Linne) and related species. It consists chiefly of the calcium salt of arabic acid.

In addition to its pharmaceutical use as a suspending agent, acacia may be employed as a demulcent to treat inflammations of the throat or stomach. It should not be combined with atropine, apomorphine, cocaine, morphine or physostigmine since oxidizing agents in the acacia partially destroy these alkaloids.

Mold grows readily in acacia mucilages; thus older preparations should be carefully inspected before they are administered. Preservatives are usually added to these preparations.

CHONDRUS, N.F. (PEARL MOSS, ROCKSALT MOSS). Chondrus is the dried plant *Chondrus crispus* (Linne) or *Gigartine mamillosa*. It is usually used in pharmaceutical preparations as a suspending or emulsifying agent, but it may also be used topically as a demulcent.

Other demulcents that may be used for purposes similar to those mentioned previously include gelatin, glycerin and glycyrrhiza (licorice).

ASTRINGENTS

Astringents are protein precipitants that may be applied locally. Their action is limited primarily to cell surfaces and the surrounding interstitial environment because they can only slightly penetrate the cell. These agents form an impermeable layer on the surface to which they are applied, but the tissue remains viable.

Astringents tend to reduce edema of inflamed tissues, and they are employed to shrink swollen membranes of the mouth, throat and intestinal mucosa. Secretions are decreased and capillary bleeding is checked.

Many commercial antiperspirants exert their effects through an astringent action. Higher concentrations of astringents are employed in styptic pencils, which are used to arrest bleeding from small skin abrasions. In excessive concentrations these agents exert a caustic effect on the skin and mucous membranes.

Since bacterial protein is also precipitated by these agents they exert an antiseptic effect, but they are not employed topically as antiseptics, however, since more effective and less irritating agents are available.

The principal astringents contain salts of zinc, aluminum, lead, iron or bismuth. Tannins, permanganates, acids, alcohols, phenols and other chemicals are also used, but they tend to have more cell penetrability than do the salts of the heavy metals, and more toxic effects may be exhibited from their use as astringents.

ALUM, U.S.P., B.P. (ALUMEN). Both the ammonium and the potassium alums are commercially available with the respective formulas of $AlNH_4(SO_4)_2 \cdot 12H_2O$ and $AlK(SO_4)_2 \cdot 12 H_2O$. They are prepared from bauxite (a hydrated aluminum oxide) and sulfuric acid with the addition of either ammonium or potassium sulfate.

In solution, alum is a powerful astringent. Its antiseptic activity is due to protein precipitation and acid liberation in solution. It is employed in astringent lotions and douches and is used especially by athletes to toughen the skin. When fused with potassium nitrate, potassium alum is quite effective as a styptic pencil.

ALUMINUM PASTE, U.S.P. This official preparation contains 10 per cent aluminum powder in a base of mineral oil and zinc oxide ointment. It is used as a protective agent upon abraded skin and around ileostomy and colostomy apertures. The protective agent remaining on the skin should be thoroughly removed before reapplication.

The mineral oil provides an emollient effect, which increases its usefulness as a protective agent. Some authorities doubt that the aluminum powder exerts a measurable astringent effect in this preparation because of its extremely low solubility ratio, and they have attributed most of the therapeutic effects of this preparation to the zinc oxide ointment it contains.

ALUMINUM ACETATE SOLUTION, U.S.P. (BUROW'S SOLUTION). Aluminum acetate solution contains approximately 1.3 per cent aluminum acetate in aqueous solution. When diluted with 10 to 40 parts water, it is useful as an antiseptic mouthwash, gargle or dressing. It is weakly astringent and for this reason is often employed in dermatology to relieve pruritus from various skin conditions.

Upon exposure to air, these solutions deteriorate, as evidenced by the formation of an insoluble precipitate, aluminum subacetate, on the bottom of the bottle. If the formation of the precipitate is minimal, the supernatant liquid may still be used. The bottle should NOT be shaken before use, however. Excessive precipitation renders the solution unfit for use.

CALAMINE LOTION, U.S.P., B.P. Calamine consists of zinc oxide powder with a small amount of ferric oxide, which imparts a pink color.

The uses of calamine are very similar to those of zinc oxide. It is prepared chiefly in lotion form and is applied to the skin for its astringent and protective effects in the treatment of sunburn, poison ivy and various dermatoses.

HAMAMELIS WATER, N.F. (WITCH HAZEL). This hydroalcoholic solution is prepared from a distillate of the twigs of *Hamamelis virginiana* (Linne). Although the preparation is frequently employed as a topical astringent and antiseptic, its therapeutic value is due almost exclusively to its alcohol content, because the minute amounts of this volatile oil that are soluble have little if any effect.

TANNIC ACID, N.F., B.P. Tannic acid is a protein precipitant obtained commercially from nutgalls, which are produced on the young twigs of *Quercus infectoria* (Oliver) and similar species. The galls are formed during the development of the gall fly from eggs deposited in young leaf buds by the adult female.

Tannic acid is frequently employed in an alcoholic solution for the treatment of bedsores, and the powder may be applied topically to burned areas. It is absorbed systemically if applied to large denuded areas and liver damage is a frequent complication of absorption.

ZINC OXIDE OINTMENT, U.S.P., B.P. Zinc oxide is a mild astringent and antiseptic and is most often applied in ointment form for protection. It is used in the treatment of skin conditions, such as eczema, impetigo, psoriasis, ulcerations and ringworm.

ZINC OXIDE PASTE, U.S.P., B.P. (LASSAR'S PASTE). Zinc oxide paste differs from the ointment in that it contains slightly more zinc oxide. This renders it less pliable and less acceptable for many skin conditions. It is used when a more resistant protective action is desired.

COUNTERIRRITANTS

Counterirritants are agents that may be applied to unbroken skin to symptomatically relieve deeper pain. They induce surface vasodilation and a feeling of warmth, which stimulate superficial nerve endings and afford relief from deep-seated pain arising in the muscles or viscera.

These agents are used in the treatment of arthritis, bursitis, neuralgia and muscle pain.

METHYL SALICYLATE, U.S.P., B.P. (OIL OF WINTERGREEN). Methyl salicylate may be obtained naturally from the leaves of *Gaultheria procumbens* (Linne) or prepared synthetically. It is found in both gaultheria and betula oils and in many other plants.

It is often applied in liniment form for the relief of deep muscle pain. Care must be taken in its use, however, because salicylates are absorbed through the skin, and toxic reactions may occur.

Methyl salicylate is a frequent cause of poisoning, especially in children, because it smells very much like wintergreen candy.

Other counterirritants used for similar purposes are mustard plaster, iodine tincture, camphor liniment and chloroform liniment.

ANTIPRURITICS

Pruritus, or itching, routinely accompanies many dermatologic disorders. It may, however, be a symptom of another systemic disease, such as liver damage, in which case circulating bile salts cause generalized pruritus. Pruritus also accompanies allergic reactions, blood disorders and various psychological disturbances. Patients should be encouraged not to scratch. Their nails may have to be cut or mittens applied to prevent formation of open areas that can become infected. Secondary bacterial infections often occur as complications of pruritus and are treated with appropriate anti-infective agents.

Many simple antipruritics are effective because of their astringent properties, and mild astringents, such as aluminum acetate solution, calamine lotion and alcohol, are routinely employed for this purpose.

Both cool and hot wet dressings are used to relieve pruritus and are often applied to the skin for prolonged periods of time in severe dermatologic conditions. Cool water alone is somewhat effective in the relief of mild pruritus. Physiological saline solution also has some antipruritic effect. Solutions of cornstarch or milk are convenient and often used home remedies.

Nursing measures can be used in conjunction with drug therapy to reduce itching. Since the dilation of capillaries increases the itching sensation, hot baths, heavy bedclothing and rubbing of the skin should be avoided. Since scratching may cause skin breakdown and secondary infection, patients' nails should be trimmed and the use of mittens, or elbow restraints on children, may be needed. Hands and fingernails should be kept clean. Specially laundered or disposable nonallergenic linen may be needed.

Aveeno colloidal oatmeal. This commercial preparation may be used as a soothing, cleansing and antipruritic agent. It is recommended for itching, hives, sunburn, poison ivy, prickly heat, diaper rash, chafing and cleansing tender or soap-sensitive skin.

When used for a sitz bath or foot or hand bath, three or four tablespoonfuls of the preparation are added per each gallon of warm water. Ordinarily one cupful is sufficient for a tub bath. Care must be taken since it makes the tub surface slippery.

After soaking in the bath for 30 minutes to one hour, the patient's skin should be patted dry with a soft towel. It may be used to cleanse the skin by sprinkling the powder into moistened hands and adding water until a creamlike consistency is obtained. In this case it is used instead of soap.

Aveeno oilated oatmeal contains liquid petrolatum and a hypo-allergenic fraction of lanolin with the colloidal oatmeal. It is used to soften and lubricate taut, dry skin.

Alpha-keri oil. Alpha-Keri oil is a commercial preparation containing a dewaxed fraction of lanolin, with mineral oil and an emulsifier. It is especially prepared for the treatment of dry skin, and it may be rubbed over the entire body or added to bath water for its moisturizing effect. When used in the bath, two to four capfuls of the liquid are added to a tub of water.

Alpha-Keri is also useful as an antipruritic agent for simple dermatologic disorders.

ANTISEPTICS AND PARASITICIDES

The drugs in these classes are discussed in detail in Chapter 8 on topical anti-infectives. Some general rules for their application may be mentioned here, however.

Before application of these agents, the skin should be thoroughly cleansed with soap and water to remove as many topical infectious agents as possible. When the cationic surface active agents, such as benzalkonium chloride, are applied topically for their antiseptic effect, special care should be taken to remove all traces of soap from the skin, since soap neutralizes these agents and renders them ineffective.

Topical antibiotics

The topical antibiotics are discussed in Chapter 9. Many of the systemically acting antibiotics may be given orally or parenterally for the treatment of topical infections. Many antibiotic ointments and solutions are available commercially as well, however. The following preparations are commonly used topical antibiotics.

Bacitracin ointment. Although too toxic

to be administered systemically, bacitracin is quite useful as a topical antibiotic. It may be sold without a prescription for application to minor cuts and abrasions and should be applied two or three times daily. Bacitracin may also be used in the form of a solution for wet dressings, or it may be applied to wounds as a dry topical powder.

CHLORTETRACYCLINE SURGICAL POWDER (AUREOMYCIN). Chlortetracycline hydrochloride is prepared commercially as a dry surgical powder for direct application to wounds. It should not be introduced into closed spaces or cavities, however. The surgical powder is nonirritating to normal skin, but it may irritate denuded or damaged tissue, in which case local application should be discontinued. Each vial contains 5 Gm. of chlortetracycline hydrochloride with diluents of starch and magnesium oxide.

NEOMYCIN OINTMENT (MYCIGUENT). Like bacitracin ointment, neomycin ointment may be purchased without a prescription for topical application. It is irritating to denuded skin, however, and application should be discontinued if redness, irritation, swelling or pain persists or increases after the ointment is applied.

POLYSPORIN OINTMENT. This ointment contains both polymyxin B sulfate and bacitracin in a soluble ointment base. It may be purchased without a prescription for topical application.

NEOSPORIN OINTMENT. Neosporin ointment contains polymyxin B sulfate, bacitracin and neomycin in a soluble ointment base. This combination of three antibiotics is much more effective in combating topical infections than any one used singly. It may be purchased without a prescription. This combination is also prepared as a lotion, which may be more convenient to use in some dermatologic conditions.

NYSTATIN (MYCOSTATIN). Nystatin is prepared in both powder and ointment forms for topical application. In each case the preparations contain 100,000 units per Gm.

This antibiotic is particularly useful in the treatment of yeast and fungal infections and is specific therapy for all localized forms of moniliasis. Symptomatic relief is rapid and

often occurs within 24 to 72 hours after initiation of treatment.

The oral suspension of nystatin is often applied topically to the oral mucous membranes for the treatment of thrush. There need be no concern about swallowing the suspension since it may be administered orally for systemic use as well.

AMPHOTERICIN B LOTION (FUNGIZONE). Amphotericin B is quite useful in topical antifungal therapy and is prepared commercially in the form of a tinted aqueous lotion vehicle. The lotion is quite well tolerated by patients of all ages including infants, even when therapy must be continued for many months. It is usually not irritating, and very few cases of sensitivity have been reported.

DRUGS USED IN THE TREATMENT OF PSORIASIS

Psoriasis is a chronic, scaling skin condition that is characterized by well-circumscribed, slowly enlarging lesions most often on the scalp, above the elbows and knees, on the back and the anogenital area. The cause is unknown, but some investigators believe it to be of autoimmune origin.

Drug therapy does not cure psoriasis, but in many instances it alleviates the condition considerably. Topical medication is directed toward removal of the loose, epidermal scales over the lesions. Many preparations are keratolytic agents and may irritate the skin excessively if left on for a prolonged period of time. Preparations used in this way include 2 per cent salicylic acid with 10 per cent liquor carbonis detergens in ointment form, 5 per cent crude coal tar ointment or Baker's P & S liquid (for scalp lesions). In addition, topical corticosteroid preparations are beneficial. The dressings in this case are usually applied at night and covered with plastic wrap to provide an occlusive dressing.

Ultraviolet irradiation of affected areas is often quite helpful. It may be used alone or in combination with one of the keratolytic ointments previously described. The combination of irradiation and topical medications may cause regression of lesions that are resistant to other forms of therapy.

In addition, medicated cleansing agents may be used for adjunctive therapy to provide cleansing action with mild keratolytic activity. Polytar soap, Polytar shampoo and Polytar bath are three cleansing agents that contain juniper tar, pine tar, coal tar solution, polyunsaturated vegetable oil and a water-dispersible form of crude coal tar.

ANTIMETABOLITES

The mechanism of action of the antimetabolites in the treatment of psoriasis is not fully understood, but oral therapy with these antineoplastic drugs has produced excellent results. In addition to methotrexate, other agents, such as aminopterin sodium, mercaptopurine and thioguanine, have been employed, but they offer no particular advantages over methotrexate therapy.

METHOTREXATE. This folic acid inhibitor, in addition to being useful oral therapy for cancer, is effective in the treatment of psoriasis. It should not be employed until therapy with topical corticosteroids and other agents has proved ineffective, since it has an appreciable number of toxic side effects when taken over a period of time.

> **TOXICITY.** Since methotrexate has a very low therapeutic index, patients receiving therapy must be under constant supervision. The signs of toxicity are associated with folic acid deficiency and include bone marrow depression with leukopenia or thrombocytopenia as well as liver and kidney damage. Ulcerations of the oral mucosa, gastrointestinal disturbances, alopecia, precipitation of latent diabetes and temporary sterility may also result from the use of this drug. See Chapter 20 for a further discussion of toxic effects and nursing implications.

> **DOSE.** 2.5 to 5 mg. orally daily for six to ten days. After a rest period of one week the dose may be repeated as

necessary if toxic symptoms are minimal.

DRUGS USED IN THE TREATMENT OF ACNE

Acne is basically a disease of hypersecretion of sebum, which mixes with the keratin material of the external layer of epidermis forming keratin plugs. These plugs, combined with exogenous materials on the skin surface, form blackheads. Secondary infection of the blocked sebaceous gland produces the more severe pustular form of acne, which can leave permanent disfiguring scars.

The cause of acne is unclear, but it is suspected that hormonal imbalance may play a part, since the disease characteristically occurs at puberty. The general health of the individual is important, as are diet and cleanliness of the skin surface. The nurse can play an important role in providing emotional support and encouragement, as well as providing instructions in general health measures and hygiene.

Various systemic medications have been given clinical trial in the treatment of acne. The oral antibiotics are quite effective in small doses, but the risk of untoward effects often precludes their use for the duration of the skin eruptions. X-ray irradiation has been used successfully in some cases, but again it may not be employed for long periods of time.

Although local medications are only palliative therapy, they are usually the procedures of choice for acne. The skin should be thoroughly washed three or four times daily and followed by application of a lotion or cream with a drying or peeling effect.

CLEANSING AGENTS

BRASIVOL. This scrub-cleanser for the treatment of acne contains hexachlorophene, detergents and abrasive particles of fused synthetic aluminum oxide. Four types of Brāsivol are available, ranging from Brāsivol Base, which contains no scrub particles, to Brāsivol Rough, which contains the largest particles. The product used depends upon the sensitivity of the skin and the extent of the acneiform lesions. Ordinarily patients use the preparation with the smallest particles initially and progress to the one with the largest particles.

ACNE-AID DETERGENT SOAP. This soap is a blend of non-irritating detergents and fatty acids that produce an alkaline pH in solution. It should be used in warm water and the lather massaged into the skin with the fingers or a complexion brush. It is not a keratolytic agent, but is formulated exclusively to remove excess skin oil without undue irritation from strong detergents or perfumes found occasionally in toilet soaps.

PEELING LOTIONS AND CREAMS

Many commercial preparations that induce peeling of the skin are available. Often they are flesh colored so that they may be worn in the place of make-up base. Following are only a few of the preparations that may be used for this purpose.

ACNE-AID CREAM. This tinted cream contains sulfur, resorcinol, hexachlorophene and parachloro-meta-xylenol in a water-miscible base. It should be applied to the skin three or four times daily following cleansing.

BENOXYL LOTION. This lotion, which contains 5 per cent benzoyl peroxide, forms an invisible coating on the skin that aids in the desquamation of surface epithelium. It should be applied several times daily following cleansing.

Other preparations that may be used for this purpose are White lotion, Vleminckx solution, and 0.5 per cent salicylic acid and 5 per cent resorcinol in 70 per cent ethyl alcohol solution. All peeling agents should be applied with care, avoiding sensitive areas, such as the eyelids, mouth and neck, since these areas are readily irritated.

KERATOLYTICS

Many topical counterirritants and rubefacients are keratolytics if used in sufficiently high concentration. This local action causes the tissue cells to swell, then soften and desquamate.

TABLE 15 Commercial Anti-acne Preparations

PRODUCT	DOSAGE FORM	SULFUR	RESORCINOL	SALICYLIC ACID	HEXACHLORO-PHENE	OTHER INGREDIENTS
Acne Aid	cream	2.5%	1.25%	—	0.625%	para-chloro-meta-xylenol 0.375%
Acnederm	lotion	5% (dispersible)	—	—	—	bithionol 1% zinc sulfate 3% zinc oxide 10%
Acne-Dome	cream and lotion	4%	3% (mono-acetate)	—	1%	—
Acne-Dome	cleanser	2%	—	2%	1%	emulsifiers lubricants preservatives
Acnomel	cream	8%	2%	—	0.25%	alcohol 11%
Acnomel	cake	4%	1%	—	0.25%	—
Acnycin	cream	5%	2%	—	0.5%	tyrothricin* zinc oxide*
Bensulfoid	lotion	6%	2%	—	0.5%	zinc oxide 6% alcohol 12% powder consists of 33% sulfur in bentonite
Brasivol	cleanser	—	—	—	1%	aluminum oxide in neutral soap and detergents (fine, medium and rough)

*Quantitative amounts not shown on product examined.

Table 15 *continued on opposite page.*

TABLE 15 Commercial Anti-acne Preparations (*Continued*)

PRODUCT	DOSAGE FORM	SULFUR	RESORCINOL	SALICYLIC ACID	HEXACHLORO-PHENE	OTHER INGREDIENTS
Bradac	stick	1% (colloidal)	—	—	1%	fused aluminum abrasive in detergent base alcohol 30%
Cenac	lotion	8% (colloidal)	2%	—	0.25%	
Collo-sul	cream	2% (colloidal)	—	—	—	emulsion base
Comedab	stick	2%	1%	—	1%	detergent base
Fostex	cream and cake	2% (micro-pulverized)	—	2%	1%	Sebulytic (surface active cleanser in cream)
Ionax	aerosol	—	—	—	—	polyoxyethylene ethers benzalkonium chloride 0.2%
Klaron	lotion	5% (precipitated)	—	2%	0.5%	alcohol 13.1%
Komed	lotion	—	1%	1%	—	sodium thiosulfate 2% isopropyl alcohol 25% menthol* camphor* colloidal alumina
Liquimat	lotion	5%	—	—	—	alcohol 22%
Pernox	cleanser	2%	—	1.5%	1%	polyethylene granules Sebulytic (surface active cleanser)
pHiso Ac	cream	6% (colloidal)	1.5%	—	0.3%	alcohol 10%
Postacne	lotion	2% (colloidal)	—	—	0.5%	alcohol 29%
Proseca	cleanser	4%	—	—	1%	Liposec (poly-oxyethylene lauryl ether) 3% surface active cleansers alcohol 32%
Resulin	lotion	8%	4%	—	—	also available in ½ strength
Resulin	ointment	4%	2%	—	—	zinc oxide* talc* bentonite* iron oxides* washable cream base
Rezamid	lotion	5% (colloidal)	2%	—	0.5%	parachloro-metaxylenol 0.5% alcohol 28.5%
Secomat	lotion	5%	—	—	—	alcohol 25.2%
Sulforcin	cream and lotion	5% (dispersible)	3% (mono-acetate)	—	—	—
Vanoxide	lotion	—	—	—	—	chlorhydroxy-quinoline 0.25% benzoyl peroxide 5% calcium phosphate*

*Quantitative amounts not shown on product examined.
From the Journal of the American Pharmaceutical Association, Vol. N56, September, 1966.

Keratolytic activity is quite useful for the removal of warts, for corns, some dermatoses, acne and some fungal infections, such as athlete's foot.

SALICYLIC ACID, U.S.P., B.P. Unlike its salts and esters, salicylic acid is not used internally because of its locally irritating effect on the gastrointestinal mucosa. When it is applied locally to the skin, salicylic acid has a slight antiseptic action with a marked keratolytic effect. It is painless under ordinary circumstances and should be applied for a period of time for its full effect on thickened keratin.

Petrolatum should be applied to the normal skin surrounding the area to be treated with salicylic acid in order to prevent excessive irritation from the keratolytic agent. Contact with the eyes should be avoided since corneal damage may result. Salicylic acid is usually applied as collodion, lotions or ointments.

CONCENTRATION. 2 to 20 per cent.

SILVER NITRATE, U.S.P., B. P. In solution, silver nitrate is used as a caustic, antiseptic, germicide and astringent. It is also used to cauterize wounds and to speed the removal of warts, calluses, etc. In weaker solutions it is occasionally employed for irrigation of the bladder and uretha.

Since silver nitrate is especially effective against gonococci, most state laws require that a few drops of 1 to 2 per cent silver nitrate solution be dropped in the conjunctival sac of newborn infants to prevent ophthalmia neonatorum.

Silver nitrate is prepared in the form of caustic pencils and sticks that are used to cauterize various topical wounds, such as shaving cuts. It should be moistened with water before use. These applicators should not be used to cauterize the throat, however, since deaths have resulted from swallowing a silver nitrate impregnated cone. It is also used in dilute solutions as a germicide in the treatment of burns. Silver nitrate is discussed further in Chapter 8.

CONCENTRATION. 1:10,000 solution for bladder irrigation. 1 to 2 per cent solution in the eye. A 75 per cent concentration in caustic pencils.

ESCHAROTICS OR CORROSIVES

Escharotics produce death and sloughing of undesirable tissue. They may be employed to cauterize excessive scar or granulation tissue or to remove skin blemishes, birthmarks and other disfigurations.

Freezing is usually the method of choice for escharotic activity since it rarely leaves a scar and is a relatively painless procedure. Solid carbon dioxide (dry ice), liquid nitrogen and ethyl chloride have all been employed for this purpose.

Liquefied phenol has been applied to the face by rather unscrupulous operators to remove wrinkles. Even heavily wrinkled skin sloughs, leaving a smoother and more youthful complexion, but the amount of phenol that removes wrinkles is dangerously close to the amount that causes serious burns; the use of this compound for cosmetic purposes, therefore, is strictly prohibited.

QUESTIONS FOR DISCUSSION AND REVIEW

1. What topical preparation could be applied for the following dermatologic conditions:

a.	corns	e.	small shaving cuts
b.	warts	f.	diaper rash
c.	eczema	g.	heat rash
d.	bedsores	h.	dry skin

2. Define:
   a. astringent   d. antiperspirant
   b. demulcent   e. absorbent
   c. keratolytic

3. Are all ointment and cream bases equally effective when applied to both skin and mucous membranes? Explain the difference in absorption that may be expected when a drug is applied.

4. What is the basis for the application of topical drugs in the treatment of psoriasis? Are these agents curative?

5. Why are topical agents used in acne? Are these drugs curative?

6. What is the difference between curative and palliative drug therapy? Give an example of a topical drug that is both.

BIBLIOGRAPHY

Blank, I. H.: Action of emollient creams and their additives. *J.A.M.A., 164*:413, 1957.

Bozian, M. W.: Nursing care of patients having dermatologic conditions. *Amer. J. Nurs., 52*:873, (July) 1952.

Carney, R. G.: Topical use of antibiotics. *J.A.M.A., 186*:464, 1963.

Claudia, M., Sr.: TLC and sulfamylon for burned children. *Amer. J. Nurs., 68*:755, (April) 1968.

Demis, D. J. and Gass, H.: Treatment of psoriasis, lichen planus, seborrheic dermatitis. *Mod. Treatm. 2*:873, (September) 1965.

Rodman, M. J.: Drugs for treating skin infections. *R.N., 28*:77, (February) 1965.

Rodman, M. J.: Drugs used in skin diseases. *R.N., 31*:53, (March) 1968.

Rothman, S.: Drugs in cosmetics. *J.A.M.A., 178*:38, 1961.

Shafer, K. N., et al.: *Medical-Surgical Nursing.* 5th Ed. St. Louis, C. V. Mosby Co., 1971.

Shaw, B.: Current therapy for burns. *R.N., 34*:33, (March) 1971.

Smith, D. W., et al.: *Care of the Adult Patient.* 3rd Ed. Philadelphia, J. B. Lippincott Co., 1971.

Wechsler, H. L.: Psoriasis. *Amer. J. Nurs., 65*:85, (April) 1965.

Chapter 19 Drugs that Affect the Kidney and Body Fluid Composition

Important Concepts Discussed

1. *Normally the body maintains a homeostasis of body fluids. Water intake and output are delicately balanced.*

2. *Urine is produced by filtration of blood in the kidney glomeruli and subsequent partial reabsorption of the filtrate in the convoluted tubules.*

3. *Diuretics increase urine output by decreasing reabsorption of the filtrate in the convoluted tubules of the kidney.*

4. *Pharmacologic agents may be used to restore normal body fluid composition or to alter the cellular environment for therapeutic purposes.*

5. *Nursing observations should be directed toward evaluation of diuretic effects as well as indications of fluid and electrolyte disturbances.*

6. *Drug therapy and nursing intervention should be related to the total therapeutic regimen and the underlying pathophysiological condition of the individual patient.*

There is a fundamental rule that the organism maintains itself in equilibrium between ingestion and excretion of fluids. Adequate knowledge of the kidney and excretory functions as well as the roles of water balance and electrolyte balance is necessary before one can understand the methods by which drug therapy can correct or alleviate malfunctioning in this area.

WATER BALANCE

When the output of water from the body exceeds water intake, the body is in a negative water balance. This imbalance, which leads to dehydration, occurs characteristically in diarrhea, failure to drink an adequate amount of fluid and excessive perspiration. Conversely, a positive water balance occurs when the intake of water exceeds the output.

Positive water balance may occur during physiological growth or pregnancy, and it is believed to be a factor in muscular hypertrophy. Ordinarily, however, the healthy body maintains itself in a close water balance.

Water is furnished to the body by ingestion of fluids and water-containing foods as well as by metabolic oxidation of the hydrogen portion of food or body tissues. The average amount of water needed daily by an adult under conditions of typical temperature, humidity, diet and daily habits is 2500 ml.

Water is lost from the body chiefly in the urine, although larger amounts may be lost through the skin when there is excessive perspiration. Other important vehicles of water loss are expired air and feces. The latter may become a major factor in diarrhea or continual use of laxatives. The amount of water loss through the lungs and skin varies greatly with temperature, humidity and the amount of exercise performed.

Water may be lost through the skin by insensible perspiration, which occurs through moist skin by diffusion, or by sensible perspiration, which involves secretion of the sweat glands. Sweat, or sensible perspiration, consists chiefly of a weak, aqueous solution of sodium chloride, urea, potassium and lactic acid. The sodium may vary between 200 and 500 mg. per hundred ml., the pH between 4.2 and 7.5 and the specific gravity between 1.002 and 1.003. It is possible to lose 3000 ml. of water through the skin in 24 hours when both systems are active. A loss of 2000 ml. by sensible perspiration may include a loss of 10 Gm. of sodium chloride. For this reason, salt intake should be augmented in warm weather to avoid a serious electrolyte imbalance.

THE KIDNEYS

The basic function of the kidneys is to maintain the plasma volume and the total water content of the body. In addition, they regulate the osmotic pressure of body fluids by maintaining an optimal balance of the electrolytes in the plasma.

Body fluid concentrations of sodium, potassium, calcium, phosphorus and magnesium are maintained at constant levels by selective kidney excretion. Other substances, such as glucose, hormones and some vitamins, are excreted only if the threshold concentration in the blood is exceeded. In addition, waste products of metabolism, such as urea and creatinine, are excreted. In renal disease, the extent and duration of kidney damage can readily be assessed by measuring blood levels of urea or creatinine. Unless the kidney is damaged, it does not excrete proteins.

By altering the acidity and electrolyte balance of excreted urine, the kidneys aid in the regulation of the acid-base equilibrium of the body. This equilibrium is rapidly upset in kidney failure, and drugs that otherwise would cause no shift in the acid-base balance can cause serious metabolic disturbances in the event of kidney malfunctioning.

There are more than a million functional units, or nephrons, in each kidney. Each nephron is composed of a glomerulus (a tuft of capillaries enclosed in a two-layered cuplike structure called a Bowman's capsule) and a long convoluted tubule that terminates in a collecting duct. The proximal convoluted tubule begins at the glomerulus, extends to the loop of Henle, which widens into the distal convoluted tubule, and finally empties into the collecting duct.

The kidney is grossly divided into two layers: the outer, or cortex, and the inner portion, the medulla. The glomeruli and most of the tubules lie within the cortex, whereas the loops of Henle and the collecting tubules are mostly in the medulla. The ducts terminate in the renal pelvis, which is drained by the ureter into the bladder.

KIDNEY PHYSIOLOGY

Blood enters the kidney via the renal artery. This large vessel is subdivided into progressively smaller branches to the point at which there is one afferent arteriole for each glomerulus. Within Bowman's capsule the afferent arteriole divides into an intertwined group of tiny capillaries that recon-

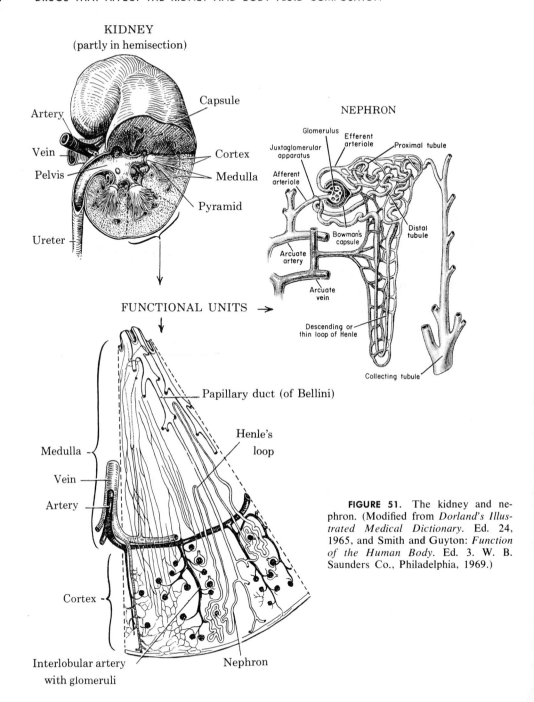

KIDNEY
(partly in hemisection)

NEPHRON

FUNCTIONAL UNITS →

FIGURE 51. The kidney and ne-phron. (Modified from *Dorland's Illustrated Medical Dictionary*. Ed. 24, 1965, and Smith and Guyton: *Function of the Human Body*. Ed. 3. W. B. Saunders Co., Philadelphia, 1969.)

verges to form the efferent arteriole, which leads from the capsule.

Within Bowman's capsule, blood filtrate, consisting chiefly of water and ions, passes across the capillary membrane and the inner lining of the capsule and enters the proximal convoluted tubule. Filtration occurs primarily because the capillary blood pressure exceeds the osmotic pressure, which would tend to hold fluid within the capillary. The net flow of fluid from the blood into Bowman's capsule is about 125 ml. per minute.

Much of this filtrate is reabsorbed into the blood as it passes through the proximal and distal convoluted tubules. This reabsorption is due primarily to the increased osmotic pressure of the blood in the capillaries surrounding these tubules as a result of fluid loss from the blood in the glomerulus, but additional fluid is resorbed because of tubular cell work. The tubular cells, by energy-expending enzymatic processes, can selectively remove substances from the tubular filtrate and return them to the blood. This active reabsorption often occurs against the osmotic gradient. Similarly, active tubular secretion can occur, and substances may be secreted into the tubular filtrate from the blood by action of these cells.

The importance of active reabsorption may be seen when diuretic agents such as the mercurials are administered, because these drugs act primarily on the tubular enzyme system to prevent active tubular transport of fluid and electrolytes back into the blood.

Because of the efficient functioning of the tubular transport system, only about 1 ml. of each 125 ml. filtered in the glomerulus per minute is actually excreted in the urine.

GLOMERULAR FILTRATION

If a substance is filtered through the glomerulus and is neither reabsorbed nor secreted by the tubules, it is possible to calculate the glomerular filtration rate simply by measuring the amount of the substance excreted in the urine per minute. Inulin is a polysaccharide that is neither reabsorbed nor secreted by the tubules, and it may be effectively used to measure the glomerular filtration rate. By use of this method, the glomerular filtration rate of 125 ml. per minute was derived. The renal clearance (or amount of substance excreted by the kidneys per minute) for inulin would then be 125. A substance with a renal clearance of 75 would be 60 per cent $\left(\dfrac{75}{125}\right)$ excreted in the urine, leaving 40 per cent to be reabsorbed by the capillaries.

ACTIVE TUBULAR SECRETION

Active tubular secretion may occur, as previously described, by enzymatic proc-

esses within the tubular cells. Renal clearance values greater than 125 would indicate that the substance, in addition to being filtered at the glomerulus, is actively secreted by the tubular cells. Some substances are secreted by the tubular cells only when they reach dangerously high levels in the blood. Under ordinary circumstances the glomerular filtration rate is sufficient to remove them from the blood.

REGULATION OF URINE VOLUME

The volume of urine excreted daily varies greatly and is largely under the influence of a posterior pituitary hormone, ADH (antidiuretic hormone). In circumstances that increase the osmotic pressure of the blood, such as dehydration or ingestion of excessive salt, the osmotic pressure-regulating center in the hypothalamus is stimulated and causes release of ADH.

This hormone greatly increases water reabsorption in the distal convoluted tubules; a decreased volume of highly concentrated urine is excreted in an attempt to conserve water and to restore the normal osmotic pressure of the tissue fluids.

REGULATION OF pH

The pH of the blood and tissue fluids must remain between 7.35 and 7.45, or serious systemic disturbances occur because of metabolic acidosis or alkalosis. The pH of the urine may vary easily from 4.8 to 8.0; excessive amounts of acid or base are readily excreted via the kidneys. Base is excreted primarily as bicarbonate, and hydrogen ions may be excreted as the ammonium ion or in the form of NaH_2PO_4.

DIURETICS

Diuretics are drugs that promote sodium and water excretion, and thus relieve the body of excessive extracellular fluid and edema. Diuretics may be divided into two general classes:

1. Physiologic diuretics, which increase the filtered load of sodium and chloride ions

or antagonize tubular reabsorption of sodium and chloride by means such as increasing the osmotic pressure of the tubular filtrate.

2. Pharmacologic diuretics, which are potent inhibitors of tubular reabsorption.

Physiologic Diuretics

The physiologic diuretics, because of their limited effectiveness in removing excessive extracellular fluid, are most useful as supplements to diuretic therapy with pharmacologic agents.

COLLOIDS

Colloids are diuretics solely because of their large particle size. These substances are not able to pass freely from the blood vessels to extracellular fluid; in order to equalize the osmotic pressure, fluid is drawn into the blood vessels from the extravascular spaces. This in turn increases blood volume and subsequently increases the glomerular filtration rate.

Diuresis based on increased glomerular filtration rate presupposes that the body is not able to reabsorb the increased amount of glomerular filtrate. This is not always the case, however, and these agents are quite unpredictable and relatively ineffective as diuretics.

Colloids such as albumin, dextran and gelatin have been used in the past as diuretic agents.

XANTHINE DIURETICS

The xanthines, caffeine, theobromine and theophylline, all have diuretic activity. Theophylline is the most potent of the three in this respect, and it is used chiefly in the form of a solubilized ethylenediamine salt.

THEOPHYLLINE ETHYLENEDIAMINE, U.S.P., B.P. (AMINOPHYLLINE). In addition to the previously mentioned uses of theophylline as a smooth muscle relaxant and myocardial stimulant, this drug has also been employed as a diuretic. Its mechanism of action is unknown, but it is believed to act primarily by dilating the afferent glomerular arterioles, allowing more blood to pass into the glomerular capillaries and subsequently increase the glomerular filtration rate. There is also an increased rate of sodium chloride excretion.

Theophylline is most useful as an adjunct to therapy with other diuretic agents, and it is often combined with digitalis and the mercurial diuretics in the treatment of congestive heart failure and cardiac edema. It is most effective as a diuretic when administered intravenously.

TOXICITY. Central stimulation, hyperexcitability, restlessness, leading to delirium and convulsions in overdosage. Cumulative effects may occur if doses are given more frequently than every 8 hours. Rapid intravenous administration may produce sudden and severe hypotension, ventricular fibrillation or cardiac arrest. For this reason the more concentrated intramuscular preparation containing 500 mg./2 ml. must never be used in place of the intravenous preparation containing 500 mg./20 ml. This intravenous dose must be administered very slowly. Oral administration may cause discomfort, nausea or vomiting.

DOSE. Oral—100 to 500 mg. three or four times daily. I.M.—500 mg. as required. I.V.—250 to 500 mg. injected slowly as required.

ACIDIFYING AGENTS

The acid-forming salts exert their diuretic effect by producing mild systemic acidosis. The kidneys, in an attempt to compensate and maintain a constant acid-base balance, excrete increased amounts of acidic ions accompanied by an increased amount of water. Only one acidifying agent, ammonium chloride, is currently used as a diuretic.

AMMONIUM CHLORIDE, U.S.P., B.P. Ammonium salts are acidifying agents because of the release of hydrogen ions following their conversion to urea in the liver. These hydrogen ions are incorporated into the bicarbonate buffer system, with a shift in the equilibrium toward the formation of carbonic acid. Carbon dioxide is excreted via the lungs to eliminate the excess carbonic acid from the body, and the sodium, which was formerly in the form of sodium bicarbonate, is excreted by the kidneys along with the chloride ions released during the degradation of ammonium chloride. It is during this excretion of sodium chloride by the kidneys that diuresis occurs. Within a few days, however, the kidney tubule cells are able to synthesize enough ammonia ions to excrete hydrogen ions in the form of the ammonium ion. When ammonium ion is excreted, it may replace sodium in the tubular filtrate, and body sodium stores may again be replenished.

Ammonium chloride is of little value as a diuretic after two or three days of administration. If the urine pH remains acidic, the drug is probably still effective. It is usually combined with the mercurials to potentiate their action

TOXICITY. Oral administration is usually in the form of enteric-coated tablets because of the gastric irritation, nausea and vomiting that may be produced by uncoated tablets. Ammonium chloride is contraindicated in kidney disorders, because of the possibility of producing uncompensated metabolic acidosis. Rapid intravenous injection may produce bradycardia, dyspnea and muscle twitching. It is usually diluted in at least 500 ml. of intravenous fluid when administered in this manner. Toxic effects are treated by the intravenous administration of sodium lactate or sodium bicarbonate.

DOSE. 4 to 12 Gm. daily orally or I.V.

Steroid antagonists

The steroid antagonists are competitive inhibitors of aldosterone, an adrenal cortical hormone that causes sodium retention and potassium excretion by the distal tubular cells.

Spironolactone, U.S.P., B.P. (Aldactone). Spironolactone, the only aldosterone inhibitor used in therapy at present, is an orally effective agent that increases sodium excretion as long as a sufficient amount of sodium is presented to the tubular cells and sodium is being reabsorbed by the action of aldosterone. It would obviously be of no benefit in an adrenalectomized patient.

spironolactone

Although spironolactone is only moderately effective when used alone, it is quite useful in combination therapy and is often administered with the thiazide diuretics to potentiate their diuretic activity but more important, to counteract the excessive potassium excretion that occurs with thiazide therapy.

Spironolactone is used in the treatment of cardiac edema, cirrhosis with ascites, the nephrotic syndrome and hypertension. Spironolactone has a specific, but unknown, antihypertensive action that is more potent than could be expected from its diuretic activity alone.

TOXICITY. Serum electrolyte balance is not usually disturbed except in patients with primary hyperaldosteronism. Sodium depletion may occur in liver failure with ascites because of the excessive excretion of sodium from the mobilization of ascitic fluid. Potassium retention is occasionally a problem when spironolactone is administered alone over a long period of time. It is contraindicated in renal diseases. Other side effects include headache, confusion, dermatitis, drowsiness, ataxia and abdominal pain.

DOSE. 100 mg. orally daily in four divided doses.

ALDACTAZIDE. Aldactazide is a commercially available tablet containing hydrochlorothiazide (25 mg.) and spironolactone (25 mg.). By combining these two drugs, more diuresis can be obtained than from either drug administered singly.

> **DOSE.** One tablet orally four times daily.

OSMOTIC DIURETICS

These substances are filtered by the glomeruli, but they are not completely reabsorbed by the tubular epithelium. They increase the osmotic pressure in the tubular filtrate, retaining water in the tubules and increasing urine flow. They have only limited use as diuretic agents because they are considerably less potent than the newer synthetic drugs.

UREA, U.S.P., B.P. (UREVERT). Although urea is a moderately effective osmotic diuretic when administered orally or intravenously, it is used only infrequently for this purpose since more potent and predictable drugs are available.

Urea is used clinically almost exclusively to reduce cerebral edema following trauma or hemorrhage, and it may be used routinely during intracranial surgery. Extravasation of this solution causes serious sloughing of tissue; it should be administered with care and the site of infusion checked carefully.

> **TOXICITY.** Headache, thrombophlebitis, thrombosis of the superficial and deep veins may occur even without extravasation of the solution and in sites far from the site of administration.

> **DOSE.** 40 to 90 Gm. intravenously as a 30% solution in 10% dextrose in water.

GLUCOSE, U.S.P. If the renal threshold of glucose is exceeded, it remains in the tubular filtrate, holding increased amounts of water and resulting in increased urine volume. Sodium and chloride excretion is slightly increased because of the increase in urine formation. Glucose is only moderately effective as a diuretic and is not used extensively at present.

> **TOXICITY.** Renal damage due to hyperglycemia.

> **DOSE.** 50 ml. of a 50% solution I.V.

Pharmacologic Diuretics

Pharmacologic diuretics in general are considerably more potent than physiologic diuretics because as they modify kidney function by inhibiting tubular ion reabsorption.

CARBONIC ANHYDRASE INHIBITORS

These diuretics inhibit the enzyme carbonic anhydrase, blocking the catalysis of the reaction:

$$CO_2 + H_2O \xrightarrow{C\text{-}A} H_2CO_3$$

Since the complete equilibrium involving this reaction is:

$$CO_2 + H_2O \underset{C\text{-}A}{\rightleftharpoons} H_2CO_3 \rightleftharpoons H^+ + HCO_3^-$$

when the enzyme carbonic anhydrase is inhibited, there is a tendency NOT to form carbonic acid and a consequent inavailability of the bicarbonate ion.

The bicarbonate ion, when present in the tubular fluid, conserves sodium by exchanging the sodium ion in the urine for hydrogen ion from the blood. The bicarbonate buffer system is necessary to maintain a stable acid-base balance in the body fluids.

When few hydrogen ions are available for sodium exchange, sodium is excreted in urine with the bicarbonate ion. Urine volume is proportionately increased when increased amounts of sodium bicarbonate must be excreted. Excessive excretion of bicarbonate depletes the basic reserve of the body, however, and a proportionate amount of carbon dioxide must be exhaled through the lungs to maintain a proper proportion of the buffering elements in the body.

In addition to their diuretic effects, the carbonic anhydrase inhibitors are beneficial in glaucoma, since this enzyme is needed for the formation of the intraocular fluid, aqueous humor. When carbonic anhydrase is inhibited, the formation of aqueous humor is appreciably decreased.

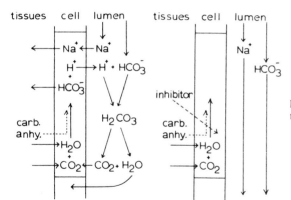

FIGURE 52. Action of carbonic anhydrase inhibitors on the excretion of sodium and bicarbonate in the urine.

ACETAZOLAMIDE, U.S.P., B.P. (DIAMOX). Acetazolamide, an analog of the sulfonamide drugs, is a carbonic anhydrase inhibitor without the antibacterial activity of the sulfonamides.

When acetazolamide is used alone, a tolerance is developed to its diuretic activity within a few days; it produces metabolic acidosis and the body becomes refractory to it by manufacturing increased amounts of ammonia in the tubular cells, which can then combine with the excess hydrogen ion, allowing sodium to be reabsorbed into the blood.

The exact site of action of this agent is not fully known. It has been shown to act in the proximal tubules, but it probably also acts along the length of the nephron tubule.

Acetazolamide is used in the treatment of cardiac edema, in preeclampsia, for premenstrual edema and as an adjunct in the treatment of glaucoma. It is moderately successful in controlling seizures in selected cases of grand mal and petit mal epilepsy that are refractory to other forms of therapy.

A duration of action of 8 to 12 hours is obtained following oral administration.

> **TOXICITY.** Drowsiness, mild paresthesias, excessive sodium or potassium loss, metabolic acidosis. It is contraindicated in nephritis, Addison's disease and liver disease.

> **DOSE.** Oral—250 to 500 mg. daily. I.V. —5 mg./kg. of body weight daily.

DICHLORPHENAMIDE, U.S.P., B.P. (DARANIDE). Also a carbonic anhydrase inhibitor, dichlorphenamide is much more potent than acetazolamide. The actions and side effects resemble those of other carbonic anhydrase inhibitors.

> **DOSE.** 25 to 100 mg. orally daily.

ETHOXZOLAMIDE (CARDRASE). The potency of ethoxzolamide is midway between that of acetazolamide and dichlorphenamide. Toxic effects resemble those of acetazolamide.

> **DOSE.** 62.5 to 125 mg. orally per day on alternate days.

THIAZIDE DIURETICS (BENZOTHIADIAZINE DIURETICS)

Although these drugs are carbonic anhydrase inhibitors, this activity is too weak to account for their entire diuretic effect.

The thiazides act directly on the kidney tubules, increasing excretion of sodium, chloride, bicarbonate and potassium. Chloride excretion is proportionately greater than bicarbonate excretion. There is therefore a tendency for hypochloremic alkalosis to occur upon prolonged therapy with these agents. It is believed that they exert their primary effect on the distal tubular ion exchange.

Thiazide diuretics are useful in the treatment of cardiac edema, particularly in patients who have become refractory to other diuretics. They are employed in the treatment of preeclampsia, premenstrual edema and sodium retention and edema associated with corticosteroid therapy.

In addition to mobilizing extracellular

fluid, the thiazides exert antihypertensive activity beyond that which could be explained by diuresis. They are not hypotensive in patients with normal blood pressure, but if given to hypertensive patients they lower blood pressure when used singly and potentiate the action of other antihypertensive agents in combination therapy. The precise mechanism of action in this regard has not as yet been determined.

TOXICITY. Hypochloremic alkalosis, cardiac arrhythmias and increased sensitivity to digitalis due to lowered potassium levels may occur. (Potassium depletion may be minimized by the inclusion of high potassium foods, such as oranges or bananas, in the diet.) Sodium and chloride depletion may become severe in patients on both restricted salt intake and thiazide therapy. Thiazides should be administered with caution to patients with hepatic cirrhosis or a history of liver malfunction. Uric acid excretion is diminished following thiazide administration, and a few attacks of gout have been precipitated during therapy.

Occasionally thrombocytopenia, leukopenia, agranulocytosis and aplastic anemia have been reported, along with gastrointestinal discomfort, dizziness and paresthesias.

CHLOROTHIAZIDE, N.F., B.P. (DIURIL). The first thiazide diuretic to be synthesized, chlorothiazide decreases the reabsorption of sodium, potassium and chloride ions, thus resulting in an increased urine output. It is less effective than the mercurial diuretics, however.

Chlorothiazide is used in the treatment of cardiac edema, hepatic cirrhosis, premenstrual edema and preeclampsia.

Oral administration is very effective; the parenteral form is reserved for instances in which the patient is unable to tolerate oral administration.

DOSE. Oral—0.5 to 1 Gm. once or twice daily. I.V.—0.5 to 1 Gm. as required.

chlorothiazide

HYDROCHLOROTHIAZIDE, U.S.P., B.P. (HYDRO-DIURIL, ESIDRIX, ORETIC). By hydrogenation of the parent compound, hydrochlorothiazide is rendered 10 times as potent as chlorothiazide, and it may thus be administered in smaller doses. Action and side effects are similar to those of chlorothiazide. It is available only for oral administration.

DOSE. 25 to 100 mg. orally once or twice daily.

BENDROFLUMETHIAZIDE (NATURETIN). By further alterations in the structure of chlorothiazide, it was possible to synthesize this compound, which is considerably more potent than hydroclorothiazide. Since bendroflumethiazide is more slowly metabolized than are many other thiazides, in some instances it may be administered in only one daily dose.

DOSE. 2.5 to 5 mg. orally daily.

FLUMETHIAZIDE (ADEMOL). The potency, action and effects of this fluorinated derivative of chlorothiazide are approximately the same as those of the parent compound.

DOSE. 0.25 to 1 Gm. orally daily.

HYDROFLUMETHIAZIDE, B.P. (SALURON, NACLEX). This hydrogenated derivative of flumethiazide bears the same relation to the parent compound that hydrochlorothiazide bears to chlorothiazide. There is also a tenfold increase in potency with this analog.

DOSE. 25 to 200 mg. orally daily.

METHYLCLOTHIAZIDE (ENDURON). Methylclothiazide is quite useful in the control of hypertension and may be administered alone or in combination with other agents for this purpose. Its diuretic action and side effects are similar to those of hydrochlorothiazide.

DOSE. 2.5 to 10 mg. orally daily.

TRICHLORMETHIAZIDE (METAHYDRIN, NAQUA).
This thiazide derivative has no particular advantage over the other available agents other than that it may be administered in slightly smaller doses. It may be used alone or in combination with other agents in the treatment of hypertension. Potassium loss may be slightly less with this agent than with some of the other thiazides.

DOSE. 2 to 4 mg. orally daily.

POLYTHIAZIDE (RENESE). Polythiazide is quite similar in action to trichlormethiazide. It may likewise produce less potassium loss than other thiazides.

DOSE. 1 to 4 mg. orally daily.

BENZTHIAZIDE (EXNA). The action and effects of benzthiazide are similar to those of hydroflumethiazide.

DOSE. 50 to 200 mg. orally daily.

CYCLOTHIAZIDE (ANHYDRON). Although the dosage of this drug may be smaller than for most thiazides because of its greater potency, it differs little in action and effects from the others.

DOSE. 1 to 2 mg. orally daily.

MERCURIAL DIURETICS

The mercurials were incidentally discovered to increase urine flow while they were being clinically tested in the treatment of syphilis. They are the most potent diuretic agents available. They were the mainstay of diuretic therapy until the early 1950's, at which time orally effective synthetic compounds became available.

They are generally believed to act in both the proximal and the distal tubule cells where the mercury ion is believed to replace sulfur in the sulfhydro enzyme molecule, thus interfering with enzyme transport necessary for the reabsorption of sodium ions. These agents increase potassium secretion either directly or indirectly by providing more sodium to exchange for potassium at the tubules. In any case, prolonged therapy is likely to produce hypokalemia if potassium levels are not carefully monitored during therapy.

Increased sodium, chloride and potassium excretion necessitates an increased urine volume; edematous fluids are thereby mobilized and excreted.

Because acidic urine is required for optimal activity of the mercurials, they are often administered in conjunction with acidifying diuretics, such as ammonium chloride. Any substance that tends to make the urine alkaline interferes with the diuretic action of the mercurials.

Although the mercurials are well absorbed when administered parenterally, they are only poorly absorbed from the gastrointestinal tract. Only one oral form is commercially available. The diuretic effect of these agents begins within a few hours following parenteral administration, reaches its peak in six to eight hours and has a duration of action of approximately 24 hours. They therefore should be given before noon so that the peak diuretic action does not occur at night.

The mercurials may be used in the treatment of cardiac edema, nephrosis and cirrhosis with ascites. They are not usually used for conditions in which only mild or moderate diuresis is required, because the orally effective agents are more convenient in these instances and are accompanied by less severe side effects.

TOXICITY. Unfortunately, the toxic effect of the mercurials is not confined to the sulfhydro enzymes of the renal tubules; enzyme interference occurs in other parts of the body as well. They are contraindicated in acute nephritis, ulcerative colitis, malignant hypertension, and should be used with caution in subacute and chronic kidney disorders. Since kidney damage may result from prolonged administration of mercurials, regular urinalyses should be performed and the mercurials discontinued if albumin, casts or blood cells appear in the urine. Cardiac effects occur following parenteral administration of the mercurials. They therefore should be administered with caution to patients susceptible to arrhythmias. Sudden cardiac fatalities have been reported following intravenous injections of these agents.

Sensitivity reactions include stomatitis, gastric distress, vertigo, febrile reactions, itching, dermatitis and agranulocytosis. Hypochloremic acidosis may result occasionally following prolonged diuresis with the mercurials because of excessive chloride loss.

With the exception of chlormerodrin, which is absorbed moderately well following oral administration, the mercurial diuretics must be administered parenterally. When administered subcutaneously or intramuscularly, edematous areas should be avoided since absorption of the drug will be impeded.

MERSALYL, N.F., B.P. (SALYRGAN). Mersalyl, the original mercurial diuretic, was at first administered both orally and parenterally, but since it is very poorly absorbed from the gastrointestinal tract, its use is essentially restricted to parenteral administration.

> **DOSE.** 100 mg. I.M., I.V. or subcutaneously once or twice weekly.

MERSALYL SODIUM AND THEOPHYLLINE, N.F., B.P. (SALYRGAN-THEOPHYLLINE). The combination of mercurial with xanthine diuretics is quite effective therapy. This preparation contains 100 mg. mersalyl and 50 mg. theophylline per ml.

> **DOSE.** 1 ml. I.M., I.V., or subcutaneously once or twice weekly.

MERALLURIDE INJECTION, U.S.P. (MERCUHYDRIN). Meralluride injection is often the mercurial of choice in the treatment of edema of congestive heart failure. It is most effective when administered intramuscularly; the intravenous route is considerably more dangerous because of the possibility of precipitating untoward reactions. Subcutaneous injection may cause pain and sloughing of tissue.

> **DOSE.** 1 to 2 ml. I.M., I.V. or subcutaneously once or twice weekly.

MERCAPTOMERIN SODIUM, U.S.P. (THIOMERIN). Mercaptomerin may be administered intravenously with somewhat less risk than can many of the other mercurial diuretics, since it is somewhat less prone to cause cardiac arrhythmias. If possible, it should be administered intramuscularly, however. Intravenous administration is necessary only for cardiac failure and pulmonary edema. Administration, particularly by the intravenous route, should be immediately discontinued if flushing of the face, fever, chills or urticaria develops since these are symptoms of serious sensitivity reactions to this drug.

Mercaptomerin should be refrigerated, and turbid or discolored solutions should not be used.

> **DOSE.** 0.2 to 2 ml. I.M., I.V. or subcutaneously daily.

MERCUMATILIN SODIUM (CUMERTILIN SODIUM). This combination of mercury and theophylline has an effectiveness comparable to that of mersalyl sodium and theophylline. It is administered parenterally primarily for the treatment of cardiac edema. One ml. contains 132 mg. mercumatilin with 50 mg. theophylline.

> **DOSE.** 1 ml. I.M. once or twice weekly.

CHLORMERODRIN, N.F. (NEOHYDRIN). Chlormerodrin is the drug of choice if a mercurial diuretic is to be administered orally. It is absorbed fairly well, but gastrointestinal symptoms occur in about 10 per cent of patients. It is sometimes administered with intermittent parenteral diuretics for potentiation of its action. Each tablet contains 18.3 mg. chlormerodrin (equivalent to 10 mg. mercury).

> **DOSE.** 18.3 to 36.6 mg. orally daily.

Miscellaneous Diuretics

ETHACRYNIC ACID (EDECRIN). Ethacrynic acid is a new diuretic compound that acts primarily on the ascending limb of the loop of Henle and on the proximal and distal portions of the tubule. Reabsorption of sodium and chloride is inhibited the entire length of the nephron tubule. Unlike thiazides, this compound does not effect an exchange of potassium for sodium in the distal tubules. Excessive potassium depletion does not occur. Because the effect is independent of the body acid-base balance, tolerance does not readily occur.

Water and electrolyte excretion may be several times greater than with thiazide diuretics and requires careful observation by the nurse and physician. The onset of action occurs within 15 minutes of intravenous injection and within 30 minutes following oral administration. Peak activity occurs in two hours, and the duration of action is six to eight hours.

Ethacrynic acid is useful in the treatment of patients refractory to other diuretics, in acute pulmonary edema, congestive heart failure, nephrotic syndrome, hepatic cirrhosis with ascites and other edematous states. Although it may be administered to children, it is generally believed to be too potent to administer to infants.

TOXICITY. It is contraindicated in anuria, increasing azotemia and progressive renal disease. It should be administered with caution to patients with advanced hepatic cirrhosis. It may produce diuresis too efficiently, with mobilization of too much fluid from extracellular tissues, resulting in hypotensive episodes and electrolyte depletion. It should always be administered in gradually increasing doses in order to assess the individual's response to the diuretic activity. Thrombophlebitis may occasionally occur following intravenous administration. Attacks of gout have been precipitated during therapy due to decreased uric acid secretion.

DOSE. Oral—50 mg. the first day, then increasing in 25 or 50 mg. increments until satisfactory diuresis is obtained. Maintenance dose may be as large as 400 mg. daily. I.V.—50 mg. (0.5 to 1 mg./kg. body weight). Usually only one dose is necessary, and the patient may be transferred to oral therapy. If a second I.V. dose is required, a new injection site should be chosen to minimize the possibility of thrombophlebitis.

FUROSEMIDE (LASIX). Like ethacrynic acid, this agent exerts diuretic effects on the ascending limb of the loop of Henle as well as on the proximal and distal tubules.

Onset of action following oral administration is within one hour, the peak effect occurs within the first or second hour and the duration of action is six to eight hours. This predictability of response is quite advantageous in diuretic therapy.

Like ethacrynic acid, furosemide is effective in refractory edema, in the presence of depressed glomerular filtration rates, in both acidosis and alkalosis and in the presence of electrolyte imbalance. Its uses and effects are quite similar to those of ethacrynic acid.

TOXICITY. Electrolyte depletion, skin reactions, blurred vision, postural hypotension, nausea, vomiting, diarrhea, weakness, fatigue, lightheadedness, muscle cramps, thirst and urinary frequency. A few cases of blood dyscrasias have been reported. Like ethacrynic acid, furosemide may precipitate attacks of gout.

DOSE. Oral—40 to 80 mg. daily. I.M., I.V.—40 mg. as necessary.

CHLORTHALIDONE (HYGROTON). The pharmacologic action of chlorthalidone closely parallels that of the thiazide diuretics. It causes sodium, chloride and potassium excretion, and like the thiazides, it may necessitate potassium replacement if therapy is prolonged. It is effective as an adjunct in the treatment of hypertension.

TOXICITY. Lightheadedness, nausea, vomiting and weakness, abdominal cramps, epigastric distress and skin rash. Potassium levels should be carefully monitored during therapy.

DOSE. 50 to 100 mg. orally daily.

QUINETHAZONE (HYDROMOX). The action and effects of quinethazone closely resemble those of the thiazide diuretics. It may be used for the treatment of mild to moderate edema and as an adjunct in the treatment of hypertension.

> **TOXICITY.** Dermatoses, nausea, vomiting, weakness, dizziness. Potassium levels should be monitored during therapy.
>
> **DOSE.** 50 to 100 mg. orally daily.

TRIAMTERENE (DYRENIUM). Triamterene is an orally administered agent that inhibits the exchange of sodium for potassium in the distal tubule independent of aldosterone. Potassium excretion is thus decreased. It is quite effective when given in combination with thiazide diuretics, since the potassium-conserving properties of this drug tend to balance the potassium depletion that regularly occurs with the thiazides. The tendency of this compound to preserve potassium is very important and useful in the treatment of digitalized patients, in whom potassium depletion may cause serious sensitization to digitalis.

Triamterene is used in the treatment of cardiac edema, cirrhosis with ascites, the nephrotic syndrome and preeclamptic states. It is also useful in steroid-induced edema due to electrolyte imbalance and sodium retention, and edema due to secondary hyperaldosteronism.

> **TOXICITY.** Triamterene is contraindicated in progressive kidney diseases and should be used with caution in the presence of liver failure. Nausea, vomiting, gastric distress, weakness, headache, dry mouth and skin dyscrasias have occurred during therapy.
>
> **DOSE.** 100 mg. orally once or twice daily.

AMISOMETRADINE (ROLICTON). Amisometradine is a pyrimidine derivative that has diuretic effectiveness between that of the xanthine derivatives and the mercurial diuretics. It inhibits the reabsorption of sodium ions by the distal tubular cells of the kidney.

Amisometradine is useful as adjunctive therapy in the treatment of cardiac edema, nephrosis and whenever mild to moderate diuretic action is desirable.

With continued administration, most patients tend to become refractory to this diuretic; it is most useful when employed in combination therapy.

> **TOXICITY.** Gastric irritation, nausea and vomiting.
>
> **DOSE.** 400 mg. orally four times daily.

Nursing Implications in Care for Patients Receiving Diuretics

In caring for the patient who is receiving a diuretic, the nurse should consider the underlying pathophysiology of the individual patient, and the type of action and desired effect of the diuretic used. Nursing observations should include evaluation of diuretic effect as well as side effects.

Since fluid loss is reflected in weight loss, the patient should be weighed before diuretic therapy is begun, and then his weight should be checked daily until the effect has stabilized. Weight checks two or three times a week are often continued throughout diuretic therapy.

There should be evidence of fluid loss based on the relief of the symptoms experienced by the patient before therapy was begun. The patient with left-sided heart failure should show indications of decreased dyspnea and rales, or other signs of pulmonary edema. A decrease in visible edema, such as in dependent areas in legs, feet and sacral area, should be evident in the person with right-sided heart failure. In the patient with ascites, the daily measurement of the abdominal girth may help to indicate relief.

Vital signs, especially the blood pressure, should be checked frequently, since the loss of fluid from the intravascular space may cause a decrease in blood pressure.

Accurate recording of the patient's fluid intake and output is essential in evaluating diuretic effect and fluid balance. The sodium intake of the patient may be restricted to some degree, and fluid intake may be restricted to decrease sodium and fluid retention.

Since most diuretics have the potential of disturbing the fluid and electrolyte and/or acid-base balance, the nurse should know the signs, symptoms and implications of the disturbance that is most likely to occur with the particular diuretic being used. When serum potassium levels are likely to be lowered by the action of a particular diuretic, the patient usually receives potassium supplements. These may be administered either in the form of a drug or by increasing the dietary intake of potassium-containing foods such as bananas or orange juice. Because imbalance of potassium can seriously affect cardiovascular function, the nurse should observe laboratory test results and the patient's symptoms indicating impending electrolyte imbalance. Patients who are also receiving digitalis glycosides should be carefully observed because of the increased sensitivity of the myocardium to digitalis when hypokalemia is present.

The time at which a diuretic is administered should be considered in relation to the length and peak of diuretic action of the particular drug. Whenever possible, administration should be scheduled so that the peak of diuretic action does not occur during the patient's sleeping hours.

The patient receiving a diuretic should be told that he will be experiencing increased urination. Bedpans and urinals should be readily available to the patient who must remain in bed.

Patients who are on diuretic therapy at home should be instructed in the correct administration of the drug, the importance of dietary prescriptions and the signs and symptoms he should report to his physician. Patients should be advised not to use salt substitutes without their physician's permission, since the substitutes are usually contraindicated if the patient has renal disease.

DRUGS USED IN THE TREATMENT OF GOUT

Gout is manifested by recurrent attacks of acute arthritic pain and swelling, usually involving a single joint, often the big toe. Gout is almost invariably associated with increased blood levels of uric acid, but these increased levels are apparently well tolerated by some individuals without symptoms or discomfort.

The swelling, erythema and pain of gout are associated with the deposition of needle-shaped microcrystals of monosodium urate monohydrate in the synovia of the joints or elsewhere in the body, and as tophi on the skin.

Acute attacks of gout may be temporary, but they may develop into the chronic form of the disease in which crystalline deposits become permanent and encysted and cause permanent disability. Low temperatures precipitate the urate crystals, which explains why the peripheral joints are almost exclusively involved in this disease.

Obese, overly well-fed individuals seem especially prone to attacks of gout but there is evidence of genetic predisposition in many hyperuricemic individuals. Attacks may also be precipitated by drug therapy (e.g., pyrazinoic acid, thiazides, furosemide and ethacrynic acid), chronic renal insufficiency and malignancies of the blood-forming tissues due to the rapid turnover of nucleic acids with the resultant increase in purine metabolism to uric acid.

Acute gouty arthritis may be treated with anti-inflammatory agents, such as colchicine, phenylbutazone or corticosteroids; hyperuricemia is specifically attacked with agents that promote urinary excretion of uric acid, such as probenecid or the salicylates; or the formation of uric acid from purine may be prevented by the use of an enzyme inhibitor, allopurinol.

Promotion of the patient's comfort is the main nursing goal during the acute attack of gout. The patient should be on complete bedrest with the affected joints in the position of comfort, usually a semiflexed position. Bed cradles should be used to keep the weight of the bedclothes off the affected area. Fluids should be forced especially when uricosuric therapy is begun, in order to prevent the precipitation of uric acid crystals in the urine.

After the acute attack has subsided, the goal becomes that of preventing a further attack. In addition to drug therapy, a diet low in purines is prescribed. Moderation in exercise is usually advised. Patients should also be advised to avoid fatty foods and alcohol, which may precipitate an acute attack.

PROBENECID, U.S.P., B.P. (BENEMID). Although probenecid is of little use in the relief of acute attacks of gout, it is often used in the prevention of recurrent attacks because of its uricosuric properties. Probenecid therapy should not be started during acute attacks of gout since it first prevents excretion of uric acid, and then prevents its reabsorption by the kidney tubules.

Probenecid should not be used with the salicylates, since the uricosuric ability is thereby inhibited.

probenecid

TOXICITY. Because precipitation of uric acid may occur in the kidney tubules, the urine should be made alkaline by adjunctive therapy, and large quantities of fluids should be ingested during therapy. Gastric irritation and skin reactions may occur.

DOSE. 500 mg. orally daily for one week, then the dose may be gradually increased to a maximum of 2 Gm. daily if necessary.

COLCHICINE, U.S.P., B.P. Although colchicine is extremely effective as an anti-inflammatory agent in the treatment of acute attacks of gouty arthritis, it is of little or no benefit in the treatment of other inflammatory conditions. Colchicine is not a uricosuric agent, and it is of no benefit in lowering serum acid levels. Its mechanism of action is unknown.

Colchicine is readily absorbed following oral administration. It is prepared for intravenous administration, but it may not be given intramuscularly or subcutaneously because of its locally irritating effects.

To be effective, colchicine must be given promptly at the first indication of an oncoming attack of gout, and the dosage must be adequate. Ordinarily the dose is gradually increased to the point at which the first toxic effects occur—usually diarrhea—then lowered slightly.

TOXICITY. Gastric irritation, nausea, vomiting, diarrhea. Interference with cell division of rapidly growing tissues, such as the gastrointestinal epithelium, and blood-forming tissues may result in melena or blood dyscrasias. Kidney damage may occur, resulting in oliguria or hematuria. When evidence of these serious toxic effects occurs, administration of colchicine should be immediately discontinued.

DOSE. Orally—0.6 to 1.2 mg. initially, followed by 0.6 mg. hourly until the pain is relieved or until nausea, vomiting or diarrhea is produced. I.V.—4 ml. followed by 1 ml. every six hours to effect.

PHENYLBUTAZONE, N.F. (BUTAZOLIDIN). Phenylbutazone is an anti-inflammatory agent (see Chapter 11) that is effective in the treatment of gouty arthritis. It has the double advantage of being effective in the alleviation of acute attacks of gout, along with the ability to function as a uricosuric agent. Phenylbutazone also causes sodium retention. Salt intake and serum sodium levels must be monitored closely during therapy.

Many patients are not able to tolerate the untoward effects of this drug. It is not used routinely in the treatment of gout, but it is usually reserved for patients who have not responded to other agents.

TOXICITY. Nausea, vomiting, diarrhea, hepatitis, kidney damage, dermatoses, hypertension and psychotic episodes have been observed. The most serious effect, however, is the tendency to cause severe and even fatal blood dyscrasias.

Peripheral blood smears should be taken regularly during therapy. Peptic ulcers occur frequently with administration, and perforation is occasionally a problem.

Phenylbutazone is contraindicated in patients with cardiac insufficiency, a history of peptic ulcer, blood dyscrasias or hepatic or renal dysfunction.

DOSE. 300 to 600 mg. orally initially in three or four divided doses, then 100 to 200 mg. daily.

OXYPHENBUTAZONE (TANDEARIL). Oxyphenbutazone was originally synthesized with the hope that it would be more specific than phenylbutazone in the treatment of gout and associated inflammatory conditions, but have fewer serious side effects. This has not proven to be the case clinically, however, and oxyphenbutazone resembles phenylbutazone almost exactly in action, effects and toxic reactions.

DOSE. 300 to 600 mg. orally initially in divided doses, then 100 to 200 mg. daily.

ALLOPURINOL (ZYLOPRIM). Allopurinol, only recently released for clinical use in the treatment of gout, is effective in the prevention and treatment of gouty arthritis because of its metabolic inhibition of the enzyme xanthine oxidase, which is necessary for the formation of uric acid from purine.

It is currently the drug of choice in the treatment of gouty arthritis in patients who are resistant to or intolerant of uricosurics, in gouty patients with recurrent uricolithiasis or otherwise impaired renal function and in the prevention of attacks of gout during accelerated purine metabolism in neoplastic diseases.

TOXICITY. Because acute attacks of gout may be precipitated during the first months of therapy, colchicine is often prophylactically administered with allopurinol at the onset of therapy. Dermatoses, fever, nausea, vomiting, diarrhea and intermittent abdominal pain have occurred during therapy. Leukopenia and peripheral neuritis have been noted in a few cases.

DOSE. 100 mg. orally three times daily after meals. Maximum recommended dose is 800 mg. daily.

ALKALIZING AGENTS

Alkalizing agents are used to treat acidosis, a condition caused by depletion of bicarbonate, which is the basic reserve of the blood. In many cases, alkalizing agents may be taken orally, but in more severe cases they may be injected intravenously. Caution must be taken in administering these drugs, because an overdose leads to an equally serious condition, alkalosis.

SODIUM BICARBONATE, U.S.P., B.P. (BAKING SODA). Sodium bicarbonate is used for its alkalizing effects in the treatment of acidosis and for alkalizing urine. Sodium bicarbonate is a systemic antacid that quickly neutralizes gastric hydrochloric acid and gives rise to systemic alkalosis. It is often given routinely with the sulfonamide drugs to render the urine alkaline and thus to reduce the risk of crystalluria.

Intravenous preparations are unstable when exposed to heat or air.

DOSE. 4 Gm. orally initially, followed by 1 to 2 Gm. every 4 hours.

SODIUM CITRATE, U.S.P., B.P. Upon entering the body, sodium citrate is converted to sodium carbonate, which appears in the urine. It is used to alkalize the urine and to restore the body's bicarbonate reserve. A diuretic action is noted upon administration of sodium citrate because water must accompany the salt in the urine.

TOXICITY. When given in excess, sodium citrate may produce alkalosis and may cause tetany or depression of the heart because of removal of calcium ions from the blood.

DOSE. 1 to 2 Gm. orally every 2 to 4 hours.

SODIUM LACTATE, U.S.P., B.P. One liter of $\frac{1}{6}$ molar sodium lactate solution is equivalent in acid-neutralizing effect to 340 ml. of 5 per cent sodium bicarbonate solution. The complete conversion of sodium lactate to bicarbonate requires one to two hours.

Sodium lactate is used in the treatment of acidosis due to sodium deficiency resulting from diarrhea, vomiting, starvation, uncontrolled diabetes mellitus, acute infections or renal failure. It should be administered with caution to prevent metabolic alkalosis.

> **TOXICITY.** Sodium lactate should not be used in acidosis associated with congenital heart disease with persistent cyanosis, and it is contraindicated in patients with respiratory alkalosis.

> **DOSE.** 60 ml. of the ⅙ molar solution/kg. of body weight I.V.

AMMONIA DETOXICANTS

Ammonia detoxicants are useful and even lifesaving in acute and chronic hepatic failure. In these conditions, the liver is unable to metabolize ammonia into urea, with resultant greatly increased serum ammonia levels in which the patient becomes comatose, moribund and exhibits the characteristic flapping tremor when the wrist is hyperextended quickly. A sharply decreased protein intake should accompany therapy with ammonia detoxicants, along with vigorous oral antibiotic therapy and cathartics to reduce the number of urea-splitting microorganisms in the gastrointestinal tract. No ammonium salts (such as ammonium chloride) should be administered to a patient with liver failure. Thiazide diuretics are equally dangerous since the release of ammonia occurs when they are metabolized.

ARGININE HYDROCHLORIDE (R-GENE); ARGININE GLUTAMATE (MODUMATE). Both arginine and glutamic acid are effective in reducing blood ammonia content, presumably by accelerating urea formation from ammonia through modifications in normal metabolic pathways of urea synthesis.

Although arginine tends to produce systemic acidosis, glutamic acid tends to produce alkalosis, and these two agents combined in arginine glutamate result in ammonia-reducing activity with minimal effect on the acid-base balance of the body.

Arginine derivatives are useful in the treatment of ammonia intoxication due to hepatic failure, but they are not recommended for the management of liver disorders in which blood levels of ammonia are not elevated because they produce no changes in the liver.

> **TOXICITY.** Because acidosis may occur with arginine hydrochloride, it should be administered with extreme caution to patients with kidney as well as liver disorders. Arginine elevates blood urea, creatine and creatinine levels. In kidney malfunction, therefore, these metabolic byproducts may reach toxic levels. Rapid infusion of both arginine derivatives may produce vomiting. Occasional irritation at the infusion site has been reported.

> **DOSE.** 20 to 25 Gm. I.V. every 8 to 12 hours.

SODIUM GLUTAMATE (GLUTAVENE). Sodium glutamate, when administered alone, lowers blood ammonia levels by combining with the free ammonia to form the amide derivative, glutamine.

> **TOXICITY.** Systemic alkalosis may be produced. Electrolyte disturbances, resulting particularly in decreased serum levels of potassium, chloride and sodium, may occur and should be monitored carefully. Nausea, vomiting, flushing, excessive salivation and hyperventilation may occur following intravenous infusion. Like arginine, this drug should be administered with extreme caution to patients with renal dysfunction.

> **DOSE.** 1100 ml. of dilute solution I.V. over four hours.

REPLACEMENT SOLUTIONS

Blood is the best replacement for blood loss. However, there are times when a fresh blood supply is not available, or when the patient suffers from a fluid or electrolyte loss rather than from a loss of blood solids. Replacement solutions may then be administered orally or intravenously. They may be merely solutions of electrolytes, or a sugar, such as dextrose or fructose, may be added as a food supplement.

DEXTRAN, U.S.P. (EXPANDEX, GENTRAN, PLAVOLEX). Dextran, a polymer of glucose, has a molecular weight ranging from 25,000 to 200,000. It is used intravenously in the form of a 6 per cent solution in isotonic sodium chloride to increase the plasma volume and aid in the maintenance of blood pressure. It is not intended to be a substitute for whole blood or its derivatives, which are necessary to restore proteins to the blood.

A decrease in total serum protein and hematocrit values for 6 to 24 hours following injection of dextran is a characteristic effect due to the dilution of body fluids with this solution. When administered to patients in shock, dextran increases plasma volume, venous pressure and cardiac output.

TOXICITY. Although antigenic reactions have been noted following administration of dextran, it has a low incidence of side effects since it is slowly metabolized to usable glucose. Bleeding time may be prolonged and should be observed for, even after infusion has been completed.

DOSE. 500 ml. of a 6 per cent solution I.V. The rate of flow must be determined by the physician because of the danger of pulmonary edema.

SODIUM CHLORIDE, U.S.P., B.P. Sodium chloride in the form of isotonic, hypotonic or hypertonic solutions is employed to replace sodium and chloride ions lost from the body.

Isotonic sodium chloride solution, which has the same osmotic pressure as body fluids, contains 0.9 per cent sodium chloride. It is often given as an intravenous infusion. Hypotonic sodium chloride is used occasionally for the initial treatment of extracellular fluid volume deficit with an increased osmolar concentration. The hypertonic solution is used for the treatment of a volume deficiency with a reduction in osmolar concentration.

Dextrose is often combined with physio-logic saline solution, but since it is readily metabolized, it does not permanently increase the osmotic pressure of the body fluids, even if the solution is quite hypertonic when administered. A solution of 5 per cent dextrose in water is approximately isotonic with body fluids.

Enteric-coated sodium chloride tablets are ordinarily employed to replace summertime salt loss because this form tends to reduce gastric irritation produced by the direct contact of a concentrated salt solution with the gastric mucosa.

TOXICITY. Sodium chloride must be used with caution in the presence of congestive heart failure, circulatory insufficiency, kidney dysfunction or hypoproteinemia. It is administered by mouth whenever possible, but the oral route may be deleterious in cholera and in severe infantile diarrhea. Administration of too much sodium chloride may result in serious electrolyte disturbances with resulting retention of water, loss of potassium and aggravation of existing acidosis.

DOSE. The dose of sodium chloride and all intravenous replacement solutions is highly individualized, depending on the desired amount of electrolyte to be administered.

Oral—1 Gm. one to three times daily. I.V.—Solutions ranging from 0.2 to 3 per cent administered as necessary.

RINGER'S INJECTION, U.S.P. (ISOTONIC SOLUTION OF THREE CHLORIDES). Ringer's injection has an electrolyte content that more closely resembles body fluids than does isotonic sodium chloride solution. It is used for about the same purposes as isotonic sodium chloride solution, but it produces less sodium retention and edema in hypoproteinemic patients than does sodium chloride solution.

Each liter contains 8.6 Gm. sodium chloride, 0.3 Gm. potassium chloride and 0.33 Gm. calcium chloride.

RINGER'S INJECTION, LACTATED, U.S.P.; COMPOUND SODIUM LACTATE INJECTION, B.P. (HART-

TABLE 16   Common Disturbances of Body Fluid and Electrolyte Balance

DISTURBANCE	COMMON CAUSES	OBSERVE FOR:	TREATMENT AND NURSING IMPLICATIONS
Hypernatremia	Renal failure Diarrhea Rapid I. V. saline infusion Tracheobronchitis	Oliguria, central nervous system Dried mucous membranes High specific gravity of urine Elevated serum sodium	Treatment of underlying cause Careful regulation of I. V. rate Low sodium diet Observe for congestive heart failure, pulmonary edema, elevated blood pressure
Hyponatremia	Decreased sodium intake Excessive perspiration Intestinal loss of sodium from vomiting, gastric suction Renal disease Diuretics Adrenal insufficiency Excessive intake of water	Abdominal cramps, diarrhea Signs of shock Signs of dehydration Low serum sodium Low specific gravity of urine Low Na and Cl in urine	Treatment of underlying cause Oral salt tablets may be needed when excessive perspiration occurs Intravenous infusion of isotonic / hypertonic saline solution Can lead to hypokalemia and other electrolyte disturbances
Hyperkalemia	Renal failure or insufficiency Burns, adrenal insufficiency Rapid I. V. infusion of solution containing potassium	Oliguria or anuria Diarrhea, intestinal cramps Weakness, slow pulse Lowered blood pressure EKG changes and arrhythmias Elevated serum potassium	Can lead to cardiac arrest: have emergency drugs and equipment available Calcium gluconate I. V. Insulin and glucose I. V. Dialysis Exchange ion resins orally or rectally
Hypokalemia	Loss of intestinal fluids Diabetic acidosis, starvation Burns	Muscle weakness and tremors Paresthesias, flaccid paralysis Disorientation, anorexia Abdominal distention EKG changes Low sodium potassium	I. V. infusion with potassium chloride Dietary supplements (bananas, orange juice, Coca-Cola) Oral supplements (e.g., Kaon Elixir or potassium chloride) Can cause cardiac arrest: have emergency drugs and equipment available Sensitizes myocardium to effect of digitalis—observe for signs of digitalis toxicity
Hypocalcemia	Hypoparathyroidism Pancreatitis, peritonitis Intestinal fistulas, burns Massive subcutaneous infection Excessive absorption of citrated blood	Carpopedal spasms Muscle cramps Tingling of extremities Tetany, convulsions Positive Chvostek sign Low serum calcium Negative Sulkowitch urine test	Treat underlying cause Oral administration of calcium lactate or galactogluconate Increased dietary calcium Slow I. V. administration of calcium gluconate
Hypercalcemia	Hyperparathyroidism Excessive vitamin D when used in arthritis myeloma, and hyperparathyroidism	Hypoactive muscles Flank and bone pain Bone cavities on X-ray Elevated serum calcium Positive Sulkowitch urine test EKG changes Pathologic fracture	Treat underlying condition or cause Can cause undue myocardial relaxation and cardiac arrest by increasing effect of potassium on heart Check other drugs and diet for calcium content

MANN'S SOLUTION). By addition of sodium lactate, this solution reduces the preponderance of chloride found in Ringer's injection and more closely resembles normal body fluids. It is indicated in practically all cases of dehydration in which mild acidosis is present, in supportive therapy and in electrolyte deficiencies.

Each liter contains 6.0 Gm. sodium chloride, 0.3 Gm. potassium chloride, 0.2 Gm.

calcium chloride and 3.0 Gm. sodium lactate.

ORAL REPLACEMENT SOLUTIONS

Hypokalemia, or potassium deficiency, may occur under a variety of conditions, including prolonged intravenous feeding without potassium supplementation, diseases such as sprue in which absorption is greatly decreased, conditions in which there is excessive loss of potassium, such as diuresis with thiazides, renal disease, prolonged vomiting or diarrhea, or prolonged administration of corticosteroids. In a few rare congenital conditions, such as familial periodic paralysis, serum levels of potassium are decreased because of increased removal of potassium from the serum into tissue cells.

Symptoms of hypokalemia include anorexia, nausea, muscle weakness, depression, shallow respirations, irregular pulse, hypotension and alterations in the electrocardiogram tracing. It is especially important to maintain physiologic levels of potassium when the patient is receiving digitalis, since decreased serum levels greatly potentiate the effects of digitalis and may even result in cardiac arrest.

Potassium may be administered orally as well as intravenously for the treatment or prevention of hypokalemia. Foods high in potassium content, such as oranges and bananas, may be given as dietary supplements.

TABLE 17   Common Disturbances of Acid-Base Balance

DISTURBANCE	COMMON CAUSES	OBSERVE FOR:	TREATMENT AND NURSING IMPLICATIONS
Respiratory Acidosis	Any decrease in expiration of carbon dioxide as in pneumonia, congestive heart failure asthma, suppression of respiratory center by drugs or disease Excessive breathing of carbon dioxide	Tachycardia, cyanosis, disorientation, weakness, coma, respiratory embarrassment Urine pH below 6.0 Plasma pH below 7.35 Plasma bicarbonate above 29 mEq/L. (25 in child) Elevated pCO_2 and serum sodium Normal or low serum chloride	Treat underlying conditions or cause Assess respiratory rate, depth, volume report and decrease Insure clear airway Observe for electrolyte disturbances Cautious use of oxygen
Respiratory Alkalosis	Increase in rate and depth of breathing as in: fever, anxiety, hysteria, intentional overbreathing, anoxia from high altitudes, central nervous system disease	Unconsciousness, convulsions, tetany Urine pH above 7.0 Plasma bicarbonate below 25 mEq/L. (20 in child) Low plasma pCO_2	Treat underlying cause or condition Observe rate, depth, character of respirations Observe for other electrolyte disturbances Precautions for convulsions
Metabolic Acidosis	Excess I. V. saline infusion Thyrotoxicosis, systemic infection Any condition causing use of fats and protein in place of carbohydrate (e.g., diabetes mellitus, starvation—drug toxicity: salicylates, ammonium chloride, paraldehyde) Excess loss of intestinal fluids Renal disease	Rapid, deep breathing, weakness Malaise, stupor, coma Urine pH below 6.0 Plasma bicarbonate below 25 mEq/L. (20 in child) Plasma pH below 7.35 Decreased pCO_2	Treat underlying cause I. V. sodium bicarbonate (or p.o.) I. V. glucose to provide carbohydrate I. V. fluids Maintain adequate airway so that carbon dioxide can be exhaled Observe urine output
Metabolic Alkalosis	Excess ingestion of sodium bicarbonate Vomiting and loss of HCl Potassium deficiency from diuretic therapy	Hypertonic muscles, tetany Slow shallow respirations, irregular pulse Delirium, personality changes Urine pH above 7.0 Plasma pH above 7.45 Plasma bicarbonate above 29 mEq/L. (25 in child) Increased pCO_2	Treat underlying cause Slow I. V. ammonium chloride possible (or p.o.) I. V. physiologic saline Potassium replacement if needed Observe for electrolyte imbalance

POTASSIUM GLUCONATE (KAON). Although this flavored preparation has a rather unpleasant, salty aftertaste, it produces little or no gastric distress upon oral administration and may be administered routinely as an oral potassium supplement. It contains 20 mEq. potassium per 15 ml. solution, which should be given well-diluted in order to prevent a saline cathartic effect.

DOSE. 30 ml. (40 mEq.) orally daily.

POTASSIUM TRIPLEX. This oral solution contains equal parts each of potassium acetate, potassium bicarbonate and potassium citrate and provides 15 mEq. potassium per 5 ml. of solution. It may be used prophylactically and postoperatively for oral potassium replacement therapy. The unpleasant taste is minimized if the solution is administered in fruit juice or broth.

DOSE. 5 ml. (15 mEq.) orally three times daily.

IRRIGATING SOLUTIONS

The solutions in this category are used topically; although they may enter body orifices for irrigating purposes they are not intended to cross body membranes or to be taken internally since many are quite toxic.

ACETIC ACID, U.S.P., B.P. Acetic acid may be used as a bladder irrigation solution in conditions involving hemorrhage or cystitis. The low pH of this solution renders it valuable as an antiseptic, especially when ammonia-forming bacteria are present. It is also of value in the dissolution of bladder calculi.

CONCENTRATION. 0.25 to 1 per cent solution.

MAGNESIUM AND SODIUM CITRATES (SUBY'S SOLUTION "G"). Magnesium and sodium citrates solution is used for bladder irrigation, especially in patients with permanent catheters, to dissolve urinary calcium composed of calcium phosphate, calcium carbonate or magnesium ammonium phosphate.

The solution contains 32.3 Gm. citric acid, 3.8 Gm. magnesium oxide and 4.4 Gm. sodium carbonate per 100 ml.

RENACIDIN. Renacidin is a powder used to prepare buffered acidic solutions which are employed to irrigate indwelling urethral catheters for the purpose of preventing the formation of urinary calculi. It is not used to dissolve calculi composed entirely of oxalates, urates, uric acid or cysteine, since the solution cannot dissolve these salts; it is useful in preventing their formation, however.

TOXICITY. Use of the solution should be discontinued if pain or a burning sensation occurs. Death may result if the solution is instilled above the bladder into the ureters or kidneys; thus it is contraindicated for this purpose. It is likewise contraindicated for use in the treatment or prevention of biliary calculi.

CONCENTRATION. 5 to 10 per cent solution.

PERITONEAL DIALYSIS SOLUTIONS (DIANEAL, INPERSOL, PERIDIAL). Although peritoneal dialysis involves minor surgery, it is a relatively simple method for removing toxic substances from the blood. It is used to treat poisoning in cases in which toxic compounds have been ingested, to remove metabolites in renal failure and to correct certain electrolyte and fluid imbalances.

In peritoneal dialysis the dialyzing fluid is allowed to remain in contact with the peritoneal membrane, which it crosses by osmosis and diffusion.

The composition of the solutions used resembles the electrolyte composition of blood plasma except that potassium is omitted in most formulae because dialysis is often performed to correct hyperkalemia. Peritoneal dialysis with solutions containing 1.5 per cent dextrose may be indicated in the treatment of acute renal failure, uncontrolled hyperkalemia and oliguria in the presence of a rapid catabolic rate, overhydration or clinical deterioration in spite of good conservation therapy. It may also be indicated in renal failure of obscure origin when additional time is required to determine the cause of the failure.

A solution with identical concentration of electrolytes but with 7 per cent dextrose is used when dialysis is performed for the relief of intractable edema.

Peritoneal dialysis requires 24 hours to remove the amounts of metabolites that can be removed in six hours with the artificial kidney; nevertheless, in the absence of critical uremia, dialysis is often preferred to the artificial kidney.

In peritoneal dialysis, a trochar is inserted into the peritoneum through a stab wound incision in the mid-abdomen, 3 to 10 cm. below the umbilicus. This catheter is then connected to tubing which connects it to the dialyzing bottle. Two liters of dialyzing solution, which have been warmed to body temperature, are allowed to run in rapidly, usually within ten to twenty minutes. The flow should be steady. If it is not, this may indicate displacement of the catheter or blockage of the catheter by a clot. If siphoning is to be used to remove the fluid, it is essential that the flow be stopped before the infusion bottle is completely empty.

The fluid remains in the peritoneal cavity for 30 to 60 minutes. The fluid is then allowed to flow out; the output flow should be approximate in volume to the amount instilled. Firm pressure to the lower abdomen, or having the patient lift his head from the pillow, may help to increase outflow by increasing the intraperitoneal pressure. The outflow fluid is usually straw-colored, but may be blood-tinged initially.

The cycle is then repeated continuously for 12 to 36 hours. A total of 30 to 50 liters is usually exchanged.

The blood pressure and pulse should be carefully and frequently monitored especially during the initial exchanges. Hypotension may result from excess fluid loss, and arrhythmias may occur from changes in electrolytes.

Abdominal pain may occur at the end of inflow or outflow, but severe pain may indicate infection or the build-up of fluid and pressure in the peritoneal cavity due to incomplete drainage and should be reported to the physician.

The patient should be observed for respiratory difficulty which may be caused by pressure on the diaphragm. Slight elevation of the head of the bed may be helpful, but severe dyspnea should be reported. The patient should also be observed for bleeding, shock or leakage of fluid around the incision site.

Accurate recording is essential and should include: the amount and type of solution infused and returned; time of inflow and outflow; the number of exchanges; amount and type of other intake and output (oral, I.V., urinary drainage, etc.); weight of the patient before and after and any medications such as antibiotics or heparin added to the dialyzing solution.

Other supportive and preventive nursing measures are essential. The patient may be turned between exchanges, when fluid has been drained and before the next infusion. Nursing care should also include: Coughing and deep breathing; adequate oral fluid and nutritional intake unless contraindicated; skin and mouth care; active and passive exercise and explanation and psychological support.

A typical dialysis solution contains 142 mEq. sodium, 101 mEq. chloride, 3.5 mEq. calcium, 1.5 mEq. magnesium, 45 mEq. lactate, 1 mEq. bisulfite and 15 Gm. dextrose per liter.

ION EXCHANGE RESINS

Ion exchange resins are compounds administered orally to selectively remove ions from the gastrointestinal tract. Although they are intended to be specific, side effects occasionally result from removal of additional electrolytes.

SODIUM POLYSTYRENE SULFONATE, U.S.P. (KAYEXALATE). Sodium polystyrene sulfonate is a synthetic resin used in the treatment of hyperkalemia. In the gastrointestinal tract, sodium ions are exchanged for potassium, and the potassium resin is excreted in the feces. (One gram of resin is able to exchange about 3.1 mEq. of potassium.) Ordinarily, an osmotic laxative, usually 70 per cent sorbitol solution, is administered orally with the resin to hasten passage through the tract. It may also be given rectally as a retention enema. 30 Gm. is suspended in 200 ml. of 1% methylcellulose solution, 10% dextrose solution or 25% sorbitol solution. It should be retained for 6 to 10 hours, and then followed by a cleansing enema.

This resin is most useful in the treatment of hyperkalemia associated with kidney failure, but it may be used whenever it is desirable to lower potassium levels. It is ordinarily administered as an adjunct to other measures aimed at reduction of potassium levels, such as restriction of potassium intake, control of acidosis and an adequate caloric intake.

TOXICITY. Serious potassium deficiency may occur if the resin is administered in overdose or for prolonged periods of time. Potassium serum levels should be monitored daily during administration. Anorexia, vomiting and hypocalcemia may occur.

DOSE. 15 Gm. orally one to four times daily with 10 to 20 ml. of 70 per cent sorbitol solution.

CARBACRYLAMINE RESINS (CARBO-RESIN). Carbacrylamine resins are a mixture of cation and anion exchangers that are useful in the oral therapy of hypernatremia. They are most useful in sodium retention due to kidney dysfunction, but they may be used as adjunctive therapy in the treatment of congestive heart failure, cirrhoses with ascites and the nephrotic syndrome.

Diuretic therapy and restriction in sodium intake should accompany therapy with these resins.

TOXICITY. Hyponatremia, hypocalcemia, systemic acidosis, gastric discomfort, anorexia, nausea, vomiting and fecal impaction.

DOSE. 16 Gm. in 6 oz. of fluid orally three times daily.

CHOLESTYRAMINE RESIN (CUEMID). Cholestyramine resin is a basic anion exchange resin that is administered orally to aid in the removal of bile acids from the gastrointestinal tract.

It is indicated as an adjunct in the treatment of pruritus associated with cholestasis, which is due to the increased concentration of bile acids in the blood and is an extremely uncomfortable though minor complication of hepatic disorders.

TOXICITY. Hypochloremic acidosis, hypoprothrombinemia due to an induced vitamin K deficiency, hypocalcemia, osteoporosis, diarrhea, nausea, constipation and impaired absorption of food and other orally administered medications.

DOSE. 4 Gm. orally three times daily for at least two weeks, then increased to 16 Gm. daily if necessary.

SALT SUBSTITUTES

SODIUM-FREE SALT (CO-SALT, DIASAL, NEO-CURTASAL). A number of other salts may be used as seasoning agents for patients with sodium restricted diets, particularly in the treatment of congestive heart failure, hypertension, arteriosclerosis, toxemias of pregnancy, steroid therapy and edema resulting from sodium imbalance. They usually contain potassium chloride, other potassium salts, glutamic acid and other agents to enhance flavor.

TOXICITY. Sodium-free preparations should not be used in the presence of severe renal insufficiency accompanied by oliguria or anuria or elevated sodium and potassium serum levels. They should be used with caution in mild renal insufficiency. Patients should be advised to obtain their doctor's permission before using salt substitutes.

DOSE. As desired.

GUIDE FOR NURSING ASSESSMENT OF A PATIENT RECEIVING A DIURETIC

I.   Why is the patient receiving a diuretic? What is the underlying pathophysiology resulting in the need for a diuretic?

II.   What is the action or mechanism of the diuretic? Is sodium restriction necessary or ordered? If so how great? Is fluid restriction also necessary?

III.   Administration: When it is administered—does peak of action interfere with sleep? If given I.M., are sites rotated? Are areas where edema is present avoided?

IV.   Observation for effect: Is there any reduction of edema in the legs, ankles, sacral area or other dependent areas of the body? Is there any decrease in dyspnea and/or rales in lungs? Has there been any weight loss? Has urinary output increased relative to intake? Has the abdominal girth decreased?

V.   Observation for side effects: Does the patient have any signs and symptoms of fluid and electrolyte imbalance, especially the particular imbalance that is apt to result from this particular diuretic? Are potassium supplements (drug or dietary) needed? What other drugs is the patient receiving which may affect this drug's action? What diseases and conditions may affect or be affected by this drug's action on the patient (e.g., diabetes, patient receiving digitalis)?

VI.   What are the patient's learning needs? Does the patient understand the purpose of the drug? Does he understand that urination will be increased and when it will occur? Does he know that his urine is to be measured and recorded? If the patient is taking the diuretic at home, does he understand when to take the drug, the fluid and sodium restrictions, potassium supplements, signs and symptoms he should report to the physician?

QUESTIONS FOR DISCUSSION AND REVIEW

1.   What symptoms would you expect in a patient who has had a negative water balance for five days?

2.   Why should salt tablets be taken during a hot summer?

3.   Explain osmosis. How does it apply to kidney function?

4.   What symptoms would the patient experience from an overdose of a mercurial diuretic?

5.   Define or explain:
   a.   renal clearance
   b.   glomerular filtration
   c.   hypokalemia
   d.   renal threshold
   e.   ion exchange resins
   f.   nephrosis

6. Explain the mechanism of action of the antidiuretic hormone (ADH).

7. Explain the procedure used for peritoneal dialysis. What is the difference between this procedure and the use of the artificial kidney? When is each used? What observations should the nurse make? What are her responsibilities?

8. Which diuretics are apt to cause the following: What are symptoms of each?
    a. hypokalemia
    b. hyperkalemia
    c. hyponatremia
    d. metabolic acidosis
    e. metabolic alkalosis

9. Select a patient who is on diuretic therapy. Outline a teaching plan for that individual patient.

BIBLIOGRAPHY

Abbott Laboratories: *Fluid and Electrolytes*. Chicago, The Laboratories, 1967.

AMA Drug Evaluations. Chicago, American Medical Association, 1971.

Brunner, L. S., et al.: *Textbook of Medical–Surgical Nursing*. 2nd Ed. Philadelphia, J. B. Lippincott Co., 1970.

Burgess, R. E.: Fluids and electrolytes. *Amer. J. Nurs., 65*:90, (October) 1965.

Dent, M. J.: Administration of diuretics. *Nurs. Mirror, 128*:41, (June 27) 1969.

Early, L. E.: Diuretics. *New Eng. J. Med., 276*:966, (April) 1967.

Early, L. E. and Orloff, J.: Thiazide diuretics. *Ann. Rev. Med., 15*:149, 1964.

Evarts, C. M.: Low molecular weight dextran. *Med. Clin. N. Amer., 51*:1285, 1967.

Falconer, M. W., et al.: *The Drug, the Nurse, the Patient*. 4th Ed. Philadelphia, W. B. Saunders Co., 1970.

Goodman, L. S. and Gilman, A.: *Pharmacological Basis of Therapeutics*. 4th Ed. New York, Macmillan Co., 1970.

Gorlin, R.: Mercurial diuretics and edema. *J.A.M.A., 192*:468, 1965.

Goss, C. M. (ed.): *Gray's Anatomy of the Human Body*. 28th Ed. Philadelphia, Lea and Febiger, 1966.

Goth, A.: *Medical Pharmacology*. 3rd Ed. St. Louis, C. V. Mosby Co., 1968.

Govoni, L. E. and Hayes, J. E.: *Drugs and Nursing Implications*. 2nd Ed. New York, Appleton-Century-Crofts, 1971.

Grollman, A.: Diuretics. *Amer. J. Nurs., 65*:84, (January) 1965.

Heller, H.: Toxicity of diuretics. *Practitioner, 194*:56, 1965.

Lapides, J., et al.: Clinical signs of dehydration and extracellular fluid loss. *J.A.M.A., 191*:413, (February) 1965.

Levitt, M. F. and Goldstein, M. H.: Mercurial diuretics. *Bull. N. Y. Acad. Med., 38*:249, 1962.

Liddle, G. W.: Aldosterone antagonists and trimeterene. *Ann. N.Y. Acad. Sci., 139*:466, 1966.

Lowe, C. A.: Principles of parenteral fluid therapy. *Amer. J. Nurs., 53*: 963, 1953.

Metheney, N. and Snively, W.: *Nurses' Handbook of Fluid Balance.* Philadelphia, J. B. Lippincott Co., 1967.

Milne, M. D.: Renal pharmacology. *Ann. Rev. Pharmacol., 5*:119, 1965.

Moravec, D. F.: When in doubt—ask the pharmacist about the action of drugs. The thyroid and diuretic drugs are discussed. *Hosp. Manage., 106*:69, (November) 1968

Mudge, G. H.: Renal pharmacology. *Ann. Rev. Pharmacol., 7*:163, 1967.

Nash, H. L., et al.: Cardiorenal hemodynamic effects of ethacrynic acid. *Amer. Heart J., 71*:153, 1966.

O'Neil, M.: Peritoneal dialysis. *Nurs. Clin. N. Amer., 1*:309–323, (June) 1966.

Pitts, R. F.: *Physiology of the Kidney and Body Fluids.* Chicago, Year Book Medical Publishers, Inc., 1963.

Reed, G. M., and Sheppard, V. F.: *Regulation of Fluid and Electrolyte Balance.* Philadelphia, W. B. Saunders Co., 1971.

Schneider, W. J. and Boyce, B. A.: Complications of diuretic therapy. *Amer. J. Nurs., 68*:1903, 1968.

Snively, W. D., Jr.: Toward a better understanding of body fluid disturbances. *Nurs. Forum, 3*:60, 1964.

Stahl, W. M.: Effect of mannitol in the kidney: changes in intrarenal hemodynamics. *New Eng. J. Med., 272*:381, 1965.

Voda, A. M.: Body water dynamics—a clinical application. *Amer. J. Nurs., 70*:2594, (December) 1970.

Walker, W. G.: The clinical use of furosemide and ethacrynic acid. *Med. Clin. N. Amer., 51*:1277, 1967.

Walker, W. G.: Indications and contraindications for diuretic therapy. *Ann. N.Y. Acad. Sci. 139*:481, 1966.

Watkins, F. L.: The patient who has peritoneal dialysis. *Amer. J. Nurs., 66*:1572, (July) 1966.

Chapter 20 Antineoplastic Agents

Important Concepts Discussed

1. *Neoplastic diseases are produced by uncontrolled cell division.*

2. *Antineoplastic drugs inhibit cell division or poison rapidly multiplying cells.*

3. *No known pharmacologic agent is a completely effective cure for cancer; at best remissions of the disease are obtained for relatively short periods.*

4. *Cytotoxic effects and rapidly acquired resistance to antineoplastic drugs limit their effectiveness in the treatment of cancer.*

5. *Nursing measures to alleviate the unavoidable side effects of these drugs are essential.*

6. *The psychological and emotional support of the patient during the therapy is an important aspect of the nursing care.*

Since cancer now accounts for one of every seven deaths in the United States, the search for more effective treatment of this disease has attained greater proportions than ever before.

The causes of cancer are at best poorly understood. Papanicolaou's discovery and the subsequent development of cytological studies have shown that, at least with cervical cancer, the cellular appearance changes years before the appearance of invasive cancer with metastases. Improved public education in the importance of yearly Papanicolaou smears of the cervical mucosa has done much to decrease mortality from this common form of female carcinoma.

The notion that cancer originates in a single cell that suddenly grows wild is now being replaced by the theory that there may be many foci, and indeed a large part of the tissue or organ of origin may be involved in various precursor stages long before the disease is discovered. This theory has been furthered by studies of the bronchial epithelium in cigarette smokers, which have shown that aberrant changes in the cells of the epithelium are present much more commonly than in nonsmokers. There is also the factor of individual susceptibility to cancer, which may be based on genetic or inherited factors. The reasons many persons can smoke cigarettes for 40 or 50 years without developing cancer, if indeed the tars in cigarette smoke are proved to be the causative factor, will have to be explained on the basis of some as yet undiscovered genetic or environmental factor.

The ultimate control of cancer, as for any disease, is in its prevention. Studies of the natural occurrence of cancer have already demonstrated many ways to prevent the disease. The greatly increased incidence of cancer of the scrotum among chimney sweeps, bladder cancer among aniline dye workers, skin cancer among individuals such as sailors and farmers who are exposed to excessive amounts of sunlight and dentists who get carcinoma in the fingers that they use to hold x-ray film in the mouth have given many clues to the possible causative factors of cancer.

Since 1911 when Rous showed that cell-free filtrates of chicken sarcoma produce tumors in other chickens, research has been directed toward a viral etiology of tumors in man. It seems likely that some types of carcinoma in humans may be produced by viruses, but many believe these are in the minority partly because of the lack of evidence for contagious forms of cancer. It is probable that cancer is a spectrum of many diseases with a variety of predisposing causes.

Surgery and radiation have long been the primary weapons used against cancer, but because of delayed diagnosis and early metastases of many tumors, the incidence of five-year survival is still alarmingly low.

This potentiality for early infiltration of cancer has led workers to search for a pharmacologic agent that could attack cancer at any site in the body. The effectiveness of antineoplastic drugs at present is still somewhat limited. Apparent total regression of some tumors, however, has occurred following drug therapy.

In general, the antineoplastic agents are cytotoxic. Cancer cells divide rapidly. They therefore have a higher metabolic rate and are dependent upon their environment for a constant supply of nutrients and the materials necessary to replicate their nucleic acids in order for mitotic cell division to take place. Many antineoplastic agents are directed toward inhibiting this cell division. This property also accounts for their high incidence of toxic effects, however, since the body has many tissues that of necessity must divide and replicate fairly rapidly. The early effects of drug toxicity become evident first in these rapidly proliferating tissues, such as the bone marrow, lymphoid tissue, gastrointestinal epithelium, oral mucosa, gonads and hair follicles.

In order to obtain optimal systemic response to the antineoplastic drugs, they are often given to the point of systemic toxicity, so that the effective dose and the toxic dose may overlap, in the hope that the tumor cells will recover more slowly than will the non-malignant cells. Nursing measures to alleviate the discomfort of the side effects are important to the success of the therapy.

No antineoplastic drug is effective against all types of cancer, and none is capable of uniformly and predictably inducing a remission in any specific neoplasm. Although a considerable amount of scientific data has been acquired regarding the susceptibility of various tumors, drug therapy must of necessity be trial-and-error in many cases. At most, these drugs must be considered to be palliative rather than curative agents, and the apparent cures obtained with a few of these drugs must be considered to be a happy exception to the rule. In most cases, resistance develops to the drug long before the tumor is brought under adequate control.

CLASSIFICATION OF ANTINEOPLASTIC DRUGS

The drugs used in the treatment of malignant disorders may be classified into five general groups:

1. *Alkylating Agents*—which transfer alkyl groups (side chains) to molecules within the cells. They probably attack the nucleoproteins that are essential for cellular metabolism and cell division.

2. *Antimetabolites*—which interfere with normal metabolism of cells because they are structurally similar to substances required for metabolic processes.

3. *Hormones*—which inhibit growth of tumors of the reproductive organs by creating an unfavorable environment. They are also used as an adjunct to therapy for other neoplasms.

4. *Radioisotopes*—which destroy or inhibit cells by radioactive particle emission.

5. *Miscellaneous drugs*—which include antineoplastic agents that do not fit into any of the specific classes.

SPECIAL METHODS OF ADMINISTRATION

Methods of administering antineoplastic drugs have been developed to allow large doses to be given at the cancer site and to reduce the systemic side effects produced by these drugs. One method is local perfusion of the involved area by the drug. In perfusion, the arterial supply and venous return of the involved area, i.e., femoral artery and vein of the lower extremity, are separated from the systemic circulation. The antineoplastic drug is then perfused into the artery through the local circulation to the cancerous area. After administration is completed, the local circulation is then rejoined to the systemic circulation.

Another method is intra-arterial infusion. A catheter is placed into the artery that supplies the cancerous area. The antineoplastic drug is then administered by infusion. Because of the greater pressure of the arterial blood, fluids do not flow into the arterial circulation by gravity as they do in intravenous infusion. A special pump forces the fluid and drug into the artery. The physician sets the rate at which the pump functions, but the nurse should check it frequently.

Several serious complications can occur with intra-arterial infusion. Hemorrhage from the artery can be a rapid and serious complication, in which case pressure should be applied until the physician arrives. An air embolus is another serious complication. The infusion fluid should never run through completely, and the tubing should be clamped if an air bubble is discovered. Because hemorrhage occurs if tubing is disconnected between the pump and the patient, the physician should be notified if the tubing contains an air bubble. The tubing should also be checked frequently for kinks. The patient with an intra-arterial catheter requires constant supervision in order to prevent and detect possible complications. Vital signs should be checked frequently.

ALKYLATING AGENTS

The primary reaction of alkylating agents is the replacement of the hydrogen ion in a reacting substance with an alkyl group. The alkylating agents are chemically unstable because of the formation of carbonium ions; the injectable forms must be reconstituted just before administration. In the body, the unstable carbonium ions react readily with groups, such as amines, hydroxyl and phosphate groups, that are found in many enzymes and other substances essential for normal as well as abnormal cellular growth. These agents have a high degree of toxicity in the human body.

The exact site of action within the cell has not been accurately determined, but the alkylating agents are believed to react primarily with the nucleoproteins of the cell and selectively with the phosphate groups of deoxyribonucleic acid (DNA), producing an altered chemical compound that is unable to replicate satisfactorily to permit cell division. The alkylating agents produce a biochemical response similar to that of irradiation of living cells.

The alkylating agents are used primarily in neoplasms of hematopoietic and reticuloendothelial tissues and induce remissions in some cases of lymphosarcoma, Hodgkin's disease, chronic myelogenous and lymphatic leukemias, polycythemia vera and mycosis fungoides.

MECHLORETHAMINE HYDROCHLORIDE, U.S.P., MUSTINE INJECTION, B.P. (NITROGEN MUSTARD, MUSTARGEN). An analog of the poisonous mustard gas used in World War I, mechlorethamine is a polyfunctional agent that is most effective as an adjunct to x-ray therapy

$$H_3C-N\begin{array}{c} CH_2CH_2Cl \\ CH_2CH_2Cl \end{array}$$

mechlorethamine hydrochloride

of inoperable or widely metastatic carcinoma and in Hodgkin's disease, lymphosarcoma, bronchogenic carcinoma, chronic lymphatic and myelocytic leukemias and mycosis fungoides.

In addition to the intravenous route, mechlorethamine may be used for intracavitary and intra-arterial administration. The route chosen obviously depends upon the site and type of malignancy. Intra-cavitary administration may be used in the treatment of pleural, peritoneal or pericardial effusions as the result of metastases. Excessive fluid is partially removed from these cavities prior to instillation of the drug. Side effects of intracavitary administration are not as severe as those noted with systemic administration, but considerable pain may be produced at the site of infusion.

TOXICITY. Mechlorethamine is an extremely toxic drug because of its uncontrolled reactivity and effects on normal as well as malignant tissues. Care should be taken when preparing this drug for administration, since it is a powerful vesicant. Nurses and doctors should wear rubber gloves when handling this drug. If contact with the skin occurs, the area should be irrigated immediately with large amounts of water.

When administered intravenously, it may produce thrombosis or thrombo-phlebitis. Extravasation causes pain, swelling, erythema, induration and sloughing, which may be minimized by prompt infiltration of ⅙ molar sodium thiosulfate solution and application of ice compresses for at least 12 hours. Normal saline may be used if sodium thiosulfate is not available.

Nausea and vomiting occur one to three hours after intravenous administration and may persist for 24 hours or more. Following intracavitary administration, the nausea, vomiting and diarrhea may persist for two or three days. In both cases, the administration of chlorpromazine alone or with a barbiturate prior to and after administration of mechlorethamine may minimize the gastrointestinal complaints.

Perhaps the most serious toxic effects are those upon the blood-forming organs. Reduction of lymphocytes occurs within hours of administration,

followed by a general decrease in the number of circulating red and white blood cells and platelets. This may be followed by multiple hemorrhages in various parts of the body and hyperuricemia due to cellular destruction. Large amounts of fluid should be ingested to prevent urate deposition in the kidneys.

The gonads are particularly susceptible to the effects of this drug; amenorrhea may follow therapy for several months. Impaired spermatogenesis, skin eruptions, weakness, drowsiness, headache, fever, tinnitus, deafness, alopecia, and in a few cases, aphasia and paresis have been observed.

Because of the toxicity and unpleasant side effects observed with this drug, it is not ordinarily employed in patients with terminal carcinoma; the beneficial effects would not be expected to outweigh the toxic symptoms.

Solutions of the drug decompose rapidly; it should be prepared immediately prior to injection and any unused portion should be discarded immediately.

DOSE. I.V.—0.1 mg./kg. daily for four successive days. Six weeks should elapse between courses to allow return of hematologic function. Intracavitary —0.4 mg./kg. of body weight.

BUSULFAN, U.S.P., B.P. (MYLERAN). The chief advantage of busulfan is that, on oral administration, it is more selective than other alkylating agents in its effect on the blood-forming cells; it is therefore used primarily in the treatment of chronic granulocytic (myelocytic) leukemia. It is not curative, but it produces remissions in a significant number of patients. It is not effective in the treatment of acute granulocytic, lymphoblastic or monocytic leukemia.

Busulfan should be stored away from light and in a tightly closed container.

TOXICITY. Depression of bone marrow may produce agranulocytosis and thrombocytopenia with concurrent hemorrhagic tendencies. These toxic effects may not become apparent for four to six months; blood counts should be taken weekly for this period. Amenorrhea, anorexia and skin reactions have been observed.

DOSE. 2 to 6 mg. orally daily until maximal hematologic and clinical improvement is attained, then the dose is reduced to 1 to 3 mg. daily.

CHLORAMBUCIL, U.S.P. (LEUKERAN). Also a potent depressant of the blood-forming tissues, chlorambucil has a slightly wider range of effectiveness than does busulfan. It is used in the treatment of chronic lymphocytic leukemia, malignant lymphomas and Hodgkin's disease. It is administered only in the form of oral tablets and should be taken one hour before breakfast or two hours after the patient's evening meal.

TOXICITY. Weekly blood counts should be taken to avoid irreversible bone marrow depression. Since the effects of this drug are potentiated following the use of other cytotoxic drugs and radiation therapy, it should not be administered sooner than four weeks after these other agents are discontinued. Gastrointestinal symptoms are uncommon with chlorambucil, but anorexia, nausea and vomiting may be observed with large doses.

DOSE. 4 to 10 mg. (0.1 to 0.2 mg./kg. of body weight) orally daily. Maintenance dose is usually 2 to 4 mg. daily.

CYCLOPHOSPHAMIDE, N.F. (CYTOXAN). Unlike nitrogen mustard, cyclophosphamide is inert when placed in contact with living cells in culture. It is theorized, therefore, that cyclophosphamide is activated in the body, probably by formation of an active ammonium ion after cleavage of the cyclic phosphorus-nitrogen or phosphorus-oxygen bonds of the molecule. Since the phosphamidase enzymes responsible for this cleavage are present in greater amounts in cancerous tissue than in normal tissue, cyclophosphamide has a somewhat selective action on tumor cells.

It is of value in the treatment of Hodgkin's disease, multiple myeloma, chronic lymphocytic and granulocytic leukemias, monocytic leukemia, breast and ovarian carcinoma, neuroblastoma and mycosis fungoides.

Since it is not a vesicant, it may be administered orally, intravenously, intramuscularly, intraperitoneally, intrapleurally or directly into the tumor. When given orally, it is preferably given on an empty stomach, unless gastric upset necessitates giving it with meals. It should not be administered to patients with preexisting bone marrow depression since the effects are additive.

TOXICITY. Serious bone marrow depression, nausea, vomiting, diarrhea, anorexia, weight loss, dizziness, blurring of vision, mental changes, fever and mucosal ulceration have been observed. Alopecia also occurs, but hair growth usually returns in two or three months, even when the drug is continued. The patient may need to be reassured.

DOSE. Parenteral—3 to 5 mg./kg. of body weight I.V. twice weekly. Oral—100 to 250 mg. daily.

THIOTEPA, U.S.P. (THIOPHOSPHORAMIDE). Thiotepa is a synthetic compound chemically related to nitrogen mustard, which releases ethylenimine radicals that affect dividing cells. It may be administered orally, intravenously, intra-arterially, intramuscularly or directly into malignant tissue in the treatment of adenocarcinoma of the breast or ovary, lymphoma and sarcoma. It has been used with varying success in chronic granulocytic and lymphocytic leukemias, in Hodgkin's disease and carcinoma of the lungs, gastrointestinal tract, genitourinary tract and central nervous system.

It has a slow onset of action, and several weeks may elapse before the results of therapy become evident. For this reason its value is limited in far-advanced cases.

The solution of the drug should be used immediately after preparation.

TOXICITY. Bone marrow depression

leading to lymphopenia, granulocytopenia and thrombocytopenia. Nausea, vomiting, anorexia, headaches, fever, allergic reactions, amenorrhea and decreased spermatogenesis may be observed. It is contraindicated in pregnancy.

DOSE. Oral—60 mg. once weekly, or less as determined by the white count. I.V.—30 mg. once weekly, or less as determined by the white count.

TRIETHYLENEMELAMINE, N.F. (TEM). Triethylenemelamine is closely related in action and effect to nitrogen mustard, its chief advantage being that it may be administered orally as well as parenterally.

TEM has been used in the treatment of chronic lymphatic leukemia and leukolymphosarcoma, Hodgkin's disease, polycythemia vera, carcinoma of the lung and mycosis fungoides.

> **TOXICITY.** Bone marrow depression, anorexia, vomiting, diarrhea, headache and weakness. The maximal evidence of bone marrow depression may not occur until two or three weeks after the last dose is administered; weekly blood counts should be taken during this time.

> **DOSE.** Oral—2.5 to 5 mg. daily. The dose should be administered with water and at least 2 Gm. ($\frac{1}{2}$ teaspoonful) of sodium bicarbonate one hour before breakfast. (Total dose should not exceed 150 mg.) I.V.—total dose of 5 to 20 mg. administered over several days.

MELPHALAN (ALKERAN, L-SARCOLYSIN). Melphalan is an orally active drug that is useful in the treatment of multiple myeloma. Its effectiveness in other neoplastic diseases is variable.

Clinical improvements are not usually evident for several weeks after initiation of treatment with this drug, but pain is often relieved long before this.

> **TOXICITY.** Severe bone marrow depression, nausea, vomiting, dermatoses, alopecia and neurologic symptoms have been observed.

DOSE. 6 mg. orally daily. Treatment should be continued for two to three weeks and then discontinued for as long as four weeks while weekly blood counts are taken. Another course of therapy may be instituted when the hematopoietic system returns to normal.

ANTIMETABOLITES

This group of antineoplastic agents includes the folic acid, purine, pyrimidine and glutamine antagonists. Because of their similarity to essential metabolites, they exert their pharmacologic effects by interference with the normal physiological actions of these metabolites in living cells. Although metabolites are more concentrated in rapidly growing and dividing cells, such as tumor cells, the side effects of antimetabolites are directly related to interference with normal metabolic processes of the body.

FOLIC ACID ANTAGONISTS

In man, folic acid *per se* is metabolically inactive. It is reduced in the tissues to tetrahydrofolic acid, which serves as a cofactor by adding one-carbon fragments to its molecule and subsequently releasing or transferring them in various metabolic synthetic processes, including the synthesis of purines and the conversion of deoxyuridine to thymidine in the synthesis of deoxyribonucleic acid.

Folic acid antagonists inhibit the enzyme that catalyzes the reduction of folic acid to the tetrahydrofolate form, and in this manner they block purine and thymine syntheses and inhibit the formation of DNA, which is essential to reproduction of tumor cells. These agents are of particular value in the treatment of leukemia. It may be that leukemic cells, because of their more active biosyntheses, are more readily affected by the deficiency of folic acid than are normal cells. Unfortunately, normal bone marrow and the rapidly dividing cells of the oral mucosa and gastrointestinal epithelium are also quite sensitive to a decrease in tetrahydrofolic acid, and toxic effects are often noted in these tissues. Calcium leucovorin, U.S.P. may be used as an antidote for folic acid antagonists. Resistance to the action of folic acid antagonists occurs eventually, and leukemic cells then become cross-resistant to other drugs in this classification.

METHOTREXATE, U.S.P. (AMETHOPTERIN). Methotrexate in 1958 accomplished the first medical "cure" of a solid malignant human tumor in the apparent total suppression of metastatic choriocarcinoma. It remains the drug of choice for this condition, but unfortunately total cures are in the minority.

It is also used in the treatment of acute lymphoblastic leukemia and produces remissions in 50 per cent of patients treated that may last many months. It is less effective in the treatment of acute monocytic and acute myelocytic leukemias. Two or three remissions may be obtained with this drug, but each succeeding remission is of shorter duration as the malignant cells eventually become resistant. It is also used in the treatment of lymphosarcoma in children and in some cases of neuroblastoma and Ewing's sarcoma in children. It is usually given orally in the treatment of these conditions, but intrathecal administration has been employed for a few selected brain tumors.

Methotrexate has been used in the treatment of psoriasis, but because of the serious toxic effects of this drug, it is reserved for severe cases in which palliative methods have proven to be unsatisfactory and the general health of the patient is good. It is also effective in the treatment of psoriatic arthritis, a common complication of this dermatologic condition. It has occasionally been used as an immunosuppressive agent following organ transplant.

> **TOXICITY.** Bone marrow depression with agranulocytopenia and thrombocytopenia. Therapy should be discontinued if bleeding occurs. Ulceration of the gastrointestinal tract, nausea, vomiting, diarrhea, anorexia, lassitude, alopecia, dermatitis and hyperpigmentation occur.

In case of an overdose of methotrexate, calcium leucovorin should be administered no later than four hours after the overdose.

> **DOSE.** As antineoplastic agent—5 to 10 mg. orally three times weekly. For psoriasis—2.5 to 5 mg. orally daily for 6 to 10 days followed by a rest period of 7 to 10 days.

PURINE ANTAGONISTS

Purine antagonists interfere with the synthesis of purines, bases necessary for the formation of nucleic acids. Only one purine antagonist, 6-mercaptopurine, is commercially available at present.

6-MERCAPTOPURINE, U.S.P., B.P. (PURINETHOL). The mechanism by which 6-mercaptopurine inhibits purine synthesis is poorly understood. It is believed to interfere in the conversion of adenine to guanine and inhibit the utilization of hypoxanthine and adenine in the cell.

It is used primarily in the treatment of acute leukemia, producing remissions in approximately one half the children treated. Fewer adult patients respond, but it is nevertheless one of the most effective agents in the treatment of adult leukemias. It is of little use in the treatment of chronic lymphocytic leukemia, Hodgkin's disease or solid tumors.

> **TOXICITY.** Bone marrow depression leading to leukopenia and thrombocytopenia. Ulceration of the mucous membranes, anorexia, nausea, vomiting and diarrhea occur, with jaundice, dermatoses, drug fever and eosinophilia. It is contraindicated during pregnancy.

> **DOSE.** 100 to 200 mg. (2.5 mg./kg. of body weight) orally daily. This dose may be doubled if no clinical response is obtained after four weeks at this dosage.

PYRIMIDINE ANTAGONISTS

Tumor cells incorporate uracil, a pyrimidine, into the ribonucleic acid molecule more rapidly than do normal tissues. Thus, by inhibiting pyrimidine formation, the growth of the tumor may be more rapidly affected than is the growth of normal tissues. The most commonly used pyrimidine antagonist is 5-fluorouracil, but other agents are under clinical investigation.

FLUOROURACIL (5-FU). Fluorouracil interferes with pyrimidine metabolism by blocking the methylation of uracil, which is necessary for the formation of thymine, an essential component of DNA (deoxyribonucleic acid); it thereby inhibits or retards DNA synthesis. In addition, it is incorporated into RNA (ribonucleic acid), forming a fraudulent RNA. These two mechanisms inhibit the growth of proliferating cells by interfering with nucleic acid replication.

Some tumors in humans are notably resistant to fluorouracil therapy, because they lack an enzyme necessary to incorporate the drug and this deficiency allows the tumor to grow uninterrupted even in the presence of massive doses of fluorouracil. The mechanism by which susceptible tumors become resistant is still a mystery, and at present can be explained only on the basis of some mutagenic change in the tumor cells.

Fluorouracil is more concentrated in tumor tissue than in surrounding healthy tissues, and because of impaired uracil catabolism, fluorouracil persists longer in some tumors than in normal tissue.

Fluorouracil is used both alone and in conjunction with surgery and x-ray therapy in the treatment of carcinomas of the breast, colon, rectum, pancreas, ovary, liver and stomach. Drug-induced remissions may last as long as a year before recurrence occurs. In some cases many repeated remissions may be obtained. Carcinoma of the lung and malignant melanoma are generally unresponsive to fluorouracil.

A new method of therapy is now being employed with fluorouracil. Rather than admitting the patient to the hospital for short-term, large dose therapy, some research centers are using transfer packs that contain 500 mg. fluorouracil with heparin in a 5 per cent dextrose solution. The transfer pack is attached to a small pressure unit similar to a sphygmomanometer cuff that adjusts the flow rate so that the volume in each package lasts 24 hours. The patient is instructed in the operation of the pressure unit and the changing of the disposable bags containing the measured dose of the drug. The metered dosage units are attached to an arterial catheter so that maximal doses of the drug may be administered directly to the tumor site. It has been postulated that a relatively small but continuous dose of fluorouracil is more effective and is accompanied by fewer toxic effects than larger doses administered over a short period of time.

TOXICITY. Anorexia, vomiting, diarrhea, stomatitis, esophagitis, alopecia, proctitis, leukopenia, thrombocytopenia and anemia occur commonly. The prospective beneficial effects of this drug must be weighed against the debilitating toxic effects in many instances before therapy is instituted.

DOSE. 15 mg./kg. of body weight I.V. for four days, or 500 mg. daily intra-arterially for a prolonged period of time.

HORMONES

The hormones used in the treatment of neoplastic diseases are believed to alter the growth pattern of hormone-dependent tumors by making the cellular environment less favorable for growth. Tumors of the secondary sex organs, such as the prostate and mammary glands, are dependent on sex hormones for their normal growth and development. When these hormones are decreased or antagonized, growth and development of the malignant cells are markedly slowed. Surgical removal of testes or ovaries results in a similar drop in hormone production and has similar effects on the growth of certain malignancies.

Prostate tumors are often treated by castration and administration of oral estrogens. Feminization does occur, but may be minimized by the administration of small doses. Mammary carcinoma is treated during the childbearing years by the administration of testosterone after mastectomy has been performed, but postmenopausal patients usually receive greater therapeutic benefits from estrogen therapy.

Corticosteroids, notably prednisone and prednisolone, have been effective in producing remissions of susceptible leukemias and lymphomas These agents are often the first employed in the treatment of acute leukemia, and they are followed by other antineoplastic agents only when the cells become resistant to their effect. They are quite effective in childhood leukemia, but they are of little benefit in the treatment of adult forms of the disease. Corticosteroids have also been employed in the treatment of Hodgkin's disease, lymphosarcoma, multiple myeloma and chronic lymphatic leukemia, but with variable beneficial effects.

TESTOLACTONE (TESLAC). Testolactone is a synthetic derivative of testosterone, the natural male hormone, and is used primarily in the treatment of advanced or metastasized breast cancer. In some cases it has been demonstrated to decrease the size of tumor masses in soft tissue, although it is of little value in altering bony metastases when present. When used in recommended doses, it does not produce masculizing changes. It is primarily recommended for postmenopausal women, but may be used in premenopausal women when ovarian function has been terminated.

TOXICITY. Dermatoses, paresthesia, nausea, vomiting and alopecia have been observed

DOSE. Oral—50 mg. three times daily. I.M.—100 mg. three times weekly.

RADIOACTIVE ISOTOPES

The use of radioactive isotopes in the treatment of carcinoma is discussed in Chapter 21.

MISCELLANEOUS ANTINEOPLASTIC DRUGS

Several antineoplastic agents that are not classified under any of the aforementioned groups of drugs will be discussed individually.

URETHAN, N.F., URETHANE, B.P. (ETHYL CARBAMATE). Urethan inhibits cell division in rapidly dividing tissues, such as bone marrow and the gastrointestinal epithelium. It has been shown under electron microscopy to produce random chromosomal breaks, which interfere with cell division. Unfortunately, there is no predilection for tumor cells, and toxic effects are observed concurrently with any beneficial effects obtained in the tumor therapy.

Urethan has been used with some success in the treatment of multiple myeloma, showing remissions in about one third of the patients treated. In addition it has been used to treat chronic myelocytic leukemia, but with variable success.

$$\begin{array}{c} NH_2 \\ | \\ CO \\ | \\ O-C_2H_5 \end{array}$$

urethan

TOXICITY. Bone marrow depression leading to leukopenia and thrombocytopenia with subsequent hemorrhagic tendencies and lower resistance to infection. Anorexia, nausea, vomiting, sedation, dizziness and liver damage have been reported.

DOSE. 2 to 4 Gm. orally or I.V. daily.

VINBLASTINE SULFATE (VELBAN). Vinblastine, a derivative of the periwinkle plant, is believed to act by interfering with metabolic pathways leading from glutamic acid to the citric acid cycle and to urea formation. It has been shown experimentally to arrest mitosis.

It relieves pain and other symptoms and is effective in the palliation of some cases of Hodgkin's disease and choriocarcinoma that are resistant to other therapy. It may be administered only intravenously for this purpose. Cellulitis and severe local reactions may occur if the drug is extravasated.

TOXICITY. Leukopenia, alopecia, anorexia, nausea, vomiting, diarrhea, stomatitis, gastrointestinal bleeding and ulceration, fever, weight loss, muscular pains and neurologic symptoms have been observed.

DOSE. One dose I.V. weekly at gradually increased increments of 0.1 mg. to 0.5 mg./kg. of body weight. When the white cell count falls to 3000, the dose should be reduced slightly and continued at weekly intervals unless more severe leukopenia occurs.

VINCRISTINE SULFATE (ONCOVIN). Like vinblastine, this agent is obtained from the periwinkle plant. It arrests mitotic cell division at the stage of metaphase, but it has not been demonstrated to have the antimetabolic activities of vinblastine. Cross-resistance between these drugs does not occur, presumably because of their different mechanisms of action.

Vincristine is indicated only for the treatment of acute leukemia in children, and it is usually not employed until resistance to most other drugs has occurred.

TOXICITY. Bone marrow depression, paresthesias of the extremities, neurologic deficits, muscular atrophy, ataxia, paralysis, nervousness, psychoses, abdominal pain, constipation, dermatoses and urinary dysfunction.

DOSE. 0.05 mg./kg. of body weight I.V. once weekly.

DEMECOLCINE (COLCEMID). This derivative of colchicine has been used experimentally in cancer chemotherapy. It is of some benefit in the treatment of chronic myelocytic leukemia, but not in the treatment of solid tumors.

TOXICITY. Bone marrow depression, stomatitis, gastrointestinal ulceration, dermatoses and alopecia occur frequently.

DOSE. 3 to 10 mg. orally daily.

DACTINOMYCIN (ACTINOMYCIN D, COSMEGEN). Dactinomycin, an antibiotic derived from *Streptomyces parvullus,* has weak antibacterial activity, but binds directly with DNA, inhibiting the synthesis of DNA-dependent RNA and slowing cellular division. It has only a slight degree of predilection for malignant tissue, however, and is extremely toxic to rapidly dividing tissues, such as bone marrow and gastrointestinal epithelium.

It may be used alone or in combination with radiation and surgery in the treatment of metastatic Wilms' tumor, carcinoma of the testes, rhabdomyosarcoma, choriocarcinoma and osteogenic sarcoma.

TOXICITY. Bone marrow depression, gastrointestinal ulceration, cheilitis, pharyngitis, nausea, vomiting, dermatoses and alopecia. These effects may not become apparent until days or weeks after the course of therapy is completed and may not become maximal before one or two more weeks have elapsed. Extravasation produces severe local tissue reactions. The drug should be injected into the tubing of an I.V. that is flowing at a rapid rate. Any unused drug should be discarded.

DOSE. 0.05 to 0.15 mg./kg. of body weight I.V. daily for a maximum of five days.

N-METHYLHYDRAZINE (NATULAN). N-methylhydrazine is a new type of cancer drug that has been proposed for use in Hodgkin's disease. It is effective in patients who would be expected to respond to nitrogen mustard and vinblastine; it does therefore not appear to offer any striking clinical advantages over these two compounds. It may occasionally produce remissions in patients who are refractory to other types of treatment, however.

TOXICITY. Leukopenia and thrombocytopenia occur frequently following the third week of treatment; the blood picture should therefore be watched carefully. Nausea and vomiting are common complaints at the onset of therapy, but these symptoms improve in most cases as therapy is continued. On some occasions phenothiazine derivatives have been used for their antiemetic effects with N-methylhydrazine, but in some cases there has been an enhancement of the central nervous system depression seen with the phenothiazine drugs.

DOSE. 30 mg./kg. of body weight orally weekly for three weeks.

PROCARBAZINE HYDROCHLORIDE (MATU-LANE). Procarbazine is a synthetic agent which has been shown to be of value in the palliative treatment of Hodgkin's disease, and has been found to be effective even in patients who have developed resistance to other forms of therapy. The mode of action of this drug is still under study, but there is evidence that it interferes with protein synthesis as well as causing some obstruction in the normal pattern of DNA and RNA synthesis. Procarbazine exhibits some secondary monoamine oxidase inhibition, thus drugs and foods with high tyramine content, such as cheese and bananas, should be avoided.

TOXICITY. It is contraindicated in patients with preexisting bone marrow depression and in pregnancy, and should be used with extreme caution in patients with impairment of liver or kidney function. Leukopenia, anemia, thrombocytopenia, nausea and vomiting occur frequently. Gastrointestinal complaints, myalgia, arthralgia, weakness and drowsiness are also noted, as are dermatoses, visual disturbances and isolated neurologic abnormalities.

DOSE. 50 to 100 mg. orally daily.

PIPOBROMAN (VERCYTE). This piperazine derivative has been found to be useful in the control of polycythemia vera, and in some instances has controlled chronic granulocytic leukemia. No significant effects have been noted when it is used in patients under 15 years of age, thus it is not recommended for this age group.

TOXICITY. Nausea, vomiting, abdominal cramps, diarrhea and skin rashes. A dose-dependent anemia and leukopenia may occur, thus blood counts should be monitored carefully during administration of this drug and it should be withheld until bone marrow recovery occurs.

DOSE. 1 to 2 mg./kg./day initially orally. Maintenance dose ranges from 10 to 175 mg. orally daily depending on patient response.

HYDROXYUREA (HYDREA). Hydroxyurea is an orally effective agent which has been shown to be of value in the treatment of malignant melanoma, resistant chronic myelocytic leukemia and metastatic ovarian carcinoma. It is believed to act by inhibiting DNA synthesis exclusively—without disturbance in RNA or protein synthesis.

TOXICITY. Contraindicated in patients with bone marrow depression. Liver and kidney function should be monitored during therapy as damage may occur. Nausea, vomiting, diarrhea, skin reactions, dysuria and alopecia have been reported. Neurologic disturbances such as hallucinations and convulsions occur rarely.

DOSE. 1.5 to 2 Gm. orally daily.

POTASSIUM ARSENITE SOLUTION (FOWLER'S SOLUTION). A one per cent solution of potassium arsenite is sometimes used as a mild suppressive in early stages of chronic myelocytic leukemia, but its activity is weak compared to other agents.

In the past potassium arsenite has also been employed in the treatment of blood dyscrasias and chronic eczema, but it has largely been replaced by other agents.

TOXICITY. Arsenic toxicity may be noted on prolonged therapy. The first signs are usually puffiness around the eyes and disturbance of the bowels. Pigmentation of the skin, gastroenteritis, hepatitis and neuritis may occur as well.

DOSE. 0.2 to 0.3 ml orally one to three times daily.

NURSING CARE OF PATIENTS RECEIVING ANTINEOPLASTIC DRUGS

The nursing care of patients receiving antineoplastic drugs involves the management of the severe side effects. The presence of these side effects is indicative of the effectiveness of therapy. A great deal of nursing skill and inventiveness is necessary to meet the needs of these patients.

Maintaining adequate nutrition and hydration may become a serious problem because of the anorexia, nausea, vomiting and ulcerations of the mouth and gastrointestinal tract produced by these drugs. Small, frequent feedings, high in carbohydrate and protein, may be helpful. Antacids and antiemetics may be needed.

The alopecia that occurs with certain drugs may be disturbing to some patients. This usually is not permanent, but hair growth may not return for a period of time. The availability and use of a wig may provide much comfort and an increased positive self-image to female patients. The impact of alopecia on the male patient should be considered, also.

Frequent and careful mouth care is essential to make the patient comfortable and to prevent infection and bleeding. A hard toothbrush should not be used; cotton swabs may be preferred. Hard candy may help to relieve the metallic taste experienced by some patients.

Because of the damage done to the bone marrow by these drugs, leukopenia may become quite severe and life-threatening. Patients should be protected as much as possible from sources of infection. Personnel and visitors with "minor colds" or any infection should not come into contact with these patients. It may be necessary to restrict visitors. Reverse isolation technique may be indicated to prevent the patient from being overwhelmed by an infection while his defense system is incapacitated. The nurse should observe carefully for early signs of infection and report them immediately.

Bleeding also presents a nursing care problem, since thrombocytopenia frequently occurs. The patient should be handled gently and observed for purpura. Stools and urine should be examined for evidence of bleeding. Vital signs should be checked frequently so that complications can be detected early. Nursing observations should also be directed toward signs that the drugs are effective. A decrease in pain or size of the malignancy if visible and increased weight, strength, and sense of well-being may be positive signs. The side effects of the drugs, however, may temporarily obscure signs of improvement.

Patients need a great deal of emotional support from the nurse as they experience many side effects, and they may be concerned with the effectiveness of the therapy in relation to their diagnosis. The nurse should consult with the physician to determine the knowledge that the patient has concerning his diagnosis and the purpose of the drug therapy. This may influence the nurse's approach to the patient as well as influence the patient's reactions to the drug side effects. The nurse should use her skills to develop a nurse-patient relationship in which the patient can freely express his fears and feelings.

GUIDE FOR THE NURSING ASSESSMENT OF A PATIENT RECEIVING AN ANTINEOPLASTIC AGENT FOR CANCER

I. Why is this patient receiving an antineoplastic agent? What type of cancer does he have and where is it located? Is the patient aware of his diagnosis? What is his understanding of the purpose of this drug? What has the physician told this patient? Is the patient aware of the inevitability of side effects? What is the understanding and attitude of the patient and his family to the therapeutic plan?

II. Is this drug being administered correctly? Is it being given correctly in relation to the patient's meals? Is it being given by the correct route and are precautions taken to insure the correct route is used? Is the drug reconstituted according to the manufacturer's recommendations? Is the drug being stored correctly?

III.   Is the drug producing the desired effect? Has the patient had any gain in weight? Has there been any regression in the size of the tumor if visible or visible on X-ray? Does the patient have less fatigue and greater strength? Does the patient have less pain? Do the results of laboratory tests indicate a lessening of cancerous activity?

IV.   What side effects is this patient experiencing and are measures being taken to alleviate them? Are there any indications of leukopenia or agranulocytosis? Has the white blood cell count decreased? Does the patient have a sore throat or fever, or other signs of infection? Is the patient being protected from sources of infection? Are reverse isolation techniques indicated? Does the patient have any evidence of bleeding? Are the vital signs taken frequently? Do any changes indicate internal bleeding? Do laboratory test results indicate a decreased platelet count or reduced clotting ability? Does the patient have purpura or petechiae on the skin? Are the stools bloody or black? Are they tested for the presence of occult blood? Is the urine smoky or red in color? Are measures taken to reduce bruising?

Does the patient have indications of increasing anemia? What are the results of laboratory tests, such as hemoglobin and hematocrit? Does the patient have increasing fatigue or dyspnea?

Is there evidence of irritation or ulceration of the mucous membranes of the gastrointestinal tract? Are there ulcerations present in the mouth? Is this interfering with the patient's nutritional intake? Is special mouth care being given frequently? Does the patient have diarrhea? Is there mucus or indications of bleeding and ulceration in the stool? Has the diarrhea produced fluid and electrolyte imbalance? Is the patient experiencing nausea and vomiting? Has an antiemetic been ordered?

Does the patient have increasing alopecia? What effect has this had on this patient? Does the patient understand the alopecia is reversible? Has the possibility of a wig been suggested to the patient or his family?

What are the patient's reactions to these effects?

V.   What are the learning and psychological needs of this patient and his family? What are the patient's and family's understanding of and attitude toward the illness, the drug therapy and the total plan of care?

Are expectations realistic in light of the information they have been given? In light of the realistic situation?

Has the expression of the patient's feelings and fears been encouraged actively by the nursing staff and other members of the health team?

QUESTIONS FOR DISCUSSION AND REVIEW

1. What recent developments in antineoplastic drugs have you read about in newspapers, current periodicals, etc.?

2. Which course of treatment is usually most effective for cancer?

3. Why do you suppose tissues eventually become insensitive to cancer drugs?

4. Define and give an example of the following:
   a. alkylating agent
   b. folic acid antagonist
   c. glutamic acid antagonist
   d. pyrimidine antagonist

5. How do each of the previous drugs function as antineoplastic agents?

6. Why do cancer drugs not affect all tissues equally?

7. What nursing measures can be taken to reduce the discomforts of side effects of the antineoplastic drugs?

8. What precautions should be taken by the nurse if a patient has leukopenia? Thrombocytopenia?

BIBLIOGRAPHY

Alston, F., et al.: Perfusion. *Amer. J. Nurs., 60*:1603, 1960.

AMA Drug Evaluations. Chicago, American Medical Association, 1971.

American Cancer Society: Hormones and chemotherapy for cancer. *Cancer, 18*:1517, 1965.

Bernstock, L.: Nitrogen mustard in the treatment of bronchogenic carcinoma. *Nurs. Times, 65*:875, (July 10) 1969.

Council on Drugs: Antineoplastic agents derived from the periwinkle plant. *J.A.M.A., 191*:749, 1965.

Craytor, J. K. and Fass, M. L.: *The Nurse and the Cancer Patient. A Programmed Textbook.* Philadelphia, J. B. Lippincott Co., 1970.

Cutler, S. J.: Trends in the management of cancer. *C.A., 18*:189, (July-August) 1968.

Donaldson, S. and Fletcher, W.: The treatment of cancer by isolation perfusion. *Amer. J. Nurs., 64*:81, (August) 1964.

Ellison, R. R.: Treating cancer with antimetabolites. *Amer. J. Nurs., 62*: 79, (November) 1962.

Fox, S. A. and Bernhardt, L.: Chemotherapy via intra-arterial infusion. *Amer. J. Nurs., 66*:966, (September) 1966.

Francis, G. M.: Cancer: the emotional component. *Amer. J. Nurs., 69*: 1677, 1969.

Govoni, L. E. and Hayes, J. E.: *Drugs and Nursing Implications.* 2nd Ed. New York, Appleton-Century-Crofts, 1971.

Hiatt, H.: Cancer chemotherapy, present status and prospects. *New Eng. J. Med., 276*:157 (January 19) 1967.

Hilkemeyer, R.: Intra-arterial cancer chemotherapy. *Nurs. Clin. N. Amer., 1*:295, (June) 1966.

Karnofsky, D. A.: Cancer chemotherapeutic agents. *C.A., 18*:72, (March-April) 1968.

Karnofsky, D. A.: Mechanisms of action of anticancer drugs at a cellular level. *C.A., 18*:232, (March-April) 1968.

Kautz, H. D., Story, R. H. and Zimmerman, A. J.: Radioactive drugs. *Amer. J. Nurs., 64*:124, (January) 1964.

Levine, L. A.: Intra-arterial chemotherapy. *Amer. J. Nurs., 64*:108 (March) 1964.

Livingston, B.: Cancer chemotherapy research. *Amer. J. Nurs., 67*:2547, (December) 1967.

Livingston, B. and Krakoff, I. H.: L-asparaginase—a new type of anti-cancer drug. *Amer. J. Nurs., 70*:1910, (September) 1970.

Lyman, M. S. and Burcjenal, J. H.: Acute leukemia. *Amer. J. Nurs., 63*:82, (April) 1963.

Moffat, E. P.: Isolated limb perfusion. *Nurs. Times, 65*:138, (January 30) 1969.

Nowak, P. A.: Nursing care in isolation perfusion. *Amer. J. Nurs., 64*:85, (August) 1964.

Schwartz, S. A. and Perry, S.: Patient protection in cancer chemotherapy. *J.A.M.A., 197*:623, 1966.

Thornblad, I.: Hormonal ablative therapy for the premenopausal patient with advanced cancer. *Nurs. Clin. N. Amer., 2*:659, (December) 1967.

Watkins, E. W. and Sullivan, R. D.: Cancer chemotherapy by prolonged arterial infusion. *Surg. Gynec. Obstet., 118*:3, 1964.

Wilson, H. E.: Leukemia. *Amer. J. Nurs., 56*:601, 1956.

Wimer, B. M. and Maycock, P. P.: Further comment on busulfan. *New Eng. J. Med., 273*:226, 1965.

Chapter 21 Radioactive Drugs

Important Concepts Discussed

1. *Radioactive elements differ from nonradioactive materials in that they emit particles or fragments from their nuclei.*

   Tissue changes and genetic mutations occur when radioactive particles pass into the body.

3. *Minor radiation damage is reversible; larger doses of radiation result in permanent cellular changes or death.*

4. *The inherent rate of decomposition of a radioactive element is measured in terms of its half-life. The amount of radiation emitted gradually decreases until it is insignificant and a stable, nonradioactive element is formed.*

5. *The nurse utilizes her knowledge of the drug's radioactive characteristics and the principles of time, distance and shielding in planning her nursing care.*

The application of radioactive elements to medicine has been one of the most significant and beneficial results of the atomic age. The possibilities for the employment of radioisotopes to the study and diagnosis of diseases have barely been explored.

Radioactivity denotes the inherent ability of certain atoms to decompose spontaneously into other atoms The nucleus alone is involved in the decomposition. The instability of these nuclei depends on a number of factors among which are the number of neutrons and protons in the nucleus and the nature of the basic force of energy related to the meson, which holds the nucleus together. The nature of this force is only beginning to be understood, and its relation to the other basic forces in the universe, such as electromagnetism and gravitation, is unknown.

When an unstable nucleus decomposes, energy is released by the ejection of one or more charged particles of matter or electromagnetic waves. The nucleus continues to decompose until a stable nonradioactive element is reached. In the case of radium, the decomposition proceeds through transitional elements until the final product, lead, is reached.

Three major types of charged particles can be ejected from the nucleus:

Alpha (α) particles—which are helium nuclei of atomic weight 4, containing 2 protons and 2 neutrons, thus having an electrical charge of $+2$.

Beta (β) particles—which are high-speed electrons having an electrical charge of -1.

Positrons ($\beta+$)—which have the mass of an electron but a charge of $+1$.

All three particles can be ejected with various energies quantitated by the physicist in terms of a unit of energy called million electron volts, often abbreviated Mev. The range or penetrability of a particle through matter is directly related to the numerical value of the Mev. The greater the Mev, the greater is the penetrability of the particle.

In addition to the particles, electromagnetic waves, called gamma (γ) rays or photons, may be emitted from radioactive nuclei. These are identical to x-rays, with the exception that gamma rays emitted from radioactive nuclei usually have greater energy than do diagnostic x-rays. The energy of gamma rays is also given in Mev.

HALF-LIFE

All radioactive isotopes have an inherent rate of decomposition or decay. There is no known means of hastening or slowing this process. The isotope C^{14} has a half-life of 5570 years, after which time its radioactivity is only half of the original measurement. After another 5570 years, the radioactivity is again reduced by half, and so forth until there is virtually no measurable activity remaining in the element.

Radioactive elements vary greatly in length of half-life; e.g., I^{131} has a half-life of 8.08 days; for Na^{24} it is 14.8 hours and K^{40} has a half-life of 1.27×10^9 years.

The isotopic half-life, which may be abbreviated "$T\frac{1}{2}$," is significant whenever a radioactive substance is to be employed. The longer the half-life, the longer the isotope is radioactive and dangerous. When an isotope is used medicinally, the problem is slightly more complicated because the body can excrete certain radioactive isotopes whereas others, such as Ra^{226}, are stored in tissue and are not excreted. The term "biological half-life" means the time it takes the organism to excrete one half of a given quantity of radioactive material after localization has occurred. Very often the biological half-life and the isotopic half-life have to be con-

sidered simultaneously to assess the hazards involved in the use of a given agent.

The term "effective half-life" is a composite of the previous two terms and indicates the length of time it takes the radioactivity of a given isotope to diminish by one half when present in the body. The rate, as stated previously, depends on the chemical form of the radioisotope and its manner of excretion from the body.

MODE OF ACTION OF RADIOISOTOPES

When an alpha or beta particle or gamma radiation passes through matter, it ionizes the nonradioactive molecules it hits in passage. The damage caused by radiation is believed to be due to the formation of free radicals and to the ionization of the tissue, fluid and gaseous molecules in the body. The result is chaotic chemical interaction, which may lead ultimately to the death of the tissues.

RADIATION MEASUREMENT

The original unit of radiation is the roentgen (named after Roentgen, the discoverer of x-rays). The roentgen pertains to the amount of ionization caused by a given quantity of x-rays. The roentgen is equal to the quantity of x-rays or gamma rays that, if absorbed by 1 Gm. of tissue, imparts 97 ergs of energy to the tissue.

The rad is a more recent unit of radiation dosage that can be used for any type of radiation, be it alpha, beta, gamma or x-rays. It is a slightly larger unit than the roentgen—the amount of ionizing radiation that imparts 100 ergs of energy to 1 Gm. of matter.

Various complex formulas are available for computing the radiation dosage to a given tissue when the activity of the isotope is in curies or fractions of a curie. A curie, formerly the amount of radon in equilibrium with 1 Gm. of radium, is currently defined as the quantity of any radioactive species (radioisotope) undergoing exactly 3.700×10^{10} disintegrations per second.

Exact amounts of radiation are very difficult to compute and further discussion is not of practical value in this text. Most important is that radiation exposure varies inversely to the square of the distance from the source. Thus, a person standing 2 ft. from a radioactive substance would receive only one quarter as much radiation as a person standing 1 ft. away. Often the radiation is computed as roentgens or rads per hour at a distance of 1 cm. or 1 meter from the source.

PENETRABILITY OF THE VARIOUS TYPES OF RADIATION

The alpha particle, being a heavy, charged particle, has very poor penetrability through matter. It penetrates to a depth of approximately 7 microns, which means that it may easily be stopped by the dead epithelial layer on the surface of the skin. Alpha particle emission from a source inside the body poses a more serious problem, however, because considerable tissue damage may occur in a very small area. This can be particularly serious with elements, such as radium, that concentrate in the bone marrow and emit alpha particles.

The beta particle penetrates much deeper than the alpha, owing to its smaller mass and charge. It may penetrate about 5 mm. and though this poses no serious threat if the source is outside the body (other than causing beta ray burns), internal emission of beta rays can cause much damage.

X-rays and gamma rays have no mass and no charge and can freely penetrate matter. Their range through matter is great and depends upon their energy. Tables are available to indicate what thickness of lead reduces radiation by half when the energy of the gamma ray is known in Mev. Theoretically, however, it is never possible to reduce the exposure to zero. The damaging effects of these electromagnetic waves are distributed over a much larger volume than with alpha and beta particles. They can effectively interact with tissues in widely divergent areas of the body, although directed to only one area. Thus, they may be a serious health hazard even when present in the proper dosage. On the other hand, since the penetrability of these rays is so great, they may pass through the body without hitting a single molecule.

All things being considered, beta particles seem to constitute the greatest local hazard

to the body because they produce a large amount of ionization in a small volume. In addition, all the energy is absorbed by the tissues.

NURSE'S ROLE IN CARING FOR PATIENTS RECEIVING RADIOACTIVE DRUGS

In caring for a patient receiving any radioactive drug, the nurse needs to know certain facts about the drug used in order to protect herself and others from overexposure to radiation. She needs to know the type of ray emitted. Alpha and beta rays are considered to be blocked by the patient's body. If the substance emits gamma rays special precautions need to be instituted.

Knowledge of the half-life of the drug enables the nurse to know when precautions may be discontinued. For example, radioactive gold has a half-life of about three days. In three days, one half of its radioactivity is gone; in another three days three fourths of its activity is gone. Precautions are necessary for at least six days.

Knowledge of the biological activity and behavior of the radioactive substance is also needed. The nurse needs to know where the drug is concentrated and how rapidly it is excreted from the body. For example, radioactive iodine is concentrated in the thyroid gland and is excreted by the kidneys and skin. Precautions are therefore indicated in relation to the disposal of urine and linens.

The amount or dosage given may also influence the action to be taken. Diagnostic doses, such as in I^{131} uptake test, are usually smaller than therapeutic doses intended to destroy tissue cells. A diagnostic dose of a drug may not require any special precautions, whereas a therapeutic dose of the same drug requires precautions.

Substances emitting gamma rays require the nurse and other personnel to protect themselves from overexposure to radiation. The precautions involved with radiation depend upon the length of exposure, distance, and shielding.

The amount of time spent by persons in the vicinity of a gamma-emitting substance should be minimal. The person involved in the care of the patient should have a dosimeter or other means by which the amount of radiation she receives in a day is measured. It is usually necessary to rotate personnel who care for these patients to prevent overexposure of one person.

Distance is another means by which personnel can easily protect themselves from radiation. The further a person is from the source of radiation, the less radiation he receives. This means that the nurse can talk with the patient from the doorway rather than right at the bedside. The psychological and emotional support of the patient should not be neglected because of fear and ignorance of personnel. Visitors should not be restricted completely because of the radiation danger, but they should take advantage of the time and distance factors.

Shielding is another method to help protect a person from gamma rays. Radioactive materials are usually transported in lead containers. Radiologists, x-ray technicians and those more constantly exposed to gamma rays use lead aprons as a shield. A certain amount of shielding can be accomplished by using the patient's body as a shield. For example, in transporting a patient with a pelvic radium implant, walking at the head of the stretcher provides the nurse with more protection from radiation than if she walked at the patient's side, near the pelvic area.

When any question arises as to the nature of the drug or precautions necessary, the radiologist or isotope laboratory should be consulted. Each hospital usually has specific procedures to be followed with respect to care of linens, excreta, accidents, etc.

NATURAL RADIOACTIVE ELEMENTS

RADIUM (Ra^{226}). In some medical situations, particularly gynecology, radium needles are still imbedded in certain organs to deliver a dose of gamma radiation to a small volume of tissue. The half-life of radium is 1580 years, and during its decomposition, alpha particles and gamma rays are emitted. The end product is lead.

Full radiation precautions are needed. The position of the insert should be checked frequently. Bedpans and linen should be checked to be sure the insert has not come out.

CARBON (C^{14}). C^{14} is the natural radioactive element that in minute quantities contaminates nonradioactive C^{12}. The C^{14} content of organic matter remains fairly constant during the life of the organism. After the organism's death, the C^{14} content decreases slowly by radioactive decay. Thus, measuring the C^{14} content of organic matter is an ingenious method of dating ancient objects. This method has been extremely useful to the archeologist and historian.

POTASSIUM (K^{40}). K^{40} is another radioactive element normally present in living tissue. The amount found in the body is extremely small and constitutes no health hazard.

THE RADIOISOTOPES

Dosage of radioisotopes is in millicuries or microcuries. Careful reading of the label and symbols is vital. Two different strengths of the same isotope should not be kept or stored in the same location.

IODINE (I^{131}) U.S.P. Perhaps the most important and most useful radiosotope, I^{131}, which has a half-life of 8.08 days, is used in the study and treatment of thyroid disease because of the ability of the thyroid gland to capture and concentrate iodide from the blood. Since I^{131} (present as sodium iodide) is chemically indistinguishable from the natural nonradioactive iodide, the thyroid gland picks it up with the other iodides. Within only a few minutes after injection of radioiodide, labeling is found in the iodotyrosines of thyroglobulin. Thyroxine and triiodothyronine are quickly formed. Because gamma rays are emitted from the isotope in the process of decay, one can detect the I^{131} by means of a scintillation detector held at the surface of the body. The rate of I^{131} uptake can be determined as well as the localization and distribution of the isotopes in the gland. The following drugs affect the uptake of I^{131} and interfere with the accuracy of the test:

Iodine preparations in any form for external or internal use, including asthma, cough and vitamin preparations containing iodine
Contrast media for x-ray examinations
Thyroid and antithyroid drugs
Para-aminosalicylic acid
Isoniazid
Benzoic acid
Cod liver oil preparations
Thiocyanates
Nitrates and nitrites
Perchlorates
Mercurials
Thiazide derivatives
Phenothiazines
Sulfonamides
Sulfonylureas
Antihistamines
Estrogens
Progesterone
Corticosteroids
Antiparasitic drugs, such as diiodohydroxyquin and iodochlorhydroxyquin
Thiopental
Phenylbutazone
Cobalt
Bromsulphalein
Suntan lotions
Resorcinol

In the event that a hyperthyroid patient is considered a poor surgical risk and cannot be adequately managed on a thyroid-blocking drug, internal destruction of the gland may be accomplished by the use of I^{131}. Definite contraindications to this use would be the known existence of pregnancy, a completely inadequate uptake of I^{131} as determined by tracer dosage, the presence of a possible malignant lesion of the thyroid (since iodide is not picked up by the thyroid in this case) and arbitrarily, if the patient is under 25 years of age.

The immediate effects of I^{131} therapy are usually minimal, consisting of mild pain, tenderness over the thyroid area and dysphagia for a few days after the administration of the therapeutic dose. Mild hypothyroidism may appear for as long as two to three months after the full effect of I^{131} treatment, but there is usually a spontaneous return to euthyroidism over the succeeding few months.

The question of carcinogenesis is often raised, probably because of recollection of the effects of the older type of externally applied x-irradiation. One group studying the problem reported only one tumor attributable to I^{131} therapy in 1500 treated patients. Other workers have obtained similar results.

In patients under 20 years of age, however, the rate is somewhat higher. Three of 18 patients in one group developed malignant thyroid nodules five to ten years after therapy. Since young, growing tissue is more apt to have the combination of features leading to malignancy, no patients under the age of 25 should be thus treated. If I^{131} therapy seems absolutely necessary in this age group, an attempt should be made to use a sufficiently large dose to destroy all thyroid tissue in order to eliminate the possibility of later neoplasms, employing replacement therapy to correct the ensuing hypothyroidism.

I^{131} may also be used to tag other iodine-containing substances to determine their respective absorption, distribution and excretion in the body.

Special precautions are not needed if the patient has received a diagnostic dose of I^{131}. If the patient should vomit the oral dose, special precautions are necessary. If the radioisotope touches skin, it should be washed promptly with soap and water. Avoid touching the vomitus, cover it with paper towels and consult the radiologist. It is usually disposed of using gloves and long forceps.

If the patient is receiving a therapeutic dose of I^{131} certain precautions are necessary. The procedure may vary from hospital to hospital, but particular precautions are taken with urine, which is usually placed in a lead container in the patient's room. Linen may require special precautions if the patient perspires heavily, vomits or contaminates the linen with sputum. The directions of the radiology department should be followed.

DOSE. I^{131} uptake: 1 to 100 microcuries orally. Therapeutic purposes: 4000 to 10,000 microcuries orally.

CHROMIUM (CR^{51}) U.S.P. Chromium in the form of chromate has a remarkable affinity for erythrocytes. After its entry into the red blood cell, almost all of it is firmly bound to the globin portion of hemoglobin.

Erythrocytes may be tagged *in vitro* with Cr^{51} and injected into the blood. The major use of radiochromium is to determine the total red blood cell volume by noting the dilution of the tagged red blood cells. Another use is in determining the quantitative blood loss from gastrointestinal bleeding by measuring the amount of Cr^{51} in the feces.

DOSE. 250 microcuries on tagged red blood cells I.V.

COBALT (Co^{60}). Co^{60} is one of the more important isotopes in clinical medicine. Because the isotope decays by emission of strong gamma radiation, it is used in teletherapy machines for the precise localized irradiation of tumor tissue. The massive machine that is necessary to shield the cobalt is built for a 1 inch cube of the material.

It is important for the nurse and patient to realize that the patient is not radioactive after this type of therapy (teletherapy) and that the markings on the skin should not be washed off because they are a guide to the radiologist in administering cobalt.

Radiocobalt is also used internally as a tracer of vitamin B_{12} metabolism. Since cobalt is a normal constituent of this vitamin, and Co^{60} in the molecule behaves chemically like nonradioactive cobalt, the metabolism can easily be traced by following the gamma emission in its route through the body. Labeled vitamin B_{12} is important in the study and diagnosis of pernicious anemia. In this disease, the vitamin is not absorbed orally and is excreted in the feces. A simpler and less time-consuming test is the serum radioactivity test performed after oral administration of the radiovitamin.

DOSE. In tests for pernicious anemia: 0.5 microcuries of tagged vitamin B_{12} orally or I.M. Also administered in varying doses by external radiotherapy.

GOLD (Au^{198}). Radioactive gold, with a half-life of 2.7 days, when injected as the colloidal metal into a serous cavity, is deposited on the tissue area and is not absorbed into the blood to any great extent. The beta particles emitted are thus confined to a small area and are useful in treating pleural and peritoneal effusions caused by malignant neoplasms.

After Au^{198} has been injected into the cavity, the patient's position should be changed frequently to insure adequate distribution within the cavity. Radiation precautions to protect personnel are necessary since gamma rays are also emitted.

Radioactive gold is deep cherry red. The nurse should therefore observe the site of injection carefully for leakage. If leakage does occur, she should notify the radiologist immediately for instruction.

Because there is a potential hazard to the patient and nursing personnel when Au^{198} is employed in therapy, all necessary precautions to avoid excessive radiation must be taken. Since the dose is high, the patient may develop radiation sickness, manifested by nausea and vomiting. Blood cell changes may also occur and lowered white cell counts as well as aplastic anemia have been reported in some patients.

DOSE. 35 to 150 millicuries by injection into closed serous cavities.

IRIDIUM (Ir^{192}). Nylon ribbons containing stainless steel cylinders (seeds) in which Ir^{192} is placed have been employed as a substitute for radium needles in the treatment of neoplasms. This newer method has the advantages of lower cost, smaller radiation sources and a better mechanical medium for holding the radiation source.

DOSE. 300 to 1000 roentgens by intracavitary radiation daily delivered at 1 cm. distance for 5 to 16 days.

IRON (Fe^{59}). Since iron is incorporated into hemoglobin, Fe^{59} can easily be detected in red blood cells and thus is extremely useful in the study of erythropoiesis. In addition, problems concerning iron turnover can be assessed by the use of Fe^{59}.

DOSE. 19 microcuries orally or I.M.

KRYPTON AND XENON (KR⁸⁵ AND XE¹³³). The gases krypton and xenon, being inert chemically under most conditions, are of value in the measurement of cardiac output and pulmonary circulatory abnormalities. Because they readily diffuse through the alveolar membranes, these gases are easily administered by inhalation and rapidly eliminated in the same manner. The time of exposure of the patient to radiation is less than if I^{131} tagged compounds, such as serum albumin, or other substances were injected to determine cardiac output.

DOSE. 25 microcuries by inhalation.

PHOSPHORUS (P³²). When administered to an organism, P^{32}, with a half-life of 14.3 days, is distributed to all tissues since high-energy phosphates play a central role in the metabolic processes of the body cells. It is also incorporated into nucleic acids.

Cells that have a high degree of metabolic activity or cells undergoing division require more phosphorus than do less active cells. Because of this relationship, P^{32} has been used in the treatment of various types of cancer. Chronic granulocytic leukemia and polycythemia vera seem somewhat amenable to this therapy.

Since all tissues of the body use phosphorus, all tissues are affected by P^{32}. If a dose is too large, serious blood dyscrasias may result, including leukopenia, thrombocytopenia and anemia.

Radiation precautions are unnecessary because only beta rays are emitted.

DOSE. 1 to 7 microcuries orally.

MERCURY (HG²⁰³). Brain tumors seem to concentrate the diuretic chlormerodrin when it is labeled with Hg^{203}. The tumor can then be located by scanning the exterior surface of the skull. This agent is also useful in kidney scanning procedures to detect and study renal disease.

DOSE. 100 microcuries orally.

SELENIUM (SE⁷⁵). Selenium has recently been used to study pancreatic function. It is incorporated in selenomethionine since this drug has a high degree of specificity for localization in the pancreas. This compound behaves physiologically like methionine and can participate in protein synthesis or enzyme formation anywhere in the body.

DOSE. 250 microcuries orally.

STRONTIUM, CALCIUM AND MAGNESIUM (SR⁸⁵, CA⁴⁷ AND MG²⁸). When administered, Sr^{85}, Ca^{47} and Mg^{28} are deposited in newly formed bone as well as distributed throughout bone mineral. They have been used to study bone lesions and metastases, scan bone and study bone metabolism in animals.

DOSE. 100 microcuries orally.

SODIUM (NA²⁴). Although it has a limited use, Na^{24} has been employed to study the total exchangeable sodium of the body.

DOSE. 100 microcuries orally.

QUESTIONS FOR DISCUSSION AND REVIEW

1. Check a physics text to determine how elements are made radioactive.
2. Why do x-rays visualize internal structures?
3. Why must drugs be given to visualize certain organs?
4. Why is the half-life important in the therapeutic use of radioactive drugs?

5. What is the difference between a natural radioactive element and a radioisotope?

6. Check the charts of patients with malignant diseases. List the drugs administered to the patient and doses used. What side effects may be expected from these drugs?

7. How can a nurse protect herself from effects of radiation when caring for a patient who has had a therapeutic dose of I^{131}?

BIBLIOGRAPHY

AMA Drug Evaluations. Chicago, American Medical Association, 1971.

Barnett, M.: The nature of radiation and its effects on man. *Nurs. Clin. N. Amer., 2*:11, (March) 1967.

Best, N.: Radiotherapy and the nurse. *Amer. J. Nurs., 50*:140, (March) 1950.

Boeker, E.: Radiation safety. *Amer. J. Nurs., 65*:111, (April) 1965.

Boeker, E.: Radiation uses and hazards. *Nurs. Clin. N. Amer., 2*:32, (March) 1967.

Croft, D. N.: Radioisotopes in clinical medicine. 1. The physics, thyroid function and treatment. *Nurs. Times, 64*:1416, (October 18) 1968.

Govoni, L. E. and Hayes, J. E.: *Drugs and Nursing Implications.* 2nd Ed. New York, Appleton-Century-Crofts, 1971.

Isler, C.: Radiation therapy. 2. The nurse and the patient. *R.N., 34*:48, (March) 1971.

Kautz, H. D., Storey, R. H. and Zimmerman, A. J.: Radioactive drugs. *Amer. J. Nurs., 64*:124, (January) 1964.

Kendall, E. B.: Care of patient with sealed sources of radioisotopes. *Nurs. Clin. N. Amer., 2*:97, (March) 1967.

Lieben, J.: The effects of radiation. *Nurs. Outlook, 10*:336, 1962.

Prosnitz, L. P.: Radiation therapy. 1. Treatment for malignant disease. *R.N., 34*:42, (March) 1971.

Rall, J. E.: The role of radioactive iodine in the diagnosis of thyroid disease. *Amer. J. Med., 20*:719, 1956.

Rummerfield, P. S. and Rummerfield, M.: What you should know about radiation hazards. *Amer. J. Nurs., 70*:780, (April) 1970.

Wagner, H. N., Jr.: Radioactive pharmaceuticals. *Clin. Pharmacol. Ther. 4*:351, 1963.

Chapter 22 Enzymes

Important Concepts Discussed

1. *Enzymes are organic compounds that are catalysts for many physiological reactions.*

2. *Some enzymes may be administered orally as replacement therapy for deficiencies in natural body enzymes.*

3. *Proteolytic enzymes may be administered therapeutically to aid wound healing by debriding wounds and reducing swelling.*

4. *Supplemental enzymes from various sources may be administered to alter physiological conditions in the body and thus aid in the management of pathological conditions.*

5. *The nurse should be observant for symptoms of an allergic reaction.*

6. *The correct route and method of administration of enzymes are essential in order to produce the intended effect.*

Enzymatic processes were used by man long before recorded history. The use of enzymes in fermenting of wines, the making of cheese, the leavening of bread and the manufacture of vinegar has an ancient origin. Even in modern times, these uses of enzymes have opened many doors for their medicinal use since much of the enzymatic research has been conducted in the laboratories of commercial breweries. The basic reactions of fermentation in a yeast culture are very similar to enzymatic processes in the tissues of animals.

The word "enzyme" means "in yeast," but it has come to refer to any number of biochemical catalysts, regardless of origin. These enzyme catalysts function in the living body just as catalysts function in any chemical process—by accelerating reactions without themselves being degraded or used up

in the process. It is believed that enzymes bind to intermediate products in the reaction, holding them in place, so to speak, for the completion of the reaction.

Normal body chemistry is extremely dependent upon the presence of enzymes. Numerous metabolic disorders, such as phenylketonuria (PKU), von Gierke's disease (glycogen storage disease) and many others are caused by the body's inability to manufacture one enzyme. The effects of this loss on the body as a whole are extensive and often totally disabling.

Nearly every step in the metabolism of nutrients and the subsequent growth and repair of body parts is dependent upon enzymes. The specificity of these enzymes is well known. An enzyme catalyzes one reaction and one reaction only; there must therefore be literally thousands of these delicate organic molecules in the body at all times.

Considerable research is devoted to the study of cellular enzymes because many complicated processes, such as the contraction of a muscle, may be divided into a series of enzyme-catalyzed reactions. Knowledge of these delicate interactions will undoubtedly open many new doors in the diagnosis and treatment of countless diseases. It is possible that even some types of cancer may be linked to aberrant enzyme activity.

Many enzymes are now used in therapy. Digestive enzymes may be administered orally in many cases to supplement deficient gastrointestinal secretions, whereas others may be injected or applied topically for specific purposes.

All known enzymes are proteins, and as such can cause allergic manifestations following administration. This causes many problems, especially when plant or animal enzymes are used in human therapy, since purification procedures are usually lengthy and expensive. The synthesis of these complicated structures is equally difficult. Their therapeutic applications at present are limited, but this type of therapy is rapidly expanding, and many more valuable products will come into use in the near future.

The nurse should be observant for symptoms of an allergic response. The patient should also be instructed to report such symptoms immediately.

When buccal administration is the route used, the patient should be carefully instructed in this method.

Plant enzymes

Bromelains (Ananase). This mixture of proteolytic enzymes is derived from the stem of the pineapple plant, *Ananus sativus.* They act on a variety of substances and generally convert proteins into smaller polypeptides and amino acids. It is postulated that the anti-inflammatory effects of bromelains are due to the digestion of fibrin with consequent increased tissue permeability.

TOXICITY. Mild diarrhea may occasionally occur following therapy. The inci-

dence of allergic reactions is quite low, however. These enzymes are contraindicated in patients receiving anticoagulant therapy, in hemophilia, severe liver or renal disease and systemic infections.

DOSE. 100,000 units orally four times daily.

Papain (Papase). Papain tablets contain extracts of proteolytic enzymes from the fruit of *Carica papaya.* These extracts reduce inflammation following injuries primarily through a proteolytic action on the unorganized fibrinous exudates that are deposited in areas of inflammation. The depolymerizing effect on the fibrin aids drainage of the inflamed area and facilitates the removal of cellular debris by the body's normal healing mechanisms. Papain may be administered also to alleviate edema following oral surgery, episiotomy, thrombophlebitis, thrombotic and postpartum hemorrhoids, stasis ulcers and instrumentation. It aids in liquefying mucoid secretions associated with respiratory disorders.

TOXICITY. The use of papain is contraindicated if anticoagulants are being administered. It is not recommended for use in generalized infections or in severe blood clotting disorders. Occasionally mild gastrointestinal disturbances and allergic reactions occur following administration, but these are infrequent. A few patients experience a tingling sensation at the site of buccal absorption.

DOSE. 10,000 to 20,000 units orally or buccally every 3 to 4 hours.

Bacterial enzymes

Streptokinase-streptodornase (Varidase). Streptokinase-streptodornase is a mixture of enzymes derived from *Streptococcus hemolyticus* cultures. Streptokinase activates plasminogen (fibrinogen), which in turn dissolves and liquefies fibrinous deposits and blood clots. Streptodornase causes liquefaction of the nucleoproteins of dead cells and pus, but it has no effect on the nucleoproteins of living cells.

The use of these enzymes is indicated in most conditions characterized by accumulation of clotted blood and fibrinous or purulent exudate. By facilitating debridement of wound areas, they enhance the action of local and systemic antibiotics. These substitutes should not be used in place of, but rather as an adjunct to, the surgical debridement and drainage of wounds, but as such they make secondary closure of inflamed areas more rapid and effective.

They may be used as an adjunct in the treatment of infected wounds, stasis ulcers, burns, empyema, sinusitis, otitis media, bronchiectasis, suppurative joint infections and osteomyelitis. They are not effective on fibrous tissues, mucoproteins or collagens and should never be used in the presence of active bleeding.

Streptokinase-streptodornase is prepared in the form of a carboxymethylcellulose jelly, which may be applied topically to wounds, or in powdered forms for topical and intramuscular administration. The tablets may be administered only buccally.

> **TOXICITY.** Streptokinase-streptodornase should be used with caution in tuberculosis since there is danger of active reopening of fistulous tracts following dissolution of fibrinous material in the walls of active tubercles. It should not be used in the presence of hemorrhage or acute cellulitis since the clotting processes and normal localizing processes may be hindered. Occasionally a pyrogenic reaction may be observed following intramuscular administration.

> **DOSE.** I.M.—5000 units streptokinase and 1250 units streptodornase twice daily. Buccal—10,000 units streptokinase and 2500 units streptodornase four times daily. Topical—In solution containing 100,000 units streptokinase and 25,000 units streptodornase in 10 ml. saline. In jelly containing 5000 units streptokinase and 1250 units streptodornase per ml.

ANIMAL ENZYMES

TRYPSIN CRYSTALLIZED, N.F. (PARENZYME, TRYPTAR). Trypsin is a proteolytic enzyme obtained commercially from the pancreas of the ox. It is effective against more proteins than is streptokinase; thus it is quite efficient in the debridement of suppurating wounds, ulcers, abscesses and fistulas. It is effective in the liquefaction of clotted blood and unorganized fibrinous exudates. It is not effective in the removal or liquefaction of fibrous tissue however.

Trypsin is used to produce liquefaction of mucoid secretions of the respiratory tract, but because it is irritating to the tissues when inhaled, its use for this purpose is somewhat limited.

It is available in powder, suspension and buccal tablet forms. One commercially prepared ointment contains both trypsin and chymotrypsin and may be applied topically for local debridement.

> **TOXICITY.** If placed in closed cavities, trypsin produces a pyrogenic effect, accompanied by release of histamine causing itching and a rash. This effect may be minimized by the administration of antihistamines. Pain and induration may be caused at the site of intramuscular injection. Allergic reactions may occasionally be observed. A sensitivity test should therefore be conducted before administration of therapeutic doses of this enzyme. It should not be applied to actively bleeding areas.

> **DOSE.** Oral and buccal—5 mg. four times daily. I.M. (deep in gluteal muscle)—5 mg. twice daily until inflammation subsides. Topical—in solution containing 4 mg. per ml. saline applied every 3 hours or as required.

CHYMOTRYPSIN, N.F. (CHYMAR, ENZEON). Like trypsin, chymotrypsin is commercially obtained from the pancreas of the ox. It is marketed as buccal and oral tablets, an aqueous solution, an oily suspension and an ointment in combination with trypsin.

Chymotrypsin may be used similarly to trypsin in the treatment of suppurating wounds, abscesses, pelvic inflammatory disease and thrombophlebitis and following oral surgery.

TOXICITY. Allergic reactions, fever and chills have been noted. A few instances of anaphylactic shock have occurred.

DOSE. I.M.—2500 to 5000 units one to three times daily. Buccal or oral—10,000 units four times daily.

ALPHA-CHYMOTRYPSIN (ALPHA CHYMAR). Alpha-chymotrypsin is a proteolytic enzyme obtained from veal pancreas that has a selective action on the zonula ciliaris of the eye without damage to surrounding structures. As such, it is of great benefit in cataract extractions and is used almost exclusively for this purpose. Care should be taken to thoroughly clean the surgical syringes and instruments to remove alcohol and other chemicals that could inactivate the enzyme. Solutions should be freshly prepared and unused portions should be discarded after four hours.

DOSE. 1 to 3 ml. of a solution containing 150 units per ml. injected behind the iris.

FIBRINUCLEASE (ELASE). Fibrinuclease is a commercial preparation containing fibrinolysin from bovine plasma and desoxyribonuclease from bovine pancreas. It is prepared in ointment form for topical application to inflamed and necrotic skin.

Fibrinolysin causes the liquefaction of fibrin, whereas desoxyribonuclease depolymerizes the nucleic acids in cellular debris and pus. It has no effect on living cells.

DOSE. 30 units fibrinolysin and 20,000 units desoxyribonuclease per oz. of ointment.

PANCREATIC DORNASE (DORNAVAC). Pancreatic dornase is a purified preparation of desoxyribonuclease obtained from beef pancreas. It quickly reduces the viscosity of inflammatory exudates by depolymerizing desoxyribonucleic acid, the material largely responsible for the character and viscosity of these exudates.

It is quite effective in the treatment of bronchopulmonary infections, such as bronchitis, bronchiectasis, pulmonary abscesses, atelectasis, asthma and emphysema, by reducing the viscosity of sputum and inflammatory exudates in these areas. It has been used as an adjunct in the treatment of cystic fibrosis and tuberculous empyema. It may be administered with or without concurrent antibiotic therapy.

When pancreatic dornase is administered by aerosol or nebulizer-oxygen tank, symptomatic relief is obtained within an hour. Clinical improvement as shown by decreased lung exudate may be observed in a few days. Positive pressure machines are superior to hand nebulizers when deep penetration of lung tissues is desired.

DOSE. 50,000 to 100,000 units by inhalation one to four times daily for one to seven days. Treatment may be resumed after an interval of a few days.

FIBRINOLYSIN (THROMBOLYSIN, ACTASE). Fibrinolysin is a proteolytic enzyme prepared by activating pooled human plasma with streptokinase. It is intended for use in the dissolution of intravascular thrombi. It may be injected intravenously for treatment of phlebothrombosis, thrombophlebitis, pulmonary embolism and other arterial thrombi. Clinical results with this compound have not been as satisfactory as were originally hoped, however, perhaps because lysis of clots occurs following complex interactions of proenzymes and enzymes, and proactivators and activators, and cannot be satisfactorily accomplished by the injection of only one enzyme.

When this compound is used, treatment should be initiated as soon as possible after a thrombus has formed. Organization of the clots makes them relatively impervious to exogenous enzymes. It is of little value after the clot has been formed for five days or more.

TOXICITY. Febrile and allergic reactions have been observed, as well as hypertension, facial flushing, chest pain and abdominal discomfort. It is contraindicated in the presence of active hemorrhage or hypofibrinogenemia, and it should be administered with caution immediately after anesthesia or surgery since endogenous fibrinolytic activity is often increased for a short time following these procedures.

DOSE. 50,000 to 500,000 units I.V. daily. The dose may be repeated in one to three subsequent days. The smaller doses are employed for venous thrombi; larger doses are used for arterial emboli.

HYALURONIDASE (ALIDASE, WYDASE). Hyaluronidase is an enzyme prepared commercially from bovine testes and administered therapeutically to hydrolyze hyaluronic acid, a polysaccharide that is a major component of the extracellular ground substance, which is a barrier to the diffusion of exogenous substances. Following the administration of hyaluronidase, it is possible to greatly increase the absorption of fluid and drugs administered subcutaneously. Large amounts of fluids may be administered by hypodermoclysis whenever intravenous administration is not feasible or possible; it is of especial advantage in pediatric therapy since intravenous administration to infants and young children is in many cases extremely difficult.

Hyaluronidase also facilitates absorption of parenteral medications, such as antibiotics, heparin and steroids, and facilitates diffusion when medications are instilled into cavities. When administered with local anesthetics, it increases the area anesthetized by as much as 40 per cent, but the duration of anesthetic effect is reduced. It has occasionally been used to increase the rate of resorption of hematomas and to permit subcutaneous administration of radiopaque dyes for x-ray examination of the urogenital tract.

Hyaluronidase should be stored in a dry place away from heat. Solutions should be prepared immediately before using; only colorless solutions should be used.

TOXICITY. Hyaluronidase should not be injected into acutely inflamed or malignant areas. Because sensitization has occurred, a test should be used prior to administration of therapeutic doses.

DOSE. 150 units in solution s.c.

QUESTIONS FOR DISCUSSION AND REVIEW

1. How do topical enzymes aid in the debridement of wounds?

2. Why would fluids be given by hypodermoclysis? How does hyaluronidase aid in their absorption?

3. What conditions would warrant the use of pancreatic dornase? What symptoms would the patient experience before administration of the drug?

4. Why would hemophilia and hepatic and renal disorders be contraindications for the use of bromelains?

5. Explain the mechanism by which chymotrypsin could produce a sensitivity reaction.

6. Review the signs and symptoms of allergic reactions. What action should be taken? What drugs and equipment should be available and why?

7. How would you explain buccal administration to a patient?

BIBLIOGRAPHY

Council on Drugs: Buccal and intramuscular use of streptokinase and streptodornase (Varidase). *J.A.M.A., 172*:701, 1960.

Council on Drugs: Enzymes proposed as systemic anti-inflammatory agents. *J.A.M.A., 188*:875, 1964.

Council on Drugs: A mucolytic agent — acetylcysteine (Mucomyst). *J.A.M.A., 190*:147, 1964.

Miller, J. M.: The proteolytic enzymes. *Amer. J. Nurs., 58*:1410, (October) 1958.

Sherry, S.: Streptokinase. *New Eng. J. Med., 280*:723, 1969.

Sherry, S.: Urokinase. *Ann. Intern. Med., 69*:415, 1968.

Tow, D. E., Wagner, H. N., Jr. and Holmes, R. A.: Urokinase in pulmonary embolism. *New Eng. J. Med., 277*:1161, 1967.

Chapter 23 Diagnostic Agents

Important Concepts Discussed

1. *Some pharmacologic agents serve as diagnostic tools by producing characteristic changes in body tissues or functions.*

2. *The function of various body organs can be determined by the rate of excretion or the concentration of certain drugs in tissues or fluids.*

3. *Alterations in normal physiology can be produced by drugs in order to determine the etiology of metabolic disorders.*

4. *Radiopaque drugs are administered to produce changes in density that permit visualization of various organs.*

5. *The nurse has an important role in the physical and psychological preparation of the patient, and in the observation of the patient's response.*

Recent advances in clinical laboratory procedures have greatly facilitated the methods for accurate diagnoses of many diseases and pathological conditions. In a nursing pharmacology text it is impossible to discuss all the laboratory procedures or tests that are performed for diagnostic purposes; instead we will confine ourselves to the tests using biological and nonbiological pharmaceutical preparations.

The nurse is usually not involved in the actual administration of most of these agents; however, she must be familiar with the agents used and the purpose of the tests in order to meet her patient's needs. She may be involved in preparing the patient physically for the test, such as withholding fluids or cleansing the bowel. Psychological preparation of the patient is important to allay his fears and misconceptions. The purpose

and procedure involved should be clearly explained to the patient.

Observations by the nurse may be important during the test and are especially important after the test is completed, since allergic responses or other side effects may occur. The nurse may also be involved in the collection of various specimens related to the particular test.

BIOLOGICAL DIAGNOSTIC AGENTS

BLASTOMYCIN, U.S.P. Blastomycin is the standardized, sterile filtrate from cultures of the mycelial phase of *Blastomyces dermatitidis*. It is used as an aid in the diagnosis of North American blastomycosis (Gilchrist's disease), which is caused by this microorganism, and in the differentiation of possible blastomycosis from tuberculosis, histoplasmosis, syphilis, sarcoidosis, silicosis, osteomyelitis, psoas abscess and other fungus infections.

In performing the test, 0.1 ml. of the diluted solution is injected intracutaneously into the forearm. The reaction should be read 24 to 48 hours after the injection. An indurated area of 5 × 5 mm. is a positive reaction, which indicates a past infection or a mild, subacute or chronic infection. A negative response may occur in acute or fulminating infections in which the body has become insensitive to the antigen.

COCCIDIOIDIN. Coccidioidin is prepared from cultures of 10 strains of *Coccidioides immitis.* Initial infections, obtained following inhalation of the spores of *C. immitis,* are often associated with the allergic dermatologic manifestation of the infection, called coccidioidal erythema nodosum.

Patients exhibiting this syndrome are frequently very sensitive to the skin testing extract; therefore it is advisable to employ very diluted preparations for the initial tests. An initial dilution of 1:10,000 is advisable; if this is negative, 1:1000 should be tried, and only if that is negative should 1:100 be used.

In a small proportion of persons, infection with *C. immitis* will not remain confined to the lungs. Under such circumstances the spores disseminate throughout the body and the patient develops coccidioidal granuloma for which the prognosis is very poor. Patients with such lesions may be insensitive to coccidioidin and may have negative skin tests even when undiluted coccidioidin is used.

The reactions to these skin tests are usually readable at 24 hours and are maximal at 36 hours. A positive reaction is an induration measuring 0.5 cm. or more.

As with tuberculin tests, a negative reaction means that the individual has not been sensitized to coccidioidin or has lost his sensitivity. A positive reaction indicates that the individual has been in contact with the fungus at some time in the past.

HISTOPLASMIN, U.S.P. Histoplasmin is the standardized sterile filtrate from cultures of *Histoplasma capsulatum.* It is employed as an aid in the diagnosis of histoplasmosis and the differentiation of possible histoplasmosis from coccidioidomycosis, sarcoidosis and other mycotic or bacterial infections, as well as in the interpretation of x-ray plates showing pulmonary infiltration and calcification.

In the test, 0.1 ml. of diluted solution is injected intracutaneously into the forearm. After 24 to 48 hours an area of induration of 5 × 5 mm. or greater is a positive reaction, indicating a past infection or a mild, subacute or chronic infection. A negative reaction may indicate no exposure or an acute, fulminating infection.

FREI ANTIGEN. Lymphogranuloma venereum skin test involves intracutaneous injection of the sterile pus from a lesion of *Lymphogranuloma venereum* and is used especially in males who develop inguinal adenitis following a primary venereal lesion, with discharging lymph nodes that heal slowly. Subclinical varieties of the disease are believed to be common, however, particularly in the female.

The late sequelae of this disease, particularly rectal stricture, are so serious that all patients with venereal disease should be given the Frei test following the acute stage of the disease.

This test is performed by injecting 0.1 ml. of the antigen intradermally. Positive reaction after 48 to 72 hours is an erythematous papule of 6 mm. surrounded by a less erythematous zone. A negative reaction may be obtained early in the course of the disease, because the reaction is not positive until two to five weeks after the appearance of the initial bubo.

MUMPS SKIN TEST ANTIGEN. Mumps skin test antigen is a suspension of killed mumps virus. The appearance of an area of erythema 1.5 cm. in diameter 24 to 36 hours after intradermal injection of 0.1 ml. of antigen indicates immunity. A negative reaction indicates susceptibility to the infection.

The vaccine is contraindicated in patients who are allergic to chicken, chicken feathers or eggs.

DOSE. Intradermal—0.1 ml. (20 complement fixing units).

TRICHINELLA EXTRACT, U.S.P. *Trichinella* extract is a preparation of dried *Trichinella* larvae, and it is used in the differential diagnosis of trichinosis.

A positive reaction to the intracutaneous injection of 0.1 ml. usually appears within 15 to 20 minutes. The formation of a wheal that exceeds that of the control wheal by 3 mm. or more, with or without pseudopodia, is a positive reaction, indicating that the patient may harbor a clinical infection with *Trichinella* or a latent or healed infection without clinical significance. Thus, a positive test is only suggestive of clinical trichinosis and should be confirmed by further clinical observations or biopsy. Occasionally a positive cross-reaction occurs in patients infected with other parasites, notably *Trichuris trichiura*.

A negative reaction may occur early in the course of the disease because the skin test does not become positive until about the second week of infection.

TUBERCULINS. Similarly to the previously discussed agents, the tuberculins are useful only in the detection of mild or chronic forms of the disease. The test may be negative in acute or fulminating infections. The concurrent presence of sarcoidosis, Hodgkin's disease or viral infections may cause a false negative skin reaction.

Old Tuberculin U.S.P., B.P. (O. T., Koch's Tuberculin). This is the sterile, concentrated culture medium in which the tubercle bacillus *Mycobacterium tuberculosis* has grown.

The Mantoux test (or Mendel's test) is performed by injecting the tuberculin intracutaneously in increasing amounts if no reaction appears. A positive reaction is a zone of redness and edema, usually with a papule at the site of injection, which reaches its height in about 48 hours.

This indicates that the individual has at some time had a tuberculous focus in his system, but it does not prove the existence of positive tuberculosis or reveal the extent of any existing infection. Chest x-rays and sputum cultures are used to check for active tuberculosis. Prophylactic doses of anti-tuberculosis drugs may be prescribed.

The Vollmer patch test utilizes an adhesive strip with two thin filter paper squares saturated with a tuberculin solution about four times as strong as the official solution and one control square. This is held in contact with the skin for about 48 hours. In susceptible persons, the area covered by the paper will be marked with follicles or papules of an erythematous base.

DOSE. 0.0001 ml. with a range of 0.00001 to 0.001 ml. intracutaneously.

Purified protein derivative of tuberculin (PPD), U.S.P., B.P. This is a sterile, product of growth of the tubercle bacillus. It is devoid of the culture medium proteins and many of the culture metabolism end-products found in Old Tuberculin. This increased purity renders it more acceptable as a diagnostic aid; it is used almost exclusively to aid in the diagnosis of tuberculosis. It is supplied in three strengths to enable administration of increasingly larger doses of the tuberculin if desired.

The skin test is read in 48 hours. Erythema and/or induration of an area greater than 0.5 cm. is considered to be positive.

DOSE. 0.00002 to 0.0002 mg. intracutaneously.

BRUCELLERGEN. Brucellergen skin test is prepared from a strain of *Brucella abortus* and is used in the diagnosis of brucellosis (undulant fever). The reaction may be read 24 to 48 hours following intradermal injection of 0.1 ml. of solution. A positive reaction is indicated by erythema, edema and induration varying from 2 to 10 cm.

A negative reaction to Brucellergen is not necessarily an indication of the absence of brucellosis, because in some individuals an allergy does not develop. The ability to detect skin sensitization depends upon the existence and continuance of the allergic state.

DIAGNOSTIC DIPHTHERIA TOXIN, U.S.P.; SCHICK TEST TOXIN, B.P. Consisting merely of an isotonic solution of diphtheria toxin, this product is employed to determine immunity to diphtheria. Since older children are more prone to exhibit unpleasant reactions after immunizing injections, only known susceptible people should be immunized. A positive reaction at the site of injection indicates susceptibility to diphtheria. Absence of reaction indicates the presence of circulating antitoxin and, hence, immunity. A positive reaction, best read on the fourth or fifth day, consists of redness and induration, which appear in 24 to 36 hours and persist four or five days. The reaction gradually disappears. Occasionally local reaction is severe and can progress to tissue necrosis.

DOSE. 0.1 ml. intradermally.

SCARLET FEVER STREPTOCOCCUS TOXIN (DICK TEST TOXIN). The Dick test toxin, a reagent used for the diagnosis of susceptibility to scarlet fever, is a sterile filtrate from a culture of a toxigenic strain of *Streptococcus pyogenes* or material obtained therefrom. When used intracutaneously, an area of redness with a slight infiltration of at least 1 cm. in diameter appears in susceptible persons within 24 hours. It is never indurated. Untoward reactions are rare.

DOSE. 0.1 ml. intracutaneously.

NONBIOLOGIC DIAGNOSTIC AGENTS

SODIUM SULFOBROMOPHTHALEIN, U.S.P. B.P. (BROMSULPHALEIN, B.S.P.). After injection of this agent, the liver removes it from the blood and excretes it into bile within 30 minutes. The patient should be fasting for 12 hours and should not have received any other dyes within the past 48 hours. The amount of sulfobromophthalein retained by the blood serum is determined colorimetrically and compared to normal performance in order to assess liver function. Less than 5% should be retained in the blood in 45 minutes.

Epinephrine should be immediately available, since severe hypersensitivity reactions may occur.

DOSE. 2 mg. of 50% solution/kg of body weight I.V.

INDOCYANINE GREEN (CARDIO-GREEN). Indocyanine green is a dye used to determine cardiac function. Standard dilutions of indocyanine green are made in whole blood and compared to aliquots of the patient's blood to determine the dilution of the dye in the blood within a specified period of time.

Since a small amount of sodium iodide is present in indocyanine green, it should not be given to patients allergic to iodides.

DOSE. 5 mg. I.V. The solution must be prepared immediately before injection.

DEHYDROCHOLIC ACID, N.F. (DECHOLIN SODIUM). Dehydrocholic acid is used chiefly to determine circulation time, the time that it takes the I.V. injection of a substance capable of stimulating a receptor organ to reach that organ in sufficient quantity to produce a response.

The arm-to-tongue method is usually used, and determination is made of the time for blood carrying dehydrocholic acid to flow from the site of injection in the antecubital vein to the taste receptors of the tongue, where it produces an immediate, marked bitter taste of short duration. Most investigators consider 8 to 16 seconds to be the normal range of the circulation time procedure.

Circulation time is usually prolonged in congestive heart failure, myxedema, polycythemia vera, some cases of complete atrioventricular block, chronic constructive pericarditis, pericardial effusion with tamponade and some cases of paroxysmal tachycardia and shock. As cardiac compensation is restored, circulation time returns to normal and is thus a guide to therapy.

The circulation time is usually shortened in hyperthyroidism, beriberi, anemia, congenital cardiac anomalies (right-to-left shunt) and abnormalities of the great vessels (reversed flow due to truncus arteriosus or patent ductus arteriosus).

In addition to measuring circulation time, dehydrocholic acid may also be used to demonstrate the reservoir capacity of the gallbladder because of its hydrocholeretic effect. The volume of bile is increased 100 to 200 per cent above the normal flow.

DOSE. 3 to 5 ml. of a 20% solution.

AZURESIN, N.F. (DIAGNEX BLUE). Azuresin, prepared by exchanging the hydrogen ions of a carbacrylic cation exchange resin with azure A, a blue dye, determines the presence of free hydrochloric acid in the stomach by a tubeless procedure. When the resin indicator reaches the stomach following oral administration, the azure A is liberated in the presence of free gastric hydrochloric acid, absorbed in the blood, and excreted in the urine in which its presence may be detected by colorimetric inspection.

The patient receives nothing by mouth after midnight and his first urine voiding is discarded. He is given 500 mg. of caffeine in a glass of water. A urine specimen is obtained in one hour and the specimen saved as a control specimen. He then swallows the dye in one fourth to one half glass of water. After 2 hours, the patient voids and the specimen is sent to the laboratory. The urine may continue to be blue or blue-green for a few days after the test. If inspection of urine voided two hours after oral administration shows the presence of 0.6 mg. or more azure A, the patient has free gastric hydrochloric acid. Less than 0.3 mg. is an indication of achlorhydria, and the presence of amounts between 0.3 and 0.6 mg. indicates hypochlorhydria.

The test results may not be valid in the presence of pyloric obstruction, severe hepatic or renal disease, abnormalities that impair intestinal absorption, vomiting, marked dehydration, urinary bladder retention or partial or total gastrectomy.

DOSE.   2 Gm. orally.

EVANS BLUE, U.S.P.   Evans blue is a diazo dye that combines firmly with plasma albumin when injected into the blood and leaves the circulation very slowly. It is used for blood volume determination because the optical density of this dye is directly proportional to its concentration. A blood sample is withdrawn before the dye is injected to serve as a control. Ten minutes after the dye is injected, another blood sample is withdrawn from a vein in the opposite arm for the reading. Colorimetric determinations are made on the blood samples.

DOSE.   0.3 mg./kg. of body weight I.V.

FLUORESCIN SODIUM U.S.P., B.P. (FLUORESCITE).   Fluorescin, which is strongly fluorescent, is used diagnostically to measure circulation time, adequacy of the blood supply and tissue viability. After rapid intravenous injections, fluorescin quickly appears in extracellular fluid and is transported to viable cells only. Fluorescin is also useful as a guide in amputations and in distinguishing between second and third degree burns, since the circulation to visible skin has been destroyed in third degree burns.

The presence of fluorescin in the circulating blood also makes possible the "string test" in localizing gastrointestinal hemorrhage. In this test, a cotton tape with radiopaque markings is swallowed. At the position of the hemorrhage, the blood, containing fluorescin, is absorbed by the tape. Following removal of the tape, the site of bleeding can be localized by the position of the fluorescence relative to the radiopaque markings.

Since only viable cells take up the dye, fluorescin is of value in establishing the viability of intestinal areas in cases of strangulated hernia. It has been reported that brain tumors take up the dye more readily than does normal brain tissue. Based on this observation, a technique has been employed to detect and localize subcortical and other tumors.

With systemic absorption, the skin may be tinted faintly yellow, but this disappears within 24 hours. The patient may experience nausea and vomiting when the dye is injected intravenously. Solutions should be freshly prepared since they can become easily contaminated with bacteria.

When fluorescin is applied to the cornea, only injured areas are stained. It is therefore useful for locating imbedded particles or trauma.

DOSE.   5 ml. or 0.7 ml./10 lb. of body weight I.V.

HISTAMINE PHOSPHATE, U.S.P., B.P.   Injections of histamine stimulate the gastric glands and thus increase the quantity and acidity of the gastric juice if the glands are able to respond. Fractional gastric analyses of gastric aspirations obtained via a naso-gastric tube are employed to determine the amount of hydrochloric acid present.

Histamine is also quite useful as a pharmacologic test for pheochromocytoma. It apparently liberates epinephrine by direct stimulation of the adrenal medulla. This test is used in patients whose blood pressure does not exceed 150/110 when they are resting; it must not be used in the elderly or in the presence of severe hypertension. In this test, 0.025 to 0.05 mg. histamine is rapidly introduced through intravenous infusion, and the blood pressure is recorded at one minute intervals for 15 minutes. When a systolic rise is 60 mm. mercury or more, and the diastolic 30 mm. or more within one to four minutes and pressures return to pre-injection levels in 5 to 15 minutes or more, the results of the test are considered positive if the elevation exceeds the cold pressor response.

histamine

TOXICITY. Large doses may produce flushing, dizziness, headache, local or generalized allergic symptoms, hypotension and abdominal cramps. Dangerous blood pressure elevation and tachycardia may result as well. Emergency drugs and equipment should be on hand.

DOSE. 0.3 to 0.5 ml. of a 1:1000 solution subcutaneously to promote gastric secretion; 0.025 to 0.05 mg. I.V. as a diagnostic test for pheochromocytoma.

BETAZOLE HYDROCHLORIDE, U.S.P. (HISTALOG). Betazole hydrochloride is an analog of histamine that may be used in place of histamine in clinical tests of gastric secretion. In the recommended dosage, betazole's stimulation of gastric secretion is equal to that obtained with the usual dose of histamine. Betazole has minimal effects on other organs and hence produces fewer side effects. It is administered I.M. or subcutaneously and the amount of secreted hydrochloric

acid is determined by fractional gastric analyses.

TOXICITY. Although reactions observed in allergic patients are less severe with betazole than with histamine, it should be used with caution in patients with bronchial asthma, urticaria or other severe forms of allergy. The most commonly observed side effect under most conditions is facial flushing.

DOSE. 50 mg. I.M. or subcutaneously.

SODIUM INDIGOTINDISULFONATE, U.S.P.; INDIGO CARMINE, B.P. Sodium indigotindisulfonate, a water-soluble dye, is useful in the diagnosis of renal function. Elimination of the dye, which begins soon after injection, is accomplished largely by the kidneys and is easy to detect since it retains its color.

At present, however, the chief application of this drug is in the localizing of ureteral orifices during cystoscopy and ureteral catheterization, since it has largely been replaced by phenolsulfonphthalein as a test of renal function.

Sensitivity tests should be done on patients with a history of allergies.

DOSE. 5 ml. of 0.8% solution I.V.

MANNITOL, N.F., B.P. Mannitol is used to measure the glomerular filtration rate because it is filtered by the glomeruli and not reabsorbed or secreted by the nephron tubules. To accomplish this, mannitol is administered intravenously so that an adequate plasma concentration can be maintained. A catheterized specimen of urine is collected at the beginning of the period, in 15 minutes and at the end of the period. Blood samples are taken for hematocrit and mannitol determinations.

The glomerular filtration rate may be calculated as follows:

$$\text{GFR in 1 minute} = \frac{U \cdot V}{P}$$

U = quantity of mannitol/ml. urine
V = volume of urine/min.
P = quantity of mannitol/ml. plasma

Normal values are 131 ± 21.5 ml./min. for men and 117 ± 15.6 ml./min for women.

DOSE. 50 ml. of 25% solution I.V.

SODIUM AMINOHIPPURATE INJECTIONS, U.S.P. (PAH). Sodium aminohippurate is used to measure effective renal plasma flow and maximal tubular secretory capacity. In addition to being filtered by the glomerulus, PAH is secreted by the tubular epithelium. 88 per cent of this compound is removed from the renal blood in man in a single circulation. The value for effective renal plasma flow is expressed as ml./min. and is normally 697 ± 135.9 for men and 594 ± 102.4 for women.

To determine the functional capacity of the tubular secretory mechanism, the plasma concentration of PAH is elevated to 40 or 60 mg./100 ml. at which the maximal capacity of the tubule cells to secrete PAH is reached. This measurement is referred to as T_mPAH or the functional tubular mass. The amount of PAH excreted by glomerular filtration is subtracted from the tubular secretion. T_mPAH is expressed in mg./min. and has a normal mean value of 77.5 ± 12.9.

DOSE. 50 ml. of 20% solution I.V.

METYRAPONE, U.S.P. (METOPIRONE). Metyrapone is a synthetic compound that selectively inhibits 11-beta-hydroxylation in the adrenal cortex. It is a test of pituitary function.

In normal individuals, metyrapone causes a decrease in plasma cortisol and its urinary metabolites. Since pituitary ACTH release depends on circulating cortisol, more ACTH is released. Continued adrenal blockade, however, causes an increase of the precursors, 11-desoxycortisol (compound S) and 11-desoxycorticosterone (DOC), which are detectable in the plasma, and their metabolites are present in urine.

Patients with reduced pituitary function lack the ability to increase ACTH production, and no significant increase in the two precursors is observed.

TOXICITY. Only transient vertigo has been observed, and it can be overcome by administering the tablets with milk. Patients with minimally functioning adrenals may develop severe adrenal insufficiency when given this drug;

suspected cases should first be tested with exogenous ACTH to determine adrenal responsiveness.

DOSE. 750 mg. orally every 4 hours for 6 doses.

TOLBUTAMIDE, U.S.P., B.P. (ORINASE DIAGNOSTIC). Tolbutamide is employed intravenously for the diagnosis of mild diabetes mellitus, pancreatic carcinoma, acute pancreatitis and functioning pancreatic islet cell adenoma.

When tolbutamide is used for the first three conditions, there is a prompt decrease in blood glucose in nondiabetic individuals, which is associated with a prompt increase in serum insulin levels 20 minutes after injection. The decrease in diabetic patients is gradual and occurs more slowly. In patients with functioning islet cell adenoma, tolbutamide has a marked and prolonged blood glucose-lowering effect associated with an excessive, prompt rise in serum insulin, resulting in a marked and prolonged blood sugar effect.

Blood determinations are compared with established standards for diagnosis of these conditions.

TOXICITY. Hypoglycemia of considerable magnitude may occur in susceptible individuals.

DOSE. 1 Gm. I.V.

PHENOLSULFONPHTHALEIN, U.S.P., B.P. (PSP). Upon use of PSP for a renal function test, the bladder must be emptied. The patient drinks 300 to 400 cc. of water about 20 minutes before PSP is injected I.M. or I.V. The urine secreted during the next two hours is analyzed colorimetrically for PSP. Urine specimens are obtained 15, 30, 60 and 120 minutes after the PSP is injected. The average normal elimination of the I.M. injection is 40 to 50 per cent the first hour and 60 to 75 per cent at the end of two hours.

TOXICITY. The excretion of the dye is diminished in the presence of cardiac failure; it should therefore be used with extreme caution in cardiac patients.

There is a danger of hypersensitivity to the drug.

DOSE. 1 ml. I.M. or I.V.

PHENTOLAMINE MESYLATE, U.S.P.; PHENTOLAMINE HYDROCHLORIDE; PHENTOLAMINE METHANESULFONATE, B.P. (REGITINE).   Phentolamine is used for the diagnosis of pheochromocytoma and is a relatively simple and accurate way of making a differential diagnosis of hypertension. The patient should be lying flat during the test. The blood pressure is measured immediately after injection and every 30 seconds for three minutes, then every minute for seven minutes.

The anti-adrenergic action of phentolamine blocks the hypertensive activity of the pressor substances emanating from a pheochromocytoma. When it is injected into an individual with an actively secreting tumor, there is usually an unmistakable fall in blood pressure. Pheochromocytoma is suggested by a prompt fall in the systolic pressure of more than 35 mm. Hg, or a fall in the diastolic pressure greater than 25 mm. Hg.

A false positive response may be obtained in patients with uremia, emotional disturbances, and those who have taken sedatives, narcotics, anesthetics, thiocyanates or other drugs. A negative response may indicate that the tumor is quiescent. In such cases, a provocative test with histamine may be considered.

TOXICITY. Tachycardia, weakness, dizziness and flushing have been noted.

DOSE. 5 mg. I.V.

EDROPHONIUM CHLORIDE INJECTION, U.S.P., B.P. (TENSILON). A very rapidly acting drug, edrophonium is helpful in the differential diagnosis of myasthenia gravis. In patients with this disease, edrophonium results in markedly increased strength that is maximal within five minutes. Because of the brief action, it is not recommended for maintenance therapy in myasthenia gravis.

TOXICITY. Edrophonium should be used with caution in patients with bronchial asthma or cardiac arrhythmias. The transient bradycardia that occurs occasionally may be prevented by administration of atropine.

DOSE. 10 mg. I.M.

NEOSTIGMINE METHYLSULFATE INJECTION, U.S.P., B.P. (PROSTIGMIN). Neostigmine is used in the diagnosis of myasthenia gravis, because there is a prompt remission of muscular weakness following its injection.

TOXICITY. Profuse perspiration, abdominal cramps, diarrhea, precipitation of micturition or strangury may occur.

DOSE. 0.5 mg. of neostigmine methylsulfate I.M. or subcutaneously.

CALCIUM IPODATE (ORAGRAFIN). Ipodate is an oral radiopaque medium for cholangiography and cholecystography. Rapid absorption from the gastrointestinal tract results in optimal concentration in the hepatic and biliary ducts in one to three hours. The course and caliber of the ducts may then be ascertained by roentgenography. Stones, strictures and anomalies may frequently be diagnosed.

TOXICITY. Nausea, vomiting and diarrhea which are reduced by decreasing the dose. Headache, dysuria, urticaria or abdominal pains may occur infrequently. It is contraindicated in combined renal and hepatic disease or severe kidney impairment. Gastrointestinal disorders inhibiting absorption or liver dysfunction causing inadequate biliary secretion of the dye are likely to result in inadequate visualization.

DOSE. 3 Gm. orally in the evening, 10 to 12 hrs. before the x-rays are to be taken.

IOPANOIC ACID, U.S.P., B.P. (TELEPAQUE). Iopanoic acid, an organic iodine compound, is administered orally as a radiopaque medium in cholecystography. It is rapidly absorbed, stored in the gallbladder and eliminated in the bile.

The patient usually has a fat-free meal the evening before and takes nothing by mouth after the tablets have been taken.

TOXICITY. Nausea, diarrhea, dysuria. It is contraindicated in acute nephritis and uremia and should not be administered when gastrointestinal disorders prevent its absorption. Since it is an iodine compound, it can cause allergic reactions. The patient should not take the entire dose at once, but rather one tablet every 5 minutes in case of allergy.

DOSE. 3 Gm. (6 tablets) orally 10 hours before x-ray is to be taken.

CONGO RED, U.S.P., B.P. An azo dye, congo red is used in the diagnosis of amyloid disease and for the management of profuse capillary hemorrhage such as occurs in septicemia and in terminal cases of leukemia.

Congo red is removed rapidly from the blood by amyloid tissue, and the rate of disappearance from the blood indicates the presence or absence of amyloid. Normally only 40 per cent disappears in one hour, but in amyloid disease 40 to 100 per cent disappears, and only traces are found in the urine. In nephrosis, there is a rapid disappearance from the blood, but the dye is excreted in the urine.

TOXICITY. Congo red may produce a thromboplastic action; intravascular clotting may result from too rapid injection or too large a dose.

DOSE. 10 to 20 ml. of 1 per cent solution I.V.

GALACTOSE. Galactose, a sugar rapidly converted to glycogen by the normal liver, is excreted unchanged in the urine in the presence of cirrhosis of the liver. It is used as a diagnostic agent for this condition.

DOSE. 40 Gm. orally.

THYROTROPIN (THYTROPAR, TSH). Thyrotropin is the thyroid-stimulating hormone secreted from the anterior pituitary. It is used to differentiate primary thyroidal myxedema from pituitary myxedema, to enhance radioactive iodine uptake in metastatic thyroid carcinoma and to provide symptomatic relief of and hasten recovery in acute thyroiditis.

The diagnostic test for myxedema is based upon the ability of the thyroid to respond to pituitary stimulation. In primary myxedema, the thyroid cannot be stimulated to function normally, whereas in pituitary myxedema, it is susceptible to stimulation.

DOSE. 10 units I.M. or subcutaneously.

BARIUM SULFATE, U.S.P., B.P. Barium sulfate is an insoluble, opaque powder used in x-ray examination of the gastrointestinal tract. Its high degree of insolubility prevents absorption, and hence no toxic effects are obtained from its use.

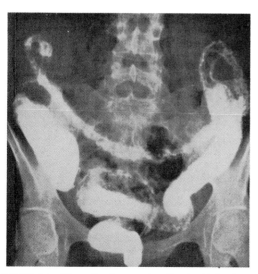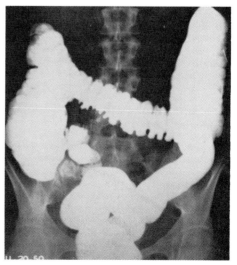

FIGURE 53. Normal colon as visualized with barium sulfate (W. L. Palmer in Cecil and Loeb: *A Textbook of Medicine.* Ed. 13. W. B. Saunders Co., Philadelphia, 1971.)

The nurse should take precautions to insure that the patient expels barium after diagnostic tests. Impaction and perforation of the bowel can occur from retained barium. Cleansing enemas are usually ordered routinely after a patient has received a barium enema. Notation should be made as to whether the barium was expelled. A cathartic and cleansing enema may be given after a patient has swallowed barium for diagnostic studies.

Barium sulfide is a toxic compound that is often fatally confused with barium sulfate. The full name of the drug should always be written out to avoid possibility of confusion.

DOSE. 200 to 300 Gm. orally.

CHLORIODIZED OIL (IODOCHLOROL). Chloriodized oil is a chlorinated and iodized peanut oil that is used as a contrast medium in the x-ray diagnosis of tumors of the spinal cord, in localization of bronchial and pulmonary lesions and in gynecology. Because of the iodine content, there is a danger of hypersensitivity.

DOSE. 1 to 20 ml. I.V. or intrathecally.

SODIUM DIATRIZOATE INJECTION, U.S.P., B.P. (HYPAQUE SODIUM). Sodium diatrizoate is used as a contrast medium in intravenous urography. It is excreted unchanged in the urine. Suitable x-ray shadows appear in 30 minutes, depending upon the adequacy of kidney function and proper preparation of the patient and injection technique.

TOXICITY. Contraindicated in advanced renal impairment with severe uremia and in severe hepatic disorders. It should be used with caution in patients with hypertension, tuberculosis, hyperthyroidism, cardiovascular disease and in patients allergic to iodine. Cardiovascular collapse and anaphylactic shock have occurred following administration of this agent.

DOSE. 30 ml. of 50% solution I.V.

IODIZED OIL, N.F., B.P. (LIPIODOL). This x-ray medium is prepared by adding iodine to unsaturated vegetable oils. It is used to visualize hollow viscera, sinus and fistulous tracts and intradural tumors. Allergic reactions may occur.

DOSE. 1 to 20 ml. instilled in hollow viscera.

IODOPYRACET, N.F. (DIODONE, DIODRAST). Iodopyracet is used as a contrast agent for excretory and retrograde pyelography.

TOXICITY. A fall in blood pressure, respiratory stimulation, flushing, nausea, vomiting, erythematous eruptions and urticaria occur on occasion. It is contraindicated in patients with advanced renal obstruction, uremia and severe liver disorders. It should be used with caution in patients with active tuberculosis or hyperthyroidism. The drug should not be used in patients allergic to iodine.

DOSE. 20 ml. instilled into the ureters.

IOPHENDYLATE, U.S.P., B.P. (PANTOPAQUE). An iodized fatty acid, iophendylate is used for myelography, especially for visualization of the lumbar region.

TOXICITY. Backache and fever have been noted. It should not be used in other body cavities, because the effects are unknown. Allergic reactions may occur.

DOSE. 2 to 5 ml. intrathecally.

PROPYLIODONE, U.S.P., B.P. (DIONOSIL). Structurally related to iodopyracet, this agent is used in bronchography. It is absorbed more slowly than iodopyracet, and gives well-defined bronchograms for 30 minutes.

TOXICITY. Propyliodone should be used with caution in patients with pulmonary emphysema or bronchiectasis. It may produce fever and joint pains, headache, sore throat, shortness of breath and skin rash. The oily suspension creates the danger of an oil embolism.

DOSE. 10 to 20 ml. of 50% solution instilled into the lungs.

Sodium acetrizoate injection, B.P. (Urokon Sodium). This agent, also an iodine substituted molecule, is used as a contrast medium for excretory urography, retrograde pyelography, nephrography, translumbar arteriography, angiocardiography and intraductal cholangiography.

dose. 25 ml. of 30% solution instilled into the ureters.

GUIDE FOR THE NURSING ASSESSMENT OF A PATIENT RECEIVING A DIAGNOSTIC AGENT

I. What does the patient understand about the test? Does he understand why the test is being done? Does he understand how the test will be done? Has he had this test done before? Does he have any misconceptions about the test? What may the results of this test mean to this patient?

II. Does the patient have any known allergies? Have they been reported and recorded appropriately?

III. Is there any special physical preparation of the patient for this test? Should food and/or fluids be withheld? Is cleansing of the bowel necessary? What instructions should be given to the patient, especially if preparation is done by the patient at home?

IV. Is there any special preparation of the drug? How is it administered? Is any special equipment needed? Is it administered by the physician or the nurse?

V. What observations should be made during the test? After the test? Are there any measures to be taken after the diagnostic agent has been given? Are specimens to be collected? When? How? Are enemas or cathartics needed to remove the diagnostic agent? What follow-up or treatment may be indicated if the results of the testing are positive?

QUESTIONS FOR DISCUSSION AND REVIEW

1. Why are diagnostic agents rather than x-rays used in the diagnoses of blastomycosis and histoplasmosis?

2. Does a positive reaction to a skin test always reveal the presence of active tuberculosis? Why?

3. Does a negative reaction to a skin test always indicate that the patient does not have tuberculosis? Why?

4. Why are tests for circulation time and venous pressure often given at the same time?

5. Under what conditions would a mannitol diagnostic test be indicated?

6.   What is pheochromocytoma? What symptoms would be exhibited by a patient with this condition?

7.   What uses does edrophonium chloride have other than that of a diagnostic agent?

8.   Check the physical preparation of the patient recommended in your hospital for:

a. upper G.I. series
b. barium enema
c. intravenous pyelogram
d. gallbladder series

BIBLIOGRAPHY

AMA Drug Evaluations. Chicago, American Medical Association, 1971.

Crocker, D. and Vandam, L. D.: Untoward reactions to radiopaque contrast media. *Clin. Pharmacol. Ther. 4*:654, 1963.

Garb, S.: *Laboratory Tests in Common Use.* 4th Ed. New York, Springer, 1966.

Hoppe, J. O.: Some pharmacological aspects of radiopaque compounds. *Ann. N.Y. Acad. Sci., 78*:727, 1959.

Monis, D.: How to have a barium meal. *Nurs. Times, 65*:577, (May 1) 1969.

Rodman, M. J.: Drugs used for diagnosis. *R.N., 22*:43, (December) 1959.

Chapter 24 Toxicology

Important Concepts Discussed

1. *Poisons are substances that injure health or cause death.*

2. *Disturbances in body chemistry are often brought about by poisons either directly or as a result of induced vomiting and diarrhea.*

3. *The absorption of a poison is delayed whenever possible to facilitate more complete removal of the noxious substance.*

4. *Educating the patient, his family and the general public in measures to prevent accidental poisoning is an important nursing function.*

Toxicology is the branch of medicine that deals with the nature, properties, effects and detection of poisons. Although the treatment of acute poisoning is not ordinarily within the nurse's responsibilities, it is nevertheless quite helpful to become acquainted with necessary measures to be taken immediately when poisonous substances are inhaled, ingested or injected.

Nearly every known substance may be a poison or exert a harmful action if administered in an unsuitable manner or in excessive doses. Many drugs, even though they may be quite innocuous when administered as prescribed, may exert dangerous or lethal effects when taken in excessive doses.

Although many cases of poisoning have been recorded in which children gained access to prescription drugs in medicine cabinets, common household items that are stored in easily accessible areas are often of even greater danger. Even though it would seem to be common sense, in spite of repeated exhortations, many families still store substances such as bleach, turpentine and ammonia in food and soft drink containers and leave them on low shelves or exposed in work areas where they are readily accessible to curious toddlers.

Many commercial poisons may be purchased quite readily, and the fact that when administered in small doses over a period of time, the symptoms produced may vary greatly or even resemble known diseases, accounts for their extensive use for homicidal and suicidal purposes. A high degree of suspicion is often the only reason for considering poisoning rather than natural causes of death.

TYPES OF POISONING

It is customary to classify poisoning as acute, subacute or chronic. Many substances are capable of producing all three types, but the arbitrary classification is based on the rate of intake of the poison, the symptoms experienced and the lethality of the effects produced. In some cases the treatment varies with the type of poisoning by one agent, but often the treatment is similar; it simply need not be as intensive if the poisoning is mild and chronic when discovered.

Acute poisoning occurs when exposure to the noxious substance is sudden and severe. For example, sudden exposure to an atmosphere containing large quantities of carbon monoxide or swallowing a toxic quantity of a cyanide preparation produces acute poisoning. The symptoms develop in a short period of time, and death may be rapid. Acute poisoning is usually caused by a single dose of a substance that is readily absorbed and has the ability to damage one or more vital body processes. Recovery from acute poisoning may be followed by the later development of serious symptoms; for instance, recovery from arsenicals may be followed after many years by malignant changes in internal organs or the development of hyperpigmented areas on the palms or soles that may later develop into skin cancer.

Subacute poisoning may result from frequent exposure to a poison over a period of several hours or days. This would be the type of poisoning that would occur following repeated, frequent exposure to insecticide sprays.

Chronic poisoning occurs from repeated exposure over a long period of time to a substance that has a tendency to accumulate in the body. Chronic poisoning occurs often in industrial areas in which a contaminated atmosphere is inhaled over months or years. Small quantities of poisons may be absorbed following repeated skin contact or after ingestion. Leadfree paints are now usually used on infants' cribs because many cases of chronic lead poisoning occurred after babies nibbled repeatedly on the paint. Arsenic readily causes chronic poisoning as do digitalis and many other agents used for medicinal purposes.

Even substances such as water can be perilous if injected into a gravid uterus, and salt ingestion may lead to serious cardiac and circulatory disturbances if ingested in excessive amounts, particularly in individuals with cardiac and renal disorders. Concentrated salt solutions, when ingested, may produce serious gastritis.

Accidental poisoning in childhood is common, especially in the preschool child, although the mortality is low (about 2 of 500 hospital admissions).

One study concluded that children who poison themselves can be divided into two groups: a small group of normal exploratory toddlers who may take poison in small amounts, merely tasting it and usually rejecting it before ingesting a harmful quantity but a larger group of children show exaggerated oral tendencies and poison themselves indiscriminately with tablets and liquids. This latter group is particularly liable to gulp the poison in lethal quantities.

Nurses frequently have excellent opportunities to teach mothers the importance of keeping cleaning solutions, shoe polish and other poisons in cabinets that are not easily reached by children. All medications should be locked in a safe place. Parents should be discouraged from telling children that medicine is candy in order to persuade them to take it. Children then think all pills are candy.

Other measures should be taken to prevent accidental poisonings. Insecticides, kerosene, paint solvents and other substances usually stored in the garage or basement should be far out of the reach of children. Lead poisoning can be avoided by using lead-free paint on children's furniture and house interiors.

Precautions should be taken in regard to prescribed medications in order to prevent accidental overdosage or poisoning. Medications intended for oral use should be kept in a separate area from those poisons and drugs intended for external use. Careful instructions on how and when medications are to be taken should be given to patients, especially the elderly. Medications should not be taken in the dark and labels should be read carefully. Patients and their families should be cautioned about the dangers of transferring chemicals or drugs into other containers, especially into one which indicates that it contains another substance. Old or unused medications should be discarded into the sewer system rather than into the trash where curious children may find them.

GENERAL ACTIONS OF POISONS

Poisons attack living organisms in two general ways:

1. Locally by irritating or destroying tissues with which they come in contact. This effect may be mild, merely producing a contact dermatitis, or it may produce severe damage to and sloughing of the tissue. This latter effect is seen primarily following contact with caustic acids and alkalis. When poisons are ingested, severe damage may occur to the tissues of the esophagus and stomach. The use of nasogastric tubes is prohibited following ingestion of these substances since the tissue may be sufficiently softened to allow perforation of the esopha-gus by the tube. Healing often occurs with extensive scarring, which may in some cases be minimized by repeated dilation of the esophagus for a long time after ingestion has occurred, but in some cases the stricture may be severe enough to necessitate removal of the esophagus and replacement with a loop of bowel. Locally irritating substances cause more serious damage when in contact with delicate tissues, such as the eye.

2. Systemically by being absorbed into the blood and carried to target tissues. The tissues and organs affected depend upon the type of poison absorbed. Usual target organ systems include the central nervous system, blood-forming tissues, circulatory system, viscera, muscle and bone.

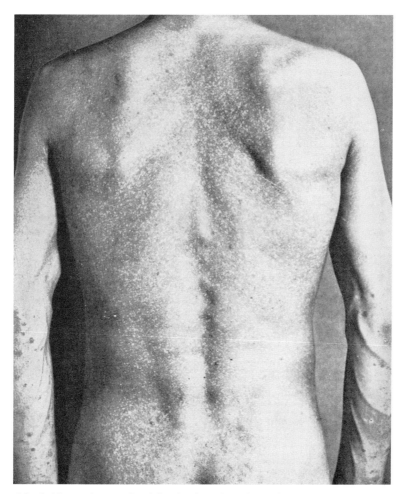

FIGURE 54.   Mottled hyperpigmentation following ingestion of arsenic. (Grollman: *Pharmacology and Therapeutics*. Ed. 6. Lea & Febiger, Philadelphia, 1965.)

Although considerable work has been carried out on the mechanisms of action of various poisons, the information is quite limited. Probably the most important mechanism of action of many poisonous substances involves interference with vital enzyme systems. The arsenicals and mercurials inhibit enzymes containing sulfhydryl groups. Cyanide inhibits cytochrome oxidase, an enzyme necessary for cellular respiration and energy production. Organic phosphorus-containing insecticides inhibit cholinesterase, thus permitting excessive amounts of acetylcholine to accumulate and interfere with bodily processes such as muscular contraction.

Carbon monoxide interferes with extracellular oxygen transport by combining with hemoglobin in lieu of oxygen. Other agents interfere with the mechanisms for cellular transport and metabolism, leading to changes in the permeability, irritability and nutrition of cells.

It is important to realize that symptomatic control of poisoning is relatively ineffective unless therapy is aimed concurrently toward causing excretion, metabolism or removal of the poison from chemical combination with a cellular component. These objectives are impossible to achieve in many instances, however, using present methods of treatment.

INTENSITY OF TOXIC EFFECT

The intensity of the toxic effect on a tissue or target organ is directly related to the concentration of the poison at the site of action. When unchanged by the administration of antidotes, this effect depends directly upon the balance between the rates of absorption, detoxification and excretion of the substance. When a poison has been taken orally, the administration of substances such as egg white, milk, powdered charcoal or even water may dilute it and delay absorption until corrective measures may be taken.

The rate at which a substance is absorbed depends upon its solubility in the medium of the stomach, the dose administered, the mode of administration and the presence of modifying substances or drugs. Absorption of an orally administered agent is slower if it is taken after a meal. Heavy metals react with protein in food, and they may be inactivated or removed from the gastrointestinal tract with fecal material. Solutions of poisons are generally more rapidly absorbed than are tablets or solid forms, merely because tablets and solids must first be dissolved.

Detoxification of a poison is ordinarily accomplished through enzymatic reactions resulting in oxidation, reduction, hydrolysis or conjugation of the material. Since most mechanisms of detoxification depend on adequate liver function, toxic amounts of a substance may readily accumulate if liver function is compromised or decreased.

Excretion of a poison may occur through the gastrointestinal tract, the kidneys, lungs or skin. If they are injured or their effectiveness is decreased, the rate of excretion of the toxic agent is also decreased. Kidney function is particularly important since many drugs are excreted in this manner.

Cumulative poisons are substances that are excreted or detoxified at rates slower than the rate of intake into the body. Digitalis is a cumulative drug, and care must be taken to take the pulse before each dose is administered. The anticoagulants, such as the coumarin derivatives, are likewise cumulative drugs. Prothrombin times must be checked during the entire time that these agents are administered.

INDIVIDUAL VARIATIONS IN SUSCEPTIBILITY

There is great individual variation in the expected response to chemicals and drugs. Children are generally more susceptible than adults, partly because of their smaller body size and rapid growth rate, and healthy individuals with normally functioning liver and kidneys would obviously be more resistant than persons with organic or metabolic disorders. Persons with pre-existing disorders of the blood-forming organs would be more susceptible to drugs with a side effect of marrow toxicity than would healthy individuals.

Sex differences occur also. Women are generally more susceptible than men. Dark-skinned individuals seem to be less susceptible to agents absorbed through the skin than are the lighter races.

GENERAL TREATMENT OF POISONING

The treatment of poisoning must be prompt and as specific as possible. Immediate general treatment is aimed toward preventing absorption of the poison and combating the effects of poison already absorbed. Following is an outline for the general emergency treatment of poisoning:

1. Call the physician or Poison Control Center immediately.

2. Attempt to identify the poison. Many commercial household items have the poisonous ingredients listed on the label. The area poison information center can often supply the list of ingredients if the trade name and manufacturer of the poison are known. Prescription drugs can readily be identified by calling the pharmacy from which they were obtained.

3. First aid measures should be followed. The absorption of orally ingested poisons should be delayed by the administration of milk, egg whites or similar substances. If the agent is not a petroleum derivative or a corrosive, emesis should be induced by administering ipecac syrup or home remedies, such as tepid salt water or soapsuds solution, or by merely touching the back of the throat with a finger or spoon handle.

4. Chemical alteration of the ingested substance may be carried out by administration of a weak alkali, such as milk of magnesia for acidic substances or vinegar if alkaline substances have been ingested. Ingestion of petroleum products should be treated by immediately administering large amounts of mineral oil to emulsify the poison and prevent its absorption.

5. Specific antidotes are given whenever possible. These are ordinarily administered by the physician upon arrival at the emergency room or poison treatment center.

6. Supportive care should be aimed at maintaining normal body temperature, giving artificial respiration when required and administering cardiac or respiratory stimulants. The patient should be kept in bed and exercise and excessive excitement should be avoided.

First Aid Treatment

The American Medical Association and the Committee on Toxicology have compiled a list of emergency or first aid measures in poisoning. Some of the major points of treatment will be discussed here.

INGESTED POISONS

1. Nonprofessional personnel should not attempt treatment of any kind if the patient is convulsing or unconscious.

2. Substances to delay absorption should be given immediately. Milk, egg white, beaten whole eggs or a suspension of flour, starch or mashed potatoes in water may be given. If no other materials are available, water alone is better than nothing, because it dilutes the poison and reduces possible local effects on the stomach lining. For children less than five years of age, one to two cups of these materials should be given. For patients over five years of age, up to one quart should be administered.

3. Universal antidote, consisting of 1 part tannic acid, 1 part magnesium oxide and 2 parts activated charcoal, should be given if available. The tannic acid component precipitates heavy metals, the magnesium oxide neutralizes acidic substances and the activated charcoal is a nonspecific adsorbent. Four to five teaspoonfuls should be administered in a glass of water.

4. Vomiting should be induced by giving emetics or touching the back of the throat with a finger or spoon unless petroleum products or corrosives have been ingested. Emetics often used include salt solution (two tablespoonfuls salt in a glass of tepid water), ipecac syrup (one to two tablespoonfuls fol-

lowed by a glass of water) or mustard (four teaspoonfuls in a glass of water).

5. Give a cathartic—sodium sulfate (one teaspoonful in half a glassful of water) or magnesium sulfate (one tablespoonful in a glassful of water).

6. Conserve body heat by wrapping the patient in blankets.

INHALED POISONS

1. The patient should be removed immediately from the noxious fumes.

2. Objects obstructing the airway should be removed, and tight clothing loosened.

3. Mouth-to-mouth resuscitation should be given immediately if there is respiratory distress.

4. Treat symptoms as they occur. If the patient is vomiting, turn his head to the side to prevent aspiration; if he is chilled or hypotensive, conserve body heat with blankets.

LOCAL CONTAMINATION

1. Clothing should be removed while applying gentle water pressure from a hose or faucet.

2. Thoroughly flush skin with water. Immersion in a tub or under a shower is preferable.

3. Chemical antidotes for acid or alkali should not be applied because the heat generated by the local reaction may cause further tissue damage.

4. If poison has splashed into the eye, the eye and surrounding mucous membranes should be flushed for five minutes with a gentle stream of water. The lids should be held apart since there is a strong reflex to close the lids when irritating substances are contacted.

REPTILE OR POISONOUS INSECT BITES

1. Immobilize the patient and make him lie down.

2. Give no alcohol or stimulating beverages.

3. Place a tourniquet between the site of the bite and the heart. The tourniquet should be sufficiently tight to impede circulation, but it should not produce severe pain, nor should arterial pulses completely disappear. Every 15 minutes the tourniquet should be loosened for one minute.

4. If possible, ice or cold water packs should be applied to the area.

5. Unnecessary movement, walking and excitement should be prohibited.

SUPPORTIVE MANAGEMENT IN POISONING

Supportive management in poisoning is aimed toward relief of symptoms that occur as a result of the poisoning. Supportive management is only an adjunct to the corrective treatment of the poisoning, but may at times be extremely important in providing for the patient's overall well-being, or it may be life-saving if severe disturbances in physiological processes have occurred as a result of the poisoning.

Severe pain, if unrelieved, may cause vasomotor collapse and serious disturbances in physiological processes. Pain may be relieved by analgesics.

Water losses should be monitored carefully and replenished as necessary. Since prolonged vomiting and diarrhea may cause serious electrolyte and water disturbances, these should be replaced by intravenous fluids if the patient is unable to take food or liquids by mouth. Excessive fluid administration, particularly by the intravenous route, should be avoided since edema and circulatory disturbances may ensue.

ACIDOSIS

Metabolic acidosis may be produced either by ingestion of substances that are metabolized to acid intermediaries or by loss of basic ions from the body as a result of prolonged vomiting, diarrhea, hyperventilation or kidney disorders. In either case the blood pH is less than the normal 7.4.

Acidosis may be treated by administering 5 Gm. of sodium bicarbonate orally every 30 minutes or intravenously in a dose of 0.25

Gm./kg. of body weight or by giving a ⅙ molar solution of sodium lactate intravenously in a dose of 20 mg./kg. of body weight until the urine become alkaline.

Central Nervous System Involvement

The central nervous system may be affected by excessive stimulation or depression following poison administration. Overdoses of central nervous system stimulants commonly produce convulsions. Although convulsions in themselves are not life-threatening, anoxia may occur if prolonged spasm of the respiratory muscles occurs. Occasionally respiratory failure may occur during the depression that follows a convulsive episode. Convulsions may be controlled by central nervous system depressants, such as ether, pentobarbital and thiopental, administered in doses necessary to control the seizures. Less severe central nervous system stimulation may result in hyperactivity, delirium or mania. These disorders may be treated by administration of paraldehyde, scopolamine, chlorpromazine or promazine.

Ingestion of excessive amounts of central nervous system depressants may result in a comatose state and respiratory depression. The administration of central nervous system stimulants as treatment for this type of poisoning has not proven entirely satisfactory, partly because it is quite difficult to calculate the correct dosage, and excessive stimulation or convulsions may occur. Drug-induced comas are now usually treated by peritoneal dialysis to remove the offending substance by diffusion through the peritoneal blood vessels. Other drugs that are occasionally used include bemegride, pentylenetetrazol, nikethamide and caffeine sodium benzoate.

Respiratory Tract Involvement

Respiratory tract involvement is often directly or indirectly a result of hypoxia during coma, convulsions or muscular paralysis. Mouth-to-mouth resuscitation should be begun immediately when respiratory function is compromised.

Local irritation of the respiratory mucous membranes may result in increased excretion of exudates and pulmonary edema. When this occurs, oxygen exchange is compromised, and death may occur. Pulmonary edema is characterized by dyspnea, rales at the bases of both lungs, cyanosis, rapid respiration and in extreme cases gurgling respiration or foaming at the mouth may occur. Pulmonary edema may be treated by the administration of oxygen by face mask, aminophylline intravenously to relieve associated bronchial constriction and morphine sulfate intravenously or intramuscularly to decrease the rate of the rapid, ineffectual respiration.

Circulatory System Involvement

Circulatory system involvement can occur quite readily from poisoning. Circulatory collapse or shock may result from cerebral anoxia due to respiratory depression, extreme pain or injury to the muscles of respiration. It is characterized by cold, pale, cyanotic facies, along with a weak, rapid pulse and hypotension.

The patient should be placed in a supine position with the feet elevated. Body heat should be conserved with blankets, but external heat should not be applied. Respiratory distress should be treated by maintenance of an adequate airway and mouth-to-mouth resuscitation if necessary. Intravenous fluids, such as plasma, whole blood, plasma substitute or normal saline, should be given along with a hypertensive agent if necessary. Hypertensive agents that may be used include:

Levarterenol bitartrate (Levophed)— dilution of 4 to 16 ml./l. at a rate of 20 to 40 drops/min.
Phenylephrine hydrochloride—5 mg. I.M. as needed.
Methamphetamine—up to 100 mg. I.V.
Metaraminol—10 mg. I.M. every hour.
Mephentermine—15 to 20 mg. I.M. every hour as needed.

Congestive heart failure may be produced by poisons that damage the myocardium.

Peripheral edema becomes evident, along with pulmonary edema, hepatosplenomegaly, elevated venous pressure and ascites. Congestive heart failure may be treated by:

Digoxin—1 mg. I.V. or orally, followed by 0.5 mg. in 4 hours, then 0.25 mg. every 4 hours as needed.

Digitoxin—0.6 mg. I.V., I.M. or orally, followed by 0.2 to 0.4 mg. every 4 hours until 1 to 2 mg. has been given.

Digitalis—0.6 Gm. orally, followed by 0.4 Gm. for two doses, then 0.1 Gm. once or twice daily.

Cardiac arrest may occur following overdosage of central nervous system depressants, asphyxia from noxious gases or as an idiosyncratic response. In cardiac arrest, the pulse and blood pressure suddenly disappear, and the heart sounds are inaudible.

External cardiac massage should be carried out immediately, with mouth-to-mouth resuscitation if necessary. Drugs that may be given as adjunctive treatment include:

Calcium chloride—2 to 4 ml. of 10% solution to improve cardiac tone.

Epinephrine—4 ml. of 1:20,000 solution I.V.

Sodium lactate—⅙ molar solution I.V.

Sodium bicarbonate—50 ml. of a 0.15 molar solution.

Genitourinary Tract Involvement

Acute renal failure may occur either as a direct result of poisons that affect the kidney, such as the arsenicals and mercurials, or indirectly as a result of erythrocyte disintegration and mechanical blocking of renal tubules, such as occurs following ingestion of naphthalene and benzene. Since one of the first symptoms of cardiovascular collapse is decreased renal output, the renal output should be carefully monitored in any severe poisoning incident. In many cases the kidney damage is reversible in time, although interim treatment may necessitate the use of an artificial kidney or peritoneal dialysis to prevent toxic accumulation of waste products.

Gastrointestinal Tract Involvement

Prolonged vomiting and diarrhea may necessitate fluid and electrolyte replacement. Since these processes are often necessary for removal of the poison, they should be allowed to continue for a time. When it is relatively certain that the poison has been removed from the gastrointestinal tract, however, vomiting may be decreased by the administration of antinauseants, and diarrhea may be decreased by the administration of adsorbents or opium derivatives.

Liver Damage

Hepatotoxic drugs or poisons, such as carbon tetrachloride, phosphorus-containing compounds, arsenicals, mushrooms, lead and similar compounds, may cause severe and irreversible liver damage. Symptoms of acute poisoning include nausea, vomiting, malaise, abdominal pain, fever, jaundice and hepatomegaly; in chronic poisoning the symptoms may be less noticeable initially, although nonetheless ominous. Symptoms of chronic poisoning include weight loss, pallor, hematemesis, jaundice, ascites and an enlarged, cirrhotic liver. Later effects may include hemorrhoids and esophageal varices.

Treatment for liver failure should include complete bed rest, with limited fluid and protein intake. A high carbohydrate diet, large doses of the B vitamins and blood transfusions should be given during convalescence.

CHEMICAL ANTIDOTES

Many antagonistic drugs used to treat overdoses of specific pharmacologic agents are mentioned with the potentially toxic drugs elsewhere in this text. Following are a few other chemical antidotes which may be used in the treatment of many kinds of poisoning.

UNIVERSAL ANTIDOTE. Universal antidote is so-called because it may be employed in the treatment of a variety of ingested poisons because of its neutralizing and precipitant properties.

After a sufficient period of time has elapsed for the universal antidote to adsorb and inactivate the ingested poison, the stomach is emptied via emesis or gastric lavage, except if the poison is corrosive.

DOSE. 4 to 5 heaping teaspoonfuls orally in a glassful of water.

DIMERCAPROL, U.S.P. (BAL). The use of arsenical gases, such as lewisite, during World War II stimulated an intense search for effective antidotes. Since the arsenic in lewisite was found to combine with the sulf-hydro (—SH) groups on enzyme molecules, an effective antidote was needed to prevent or reverse this binding. British scientists were the first to synthesize an effective compound to reverse this binding, naming it British anti-lewisite (BAL).

Although subsequent investigations have shown that this compound reverses binding by other heavy metals, such as mercury and gold, it is currently employed primarily in the treatment of arsenic poisoning.

$$CH_2-SH$$
$$|$$
$$CH-SH$$
$$|$$
$$CH_2-OH$$
dimercaprol

It does not appear to be of help in lead poisoning, and studies with other heavy metals, such as antimony and bismuth, have been inconclusive.

TOXICITY. The side effects, while at times alarming, are usually not life-threatening. Elevations of systolic and diastolic blood pressure occur frequently. The pressure begins to rise within a few minutes after injection, reaches a peak in 15 to 30 minutes and falls to normal levels within two hours. There may be local pain at the site of injection, along with nausea, vomiting, burning sensation of the mucous membranes, conjunctivitis, and a sense of constriction in the chest. These symptoms usually subside in 30 to 90 minutes.

DOSE. 2.5 mg./kg. of body weight I.M. The dose should be repeated at four hour intervals for a total of 4 to 6 injections daily for two days, then 2 doses daily for 10 days or until complete recovery.

CALCIUM DISODIUM EDETATE, U.S.P. (CALCIUM DISODIUM VERSENATE). Calcium disodium edetate readily dissolves ordinarily insoluble salts, such as barium sulfate, calcium oxalate and lead phosphate, by combining with the metallic ions to form chelates that can be readily removed by the kidneys. Since the bond formed by this agent with lead is much stronger than that formed by other heavy metal antidotes, it is the agent of choice for lead poisoning.

The affinity of the sodium salt for calcium has provided problems in the past by removing excessive amounts of calcium from body tissues and fluids. The salt in this preparation is saturated with calcium so that tissue calcium is undisturbed.

Calcium disodium edetate is useful in the treatment of acute and chronic lead poisoning, lead encephalopathy and prophylactically against symptomatic exacerbations in chronic lead poisoning. Lead deposited in bone and tissues is slowly removed by this agent.

TOXICITY. Acute tubular necrosis, particularly of the proximal convoluted

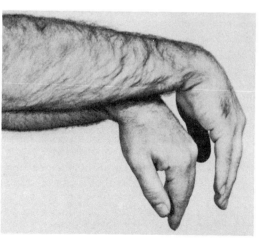

FIGURE 55. Lead palsy of the forearm extensors. (Grollman: *Pharmacology and Therapeutics.* Ed. 6. Lea & Febiger, Philadelphia, 1965.)

tubules, has been observed following therapy. In some cases, lead encephalopathy may be observed at the initiation of therapy, and it is believed that intravenous administration may promote absorption of lead from the intestinal tract and facilitate its transport to the brain.

DOSE. 1 Gm. diluted with 250 to 500 ml. of normal saline or 5 per cent dextrose in water and administered by I.V. drip over a period of one hour. This dose should be administered twice daily for five days, then after therapy is interrupted for two days, it may be followed by an additional five days of therapy if indicated. For children the dose should not exceed 0.5 Gm./30 lb. of body weight given twice daily.

Although the drug is most effective when administered intravenously, it is available in tablet form for administration in divided doses of 4 Gm. daily.

PENICILLAMINE (CUPRIMINE). Penicillamine, a degradation product of penicillin, is prepared by hydrolysis of the parent molecule. It is quite effective as a chelating agent in the treatment of copper, mercury and lead poisonings, but it is perhaps most useful in the treatment of hepatolenticular degeneration (Wilson's disease), which is a congenital, hereditary disorder characterized by a deficiency or absence of ceruloplasm, the plasma protein necessary for copper transport. When this protein is missing, copper is deposited in many tissues of the body in excessive amounts.

TOXICITY. Nausea, vomiting, anorexia, dermatologic reactions, thrombocytopenia, leukopenia and purpuric extravasations may occur. Hemorrhagic extravasation of blood may occur, particularly at sites of trauma, such as over the knees, elbows and toes. Iron deficiency may occur particularly in menstruating women and in children, since a diet low in copper is usually low in iron as well. Penicillamine diminishes iron absorption and facilitates excretion. The drug should be withdrawn if blood dyscrasias occur.

DOSE. 250 mg. orally four times daily.

DESFERRIOXAMINE (DESFERAL). Desferrioxamine is prepared commercially by removing iron from a chelate produced by the microorganism *Streptomyces pilosus*.

This drug has a specificity for iron, and it is useful in the treatment of iron poisoning and hemochromatosis, a congenital disorder in which excessive amounts of iron are stored in body organs, particularly the liver and spleen.

It is usually administered intravenously for treatment of poisoning, but it may be administered orally for long-term treatment of iron storage diseases when decreased iron absorption is desired from the gastrointestinal tract.

DOSE. 400 to 600 mg. I.V. once or twice daily.

PRALIDOXIME (PROTOPAM). Pralidoxime, a derivative of pyridine, is effective in antagonizing anticholinesterases, such as insecticides and chemical warfare agents. It may be used to counteract overdoses of drugs (anticholinesterases) given in the treatment of myasthenia gravis. It should be administered for this purpose only in a hospital, however, since respiratory failure may be precipitated by a myasthenic crisis when the drugs are inhibited.

TOXICITY. Neuromuscular blockade, weakness, blurred vision, diplopia, dizziness, headache and tachycardia have been observed.

DOSE. 1 to 2 Gm. I.V. at a rate of 500 mg./min.

POISON CONTROL CENTERS

There are more than 200 Poison Control Centers in the United States, a relatively rapid increase in number since the establishment of the first center in Chicago in 1953. Some centers are merely information centers

TABLE 18 Poisons, Signs and Symptoms and Emergency Treatment

POISON	SOURCES	SIGNS AND SYMPTOMS	EMERGENCY TREATMENT
Acetanilid	Headache remedies	Gastrointestinal disturbances; anemia; methemoglobinemia; antipyresis; collapse.	Gastric lavage; cathartics; enema; oxygen; artificial respiration; transfusions.
Acids (e.g., hydro-chloric and nitric acids)	Cleaning solutions	Pain in throat, esophagus and stomach; dysphagia; diarrhea; shock; collapse. If topical, skin is first white, then turns yellow or brown.	Give milk of magnesia, aluminum hydroxide, mild soap solution, milk or water with egg whites. Apply sodium bicarbonate solution to skin.
Ammonia	Household ammonia	Burning sensation in mouth and stomach; nausea; vomiting; abdominal pain; respiratory failure.	Give weak acids, olive oil, fluids.
Aniline dyes	Crayons, shoe polish	Apathy; dyspnea; cyanosis due to methemoglobinemia	1% methylene blue solution I.V. (2 mg./kg.); lavage with water; oxygen; blood.
Amphetamines	Stimulants, anti-obesity preparations	Irrational behavior; cerebral stimulation; shock; cardiac arrhythmias; tremors; convulsions; coma.	Pentobarbital (100 mg.) or Amytal (250 mg.) I.M.
Antihistamines	Cold compounds, anti-allergic drugs	Vomiting; convulsions; hyperpyrexia; generalized depression; hallucinations; unconsciousness.	Gastric lavage; symptomatic treatment (paraldehyde or ether during convulsions; caffeine or coramine during depressed state). Histamine 0.1 mg./kg.
Arsenic	Insecticides, weed killer, rodenticides.	Odor of garlic on breath and in stools; faintness; nausea; difficulty in swallowing; thirst; vomiting; gastric pain; oliguria; albuminuria; cold, clammy skin; "rice water stools"; collapse.	Universal antidote followed by lavage with sodium bicarbonate solution or emetic; intravenous fluids; sedation; dimercaprol (BAL). Conserve body heat.
Barbiturates	Sedatives	Somnolence; stupor; coma; respiratory and circulatory collapse.	Bemegride; fluids; oxygen; peritoneal dialysis.
Bromides	Bromo Seltzer, sedatives	Acute poisoning; stupor; ataxia; muscular weakness; collapse. Chronic poisoning: bromide acne; foul breath; gastrointestinal disturbances; depression; apathy; ataxia; muscular weakness; anemia.	Large doses of normal saline solution; diuretics (ammonium chloride or mercuhydrin).
Caffeine	Coffee, No-Doz	Gastrointestinal distress; diuresis; photophobia; premature systoles; tremors; convulsions; hallucinations.	Gastric lavage; central depressants (pentobarbital); fluids.
Camphor	Camphorated oil, moth balls.	Odor on breath; headache; excitement; delirium; convulsions.	Gastric lavage with water; sedation with barbiturates, but no opiates.
Carbon monoxide	Coal gas, illuminating gas, exhaust from motor vehicles.	Skin is cherry red; headache; dizziness; impaired hearing and vision; drowsiness; confusion; loss of consciousness; slow respiration; rapid pulse.	Move victim to fresh air; artificial respiration; mixture of 90% oxygen and 10% carbon dioxide; bed rest for 48 hours. Conserve body heat.
Carbon tetrachloride	Spot removers, some fire extinguishers, solvents	Nausea; vomiting; headache; inebriation; convulsions; coma; dark colored urine; jaundice; diarrhea; disturbance of hearing and vision.	If poison has been swallowed, lavage with 1:10,000 potassium permanganate solution. If inhaled give oxygen—carbon dioxide mixture. High protein and carbohydrate diet; fluids.

Table continues on following page—

TABLE 18   Poisons, Signs and Symptoms and Emergency Treatment—*Continued*

POISON	SOURCES	SIGNS AND SYMPTOMS	EMERGENCY TREATMENT
Chlorophenothane (DDT)	Insecticides	Headache, nausea; vomiting; diarrhea; paresthesias of lips and tongue; numbness of extremities; malaise; sore throat; tremor; convulsions; respiratory failure.	Lavage with water; saline cathartic; force fluids (tea or coffee); give calcium gluconate. Avoid fats, fat solvents and opiates. Wash skin with soap and water.
Cyanide	Rodenticides, metal polish	Odor of bitter almond oil on breath; headache; rapid breathing; dyspnea; heart palpitation; tightness in chest; cyanosis; convulsions. Death may occur within a few minutes.	Immediately after ingestion, lavage with 1:10,000 potassium permanganate solution. Inhale several amyl nitrite perles followed by 10% sodium nitrite I.V. May follow with 50% sodium thiosulfate I.V. (Principle of therapy is to form methemoglobin in blood, which combines with cyanide.) Oxygen and blood transfusion.
Ethyl alcohol	Liquors	Central depression; disturbance in gait; incoherence; excitement; stupor; coma; respiratory depression.	Excitement treated with paraldehyde, chloral hydrate or tranquilizers. Drowsiness treated with caffeine sodium benzoate, dextroamphetamine or methylphenidate. Intravenous infusions with dextrose; vitamins; artificial respiration if necessary.
Fluoride	Insecticides	Excessive salivation; abdominal pain; hematemesis; diarrhea; muscle weakness; difficulty swallowing; facial paralysis; respiratory failure; circulatory collapse.	Calcium chloride or milk orally. Lavage with 1% calcium chloride or milk.
Hydrocarbons	Kerosene, gasoline, cleaning fluids	Burning sensation in mouth, esophagus and stomach; vomiting; dizziness; tremor; muscular cramps; confusion; fever; cold, clammy skin; weak pulse; thirst; coma; respiratory failure.	Avoid lavage. Oxygen; fluids; antibiotics; saline cathartics.
Iodine	Tincture of iodine	Brown stain on lips, tongue, and in mouth; odor of iodine in vomitus; thirst, fainting; giddiness; vomiting; abdominal pain; diarrhea; shock.	Water with starch, flour or mashed potatoes. Lavage with starch or 5% sodium thiosulfate solution, milk or egg whites.
Lead	Paint	Gastrointestinal irritation; pain; vomiting; diarrhea; headache; insomnia; visual disturbances; irritability; delirium; convulsions. In chronic poisoning, "lead lines" on gums.	Gastric lavage; papaverine or calcium gluconate for relief of colic; surgery to correct encephalopathy in children. Edathamil calcium-disodium I.V. Barbiturates to control central excitation.
Lye	Drain and toilet bowl cleanser	Burning pain in mouth, throat and stomach; mucous membranes ulcerated; bloody vomitus; constricted throat; difficult respirations; cold, clammy skin; rapid pulse; violent purging; anxiety.	Emetics and lavage not recommended; give large amounts of weak acids, such as lemon or vinegar followed by demulcents such as egg whites, gruel, olive oil, salad oil. Analgesics; parenteral fluids.

Table continues on following page.

TABLE 18 Poisons, Signs and Symptoms and Emergency Treatment—*Continued*

POISON	SOURCES	SIGNS AND SYMPTOMS	EMERGENCY TREATMENT
Mercury	Antiseptics, fireworks, insect spray	Abdominal pain; vomiting; bloody diarrhea; constriction of throat and esophagus; ashen gray color of mucous membranes; circulatory collapse; kidney damage; oliguria; anuria.	Universal antidote. Lavage with copious milk, egg white or 5% sodium formaldehyde sulfoxylate, followed by sodium bicarbonate solution. Dimercaprol; fluids. Conserve body heat.
Morphine	Opium derivative	Slow, shallow respiration; pinpoint pupils; weak pulse; muscle twitching; spasm; cyanosis; coma; respiratory paralysis.	Keep respiratory passages clear; administer oxygen; nalorphine.
Nicotine	Insecticides, tobacco	Nausea; vomiting; confusion; salivation; abdominal cramps; convulsions; diarrhea; sweating; headache; weakness; perspiration; dilation of pupils; faintness; respiratory paralysis.	Universal antidote; lavage with 0.5% tannic acid or 1:5000 potassium permanganate solution; artificial respiration. Wash contaminated skin with cold water; stimulants if needed.
Paris Green (Copper arsenite + copper acetate)	Pesticides	Vomiting of green material followed by gastric and abdominal pain; diarrhea with dark and sometimes bloody stools; metallic taste in mouth; neuromuscular weakness; thirst; oliguria→anuria; cold, clammy skin; coma; convulsions; death.	Potassium ferrocyanide 10 gr. in water (to form an insoluble salt of copper) followed by lavage with sodium bicarbonate solution; demulcents (milk, egg white in water, gelatin, etc.).
Phenols	Phenol liquefied, cresol, Lysol, creosote	Corrosion of mucous membranes; pain; vomiting; bloody diarrhea; headache; dizziness; cold, clammy skin; oliguria; hematuria; unconsciousness; slow respiration; respiratory failure; dark urine.	Lavage with olive oil, egg white and milk; parenteral fluids; oxygen and carbon dioxide; analgesics. Remove from skin with 50% solution of alcohol or olive oil.
Phosphorus	Rodenticides, roach poison, fireworks, matches	Nausea; vomiting; abdominal pain; diarrhea; shock; garlic odor on breath; liver and kidney damage.	Lavage with 2% copper sulfide then 1:10,000 potassium permanganate; give fluids.
Salicylates	Aspirin, oil of wintergreen	Hyperpnea; listlessness; vomiting; dizziness; mental confusion; acidosis; hemorrhagic manifestations.	Lavage with milk or 1:10,000 potassium permanganate solution. Instill saline cathartic in stomach after lavage; oral or parenteral fluid. Watch electrolyte and acid-base balance.
Sodium hypophosphite or hypochlorite	Bleaching agents, washing powders	Vomiting; corrosive burns of lips, mouth and tongue	Gastric lavage; give fluids.
Strychnine	Cathartics, insecticides, rodenticides	Central nervous system stimulation; hyperreflexia, stiffness of face or neck; convulsions; episthotonos; death due to asphyxia.	Lavage with 1:10,000 potassium permanganate (unless convulsing). Universal antidote; barbiturates to control convulsions; keep patient in quiet room away from stimulation; oxygen.
Quaternary ammonium compounds	Zephiran, etc.	Burning pain in mouth and throat; nausea; vomiting; apprehension; restlessness; muscle weakness; collapse; coma; convulsions.	Lavage or induce vomiting, Give mild soap solution as antidote; cathartic.

from which the list of toxic ingredients of commercial preparations along with antidotes and methods of supportive treatment can be obtained by physicians treating a poisoning emergency. Other centers located in hospitals are fully equipped to treat poisoning.

The National Poison Clearing House in Washington, D.C., provides information concerning new commercial products and improved methods of treatment to all Poison Information Centers. There is a 24-hour daily service in Washington, D.C., to provide information that may not be available at local centers.

The nurse can perform a very useful service in public information by acquainting the laity with the services of the Poison Information Centers, and particularly if she is on duty in the emergency room, she should become fully acquainted with the facilities available at the regional center.

ANTIDOTE KIT

The following antidotes for the emergency treatment of poisoning should be available in all hospital emergency rooms.

Amyl nitrite pearls 0.2 mg.
Apromorphine tablets 2 mg.
Aromatic ammonia spirit
Atropine tablets 0.5 mg.
Bemegride injection 50 mg.
Caffeine sodium benzoate ampules 500 mg.
Calcium gluconate injection 10%, 10 ml.
Charcoal, activated
Chloroform
Copper sulfate crystals
Dextrose 50%, 50 ml. ampules
Digoxin injection 0.5 mg.
Dimercaprol injection (BAL), 300 mg.
Ephedrine hydrochloride capsules 25 mg.
Epinephrine injection 1:1000, 1 ml.
Iodine tincture
Ipecac syrup
Magnesia magma
Methylene blue injection 1%, 50 ml.
Metrazol injection 10%, 1 ml.
Morphine sulfate tablets 10 mg.
Mustard
Nalorphine ampules 5 mg.
Nikethamide injection 25%, 1.5 ml.
Olive oil
Pentobarbital sodium ampules 100 mg.
Potassium permanganate solution 1%
Sodium bicarbonate
Sodium nitrite ampules 2%, 10 ml.
Sodium thiosulfate ampules 30%, 10 ml.
Universal antidote
Whiskey

QUESTIONS FOR DISCUSSION AND REVIEW

1. What would you do to treat a child who had just consumed lye?
2. What first aid measures would be appropriate if fluid from a home permanent were consumed accidentally?
3. Where is the closest Poison Control Center in your community? Become acquainted with its facilities.
4. What symptoms would you expect in a drug addict who had taken an overdose of heroin? How would this poisoning be treated?
5. What secondary effects may result from prolonged vomiting? How may this be treated?

6.   What would be the course of treatment for a two year old who had swallowed a bottle of phenobarbital tablets?

7.   If a patient weighed 195 pounds, what would be: (a) The volume of his total body water? (b) His extracellular fluid volume?

8.   What measures can the nurse take to prevent accidental ingestion of poisons or drug overdosage?

BIBLIOGRAPHY

Adams, W. C.: Poison control centers: their purpose and operation. *Clin. Pharmacol. Ther., 4*:293, 1963.

Castell, D. O. and Morrison, C. C.: Management of common adult intoxications. *G.P., 33*:105, 1966.

Coleman, A. B.: Accidental poisoning. *New Eng. J. Med., 277*:1135, 1967.

Done, A. K.: Salicylate poisoning. *J.A.M.A., 192*:770, 1965.

Dreisback, R. H.: *Handbook of Poisoning.* 4th Ed. Los Altos, California, Lange Medical Publications, 1963.

DuBois, K. P. and Geiling, E. M. K.: *Textbook of Toxicology.* New York, Oxford University Press, 1959.

Gardner, A.: Prevention and first aid treatment of poisoning. *Nurs. Mirror, 129*:48, (October 17) 1969.

Henderson, I. W. and Merrill, J. P.: Treatment of barbiturate intoxication. *Ann. Intern. Med., 64*:876, 1966.

Hollister, L. E.: Overdosage of psychotherapeutic drugs. *Clin. Pharmacol. Ther., 7*:142, 1966.

Jacobziner, H.: Accidental chemical and drug poisoning in children. *G.P., 29*:110, 1964.

Keehn, R.: Home accidents resulting from gas. *Amer. J. Nurs., 55*:720, 1955.

Lawson, A. A. H.: The basic management of acute poisoning. *Nurs. Times,* October 29, 1965, p. 1475.

Long, K. R.: Pesticides—an occupational hazard on farms. *Amer. J. Nurs., 71*:740, (April) 1971.

Mark, L. C. and Papper, E. M.: Changing therapeutic goals in barbiturate poisoning. *Pharmacol. Physicians, 1(3)*:1, 1967.

Polson, C. J. and Tattersall, R. N.: *Clinical Toxicology.* Philadelphia, J. B. Lippincott Co., 1959.

Press, E.: Poison control center. *Nurs. Outlook, 5*:29, 1957.

Stewart, R. D.: Poisoning from chlorinated hydrocarbon solvents. *Amer. J. Nurs., 67*:85, 1967.

Tonyan, A.: The nurse's part in poison control. *Amer. J. Nurs., 58*:96, 1958.

Chapter 25 Drug Addiction and Habituation

Important Concepts Discussed

1. *Drug addiction is a complex phenomenon involving social, personality and pharmacologic factors, and it is at the same time a disease and a result of diseases.*

2. *Tissue changes occur when the body is repeatedly exposed to addicting drugs. The body can then function "normally" only in the presence of this drug, and severe withdrawal symptoms occur when the drug is withheld.*

3. *A high degree of tolerance may develop to narcotic analgesics. The addict then must administer larger and larger doses in order to maintain his habit.*

4. *Treatment of the narcotic addict should be attempted only when there are adequate facilities for physical and mental rehabilitation.*

The dangers of drug abuse are many. They are in no way confined to the toxic and perhaps lethal effects on the individual. The drug abuser often becomes unproductive, dissipating his available resources for drugs, neglecting his family and communal obligations, becoming dangerous and threatening the safety of others while intoxicated, as well as endangering his own life because of drug-induced toxic effects. These dangers are magnified and enhanced by the addicting as well as habit-forming nature of many drugs.

Drug addiction is a complex, phenomenon involving social, personality and pharmacologic factors, and it is at the same time a disease, a result of other diseases and a cause of criminal acts.

Three major factors that determine the "abuse potentiality" of a drug are its capacity to induce compulsive drug-seeking behavior, its toxicity, and social attitudes toward its effects and its use.

Drugs that today pose serious addiction problems have been known since antiquity, yet it is not clear when their addictive nature was first recognized. Opium preparations were used as soporific agents, analgesics, antidiarrheals and antipyretics in ancient civilizations. In all probability, these drugs were used to such an extent even in those times that individuals became physically dependent upon them.

Opiate abuse was first recognized on a worldwide scale in the middle of the nine-

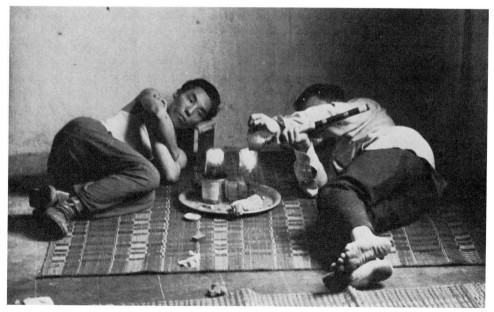

A

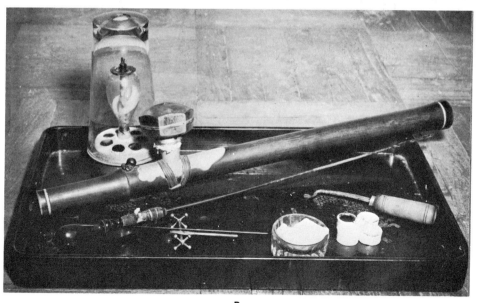

B

FIGURE 56. *A*. Opium smokers in one of the clandestine dens in Hong Kong. *B*. The apparatus of the opium smoker. (Courtesy World Health Organization. Photo by Paul Almasy.)

teenth century. Addiction, especially in China, became a serious problem at this time because of the introduction of opium smoking and the commercial exploitation of opium grown in India and sold by the East India Company. At this same time, the consumption of opium and morphine was increasing in the United States. The ready availability of these agents, the introduction of opium smoking by Chinese laborers on the West Coast and the use of morphine as a pure salt for hypodermic injection contributed to the addiction problem.

It was not until 1909, however, that the

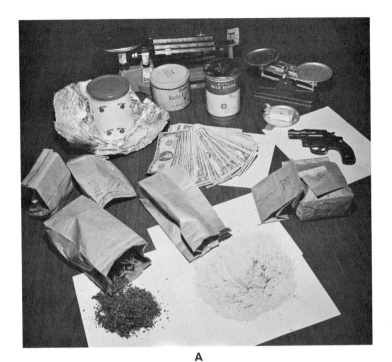

A

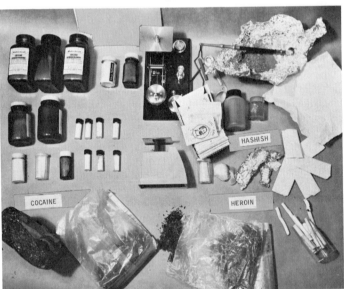

B

FIGURE 57. *A*, A quantity of marijuana and heroin seized by the Bureau of Narcotics. Note the methods of packaging these crude drugs as well as the money involved in illegal trafficking of drugs. (Courtesy U.S. Treasury Dept. Bureau of Narcotics.)

B, Examples of narcotics in various forms as well as paraphernalia involved in their use by addicts. (Courtesy U.S. Treasury Dept. Bureau of Narcotics.)

first narcotic laws were passed, which prohibited importation of opium and its derivatives except for medicinal purposes. The aim of this law was not primarily to control traffic in the United States, but rather to reconcile the official position of the United States with the aim of the American Opium Commission to suppress opium traffic in the Far East. The Harrison Narcotic Act was passed in 1914 to control domestic traffic in and the production of opium coca leaves and similar products.

Federal narcotic laws impose severe penalties for illegal possession and sale of narcotics; however, no totally satisfactory and effective means have been developed to date to cope with illegal drug traffic and addiction. Because of the extremely high profit in the illegal sale of narcotics, there seems to be no limit to the cunning and resourcefulness of the syndicates, organizations and individuals who contrive to obtain and distribute these drugs.

True drug addiction occurs when the body's cells have undergone physiological changes allowing them to function normally only in the presence of the addicting drug. Along with these physiologic changes, there are dependence and tolerance, which necessitates periodic increases in the dose.

A habit-forming drug, on the other hand, is one that may be taken periodically, but to which the dependence is largely psychological rather than physiological. Mental anguish, rather than true physical symptoms, is usually precipitated by withdrawal of these agents. Smoking and routine use of many sleeping pills are included in this classification.

The World Health Organization differentiates addicting drugs from habit-forming drugs on the basis of the following: (1) the magnitude of detrimental effects, which is less for habituation than for addiction, (2) the desire to take drugs, which is less intense in habituation and (3) the lack of physical dependence on the drug in habituation.

The compulsion to take drugs is influenced by a number of factors, such as social attitudes and individual personality characteristics. The feeling of elation produced by many agents, such as narcotic analgesics, alcohol, barbiturates and amphetamines, is especially attractive to thrill-seeking, hedonistic, addiction-prone psychopaths. Neurotic persons, on the other hand, are attracted to narcotic analgesics because they suppress anxiety, fear, suffering and pain.

A very high degree of tolerance may develop to narcotic analgesics. Clinical evidence in man indicates that several hundred times as much morphine may be required to produce comparable degrees of respiratory depression in highly tolerant subjects as in nontolerant subjects.

WHY IS COMPULSIVE DRUG USAGE UNDESIRABLE? There are a number of medical conditions in which fear, anxiety and suffering are detrimental to the health of the individual and thus justify treatment with sedatives, hypnotics, tranquilizers and analgesics. Under other circumstances, however, these emotions may serve a useful purpose, and it can be argued that their suppression may decrease the adaptive capacity of the individual and thus be undesirable.

There is yet another aspect of compulsive drug use that is of primary importance. Drugs that produce physical dependence are a powerful determinant of behavior and it may require a major part of the addict's efforts for satisfaction. In order to satisfy this artificial appetite, life-sustaining needs are partially denied and social obligations are not met, with resulting harm to both the individual and society.

TISSUE TOXICITY. All habit-forming and addicting drugs produce marked tissue toxicity when used in excessive quantities. Thus, it is not uncommon for a narcotic addict, following withdrawal and loss of tolerance to narcotics, to use excessively large doses that may result in death through respiratory depression. Excessive amounts of barbiturates and alcohol may produce similar effects.

In addition to these acute toxic reactions, some drugs produce chronic toxicity. Opiates produce very few chronic effects, whereas alcohol produces many, the most important being liver damage.

SOCIAL EFFECTS. The social and moral havoc produced by crimes and atrocities committed by addicts to secure money for their narcotic requirements is well-known. Social attitudes toward these occurrences, however, vary greatly from the wealthy suburbs to the city slums.

WHEN DOES IT START? Most addicts begin experimenting with narcotics and other drugs during their teens and early twenties. Data from the Bureau of Narcotics indicate that more than half the known addicts are under 30 years of age. Most addicts have a history of delinquency and have experimented with other drugs, such as tobacco, marijuana, alcohol, barbiturates and amphetamines, before using narcotics.

THE NURSE'S ROLE. The nurse has an important role in the education of the general public about the abuse of drugs. The dangers of self-medication should be emphasized, as well as the abuse of prescribed medications. Too often parents do not see their extravagant use of sleeping pills and diet pills as drug abuse or as part of today's drug culture.

The nurse may also serve as a resource person for parents and adolescents seeking facts about drugs and drug abuse. Misconceptions are prevalent especially about the addiction liability and the long-term effects of certain drugs. Unfortunately, a definite answer is not possible in many cases, but the nurse can provide the facts that are known at the time.

THE TYPES OF ADDICTION. Heroin, because of its potency and the high degree of euphoria produced, is the narcotic analgesic of choice for most addicts in the United States. Although it has been outlawed in this country even for medicinal use, a sufficient amount is transmitted via black market outlets to keep the country's addicts supplied. Paregoric, dilaudid and morphine are also high on the list of preference.

The drugs are usually administered intravenously, but some agents, particularly paregoric, are taken orally. Heroin is occasionally used as snuff.

In the Orient, opium smoking is still practiced, including a recent variation called "chasing the dragon" in which small quantities of heroin and barbital are heated on a piece of metal foil, and the smoke is inhaled through a straw or tube.

Following the administration of a dose of a narcotic analgesic, an inexperienced user may be nauseated, sweat profusely and have an itching sensation, which may be quite unpleasant. These reactions are followed by feelings of euphoria, tranquility and somnolence. Morphine produces a feeling of being "high" and of increased energy, which may be manifest as increased purposeful or nonpurposeful motor activity. In addition, these agents produce a variety of sensations, such as a "turning in the stomach," a feeling of warmth that may localize in the epigastrium or other parts of the body and a tingling sensation that may be likened to sexual orgasm. The importance of these changes as a substitute for sexual experience has been emphasized by those who believe that psychosexual immaturity may be an important causative factor in drug addiction.

With continued use of narcotics, tolerance first develops to the euphoria, and the dose must be increased to attain it. After a period of time the drug is taken more to maintain homeostasis than to experience the euphoric effect.

ABSTINENCE SYNDROME. If narcotics are withheld from an addict, the abstinence syndrome is precipitated. The withdrawal symptoms may also be brought about immediately by administration of a narcotic antagonist, such as nalorphine. The appearance of withdrawal symptoms from either cause is proof of addiction and may be used by law enforcement officers to determine whether a suspect is an addict.

In morphine addicts, the initial abstinence symptoms, malaise and weakness appear 6 to 12 hours after the last dose. After 12 hours, yawning, lacrimation, rhinorrhea and perspiration occur, and the patient may sleep fitfully. After 24 hours, the patient becomes increasingly restless, twitching appears and he has hot and cold flashes, chills, back and leg pains, fever, increased rate and depth of respiration, elevation of blood pressure and pupil dilation. The peak is reached at about 48 hours, and the patient is nauseated, vomits, has diarrhea, eats and drinks very little and loses weight rapidly. He lies in a fetal position and covers himself with a blanket even in hottest weather. The symptoms begin to subside in 72 hours and disappear in five to ten days, but the patient may continue to complain of insomnia, weakness, restlessness and muscle pains for several weeks.

All the more obvious signs of abstinence from narcotics seem to disappear within a six month period following withdrawal. Most addicts who spend six months or longer at the Public Health Service Hospitals at Lexington, Kentucky, and Fort Worth, Texas, appear to make an excellent adjustment, apparently losing most of their dependence on and craving for drugs and regaining their health.

There are no reliable estimates of what percentage of addicts return to narcotics upon discharge from the hospital, but it is thought to be very high. One study of patients admitted to the PHS Hospitals indicated that approximately three-fourths of the subjects on whom information was available had returned to the use of drugs. Of those who are treated, most return to drugs at least once. Several factors have been suggested as being of possible importance:

1. The environment and personality disturbances that initially predispose people to drug addiction are probably of major importance.

2. Addiction to narcotics may produce physiological and psychological alterations that are either irreversible or slowly reversible. Studies in man and rats indicate that addicts show physiological abnormalities for many months, which may make the addict particularly subject to the stresses of his environment. Addicts exhibit increased sympathetic nervous system responses for six months following withdrawal of narcotics.

3. The conditioning of the addict may be an important factor in his return to the use of drugs.

TREATMENT OF THE ADDICT. Treatment of the narcotic addict should be attempted only when there are adequate facilities for physical and mental rehabilitation. Several methods or procedures are used to minimize the withdrawal symptoms. Intravenous alcohol has been used periodically during the withdrawal period. Methadone often has been substituted for the originally addicting narcotic because it may be administered orally and has a longer duration of action than morphine. Methadone then may be decreased gradually without serious deleterious effects. During this period tranquilizers, especially the phenothiazines such as chlorpromazine, are of great value. Barbiturates, meprobamate and chlordiazepoxide also have been used.

Following the withdrawal period, every effort should be made to rehabilitate the addict and to prevent his return to the same environment and circumstances that initially led him to addiction. Very few addicts have a strong desire to discontinue drug use, however, because of their psychological characteristics. Many addicts have very little insight into their addiction and do not appear to be good candidates for psychotherapy.

BARBITURATES AND OTHER SEDATIVES. Although barbiturates may be used for inducing sleep over a period of time without causing more than habituation, they occasionally also cause addiction. Barbiturate intoxication is characterized by the same symptoms as chronic alcoholism—drowsiness, poor judgment, emotional liability, slurred speech, nystagmus, tremor and a staggering gait. A low-grade tolerance develops, but it does not usually exceed a dose of 1 to 2.5 Gm. daily. (Average range of doses is 0.03 to 0.1 Gm.)

When given therapeutically for sedative or hypnotic purposes, barbiturates are most often taken orally. The addict greatly prefers the drug by injection, however, and if no parenteral form is available, he occasionally resorts to the injection of the contents of an oral capsule. Because of the crude solution or suspension made when the fillers and diluents of the capsule are dissolved in water and the irritation from the barbiturate itself, ulcerlike sores form on the skin at the injection sites. These ulcers have a typical ap-

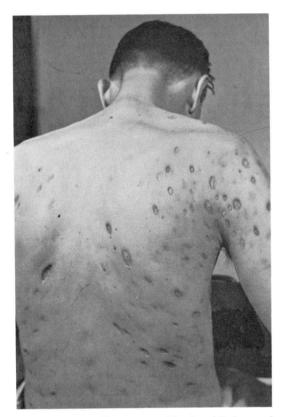

FIGURE 58. Abscess caused by the addict's use of dirty needles to administer narcotics. (Courtesy U.S. Treasury Dept. Bureau of Narcotics.)

pearance, are slow to heal and have been noted on almost every available injection surface of the body.

Abrupt and complete withdrawal of a barbiturate after chronic use results in a serious withdrawal syndrome that includes apprehension, weakness, anorexia, nausea, vomiting, disturbances in cardiovascular function, tremulousness, insomnia, grand mal convulsions and delirium associated with disorientation, delusions and hallucinations.

Every year there are approximately 3000 deaths due to accidental or intentional overdoses of barbiturates. An individual who is confused or euphoric owing to previously ingested doses may take additional doses during the night, resulting in unintentional overdosage. Likewise, alcohol combined with normally harmless doses of barbiturates may produce severe depressive reactions.

Barbiturate addiction should be treated by

hospitalization and psychotherapy followed by attempts at rehabilitation.

Since 1950, an increasing number of non-barbiturate hypnotics have been introduced into medical practice. Some have been advertised as "tranquilizers," "relaxants" or "psychotropic agents," but regardless of the name, they act on the central nervous system in a manner similar to the barbiturates, i.e., through depression of the higher brain centers. Although most problems occur when the drugs are taken chronically in doses exceeding the usual therapeutic amounts, they can cause intoxication and physical dependence that are clinically very similar to those induced by barbiturates. Such drugs include meprobamate, glutethimide, ethinamate, ethchlorvynol, methprylon and chlordiazepoxide. Each of these drugs is discussed in detail elsewhere in the text.

CENTRAL NERVOUS SYSTEM STIMULANTS. The use of central nervous system stimulants is increasing rapidly and is replacing in many cases the use of drugs such as heroin, opium and cocaine. Amphetamines are the drugs most often abused at both bootleg and unauthorized pharmacy sales. The Food and Drug Administration estimates that the volume of amphetamines being sold illegally exceeds the volume sold legally through the pharmacies of this country.

Prolonged use and preliminary dependence on amphetamines have often started through excessive use of amphetamine-containing anorexic agents. Because these substances are stimulants, depressed or exhausted individuals are made to feel "alive"; this artificial mood elevation appears to be a major factor underlying amphetamine abuse.

Tolerance develops gradually, but there continues to be some disagreement as to whether actual physical dependence or merely habituation occurs with the amphetamines. There is no question that a psychic dependence—frequently in severe form—occurs after repeated use.

Generally, the milder symptoms of amphetamine misuse are seen. These include restlessness, incessant talking, tremor, mydriasis and profuse perspiration. However, in a few instances, a drug psychosis resembling schizophrenia can occur. The symptoms usually resolve rather quickly upon withdrawal of the drug.

Users of amphetamines are prone to hallucinations as typified by the following case history published by T. C. McCormick, Jr., in *Diseases of the Nervous System:*

Unmarried white male, born in 1903. This man was hospitalized 20 times between 1946 and 1954; all occasions associated with excessive use of alcohol, amphetamines and barbiturates. When taking large doses of Benzedrine (amphetamine) he would hear voices, usually coming from his car. On several occasions he severely damaged the car, kicking and beating the fenders and hood, trying to quiet the voices. On one occasion he shot the car full of holes with a pistol and ripped out the upholstery. After a few days in the hospital without access to amphetamines, he would make a rapid recovery. Although alcohol and barbiturates were also involved, his hallucinatory experiences were most rampant when he was on Benzedrine or Dexedrine (dextro-amphetamine), and withdrawal delirium is unrecorded.

The crime rate among amphetamine users is high. These agents and all combinations thereof are controlled by the Bureau of Narcotics and Dangerous Drugs.

COCAINE. Cocaine addiction is not a serious problem in the United States, although it is quite common in South America. Chewing of the coca leaf by the Indians is extensive in the lower economic stratum to relieve feelings of fatigue and hunger. Snuffing the drug may produce perforation of the nasal septum.

Occasionally cocaine is mixed with morphine and other opiates to form a "speedball." Intravenous injection of cocaine produces a short-lived feeling of elation. Acute intoxication is characterized by symptoms of autonomic stimulation, including tachycardia, mydriasis and hypertension, and by signs of central stimulation, including hyperreflexia, tremors, muscle twitches, convulsions, delusions and hallucination. The patient suffering from cocaine paranoia may commit acts of violence.

The toxicologic symptoms of cocaine abuse are emotional lability, loss of appetite,

mental impairment and the tendency to withdraw from social contacts.

Tolerance does not develop to the effects of cocaine, nor does chronic abuse of this drug produce physical dependence. The excitant effects of cocaine can be treated readily with barbiturates.

THE HALLUCINOGENS. Hallucinogens presently circulating in the illicit drug market, such as lysergic acid diethylamide (LSD), mescaline, psilocybin, dimethyltryptamine (DMT) and methyl dimethoxy methylphenylethylamine (STP), have no legitimate medical use. Because of the apparently very pleasant distortions of perception, dream images and hallucinations, these drugs are found in illicit drug traffic circles and on college campuses with increasing and alarming frequency. Marihuana, while chemically distinct from the above drugs and consideraly less potent, is generally considered with these drugs and has the same social implications.

LSD. This drug, first synthesized in 1938, is usually taken orally either as a tablet, a crystalline powder or as a liquid which can be deposited on sugar cubes, cookies or other foods. It can be particularly dangerous in that it may be taken by unsuspecting individuals when the compound is maliciously placed on food or in drinks. A variety of effects have been reported following ingestion, including hallucinations, panic, extended psychoses and accidental suicides. These deaths are due to delusional impressions of being able to fly from a window, or a feeling of immunity from danger of various sorts. Recent studies have shown experimentally that chromosome breaks and genetic complications can occur in the offspring of laboratory animals fed LSD. The hazardous effects of this drug on the human population may not be known with certainty for years to come.

Mescaline, Psilocybin, DMT, STP. Mescaline has been used for centuries among primitive tribes for religious ceremonies. It is usually ingested orally either as the whole peyote cactus "button," chopped buttons in capsules or other forms or as a liquid extract. Taken alone, the drug has a bitter taste, thus it is often mixed with food or a beverage. Increased sensory awareness, visual imagery, anxiety, nausea and impaired coordination may occur following ingestion.

Psilocybin is obtained from certain mushrooms found originally in Central America. Like mescaline, it has been used in religious rites with very similar effects.

DMT was originally obtained from certain plant seeds found in the West Indies and South America, but it is relatively easy to synthesize and most illicit drug traffic carry the synthetic form. The effects are similar to those of LSD but larger doses are required.

STP is also prepared synthetically and has been found to be more powerful and longer acting than LSD. Some confusion has been created in illicit drug traffic circles since it has been apparent that several drugs have been sold under the name STP.

Marihuana. The extract of a resin found in the flowering tops and leaves of the cannabis plant is the intoxicating substance of marihuana. It is generally smoked in cigarette form, producing a feeling of euphoria and a dreamy state followed by a free flow of ideas. It tends to release inhibitions similar to the effect of alcohol, but may precipitate psychotic episodes and panic reactions. There are many records of crime committed under the influence of marihuana as well as under the influence of the other hallucinogens, and for this reason all the above drugs are now strictly controlled by the Bureau of Narcotics and Dangerous Drugs, and the illicit use of these drugs is considered a criminal offense.

ORGANIC SOLVENTS. Another class of compounds currently being misused, particularly by teenage boys, can be referred to collectively as the organic solvents. The most publicized abuse is with model airplane glue, which contains the solvent toluene; however, other solvents, such as cleaning fluid and gasoline, produce the same effect. The symptoms are rather similar to alcoholic intoxication and often include marked euphoria and hallucinations.

The tragic death of a 16-year-old boy illustrates the dangers of this form of drug dependence. He died of suffocation, apparently after losing consciousness from sniffing airplane glue with his head encased in a plastic bag.

One case of apparent dependence on mentholated cigarettes was reported in a middle-aged woman showing clinical signs of intoxication. It was noted that she was smoking four or more packages of cigarettes per day. When the cigarettes were withdrawn she improved. When pure menthol was administered, the same clinical symptoms appeared.

CONCLUSIONS. In closing, we may observe that drug abuse and dependence are not merely related to a few, specific chemical compounds. A wide variety of substances are involved. The rapid development of synthetic compounds and our growing dependence upon organic chemicals for industrial and household use, create a new and widespread source of potentially dangerous drugs. Present laws and means of regulation are no longer adequate to control drug dependence.

In order to deal effectively with the problem, more information is needed about the psychological needs that are alleviated by the habitual use of drugs. We must recognize a dependency continuum that ranges from simple overeating, through excessive use of daily consumed products, such as coffee, tobacco and alcohol, to the dangerous drugs and finally to narcotics. The positions of these substances in the continuum involve value judgments about which there is much disagreement.

As our society becomes more complex and the future of our world more uncertain, we may anticipate more prevalent misuse of chemical substances and greater ingenuity in finding new substances to abuse. This fact has serious implications for those who write and enforce our laws.

QUESTIONS FOR DISCUSSION AND REVIEW

1. Suppose you discovered that one of your classmates was a drug addict. What would you do?

2. Why do you think the percentage of "cures" of drug addicts is so low? What do you think could be done to improve this situation?

3. In view of the high addiction potential of morphine, is this drug safe to administer to hospitalized patients? Why?

4. Why do you think the rate of drug addiction among physicians and nurses is as high as it is? What practical means could be taken to limit drug addiction among medical personnel?

5. In what ways may the nurse aid in the prevention of drug addiction? What can the lay person do to help?

6. Conduct a panel discussion on drug addiction, including the various addicting drugs and the phases of the problem, such as medical, economic, social and psychological effects on the individual and society.

BIBLIOGRAPHY

Armstrong, J. D.: Drug addiction of alcohol type. *Amer. J. Hosp. Pharm.,* March, 1965, p. 149.

Block, M. A.: Preventive treatment of alcoholism. *Mod. Treatm., 3*:450, (May) 1966.

Bloomquist, E. R.: The doctor, the nurse and drug addiction. *G.P., 18*: 124, 1958.

Bloomquist, E. R. and Blanchard, B. H.: Drug abuse in the nursing profession. *G.P., 34*:133, 1966.

Burton, G.: An alcoholic in the family. *Nurs. Outlook, 12*:34, (May) 1964.

Byrd, O.: *Medical Readings on Drug Abuse.* Reading, Massachusetts, Addison-Wesley, 1970.

Caskey, K., Blaylock, E. V., and Wauson, B. M.: The school nurse and drug abusers. *Nurs. Outlook, 18*:27, (December) 1970.

Chafitz, M. E.: Drugs in the treatment of alcoholism. *Med. Clin. N. Amer., 51*:1249, 1967.

Childress, G.: The role of the nurse with the drug abuser and addict. *J. Psychiat. Nurs., 8*:21, (March-April) 1970.

Condon, A. and Roland, A.: Drug abuse jargon. *Amer. J. Nurs., 71*:1738, (September) 1971.

Connel, P. H.: Clinical manifestations and treatment of amphetamine-type dependence. *J.A.M.A., 196*:718, 1966.

Dansky, K. H.: Bridge to the turned on. *Amer. J. Nurs., 70*:778, (April) 1970.

Drug Abuse. 4th Ed. Philadelphia, Smith, Kline and French Laboratories, 1968.

Eddy, N. B.: The phenomena of drug dependence and drug abuse. *Amer. J. Hosp. Pharm., 22*:130, 1965.

Edwards, R. E.: Abuse of central nervous system stimulants. *Amer. J. Hosp. Pharm.,* March, 1965, p. 145.

Essig, C. F.: Addiction to non-barbiturate sedative and tranquilizing drugs. *Clin. Pharmacol. Ther.,* 5:334, 1964.

Essig, C. F.: Clinical aspects of barbiturate and sedative drug abuse. *Amer. J. Hosp. Pharm.,* March, 1965, p. 140.

Foreman, N. J. and Zerwelch, J. V.: Drug crisis intervention. *Amer. J. Nurs.,* 71:1736, (September) 1971.

Fort, J.: Comparison chart of major substances used for mind alteration. *Amer. J. Nurs.,* 71:1740 (September) 1971.

Freedman, A. M., et al.: Cyclozocine and methadone in narcotic addiction. *J.A.M.A.,* 202:119, 1967.

Garb, S.: Narcotic addiction in nurses and doctors. *Nurs. Outlook, 13*:30, (November) 1965.

Gardner, R.: Amphetamine dependence and misuse. *Nurs. Mirror, 130*:22, (March 6) 1970.

Gelber, I.: The addict and his drugs. *Amer. J. Nurs., 63*:52, (July) 1963.

Gelperin, A. and Gelperin, E. A.: The inebriate in the emergency room. *Amer. J. Nurs., 70*:1494, (July) 1970.

Gillespie, C.: Nurses help combat alcoholism. *Amer. J. Nurs., 69*:1938, (September) 1969.

Giordano, H. L.: Narcotic responsibilities of pharmacists. *J. Amer. Pharm. Ass.,* June, 1965, p. 311.

Gitlow, S. E.: Treatment of the reversible acute complications of alcoholism. *Mod. Treatm., 3*:450, (May) 1966.

Golder, G. M.: The nurse and the alcoholic patient. *Amer. J. Nurs., 56*: 436, 1956.

Golub, S.: Recognizing the drug abuser. *R.N., 32*:44, (July) 1969.

Grinspoon, L.: Marihuana. *Sci. Amer., 221*:17, (December) 1969.

Isselbacher, K. J. and Greenberger, N. J.: Metabolic effects of alcohol on the liver. *New Eng. J. Med., 170*:351, 1964.

Jacobsen, E.: Metabolism of ethyl alcohol. *Pharmacol. Rev., 4*:107, 1952.

Keating, K.: The craze for chemical comfort. *AORN J., 11*:35, (April) 1970.

Kimmel, M. E.: Antabuse in a clinic program. *Amer. J. Nurs., 71*:73, 1971.

Kramer, J. C., et al.: Amphetamine abuse. *J.A.M.A., 201*:305, 1967.

Kromberg, C. J. and Proctor, J. B.: Methadone maintenance in heroin addiction. Evolution of a day program. *Amer. J. Nurs., 70*:2575, (December) 1970.

LSD: the false illusion. Reprint from FDA Papers. Washington, D.C., U.S. Government Printing Office, July-August, 1967.

Ludwig, A. M. and Levine, J.: Patterns of hallucinogenic drug abuse. *J.A.M.A., 191*:92, 1965.

Martin, W. R.: Some clinical aspects of addiction to narcotic analgesics. *Amer. J. Hosp. Pharm., 22*:133, 1965.

McCarthy, R. G.: Alcoholism. *Amer. J. Nurs., 59*:203, 1959.

McDermott, R., Sr.: Maintaining the methadone patient. *Nurs. Outlook, 18*:22, (December) 1970.

Morton, E. L.: Nursing care in an alcoholic unit. *Nurs. Outlook, 14*:45, (October) 1966.

Nowlis, H.: *Drugs on the College Campus.* Detroit, N.A.S.P.A. Central Office, 1967.

Parry, A., McNatt, H. J. and Sahler, S.: Alcoholism and caring for the alcoholic. *Amer. J. Nurs., 65*:111, (March) 1965.

Pearson, B. A.: Methadone maintenance in heroin addiction. The program at Beth Israel Medical Center. *Amer. J. Nurs., 70*:2571, (December) 1970.

Poplar, J. F.: Characteristics of nurse addicts. *Amer. J. Nurs., 69*:117, (January) 1969.

Rodman, M. J.: Management in drug abuse and addiction. *R.N., 27*:59, (December) 1964.

Russaw, E. H.: Nursing in a narcotic-detoxification unit. *Amer. J. Nurs., 70*:1720, (August) 1970.

Sankot, M. and Smith, D. E.: Drug problems in the Haight-Asbury. *Amer. J. Nurs., 68*:1686, 1968.

Sartwell, P. E. (ed.): *Maxcy-Rosenau Preventive Medicine and Public Health.* 9th Ed. New York, Appleton-Century-Crofts, 1965.

Schultes, R. E.: Hallucinogenics of plant origin. *Science, 163*:245, 1969.

Seever, M. H.: Medical perspectives in habituation and addiction. *J.A.M.A., 206*:1263, 1968.

Soreson, K. and Fagan, R. J.: The hospitalized skid row alcoholic. *Nurs. Forum, 2*:88, 1963.

Talalay, P. (ed.): *Drugs in Our Society.* Baltimore, The Johns Hopkins Press, 1963.

Victor, M.: Treatment of the neurological complications of alcoholism. *Mod. Treatm., 3*:491, (May) 1966.

Webb, W. R. and Degerlis, I. U.: Ethyl alcohol and the cardiovascular system. *J.A.M.A., 191*:1055, 1965.

Wilmer, H. A.: Drugs, hippies and doctors. *J.A.M.A., 206*:1272, 1968.

Yolles, S. E.: The drug scene. *Nurs. Outlook, 18*:24, (July) 1970.

Index